OXFORD MEDICAL PUBLICATIONS

Audiology and audiological medicine

Volume 1

Audiology and audiological medicine

Volume 1

Edited by

H. A. BEAGLEY

Consultant Otologist and Consultant in Charge of the Department of Electrophysiology, The Royal National Throat, Nose and Ear Hospital, London
Honorary Lecturer in the Institute of Laryngology and Otology, University of London
Honorary Lecturer, Imperial College, London

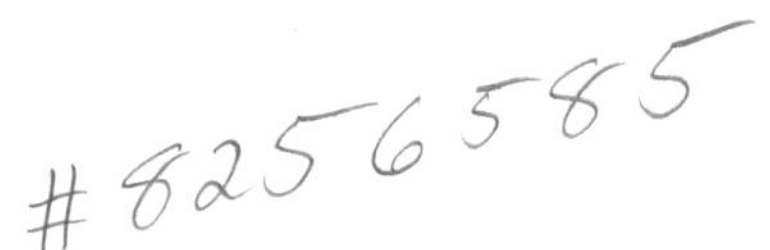

OXFORD
OXFORD UNIVERSITY PRESS
NEW YORK TORONTO
1981

Oxford University Press, Walton Street, Oxford OX2 6DP

London Glasgow New York Toronto
Delhi Bombay Calcutta Madras Karachi
Kuala Lumpur Singapore Hong Kong Tokyo
Nairobi Dar es Salaam Cape Town
Melbourne Wellington

and associate companies in
Beirut Berlin Ibadan Mexico City

British Library Cataloguing in Publication Data

Audiology and audiological medicine.
– (Oxford medical publications).
1. Hearing disorders
2. Audiology
I. Beagley, H A
617.8'9 RF290 80–41814
ISBN 0–19–261154–2

Set by Western Printing Services Ltd, Bristol
Printed in Great Britain by the Thetford Press, Norfolk.

Preface

This volume has been compiled with medical people interested in audiology primarily in view. Audiology is increasingly significant in medicine and surgery and indeed audiological medicine has recently been recognized as a medical specialty in the UK, as it is in many European countries.

The subject matter covers all clinical aspects of medical audiology. Considerable emphasis has also been placed on certain subjects where the scientific substrate is somewhat advanced with respect to routine clinical practice, but which will become steadily of greater importance. For this reason subjects such as ultrastructure of the inner ear and its innervation as well as the pathophysiology of the Eustachean tube have been treated in some detail. Other subjects treated extensively are forensic audiology and industrial audiology, noise control, and compensation, as well as psychological and psychiatric aspects of hearing loss and paedoaudiology.

Inevitably some basic subjects are dealt with in a more introductory manner. A case in point is the chapter on the psychophysics of hearing. This information is basic to many aspects of audiology and has been presented accordingly. But psychophysics is a major scientific study in its own right and those who would like to pursue this subject further are referred to the standard texts which deal with it. Similarly, no attention has been paid to the vestibular labyrinth and its disorders as this is generally considered to be a separate, if related, subject, albeit one of considerable importance.

While the uses, advantages, disadvantages, and implications of various audiological procedures have been treated in the same depth, little space has been allotted to describing, step by step, the mechanics of carrying out such tests and the book cannot be regarded as being simply a technical manual. Instead the philosophy and the rationale behind the procedures and their clinical implications are dealt with predominantly. On the other hand in the case of some of the newer procedures such as electrophysiological tests of hearing a certain amount of practical advice has been included which may prove helpful to some readers.

It is a matter of deep regret that Professor Ingelstedt died between the time that his manuscript was received and its publication in this book. Those who knew Professor Ingelstedt are aware of his significant contributions to the important matter of Eustachean tube function and his comprehensive treatment of this subject in Chapter 29 is a fitting memorial.

London HAB
March 1981

Preface

Contents

Contributors

P. W. ALBERTI
Department of Otolaryngology,
University of Toronto,
Toronto, Canada

H. A. BEAGLEY
The Royal National Throat, Nose and Ear Hospital,
London

M. V. BICKERTON
Royal National Throat, Nose and Ear Hospital,
London

J. B. BOOTH
The London Hospital,
Whitechapel,
London

M. E. BRYAN
Audiology Group,
University of Salford,
Salford

K. K. CHAO-CHARIA
Institute of Laryngology and Otology,
University of London

J. C. DENMARK
Whittingham Hospital,
Whittingham,
Preston

E. DOUEK
Hearing Research Group,
Guy's Hospital,
London

L. L. ELLIOTT
Northwestern University,
Evanston,
Illinois, U.S.A.

L. FISCH
Institute of Laryngology and Otology,
London

G. R. FRASER
Lister Hill National Center for Biomedical Communications,
National Library of Medicine,
Bethesda, U.S.A.

W. P. R. GIBSON
Royal National Throat, Nose and Ear Hospital
and Hospital for Nervous Diseases (Queen Square),
London

A. GLORIG
Otologic Medical Group Inc.,
Los Angeles, U.S.A.

D. HAYES
Baylor College of Medicine,
Houston, U.S.A.

R. HINCHCLIFFE
Institute of Laryngology and Otology,
University of London

J. D. HOOD
Medical Research Council Hearing and Balance Unit,
National Hospital for Nervous Diseases,
London

J. N. T. HUTTON
Department of Anaesthetics,
Royal National Throat, Nose and Ear Hospital,
London

S. INGELSTEDT ✠
ENT Department,
Malmö General Hospital,
Sweden

P. D. JACKSON
Institute of Laryngology and Otology,
University of London

J. JERGER
Baylor College of Medicine,
Houston, U.S.A.

H. KERNOHAN
Wall Hall College of Further Education,
Radlett, Hertfordshire

J. J. KNIGHT
Institute of Laryngology and Otology,
University of London

S. A. LERNER
Department of Medicine,
University of Chicago,
U.S.A.

G. LUCAS
Nuffield Hearing and Speech Centre,
Royal National Throat, Nose and Ear Hospital,
London

J. A. MACRAE
National Acoustic Laboratories,
Australian Department of Health,
Sydney, Australia

M. C. MARTIN
Scientific and Technical Department,
The Royal National Institute for the Deaf,
London

G. J. MATZ
Department of Surgery,
University of Chicago,
U.S.A.

L. MICHAELS
Department of Pathology,
Institute of Laryngology and Otology,
University of London

A. W. MORRISON
The London Hospital,
Whitechapel, London

V. A. MUTER
Nuffield Hearing and Speech Centre,
Royal National Throat, Nose and Ear Hospital,
London

T. NICOL
Department of Clinical Anatomy,
Institute of Laryngology and Otology,
University of London

P. D. PHELPS
Department of Radiology,
The Royal National Throat, Nose and Ear Hospital,
London

R. A. PIESSE
National Acoustic Laboratory,
Australian Department of Health,
Sydney, Australia

N. SHAH
The Royal National Throat, Nose and Ear Hospital,
London

C. A. SMITH
Department of Otolaryngology,
University of Oregon School of Medicine,
Oregon, U.S.A.

H. H. SPOENDLIN
Universitätsklink fur Hals-, Nasen- und Ohrenkrankheiten,
Innsbruck, Austria

S. D. G. STEPHENS
Adult Auditory Rehabilitation Centre,
The Royal National Throat, Nose and Ear Hospital,
London

W. TEMPEST
Audiology Group,
University of Salford, Salford

A. R. D. THORNTON
Medical Research Council Institute of Hearing Research,
Royal South Hants Hospital,
Southampton

J. TONNDORF
Columbia University,
New York, U.S.A.

M. WELLS
Department of Pathology,
Institute of Laryngology and Otology,
University of London

J. J. ZWISLOCKI
Institute for Sensory Research,
Syracuse University,
New York, U.S.A.

Section 1

Basic Sciences

1 Clinical anatomy of the auditory part of the human ear

T. NICOL and K. K. CHAO-CHARIA

The **ear** consists of the external ear, the middle ear, the inner ear, and the internal auditory meatus (Fig. 1.7).

THE EXTERNAL EAR

This consists of the auricle or pinna, the external auditory meatus or auditory canal and the outer layer of the tympanic membrane.

The auricle

Consists of a skeleton of elastic cartilage covered with thin skin. It shows depressions and elevations which are given special names (Fig. 1.1). The most prominent is the deep fossa or concha which leads into the external auditory meatus. The auricle is designed to collect sound waves and transmit them along the external auditory meatus to the tympanic membrane. Sound

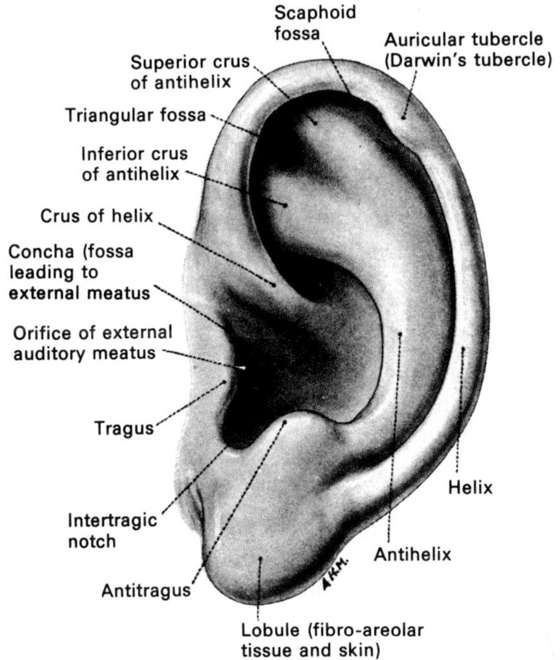

Fig. 1.1. Lateral view of the left auricle (pinna).

waves are best heard if received by the auricle at an angle of 45°. Localization of sound is also an important function of the auricle and if the auricle is removed by trauma sound reception is decreased by about 5 decibels and sound localization is also reduced.

The skin on the lateral surface of the auricle is more adherent to the perichondrium of the cartilage than on the cranial surface, therefore in any infection swelling will be more marked in the looser tissue on the cranial surface. The shape of the cartilage is shown in Fig. 1.2. It is absent in the

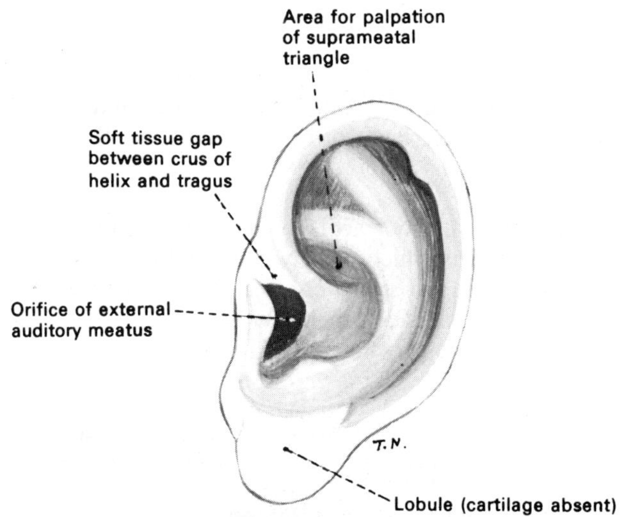

Fig. 1.2. Lateral view of the left auricle showing extent of cartilaginous skeleton.

lobule which consists only of skin and fibrofatty tissue and can be pierced for earrings. It is also absent between the crus of the helix and the tragus. The opening of the external meatus is overhung anteriorly by a flap of cartilage covered with skin and called the tragus. The cartilage of the auricle is continued inwards and is folded to form the anterior, inferior, and part of the posterior wall of the cartilaginous meatus. The *suprameatal triangle* (see p. 9) can be palpated through the concha above the crus of the helix.

The auricle is fixed to the side of the head by the skin, fusion of the perichondrium with the periosteum of the skull and by three small extrinsic muscles (see Figs. 1.3 and 1.4). These muscles have little function in man but in lower animals they can move the position of the auricle. They belong to the scalp group of muscles and arise from a downward extension of the epicranial aponeurosis. Like the scalp muscles they are supplied by nerve VII. Clinically the posterior auricular muscle may be used in a young child to find out if the *eighth nerve* is intact—electrodes are placed in the muscle and a sound is produced in the external meatus; if N. VII and N. VIII are acting normally the muscle will show contraction on the graph.

The *nerve supply* of the auricle is shown in Figs. 1.5 and 1.6.

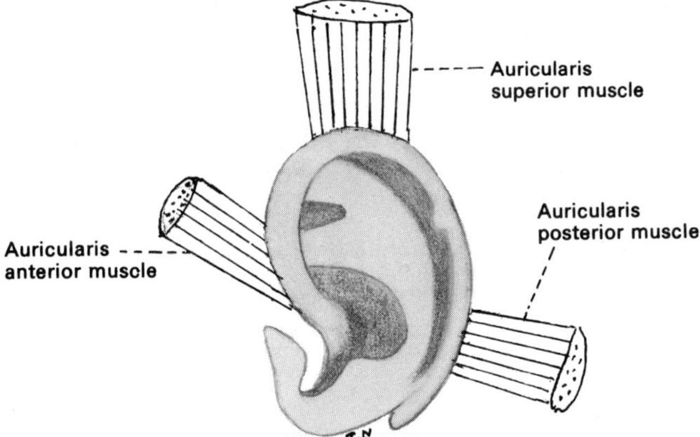

Fig. 1.3. Lateral view of the cartilage of the left auricle.

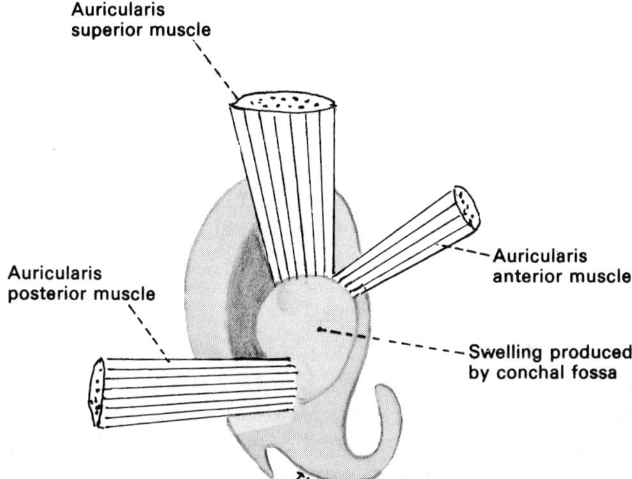

Fig. 1.4. Cartilage of the left auricle. Cranial (medial) view showing attachment of auricular muscles to auricular cartilage.

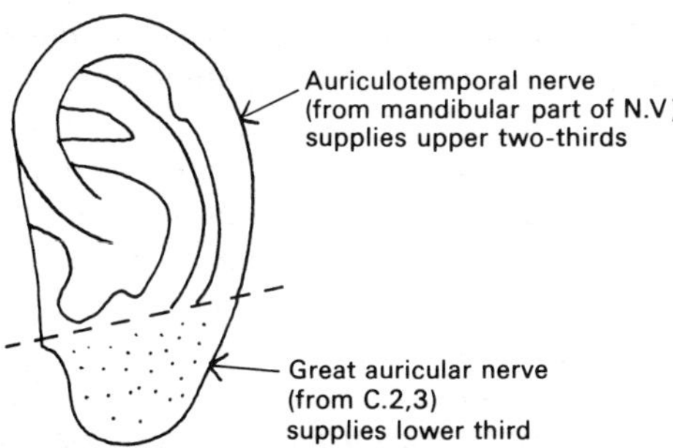

Fig. 1.5. Nerve supply to the lateral surface of the left auricle.

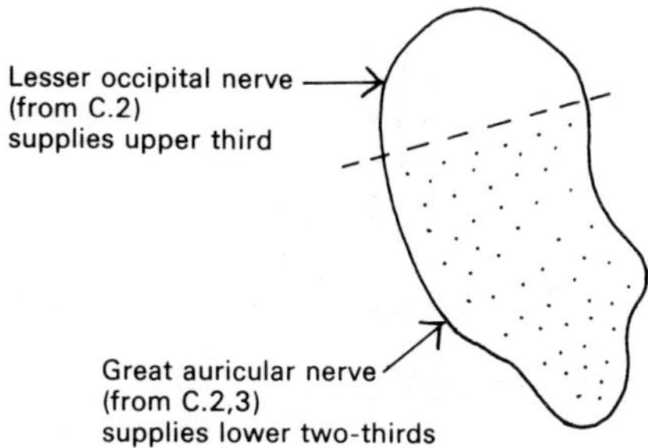

Fig. 1.6. Nerve supply to the cranial (medial) surface of left auricle.

BLOOD SUPPLY

Lateral surface—superficial temporal artery. Veins drain into superficial temporal vein. Cranial surface—posterior auricular artery. Veins drain to posterior auricular vein.

LYMPHATICS

Lateral surface—pre-auricular nodes. Cranial surface—mastoid nodes. From the lobule some lymph vessels join the nodes on the external jugular vein.

Clinically the auricle is prone to temperature variations such as frostbite because of its superficially placed vessels. Infection invading the cartilage may lead to its necrosis and also to severe pain because of the many free nerve endings.

The external meatus or auditory canal

In the adult it is 24 to 26 mm long and is directed forwards and inwards. The outer third (8 mm) of the canal is *cartilaginous* and the inner two-thirds (16 mm long) is *bony* (Figs. 1.7 and 1.8). The canal is also slightly convex upwards and the tympanic membrane lies obliquely in the adult forming an angle of 55° with the floor which is 4 mm longer than the roof. The curvature of the canal protects the tympanic membrane. If the auricle is pulled upwards and backwards it tends to straighten the meatus in the adult. Between the lower part of the membrane and the sloping inferior wall of the meatus there is a recess (the anterior recess) in which a foreign body may lodge. It is present in most mammals. The other points to note are shown in Fig. 1.8.

The narrowest point is 6 mm from the membrane but there is also a slight constriction at the junction of the cartilaginous and bony parts. The skin is closely adherent to the walls in the cartilaginous part so that a furuncle is very painful due to the increased tension in the tissue. The cartilage of the cartilaginous part gradually narrows and near the bony part it forms only the anterior wall and part of the inferior wall of the canal. Where the cartilage is absent the wall is completed by fibrous issue. The end of the cartilaginous part is attached around the margin of the bony part. Deficiencies may be

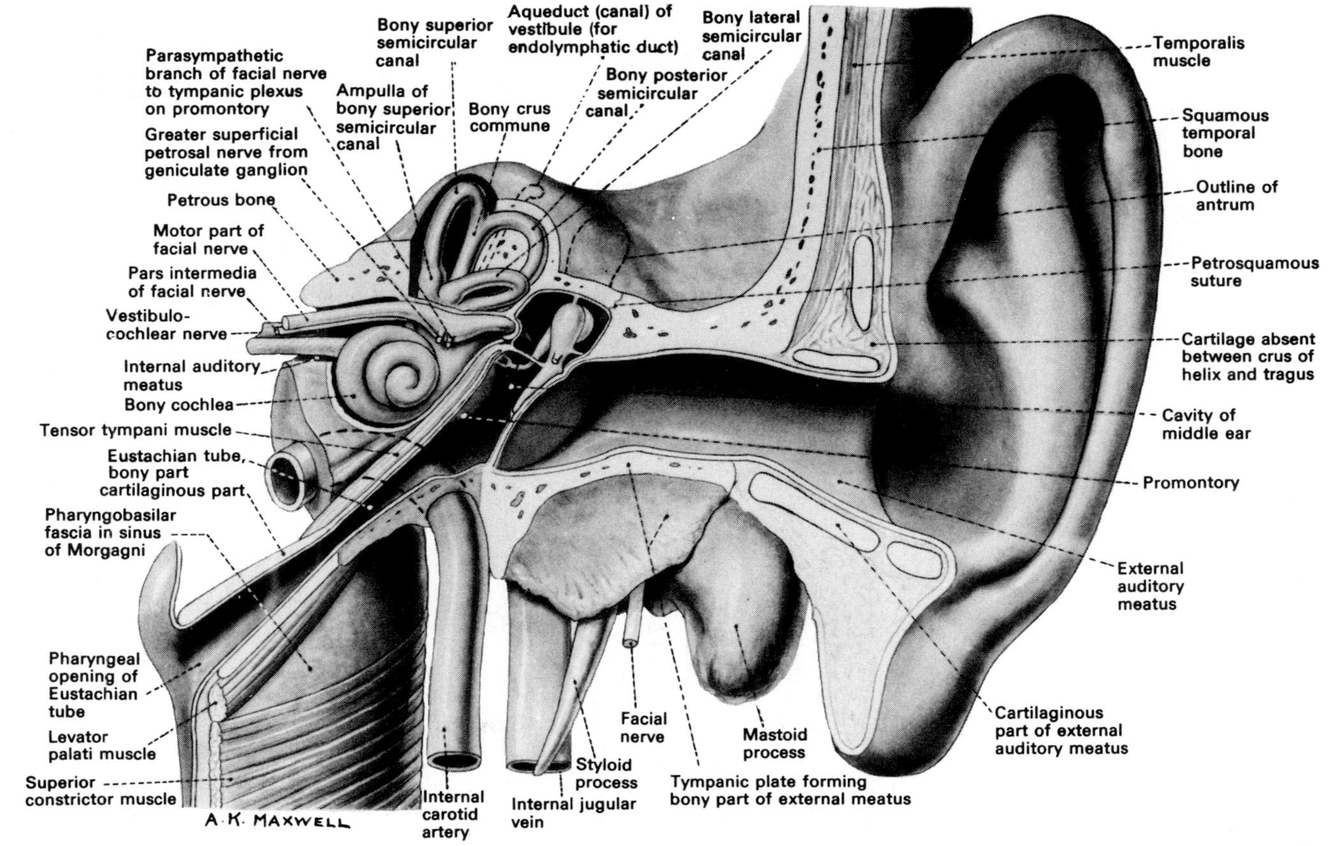

Fig. 1.7. Diagram showing left external ear, middle ear, internal ear, and internal auditory meatus.

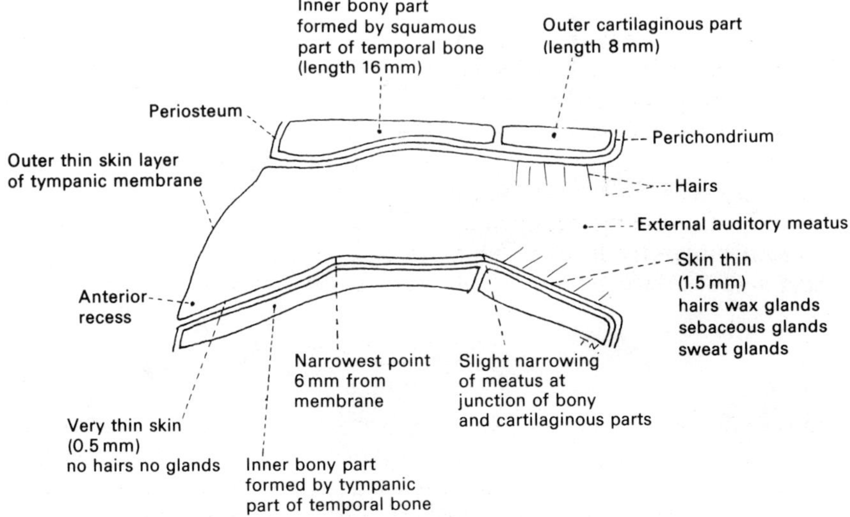

Fig. 1.8. Plan of left external auditory meatus.

present in the anterior wall of the cartilaginous part. They are called the fissures of Santorini and may provide a pathway for infection between the parotid gland and the cartilaginous meatus.

The bony part is chiefly formed by the tympanic plate which forms the anterior wall, the inferior wall, and the lower half of the posterior wall; the remainder is completed by the squamous part of the temporal bone. The inner end of the bony meatus is grooved to receive the thickened edge (called the annulus) of the tympanic membrane. The groove is called the tympanic sulcus.

At birth the tympanic part of the temporal bone is represented only by an incomplete ring of bone containing the tympanic sulcus, and the membrane is nearly horizontal. Since there is no bony meatus in the child the whole canal is shorter, the tympanic membrane is close to the surface and the stylomastoid foramen from which nerve VII emerges is unprotected since the mastoid process has not yet developed. In the child the auricle should be pulled downwards and backwards to straighten the canal since there is no bony part and the cartilaginous part is soft and partly collapsed.

When the tympanic plate grows outwards from the tympanic ring and ossifies the osteoblasts spread outwards in two streams. This may leave a foramen in the anterior wall of the bony meatus called the foramen of Hüschke. It usually closes at age six years but may remain until puberty or persist into adult life. A foreign body may lodge in the foramen or infection may pass through it into the meatus from the parotid gland. The tympanic membrane closes the inner end of the external meatus. The appearance of the outer surface of the membrane should therefore be included in a description of the external meatus—for convenience this is described on page 13.

RELATIONS OF EXTERNAL MEATUS

The inner part of the cartilaginous meatus and the anterior wall of the bony meatus are separated anteriorly by a small part of the parotid gland from the mandibular joint. Inferiorly the chief relation is the parotid gland. Posteriorly the bony meatus is separated by a thin plate of bone from the mastoid air cells. Superiorly the squamous part of the temporal bone separates the bony meatus from the middle cranial fossa.

Posterosuperiorly lies the suprameatal triangle (Macewen's triangle) which is the surface guide to the highest part of the mastoid antrum (see Fig. 1.46).

BLOOD SUPPLY

The anterior wall is supplied by branches from the superficial temporal artery (from the external carotid). The posterior wall is supplied by branches from the posterior auricular artery (from the external carotid). The inner part of the meatus is also supplied by the deep auricular branch of the maxillary artery which enters between the cartilaginous and bony parts. *Venous drainage*. The anterior part is drained by the retromandibular vein; the posterior part by the posterior auricular vein.

LYMPHATICS

Anterior wall—pre-auricular nodes on the surface of the sheath of the parotid then to the upper deep cervical nodes. Posterior wall—mastoid nodes on the mastoid process then to the upper deep cervical nodes.

NERVE SUPPLY

Anterior wall—auriculotemporal nerve (from mandibular part of N. V). Posterior wall—auricular branch of vagus (N. X).

GROWTH CHANGES

At birth the tympanic part of the temporal bone, as stated, is a thin incomplete bony ring containing the tympanic sulcus.

At six years the whole external meatus is completed, the tympanic plate from the tympanic ring has now ensheathed the base of the styloid process, the mastoid process is now well formed and the stylomastoid foramen and N. VII are now protected.

LENGTH OF EXTERNAL MEATUS

The measurements in Table 1.1 are from the external orifice along the floor of the meatus to the surface of the tympanic membrane (owing to the obliquity of the membrane the measurements along the roof would be about 4 mm shorter).

The meatus is therefore almost of adult size by the age of six.

TABLE 1.1. *Length of external meatus with age*

Age after birth	Length (mm)
2 months	16
1 year	20
6 years	24
adult	26

FUNCTIONS OF EXTERNAL MEATUS

These are as follows:

1. Because of its shape it protects the tympanic membrane and maintains a constant level of temperature and humidity.
2. It acts as a resonator which amplifies sound by 5–10 dB at certain frequencies.
3. It is self-cleansing owing to migration of the lining epithelium especially on the tympanic membrane. Migration is outwards especially along the postero superior wall of the meatus and also along the anterior wall. The rate of migration is 0.8 mm per day in the child and 0.1 mm in the adult. (For comparison the rate of growth of a finger nail is 0.05 mm per day.) The migrating cells in the outer part of the meatus become mixed with wax.
4. The formation of wax in the cartilaginous part of the meatus traps foreign material. The wax also becomes mixed with the secretory products of the sebaceous glands.
5. The anterior recess between the lower part of the membrane and the sloping inferior wall of the meatus protects the lower part of the membrane. A foreign body, however, may lodge in it.

MIDDLE EAR (TYMPANIC CAVITY)

This is the narrow cavity which lies between the tympanic membrane and the bony internal ear. It develops as an outgrowth from the first pharyngeal pouch of the developing pharynx. The stalk becomes the Eustachian tube or auditory tube, the next part dilates to form the middle ear or tympanic cavity, and at the seventh month of intra-uterine life the mastoid antrum is formed as an outgrowth from the tympanic cavity into the temporal bone. Later from the first year onwards the mastoid air cells are formed as buds from the antrum (see Fig. 1.9).

The Eustachian tube, the middle ear or tympanic cavity, the antrum, and air cells are collectively referred to as the structures of the *middle-ear cleft*.

The walls of the middle ear are formed by the structures shown in Fig. 1.10.

The lateral wall is formed by the tympanic membrane and the squamous

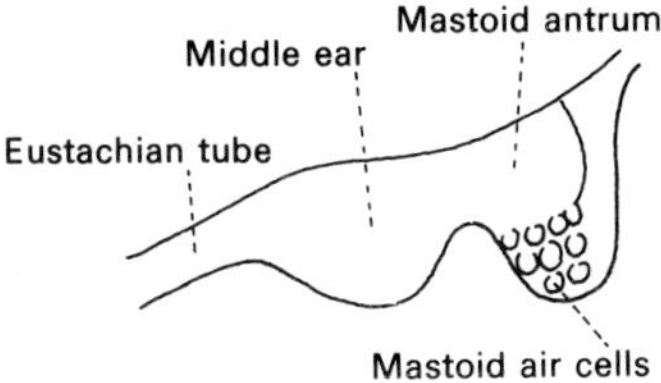

Fig. 1.9. Plan of left middle-ear (left).

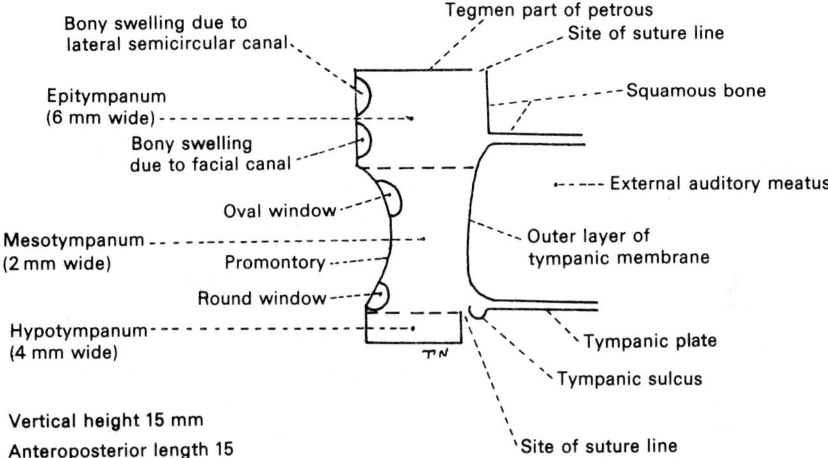

Fig. 1.10. Plan of left middle-ear cavity (all walls are formed by the petrous except the lateral wall). The dotted lines show the divisions of the middle-ear cavity.

bone above it. The other walls are formed by the petrous part of the temporal bone. The cavity is irregular in shape and is specially constricted between the tympanic membrane and a swelling called the promontory which is produced by the basal coil of the cochlea. The part of the cavity above the tympanic membrane is called the *attic or epitympanum*, the part opposite the membrane is called the *mesotympanum*, and the shallow part below the membrane is called the *hypotympanum*. The measurements are given in Fig. 1.10.

The middle-ear cavity contains three small bones called the *auditory ossicles* (Fig. 1.32). They are named from lateral to medial, the malleus, incus, and stapes. They transmit sound waves from the tympanic membrane to the oval window (fenestra vestibuli) in which is inserted the footplate of the stapes. In this way the waves are transmitted to the perilymph which is the fluid which occupies the cavity of the bony labyrinth of the inner ear. The area of the tympanic membrane is about fifteen times greater than the oval window and this, together with the mechanical effect of the ossicular chain, intensifies the sound waves eighteen times when they reach the oval window. The chain of ossicles has therefore an important part to play in the hearing mechanism.

It is believed that the malleus and incus are derived from the cartilage of the first branchial arch and the stapes from that of the second branchial arch. The dorsal ends of these arches become imprisoned in the developing temporal bone and as the ossicles develop they invaginate the lining mucosa of the middle ear, the malleus and incus from the lateral wall and the stapes from the medial wall. The invagination of the mucosa by the ossicles explains how they are covered by mucosa and also carry folds of mucosa between them and around their ligaments and tendons.

The ossicles

Should be examined before the walls of the middle ear are described since their parts are often referred to in the description. The main features of the three ossicles are shown in Fig. 1.11.

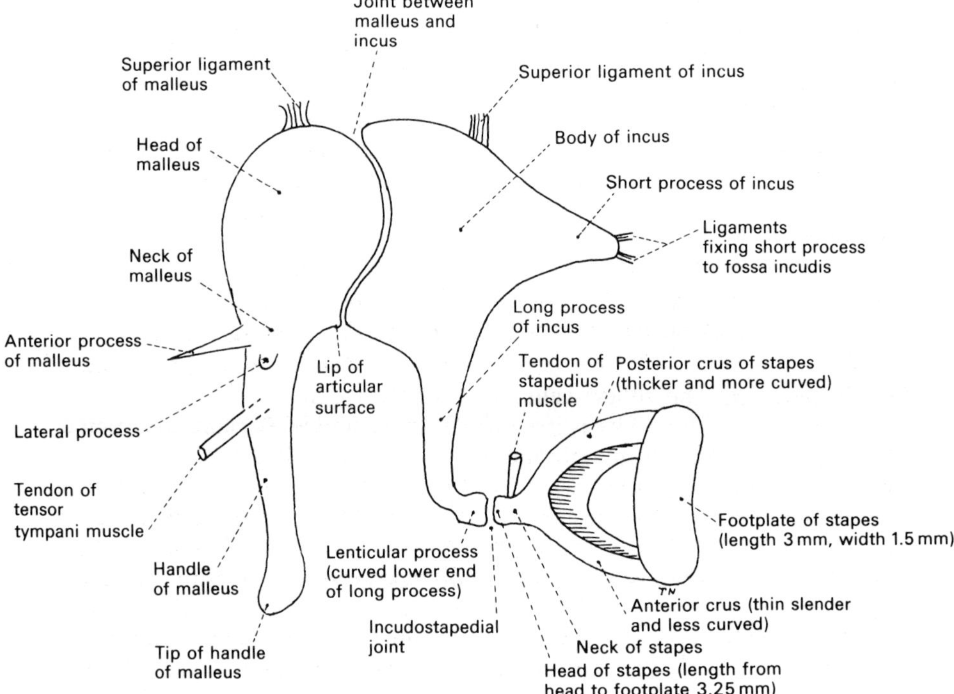

Fig. 1.11. The ossicular chain of the middle-ear cavity.

The malleus and incus are said to rotate around an anteroposterior axis formed by the anterior process of the malleus and the short process of the incus and its two ligaments. The result is that the footplate of the stapes is moved in a rocking fashion in the oval window and transmits the movements of the tympanic membrane to the perilymph in the bony labyrinth. If however the tympanic membrane is moved outwards due to inflation of the

Eustachian tube the joint between the malleus and the incus becomes lax and this prevents the stapes being pulled out of the oval window.

The joints between the malleus and incus and stapes are synovial joints. In contrast the footplate of the stapes is held in the oval window by an elastic annular ligament placed in the niche of the oval window. The niche is about 3 mm deep and the footplate of the stapes, including the niche, lies 3 mm from the utricle of the membranous labyrinth and about 4 mm from the saccule.

The ossicles are fully formed in cartilage at the 16th week of intra-uterine life. They then begin to ossify. The incus ossifies first from one centre of ossification, then the malleus from one centre. The stapes next ossifies from one centre which commences in the footplate then extends along the crura into the neck and head. The stapes begins as a ring of cartilage through which passes the stapedial artery which is a remnant of the artery of the second branchial arch. The stapes reaches its full size by the 20th week of intra-uterine life and then the stapedial artery degenerates. The ossicles are fully ossified at birth. They consist of compact bone with no Haversian systems and no marrow cavity.

The action of the middle-ear muscles is said to be protective. The tensor muscle tenses the tympanic membrane during a loud noise and the stapedius muscle holds the stapes in position and prevents it being pushed too far into the oval window, and in so doing it tilts the anterior part of the footplate outwards.

The lateral wall of the middle ear

The lateral wall is formed chiefly by the *tympanic membrane*. Above the membrane the wall is completed by the squamous part of the temporal bone and below the membrane by the petrous part.

The *structure* of the *membrane* is shown in Fig. 1.12. It is about 0.3 mm thick and consists of three layers:

1. A thin skin layer consisting only of two layers of stratified epithelium.
2. A fibrous layer which holds the malleus in position and fixes it to the skin layer. It consists of superficial fibres radiating from the handle of the malleus and a deeper layer of circular fibres especially concentrated at the periphery to form the thickened margin called the annulus which lies in the tympanic sulcus. The sulcus is deficient above (see Fig. 1.13) and ends at the level of the base of the pars flaccida of the membrane; and the fibres of the annulus are then continued to the lateral process of the malleus in the anterior and posterior malleolar folds.
3. A thin mucosa. This is part of the lining of the tympanic cavity and is covered with flattened cells.

The lateral view of the membrane is shown in Fig. 1.13. The lateral process of the malleus is a well-marked prominence and below it the handle slopes downwards and backwards. From the lateral process two folds, the anterior and posterior malleolar folds pass to the ends of the annulus and the bony margins of the notch of Rivinus. As already stated these folds contain

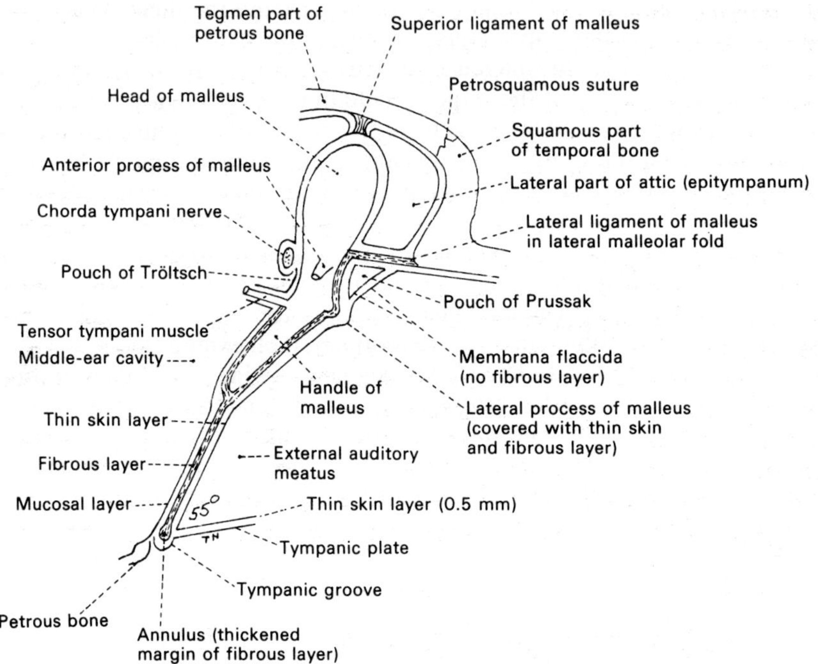

Fig. 1.12. Plan of the structure of the tympanic membrane. (The thickness of the membrane below the handle of the malleus is approximately 0.3 mm.) Left side.

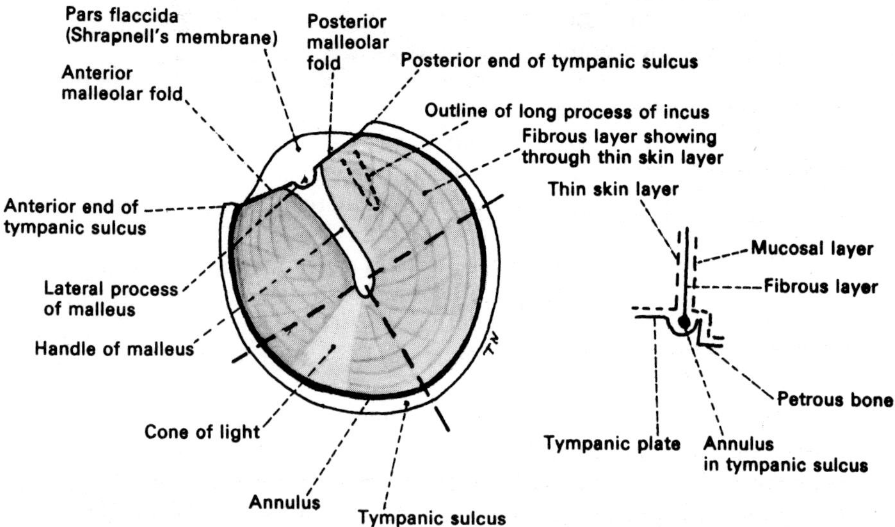

Fig. 1.13. Plan of the tympanic membrane: outer surface, left side. The insert shows the three layers of the membrane. The part of the membrane below the pars flaccida is called the pars tensa.

the terminal fibres of the annulus. Above the folds is a small triangular part of the membrane called the *pars flaccida* (Shrapnell's membrane) in which the fibrous layer is absent or very loose. The remainder of the membrane is called the *pars tensa* because of the well-developed fibrous layer. The outer surface is slightly concave and the deepest part of the concavity is just below the centre and is called the *umbo*; this is the point at which the flattened tip of the handle of the malleus is attached. The remainder of the handle is firmly attached to the skin layer of the membrane by the fibrous layer. The shadow of the long process of the incus may be seen behind the handle of the malleus and parallel to it but it is not within the membrane. The thickened margin or *annulus* of the membrane is lodged in the tympanic sulcus but can be dislocated from the sulcus at operation. The tympanic sulcus is absent opposite the pars flaccida leaving a notch called the *notch of Rivinus*. The notch is formed by the squamous part of the temporal bone and the margin of the pars flaccida is attached to it. *The cone of light* is only seen on the membrane when a reflected light is shone through the external meatus; it is the only part of the membrane at right angles to the incoming light rays.

The medial surface of the membrane is shown in Fig. 1.14. Note the

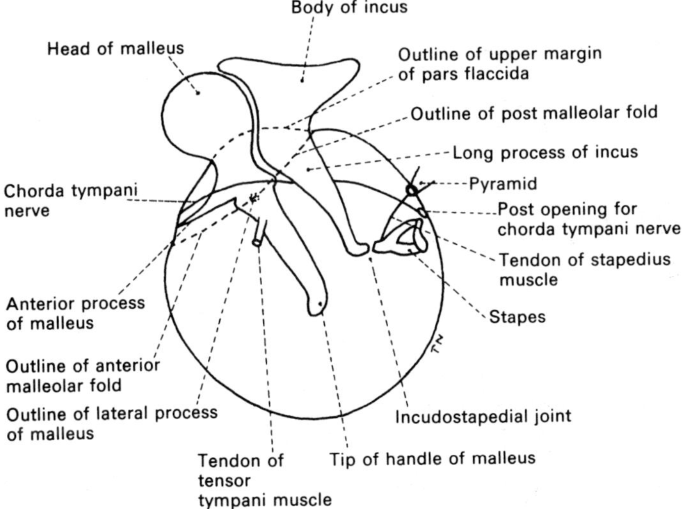

Fig. 1.14. Left tympanic membrane viewed from the medial side with the ossicular chain in position.

course of the *chorda tympani nerve*. It arises from N. VII in the facial canal 6 mm above the stylomastoid foramen and emerges into the tympanic cavity through a small foramen between the lateral and the posterior walls on a level with the pyramid. It now passes lateral to the long process of the incus then arches upwards and forwards under the mucosa of the tympanic membrane forming a fold then crosses the neck of the malleus.

The nerve now passes through the canal of Huguier in the petrotympanic fissure then grooves the spine of the sphenoid bone to enter the pterygoid region where it joins the lingual nerve.

BLOOD SUPPLY

The *blood supply* of the membrane is shown in Figs. 1.15 and 1.16.

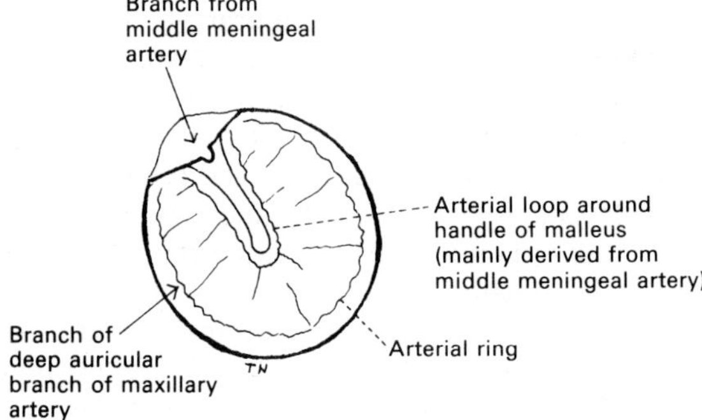

Fig. 1.15. Plan of the arterial supply of the tympanic membrane: outer surface, left side. (The vessels lie between the thin skin layer and the fibrous layer.)

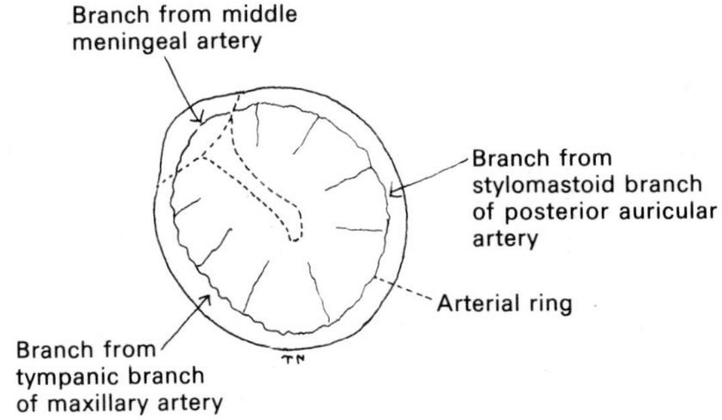

Fig. 1.16. Plan of the arterial supply of the tympanic membrane: inner surface, left side. (The vessels lie between the mucosa and the fibrous layer.)

On the outer surface (Fig. 1.15) there is an arterial ring under the thin skin layer. It is formed chiefly by the deep auricular branch of the maxillary artery. There is also an arterial loop around the handle of the malleus. This is formed by a branch from the middle meningeal artery which travels through the hiatus of the facial canal then under the mucosa and down the superior ligament of the malleus to reach the handle.

The medial surface also has an arterial ring from which branches supply the mucosa. The arteries forming this ring are shown in Fig. 1.16.

VENOUS DRAINAGE

The veins of the outer surface drain to the external jugular vein. The veins from the inner surface pass through the petrotympanic fissure to the pterygoid plexus.

NERVE SUPPLY

Outer surface: anterior half—auriculotemporal nerve (from mandibular part of N. V). Posterior half—auricular branch of N. X. Inner surface—tympanic branch of N. IX.

Medial wall of middle ear (Fig. 1.17)

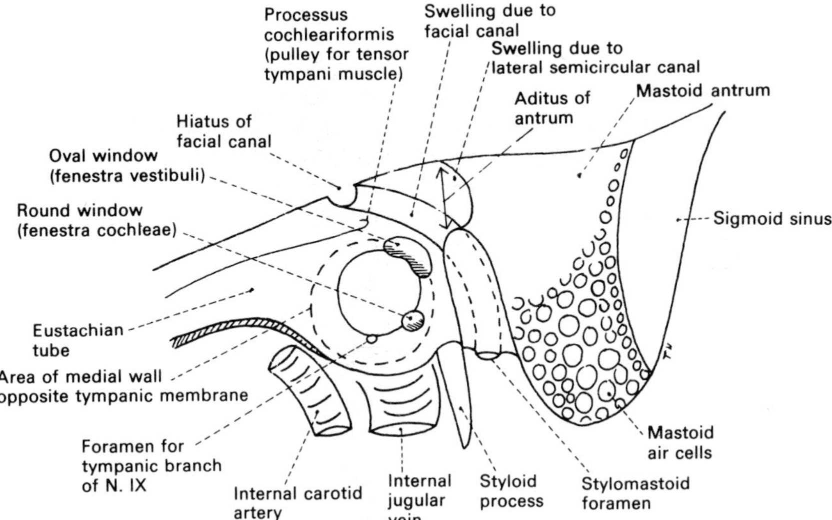

Fig. 1.17. Plan of the medial wall of the left middle ear and antrum.

This is formed by the lateral surface of the petrous part of the temporal bone. The most prominent feature is the *promontory* produced by the basal coil of the cochlea. Above and behind it is the *oval window* (fenestra vestibuli) which leads into the bony vestibule of the inner ear. The oval window is about 3 mm deep—this is called the oval niche. The lateral part of the niche receives the footplate of the stapes. The margins of the footplate and the opposing wall of the niche are covered with cartilage. The footplate is held in position by an elastic annular ligament. Below and behind the promontory is the *round window* (fenestra cochleae) which faces posteriorly and is closed by a membrane, the *secondary tympanic membrane*. This also consists of three layers—an outer mucosal layer which is part of the lining of the tympanic cavity, a middle fibrous layer, and an inner mesothelium continuous with that of the bony cochlea. The round window is also about 3 mm deep—this is called the niche of the round window and the membrane is placed about half-way along it.

When the footplate of the stapes is rocked inwards by the ossicular chain a pressure wave is transmitted to the perilymph in the bony labyrinth. This wave travels along the scala vestibuli into the scala tympani (Fig. 1.31) and finally reaches the secondary tympanic membrane which becomes convex outwards and prevents the perilymph from reaching the tympanic cavity.

Below the promontory is the opening for the tympanic branch of N. IX.

Note the extent of the medial wall which lies opposite the tympanic membrane. The part of the medial wall above the level of the tympanic membrane is the medial wall of the attic. It shows the facial canal and above this lies the bony vestibule and the bony lateral semicircular canal. Behind the attic lies the aditus which is the opening into the mastoid antrum. The lateral semicircular canal forms a swelling on the medial wall of the aditus and below this the facial canal also forms a swelling which partly occupies the floor of the aditus. The part of the facial canal in the medial wall of the attic is often called the horizontal part, but the canal in fact inclines gently downwards and backwards at an angle of 30° with the horizontal to reach the aditus; it then turns sharply downwards and descends vertically in the posterior wall of the tympanic cavity to reach the stylomastoid foramen.

It is useful to remember the structures lying opposite each quadrant of the membrane (Fig. 1.18). The quadrants are outlined by using a vertical line

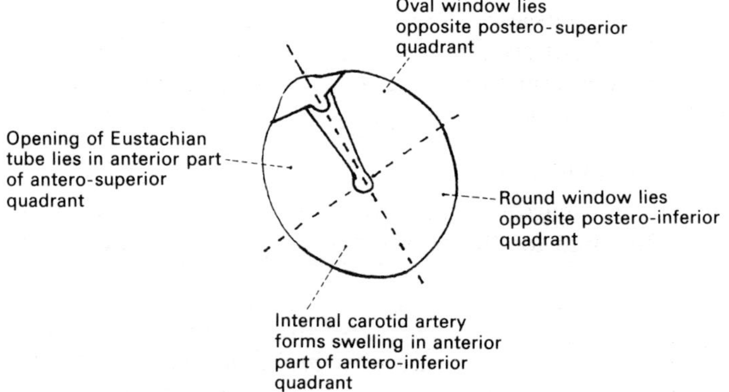

Fig. 1.18. Outer surface of the left tympanic membrane, showing the four quadrants and related structures. (The centre of the promontory lies opposite the lower end of the handle of the malleus.)

along the handle of the malleus and a horizontal line through the umbo. The middle-ear cavity is usually drained through an incision made in the anterio-inferior quadrant because this area is less vascular, not related to important structures, and lies opposite the lowest part of the cavity. The incision heals better if placed along the radial fibres of the fibrous layer of the tympanic membrane.

Posterior wall of middle ear (Fig. 1.19)

The posterior wall is narrow and shows the *aditus* in its upper third. Below this the facial canal is the most important feature; it now descends vertically

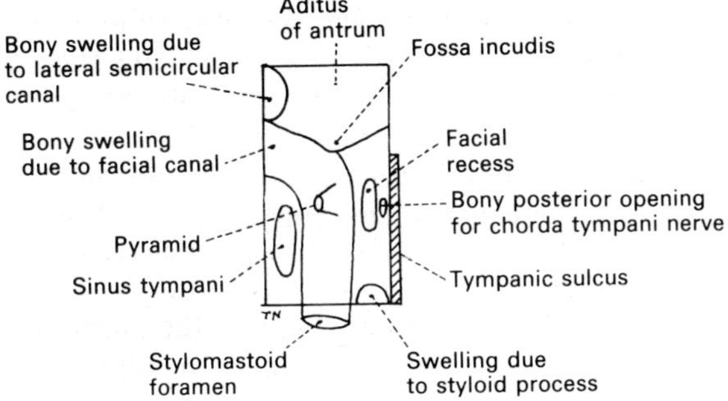

Fig. 1.19. Plan of the posterior wall of the left middle-ear cavity.

in the petrous part of the temporal bone to reach the stylomastoid foramen. Above it in the floor of the aditus is the fossa incudis to which the short process of the incus is attached by two small ligaments. On the lateral side of the facial canal there is a small recess called the facial recess; on the medial side there is another recess called the sinus tympani. Note the other points in Fig. 1.19. The pyramid is a small bony projection on the facial canal; it is hollow and from its cavity wall the stapedius muscle arises then passes through a foramen at its apex from which it runs to its insertion into the neck of the stapes. The bony opening for the chorda tympani nerve is also seen; it emerges from the lateral part of the posterior wall alongside the tympanic sulcus and lies about the level of the pyramid.

Anterior wall of middle ear (Fig. 1.20)

The anterior wall is narrower than the posterior wall. It shows from above downwards the canal for the tensor tympani muscle, the opening of the

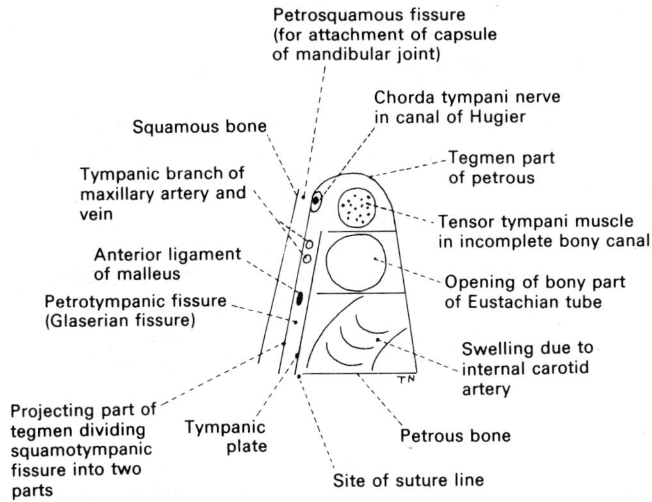

Fig. 1.20. Plan of the anterior wall of the left middle-ear cavity viewed from the inside.

Eustachian tube and below this the wall is convex owing to the internal carotid artery in its bony canal. Between the anterior and lateral walls is the petrotympanic fissure; the structures passing through it are shown in Fig. 1.20.

The structures in the anterior wall are also seen in Fig. 1.17. The bony septum between the tensor canal and the Eustachian tube ends near the oval window in a curved pulley which is called the processus cochleariformis; around it the tendon of the tensor muscle turns sharply then passes across the tympanic cavity to become inserted into the upper part of the handle of the malleus.

Roof of middle ear

This is also shown in Fig. 1.17. It is formed by the tegmen part of the petrous and shows the opening from the facial canal called the hiatus canalis facialis. At this point of the facial canal lies the facial ganglion (the geniculate ganglion) from which the greater superficial petrosal nerve is given off, then passes through the hiatus to enter the middle cranial fossa. A branch of the middle meningeal artery also enters the tympanic cavity through the hiatus. The lesser superficial petrosal nerve passes through a separate foramen lateral to the hiatus to reach the middle cranial fossa. Above the tegmen lies the temporal lobe of the brain and its membranes. The petrosquamous suture lies lateral to the roof and through it infection can pass into the middle cranial fossa. Immediately after the ganglion the facial canal turns at right angles and passes backwards on the medial wall of the attic.

Floor of middle ear

This is also shown in Fig. 1.17. It is formed by part of the petrous. The main relation is the bulb of the internal jugular vein which lies in the jugular fossa; the wall of the fossa may be very thin or deficient in places. Behind the vein is a small swelling due to the styloid process; in front of the vein lies a small part of the internal carotid artery in the carotid canal.

Mucosal folds of middle ear

These are folds of mucosa around the ossicles, ligaments, and muscles. They form spaces in which local suppuration may occur. The folds are more prominent in early childhood and gradually disappear with age.

Nerve supply of middle ear, antrum and air cells (Fig. 1.21)

A tympanic plexus is formed on the promontory by

1. The tympanic branch of N. IX (which is both sensory and parasympathetic).
2. Sympathetic branches from the plexus on the internal carotid (from superior cervical ganglion).
3. A branch from the facial ganglion (probably parasympathetic).

From the plexus branches are given off to the tympanic cavity and the Eustachian tube. The lesser superficial petrosal nerve is also given off from

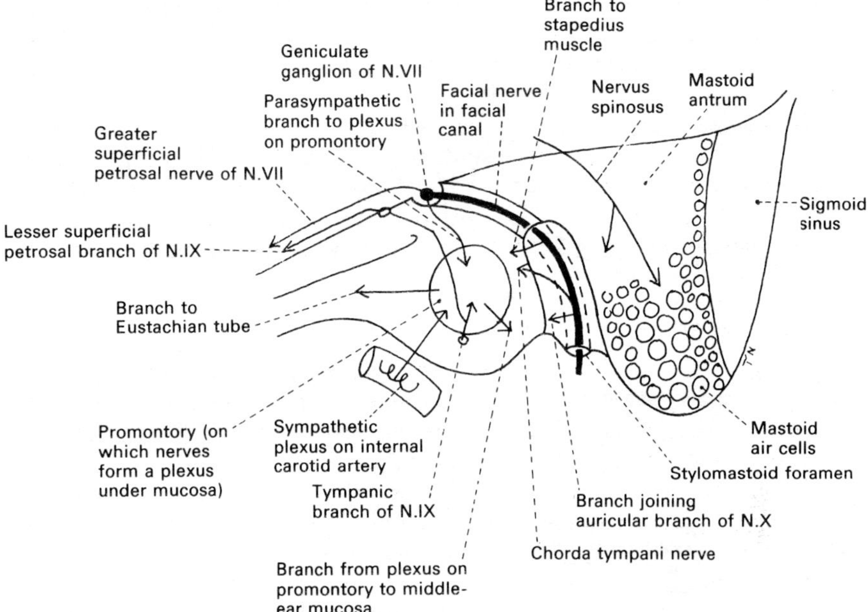

Fig. 1.21. Plan of the nerve supply to the left middle ear, antrum, and air cells. The nerves going to the promontory form a plexus under the mucosa.

the plexus; it consists of the parasympathetic fibres of N. IX which ascend over the promontory to pass through a small canal lateral to the hiatus canalis facialis; it then passes under the dura of the middle cranial fossa then through the foramen ovale to relay in the otic ganglion, and then supplies the parotid gland.

The antrum and air cells are supplied by the nervus spinosus (Fig. 1.21). It arises from the trunk of the mandibular part of N. V below the foramen ovale, then enters the cranial cavity through the foramen spinosum with the middle meningeal artery and runs under the dura.

Blood supply of middle ear, antrum, and air cells (Fig. 1.22)

ARTERIES

The main arteries are:

1. The tympanic branch of the maxillary artery.
2. The stylomastoid branch of the posterior auricular artery.

There are also smaller arteries as shown in Fig. 1.22.

VEINS

The chief drainage is probably through the petrotympanic fissure to the pterygoid plexus.

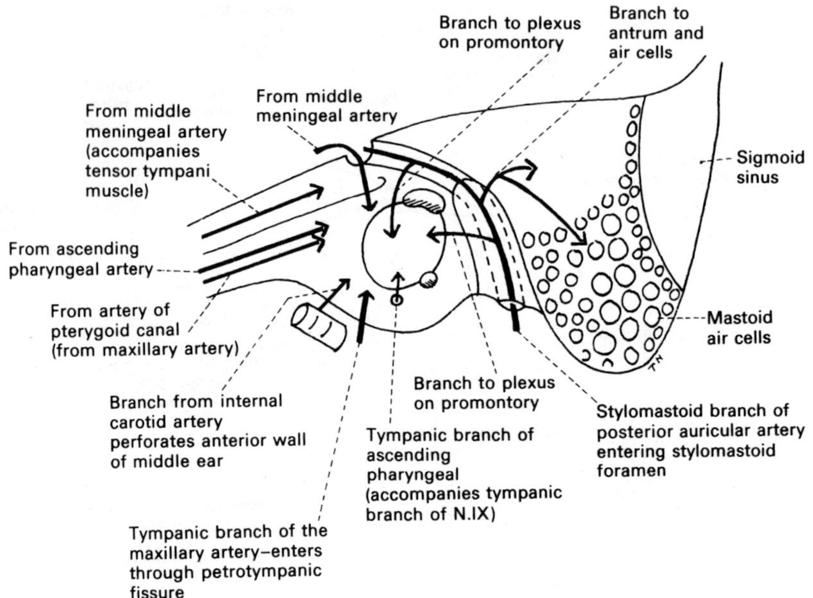

Fig. 1.22. Plan of the blood supply of the left middle ear, antrum, and air cells. The blood vessels on the promontory form a plexus under the mucosa.

LYMPHATICS

These follow the tympanic branch of the maxillary artery to the nodes inside the parotid gland.

BLOOD SUPPLY OF THE OSSICLES (FIG. 1.23)

The malleus and incus are supplied from above by a branch from the middle meningeal artery. This enters the middle ear through the hiatus canalis facialis then passes down the mucosal fold around the superior ligament of the malleus. The branches now enter the substance of the ossicles. Some branches also run around the ossicles in the mucosa. In the case of the malleus the handle is supplied by the tympanic branch of the maxillary artery. The *lenticular process* of the incus is the curved lower end of the long process. It has a poor blood supply, mainly from mucosal vessels. After stapedectomy the closure of a prosthesis around the lenticular process may reduce its blood supply and lead to necrosis of the lenticular process and separation of the prosthesis.

There is also an arterial circle supplying the head and neck of the stapes—this is formed chiefly by the stapedial artery which accompanies the stapedius tendon and arises from the stylomastoid branch of the posterior auricular artery. There is also a plexus on both sides of the footplate of the stapes—the plexus on the medial surface is supplied by the internal auditory artery; that on the lateral surface is formed by tympanic branches from the middle meningeal artery and the tympanic branch of the maxillary artery.

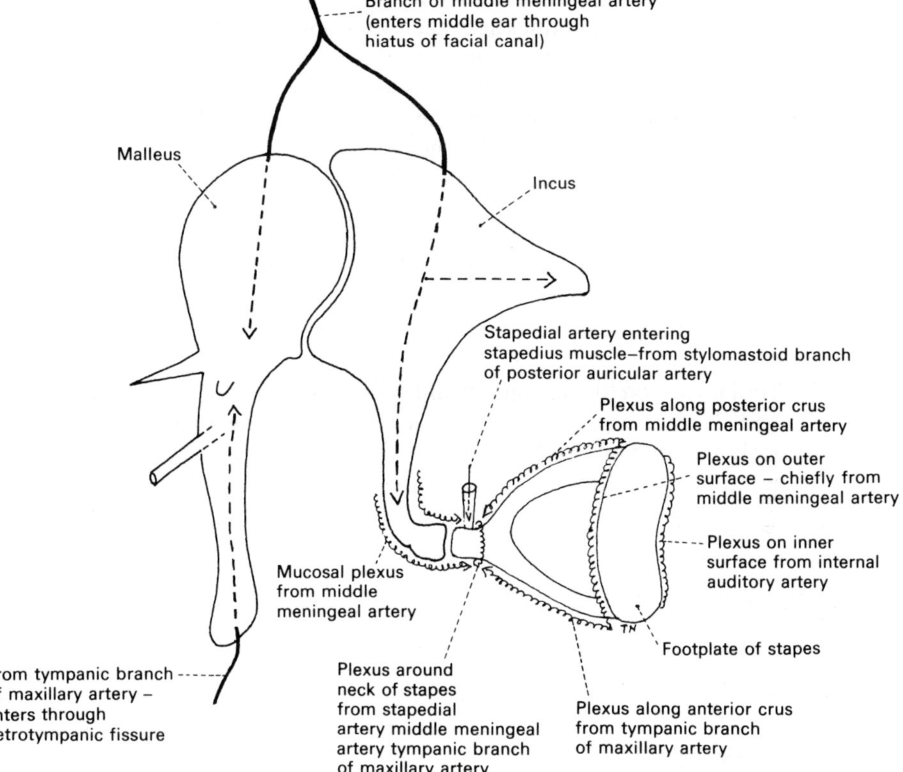

Fig. 1.23. Plan of the arterial supply of the ossicular chain in the middle-ear cavity. The vessels represented by dotted lines are inside the ossicles. The plexuses are under the mucosa.

From this lateral plexus a branch passes up each crus to join the arterial circle around the head and neck of the stapes.

THE MASTOID ANTRUM

This is one of the largest air cells in the temporal bone. Fig. 1.17. Its approximate dimensions are: anteroposterior length 10 mm; vertical height 10–15 mm; side to side width 5 mm. Anteriorly it communicates with the attic through an opening called the aditus which occupies the upper one-third of the posterior wall of the middle ear. On the medial wall of the aditus is a swelling due to the lateral semicircular canal (p. 19) and below this a second swelling due to the facial canal which also occupies part of the floor of the aditus. Below the aditus the anterior wall of the antrum is formed of bone containing the facial canal.

The lateral wall of the antrum is formed by the squamous part of the temporal bone. It is 10 to 15 mm thick in the adult. At birth it is 2 mm thick, then increases by 1 mm in thickness each year until it reaches adult proportions. On the lateral wall is the suprameatal triangle (Macewen's triangle) (see Fig. 1.46). The base of the triangle is usually formed by a prominent ridge showing a small spine called the spine of Henle. The triangle is an important guide to the antrum. It is not the surface marking of the antrum since the antrum is much larger, but in the adult it indicates the superior level of the antrum.

The medial wall of the antrum is formed by the petrous bone and in this lies the posterior semicircular canal. Sometimes a number of small veins pass through the medial wall to the subarcuate fossa and end in the superior petrosal sinus; they may carry infection into the posterior cranial fossa and cause meningitis.

The roof is formed by the tegmen and above it lies the temporal lobe of the brain and its membranes. Inferiorly it opens into the mastoid air cells. Posteriorly the antrum is related to the sigmoid sinus and commonly this is surrounded by air cells.

NERVE SUPPLY

Nervus spinosus from the mandibular part of N. V. It passes into the skull through the foramen spinosum, runs under the dura mater, supplies it, then sends a branch through the petrosquamous suture to supply the antrum and air cells from above (Fig. 1.21).

The mastoid air cells (Fig. 1.17)

These are developed as buds from the antrum, the formation of air cells being called *pneumatization*. The buds invade the mastoid part of the temporal bone from birth to puberty when the process is completed. The mastoid process, which is the part of the mastoid which projects below the level of the external meatus, does not appear until about three years of age and is said to be due to the invasion of air cells from above, plus the pull of the neck muscles. When small the mastoid part of the temporal bone and the mastoid process are almost solid but as they enlarge diploë (marrow) appears in the interior. Normally the diploë is later replaced by air cells which invade it from above downwards. Therefore the structure of the mastoid part of the temporal bone including the mastoid process may vary in the following manner:

1. It may be fully pneumatized and thus consist only of air cells, the largest cells being in the centre and extending to the tip, and the smallest arranged at the periphery. Small air cells are usually found in the posterior wall of the bony meatus; others may extend backwards around the sigmoid sinus and pass towards the area of Trautmann's triangle on the posterior surface of the petrous bone, medial to the sigmoid sinus (Fig. 1.47); others may invade the supramastoid crest; others may reach the postero-inferior angle of the parietal and perhaps also the occipital bone.

Air cells may also extend around the facial canal and around the semi-circular canals.

2. If pneumatization is incomplete it may consist of air cells in the centre surrounded by diploic spaces containing marrow or it may consist only of diploic spaces.
3. In some cases it may be sclerotic, the formation of diploë and air cells both having been arrested, for example by inflammation.

In addition to mastoid pneumatization air cells may also be found along the wall of the auditory tube and around the carotid canal extending almost to the apex of the petrous temporal. These air cells develop as buds from the tympanic cavity or the tube itself.

Normal pneumatization is usually found in 80 per cent of adults. It is interesting that air cells are usually well formed in light skulls but small and scanty in thick heavy skulls.

The function of these air cells is to provide a reservoir of air which can be used to maintain the pressure on the inner surface of the tympanic membrane if the auditory tube becomes blocked.

THE EUSTACHIAN TUBE (AUDITORY TUBE)

This connects the middle ear to the nasopharynx (Figs. 1.7 and 1.24). In the adult it is 36 mm long. It commences in the anterior wall of the tympanic cavity and is directed downwards, forwards, and medially. It consists of a bony part which is 12 mm long and a cartilaginous part which is 24 mm long. The narrowest point is where the bony and cartilaginous parts meet. The widest part is the opening into the nasopharynx. The bony part lies under the canal for the tensor tympani (Fig. 1.7) and the carotid canal runs forwards on its medial side.

The cartilaginous part inclines downwards slightly more than the bony part (Fig. 1.24) and is formed of fibrocartilage and elastic fibrous tissue. The cartilage is triangular in shape and is folded to form an incomplete tube which is completed laterally by elastic fibrous tissue (Fig. 1.25). The apex of

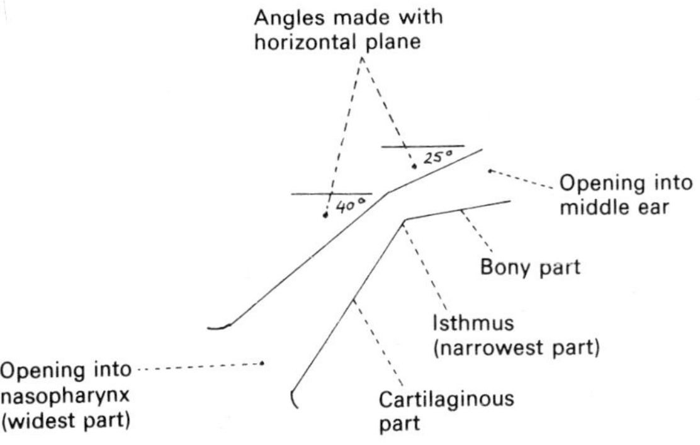

Fig. 1.24. Plan of the left Eustachian tube (auditory tube).

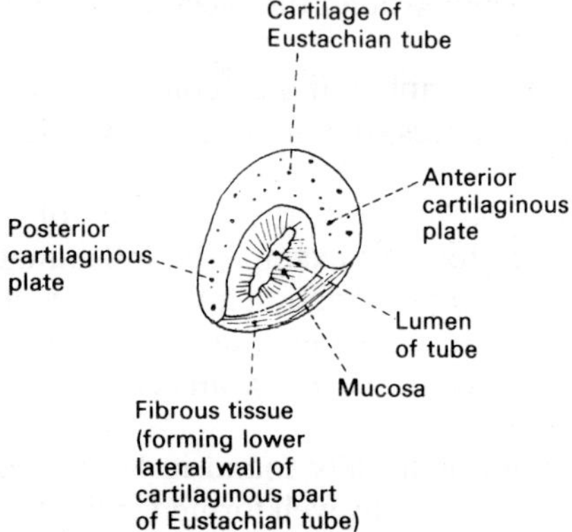

Fig. 1.25. Transverse section of the left Eustachian tube near its nasopharyngeal end. The sides of the folded cartilage are called the anterior plate and the posterior plate.

the cartilage is fixed to the bony part of the tube, while the expanded base projects under the mucosa in the nasopharynx forming a prominent margin called the tubal elevation (Fig. 1.26). The cartilaginous part is fixed to a groove on the base of the skull between the petrous and the great wing of the sphenoid (Fig. 1.27). Relations—medially lies the internal carotid artery in the petrous; laterally is the great wing of the sphenoid showing the foramen ovale, foramen spinosum, and more laterally the lateral pterygoid muscle. Two soft palate muscles become associated with the tube in this region, namely the tensor palati and levator palati and both of these have fibres of origin from the tube and also from the adjacent bone. This part of the tube

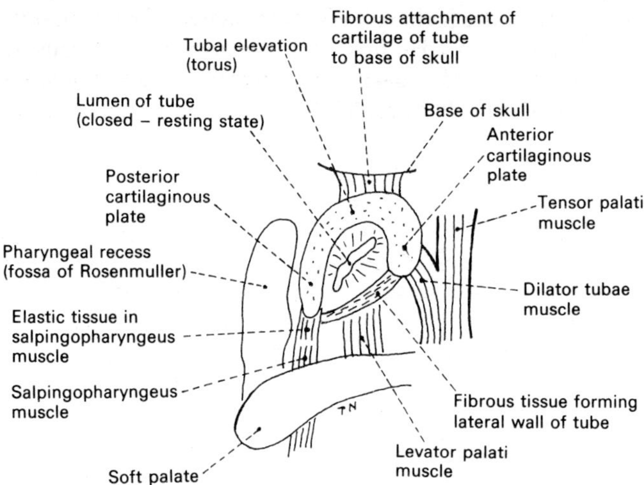

Fig. 1.26. Diagram showing the opening of the left Eustachian tube into the nasopharynx. The mucosa has been removed to show the related muscles.

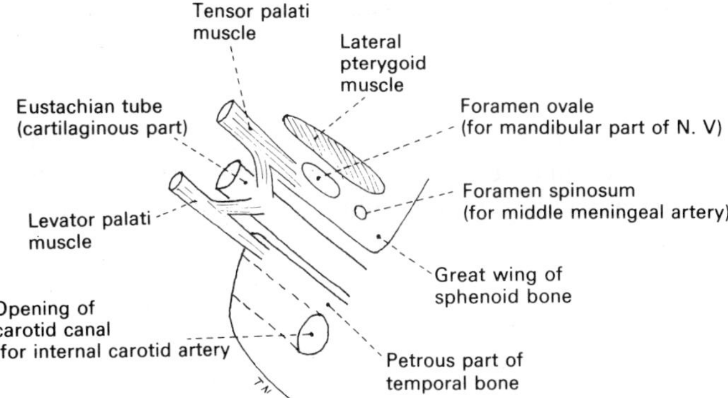

Fig. 1.27. Relations of the left Eustachian tube in its groove on the base of the skull.

can also be seen lying against the outer wall of the nasopharynx above the upper border of the superior constrictor muscle, this region being called the sinus of Morgagni (Fig. 1.7). Here it lies against the pharyngobasilar fascia (pharyngeal aponeurosis) of the pharynx which it soon pierces to open into the nasopharynx. In the adult the pharyngeal orifice lies 12 mm behind the posterior end of the inferior turbinate. The most prominent feature of the orifice is the overhanging tubal elevation which extends downwards as a prominent anterior and posterior cartilaginous plate under the mucosa on each side of the orifice (Fig. 1.26). In the floor of the orifice is a slight swelling and if the mucosa is removed it is seen to be due to the levator muscle entering the soft palate. If the mucosa is removed in front of the orifice the anterior cartilaginous plate is seen and also the tensor palati and the dilator tubae muscle joining it. From the posterior cartilaginous plate a mucosal fold is seen descending into the pharyngeal wall; this is produced chiefly by the underlying salpingopharyngeus muscle which is attached above by elastic fibres to the posterior cartilaginous plate and to the mucosal floor of the tubal orifice; inferiorly it is inserted among the pharyngeal constrictors.

The tubal orifice is usually closed except during swallowing and yawning when it allows air to enter the middle ear to maintain equality of pressure on both sides of the tympanic membrane. The tensor palati and its dilator tubae part open the pharyngeal orifice, probably assisted by the levator palati muscle. The salpingopharyngeus probably keeps the orifice closed by tonic contraction pulling down the posterior cartilaginous plate and the mucosal floor and making the opening slit like; during swallowing, when the pharynx is pulled upwards, it relaxes and allows the tube to be opened by the other muscles. In the resting state the mucosa of the side walls of the tube lie in apposition except at the upper and lower ends.

The mucosa of the tube is continuous with that of the middle ear, antrum, and air cells. The lining epithelium is columnar ciliated but this ends on the anterior wall of the middle ear. Thereafter in the middle-ear antrum and air cells the lining epithelium mostly consists of flattened non-ciliated cells.

NERVE SUPPLY

Bony part—branches from tympanic plexus. Cartilaginous part—upper part which lies in groove on base of skull is supplied by nervous spinosus branch of mandibular nerve; lower part—pharyngeal branch of sphenopalatine ganglion.

BLOOD SUPPLY

Ascending pharyngeal artery (from external carotid); middle meningeal artery (from maxillary A.); artery of pterygoid canal (from maxillary A.). Veins drain into pterygoid plexus.

GROWTH CHANGES

At birth the tube is almost horizontal. Thereafter is begins to slope downwards because of growth changes in the base of the skull. At about four years it forms an angle of about 20° with the horizontal; in the adult the slope is about 40° with the horizontal.

Growth of the tube in length is rapid; at birth the total length is 17 mm, at six years it is 30 mm, and in the adult 36 mm. Up to six years of age there is practically no bony part of the tube almost its whole length being cartilaginous; whereas in the adult one-third of the whole tube is bony.

The pharyngeal orifice is relatively wider in early childhood (six months to six years), whereas the tympanic orifice is of adult size. At birth the pharyngeal orifice is immediately above the soft palate; at six years it is 4 mm above soft palate; at twelve years it rises to 8 mm, and in adult life to 10 mm above the soft palate. These changes are due to the descent of the palate as the nasal cavities increase in height.

Middle-ear infection is thus facilitated in the child since the tube is almost horizontal, shorter and relatively wider than in the adult.

FUNCTIONS OF MIDDLE EAR CAVITY

1. It allows the transmission of sound waves via the ossicular chain to the oval window.
2. It increases the intensity of the sound waves.
3. The middle-ear cavity is an air containing cavity whereas the inner ear contains fluid. Transmission of sound waves is impeded in fluid and the middle-ear cavity helps to match this impedance.

INNER EAR

This consists of a bony labyrinth and a membranous labyrinth which lies inside the body labyrinth and contains the essential organ of hearing and the special receptors for balance.

Bony labyrinth

The bony labyrinth lies in the petrous part of the temporal bone. It consists of harder bone than the surrounding petrous and can therefore be separated by dissection. It consists of a central part called the vestibule, a coiled tube called the bony cochlea placed anteromedially, and three bony semicircular canals placed posterolaterally (Figs. 1.7 and 1.28).

A plan of the lateral surface of the bony labyrinth is shown in Fig. 1.28 and the internal appearances are shown in Fig. 1.29.

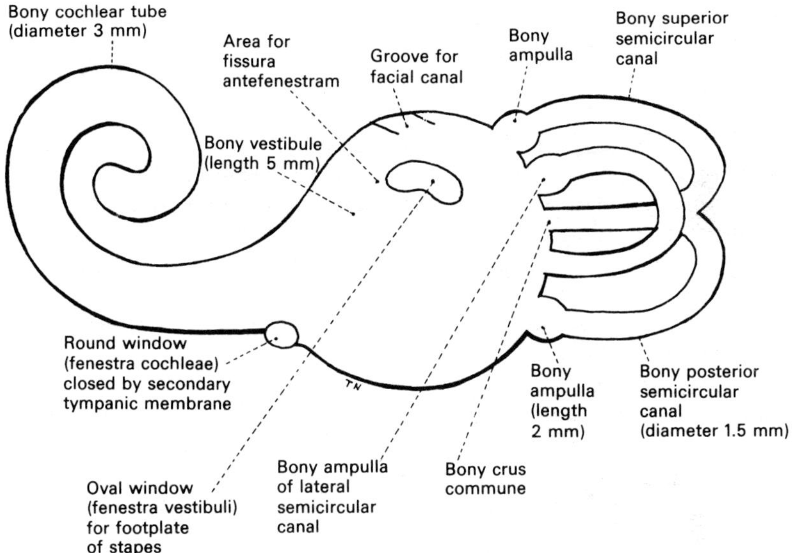

Fig. 1.28. Plan of the lateral surface of the left bony labyrinth.

SEMICIRCULAR CANALS

There are three **semicircular canals**—superior, lateral, and posterior. One end of each canal is expanded and called the ampulla. The canals are placed in planes at right angles to each other. They open by only five openings into the vestibule, since one end of the superior and posterior canals join to form a common canal called the crus commune.

VESTIBULE

The **vestibule** shows the *oval window* (fenestra vestibuli) and above it is a groove for the facial canal (Fig. 1.28). Below lies the *round window* (fenestra cochleae). In front of the oval window is the area of the *fissura ante fenestram*; this is a fissure containing fibrous tissue which becomes ossified in otosclerosis and causes the footplate of the stapes to become fixed.

The interior of the vestibule (Fig. 1.29) contains two depressions for the

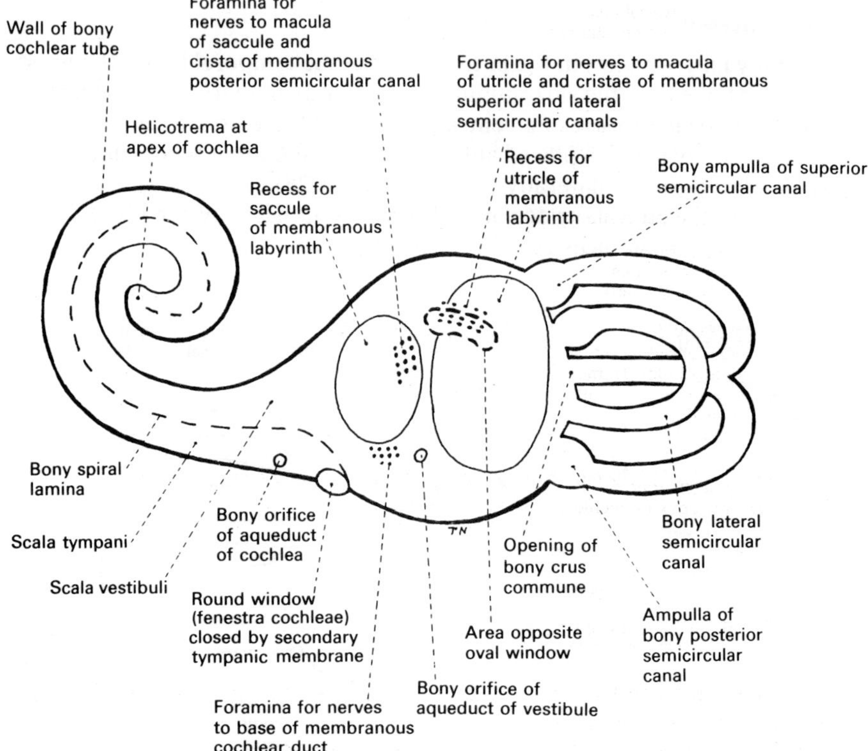

Fig. 1.29. Plan of the internal appearances of the left bony labyrinth after removal of the lateral wall.

utricle and *saccule* of the membranous labyrinth, and a small canal called the *aqueduct* of the *vestibule*.

THE BONY COCHLEA

This is cone-shaped (Figs. 1.7 and 1.30) and measures about 5 mm from base to apex. It consists of a bony tube coiled $2\frac{3}{4}$ times around a bony pillar called the *modiolus* (Fig. 1.30). The modiolus is almost horizontal when the body is in the upright position. The base of the modiolus lies against the antero-inferior quadrant of the cribriform plate at the outer end of the internal meatus. The basal coil of the tube is the widest and produces a swelling called the promontory on the medial wall of the middle-ear cavity (Figs. 1.7 and 1.32). The cavity of the tube is incompletely divided into two chambers by a bony septum called the *bony spiral lamina* (Fig. 1.29) which is attached to the modiolus. The two chambers are called the *scala vestibuli* which opens into the vestibule and the *scala tympani* which ends at the round window where it is separated from the middle ear by the secondary tympanic membrane (Fig. 1.29). At the apex of the cochlea the two scalae communicate

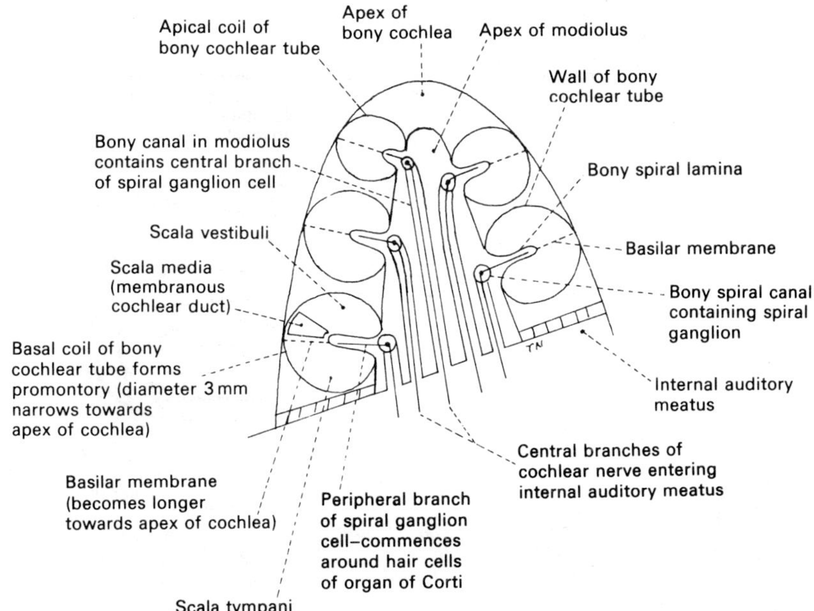

Fig. 1.30. Plan of the left cochlea. (Section along the modiolus.)

with each other; this point is called the *helicotrema* (Fig. 1.29). Near the lower end of the scala tympani is the opening of the aqueduct of the cochlea; this is a small bony canal which opens on the inferior surface of the petrous bone medial to the jugular fossa.

The membranous labyrinth

This lies inside the bony labyrinth (see Fig. 1.31). It has three parts as in the bony labyrinth:

1. Three membranous semicircular canals inside the bony canals.
2. Two sacs, the utricle and saccule, lodged in the bony vestibule.
3. The cochlear duct lying within the canal of the bony cochlea.

THE MEMBRANOUS SEMICIRCULAR CANALS

Are similar in shape to the bony canals and each has one swollen end called the ampulla. They are a quarter of the diameter of the bony canals and are held in position by fibrous bands. The membranous ampullae almost fill the bony ampullae.

THE UTRICLE AND SACCULE

The *utricle* is a sac which receives the five openings of the membranous canals. The *saccule* is a smaller sac and is joined to the cochlear duct by the narrow canal called the canalis reuniens. From both the utricle and the saccule a small duct is given off and these join to form the ductus endo-

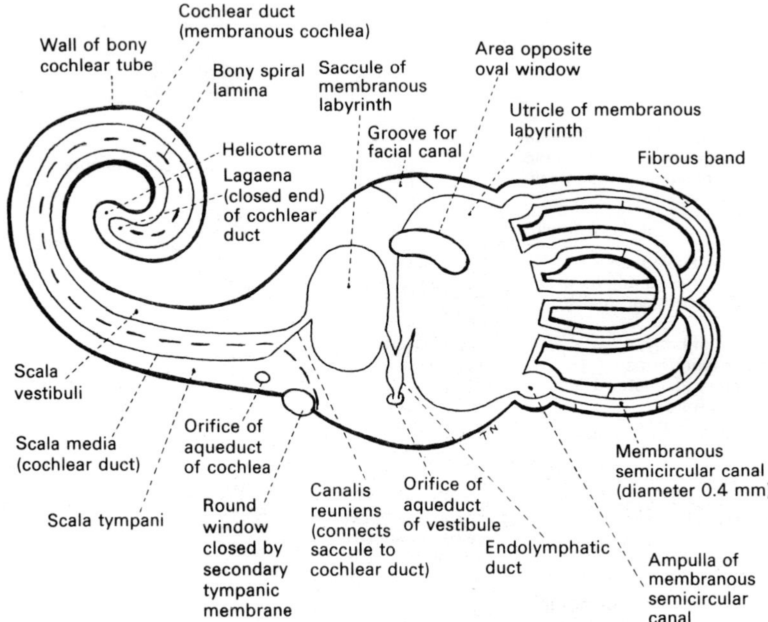

Fig. 1.31. Plan of the membranous labyrinth inside the left bony labyrinth.

lymphaticus. This passes through the aqueduct of the vestibule which is a small bony canal which passes to the posterior surface of the petrous and ends as a slit-like opening 12 mm behind the internal meatus (see Fig. 1.48). The ductus emerges through this opening and ends blindly under the dura surrounded by a plexus of capillaries. The blind end is slightly dilated and called the saccus (Fig. 1.37).

In the utricle and saccule and in each membranous ampulla part of the wall is thickened to form a vestibular receptor. In these special areas the epithelium is modified and consists of hair cells and supporting cells resting on thickened periosteum. The special receptor areas in the utricle and saccule are called the maculae and the hairs project into a gelatinous mass containing particles of calcium carbonate called *otoliths.* The receptor in each membranous ampulla also consists of hair cells and supporting cells resting on thickened periosteum; these form a small crest called the crista and the hairs project into a gelatinous mass called the cupola. The fibres of the vestibular nerve commence around these hair cells, then pierce the cribriform plate to enter the vestibular ganglion (Scarpa's ganglion) which lies in the internal auditory meatus (Fig. 1.32). They are the peripheral processes of the ganglion cells. The ganglion cells are bipolar and thus there is no relay. The central processes of the ganglion cells form the main part of the vestibular nerve which joins the cochlear nerve in the internal auditory meatus to form the vestibulocochlear nerve which enters the brain stem in

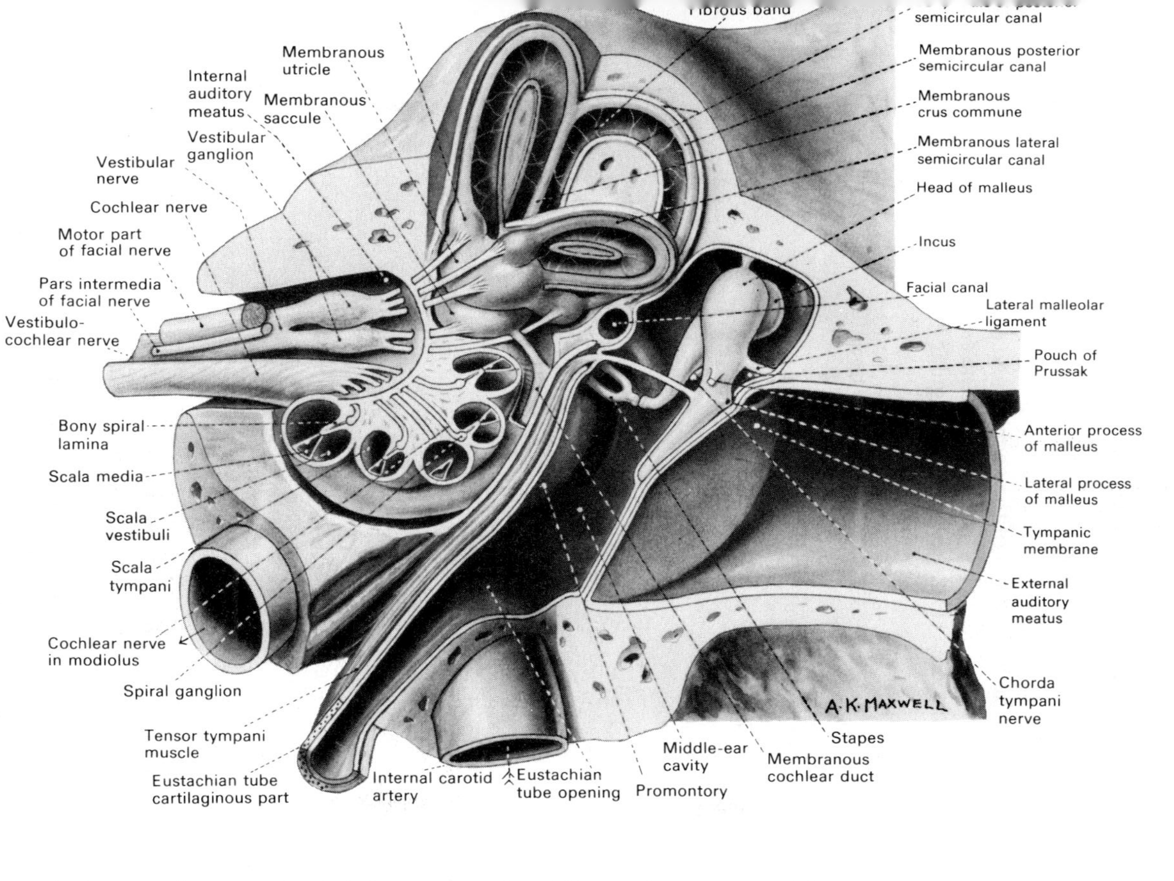

Fig. 1.32. Diagram showing part of the left external ear, the middle ear, the inner ear, and the internal auditory meatus. The inner ear has been opened to show the membranous semicircular canals, utricle, and saccule; the bony cochlea has been opened to show the membranous cochlear duct and the cochlear nerve fibres in the modiolus. The details of the structures in the internal auditory meatus are also shown including the cochlear and vestibular nerve fibres passing through the cribriform plate.

the groove between the pons and medulla. The vestibular fibres then relay in the vestibular nuclei in the floor of the fourth ventricle (Fig. 1.42).

THE COCHLEAR DUCT (THE MEMBRANOUS COCHLEA) (FIG. 1.31)
This lies in the canal of the bony cochlea and ends blindly at the apex of the cochlea. The blind end is called the *lagaena*. At the base of the cochlea the duct communicates with the saccule by the narrow canalis reuniens. When the cochlear duct is in position it lies between the bony spiral lamina and the opposite wall of the bony canal of the cochlea and completes the separation of the scala vestibuli from the scala tympani. The cavity of the cochlear duct is called the scala media (Fig. 1.31). It is triangular in section (Fig. 1.33) and

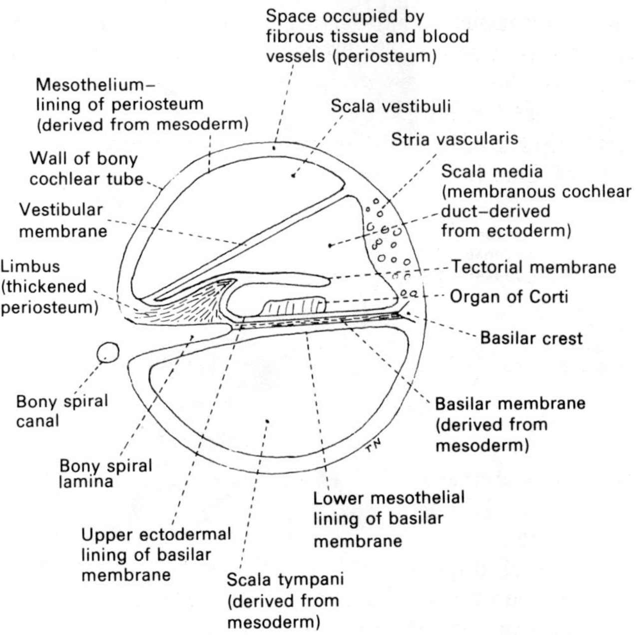

Fig. 1.33. Plan of the left bony cochlear tube and the membranous cochlear duct.

is ectodermal in origin like the brain. The roof is a very thin membrane called Reissner's membrane (the vestibular membrane). It consists of two layers of cells, one derived from the ectoderm of the cochlear duct and the other being mesothelium derived from the mesoderm. The cells of the ectoderm layer are connected by tight junctions which prevent the passage of fluid.

The outer wall consists of specially modified ectodermal epithelium which overlies a great thickening of periosteum containing many blood vessels called the stria vascularis; the epithelial cells have finger-like processes which are applied to the walls of the capillaries (Fig. 1.35).

The floor is formed by the *basilar membrane* which extends from the bony spiral lamina to a thickening of periosteum called the basilar crest. The basilar membrane consists of a substantia propria made up of numerous fibres called the auditory strings which are believed to be 24 000 in number and are embedded in a homogenous ground substance. The membrane has an average length of 30 mm in man and is about four times wider at the apex of the cochlea than at the base (Fig. 1.34). The bony spiral lamina varies in width in a corresponding manner being wider at the base than at the apex (Fig. 30). The auditory strings vibrate in sympathy with the waves of movement in the perilymph of the scala tympani.

The under surface of the basilar membrane is covered by a thin layer of vascular connective tissue and a flattened mesothelium derived from the mesoderm and continuous with the lining of the scala tympani (Fig. 1.33). The upper surface is covered with a layer of epithelium derived from the ectodermal wall of the cochlear duct. The inner zone of this epithelium becomes highly specialized to form the organ of Corti which is the receptor organ of hearing (Fig. 1.35); the outer zone remains as a layer of cubical cells called the cells of Claudius.

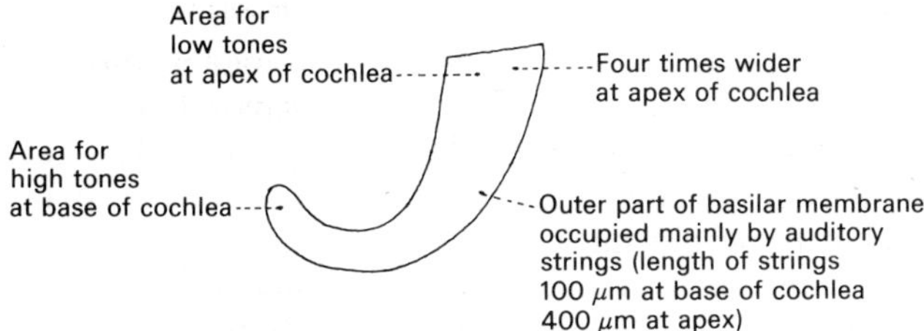

Fig. 1.34. Plan of the basilar membrane.

THE ORGAN OF CORTI

Consists of one row of inner hair cells and three or four rows of outer hair cells. The inner and outer hair cells are separated by the inner and outer rods of Corti which enclose betweem them a tunnel called the tunnel of Corti. The hair cells are also separated by supporting cells which have tight junctions around the upper ends of the hair cells and the rods; these separate the fluid around the hair cells and in the tunnel of Corti from the endolymph in the cochlear duct. The largest hairs of the outer hair cells project into the substance of an overlying membrane called the membrana tectoria which is semi-solid and has marked adhesiveness. The hairs of the inner hair cells are believed to lie free in the endolymph.

There are about one hundred hairs (stereocilia) in each hair cell. In the inner hair cells they are in two rows. In the outer hair cells, they are in three rows. Kinocilia are absent in the hair cells and are replaced in each cell by a basal body which probably directs the movements of the stereocilia.

The waves in the perilymph of the scala tympani produce the vibrations in the basilar membrane. The membrane moves up and down in waves as it vibrates and also produces waves in the endolymph of the scale media; these cause the hairs to bend and this starts the nerve impulse. The movement of the cilia of the outer hair cells may in some way affect the activity of the cilia of the inner hair cells whose afferents form the main component of the cochlear nerve. The function of the outer hair cells is not yet clear. Hair cells can survive for about eight minutes after the arterial supply is cut off or blocked. In contrast brain cells are damaged in about three minutes without oxygen. Hair cells probably survive longer by using up the oxygen in the endolymph.

The cochlear nerve

Its ganglion cells lie in the spiral ganglion and are bipolar so there is no relay in the ganglion. The peripheral processes of the cells commence around the hair cells (Fig. 1.35), then pass through the bony spiral lamina at points called the habenular openings to reach the spiral canal (Rosenthal's canal) containing the spiral ganglion. The central processes of the ganglion cells now run through the modiolus then pierce the antero-inferior quadrant of the cribriform plate and enter the internal auditory meatus as the afferent fibres of the cochlear nerve which then joins the vestibular nerve to form the vestibulocochlear nerve. They finally pass to the groove below the pons then enter the upper part of the medulla. Their central connections are shown in Fig. 1.42. The fibres on entering the brainstem separate into two groups, ventral and dorsal. The ventral fibres relay in a ventral cochlear nucleus then cross the midline and are now called the trapezoid body; some of these fibres relay in a small trapezoid nucleus then pass to the medial longitudinal bundle which connects them with the other cranial nerve nuclei.

In contrast the dorsal fibres wind around the inferior cerebellar peduncle then relay in a dorsal cochlear nucleus. The pathway is then continued as the auditory striae which pass to the midline then dip into the substance of the upper medulla to join the trapezoid body and form the chief auditory pathway called the lateral lemniscus. This ascends through the pons into the midbrain and relays chiefly in the medial geniculate body; some of its fibres also pass to the inferior colliculus which is a reflex centre in the auditory pathway. The main group of auditory fibres now pass from the medial geniculate body into the posterior part of the posterior limb of the internal capsule of the cerebral hemisphere and are now called the auditory radiation. They finally pass to the upper part of the superior temporal gyrus which is the primary auditory area or the auditosensory area (Fig. 1.43). This receives the impulses and then relays them to the secondary auditory area or auditopsychic area in the surrounding part of the superior temporal gyrus. Here it is believed they are analysed and interpreted by comparison with previously stored information and only now become what we know as hearing; this is a complex function of the cerebral cortex.

The auditory cortical area is connected to other parts of the brain but fibres also pass back to the inferior colliculus and also to the superior colliculus which is a reflex centre in the visual pathway (Fig. 1.42). The two

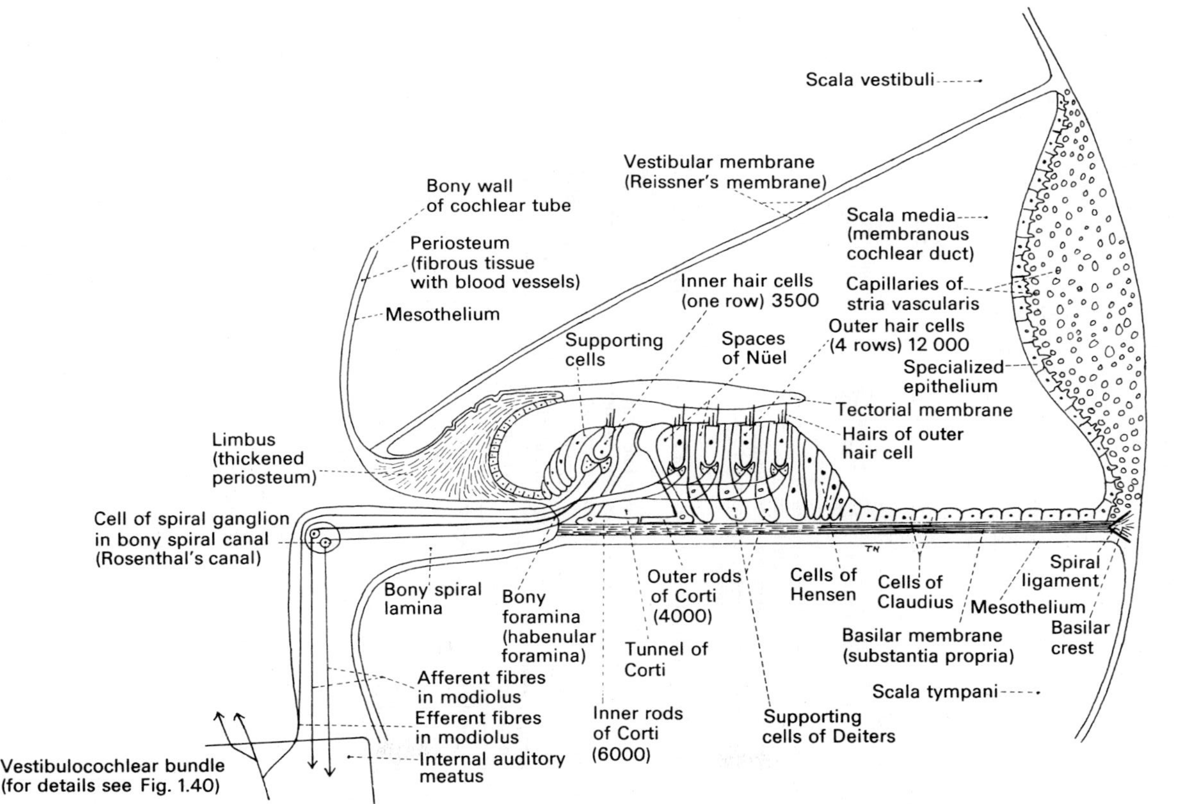

Fig. 1.35. Diagram of the organ of Corti.

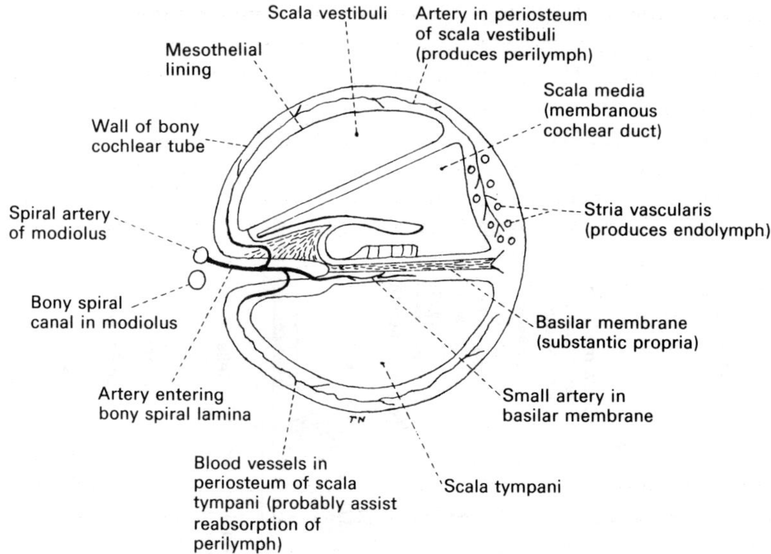

Fig. 1.36. Plan of the arteries in the wall of the bony cochlear tube.

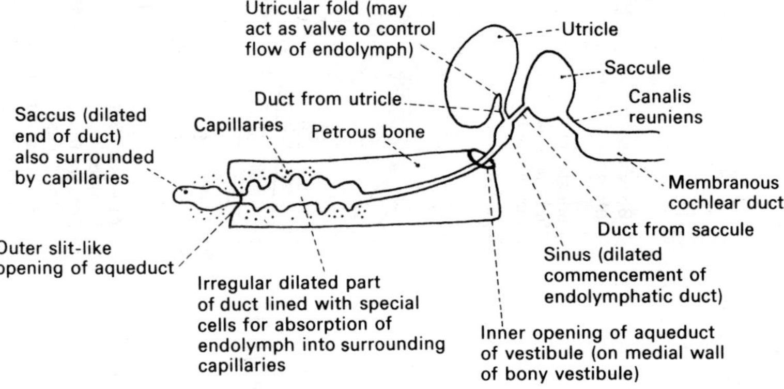

Fig. 1.37. Plan of the endolymphatic duct and sac.

colliculi are then connected to the tectospinal tract which connects them with the anterior horn cells of the spinal cord. Hearing and sight are closely connected and the tectospinal tract allows the body to be moved reflexly in response to a loud noise or a moving object seen approaching.

In man there are about 30 000 ganglion cells in the spiral ganglion. They are of two types, myelinated (type 1) and unmyelinated (type 2). It is now believed that 90 per cent of the afferent fibres in the cochlear nerve come from the inner hair cells and are the processes of the myelinated spiral ganglion cells. The inner hair cells may be compared with the cone cells in the retina; each cell has one or more nerve fibres commencing around it and these give precise and detailed information. In contrast the outer hair cells are like the rod cells in the retina; one nerve fibre conveys impulses from a number of cells and so this information is less precise. These fibres are the processes of the unmyelinated spiral ganglion cells and form about 10 per cent of the afferents in the cochlear nerve.

After destruction of the organ of Corti by ototoxic drugs or virus infections about 10 per cent of the ganglion cells in the spiral ganglion survive if the blood supply is intact. It is believed that these surviving cells are independent of the hair cells and that their peripheral processes are connected to the supporting cells of the organ of Corti. This is utilized in electrical stimulation of the cochlea in very deaf ears (cochlear implant) to produce crude hearing.

THE OLIVOCOCHLEAR EFFERENT FIBRES

These efferent fibres end around the hair cells and are believed to prevent their overaction and thus have a protective function; those to the inner hair cells come from the main superior olivary nucleus of the same side and those to the outer hair cells arise in the accessory olivary nucleus of the opposite side.

Vestibular efferents also come from the olivary nuclei. They join the cochlear efferents to form the vestibulocochlear bundle which runs with the vestibular nerve in the internal auditory meatus (Fig. 1.38). At the outer end of the meatus the cochlear efferents separate from the vestibular efferents and join the cochlear nerve to pass into the modiolus. The vestibular efferents pass to the hair cells of the vestibular receptors and are also believed to prevent overaction.

Both the cochlear and the vestibular efferents are part of the extrapyramidal system which is chiefly inhibitory in function.

HEARING LOSS

Clinically *hearing loss* is described as sensorineural or conductive.

Sensorineural hearing loss. This may be due to several causes:

1. Incomplete damage to the organ of Corti: results in deafness to certain levels of hearing frequency in the ear involved.
2. Complete damage to the organ of Corti or cochlear nuclei: results in total deafness in that ear.
3. Damage to lateral lemniscus or medial geniculate body or cortex: results in impaired hearing in both ears but more marked on the opposite side because the fibres of the cochlear nerve cross to the opposite side in the upper medulla (Fig. 1.42).

Conductive hearing loss is mainly due to damage to the ossicular chain. It is also produced by fluid in the middle ear cavity, eustachian tube dysfunction or a large perforation in the tympanic membrane. In all these cases the hearing is impaired to a varying degree but the hearing which remains is due to bone conduction producing vibrations in the skull bones which result in the production of waves in the inner ear fluids; these then stimulate the unaffected sensory neural pathway.

Noises in the ear (tinnitus) are produced by a lesion in the external, middle or inner ear or its nervous connections.

THE PERILYMPH

This is the fluid which fills all parts of the bony labyrinth. It is believed to be derived from the blood vessels in the wall of the scala vestibuli (Fig. 1.36) and reabsorbed by the blood vessels in the wall of the scala tympani and perhaps also through the aqueduct of the cochlea into the cerebrospinal fluid in the subarachnoid space. It is low in potassium and high in sodium.

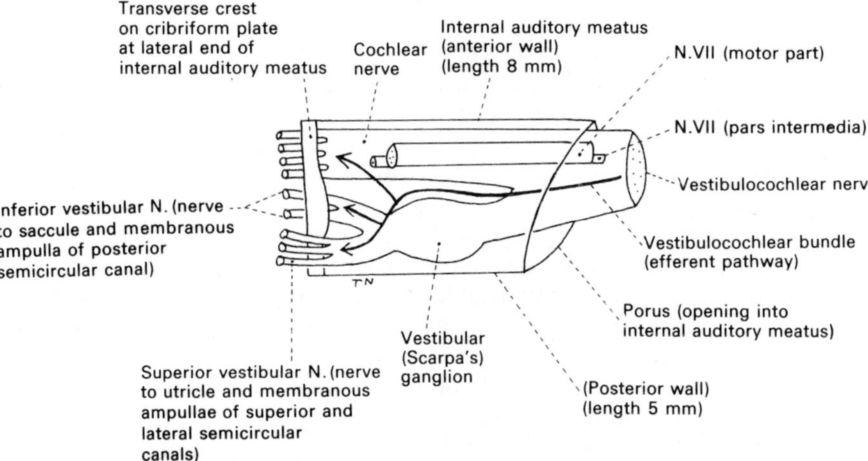

Fig. 1.38. Plan of the nerves in the left internal auditory meatus.

THE ENDOLYMPH

This is the fluid which fills all parts of the membranous labyrinth. It is a closed system. It is derived from the striae vascularis in the wall of the cochlear duct and reabsorbed by the special cells in the irregular dilated part of the endolymphatic duct and its saccus into the surrounding capillaries (Fig. 1.37). It may also be reabsorbed by the specialized epithelium of the striae vascularis. In contrast to the perilymph the endolymph is high in potassium and low in sodium and this ratio is probably maintained by the special epithelium covering the stria vascularis. The high potassium in the endolymph inhibits the passage of nerve impulses and thus allows the organ of Corti to function.

THE CORTILYMPH

This is the fluid in the tunnel of Corti. It is connected by intercellular channels with the fluid around the hair cells in the spaces of Nuel, but the tight junctions between the upper ends of the hair cells, the supporting cells

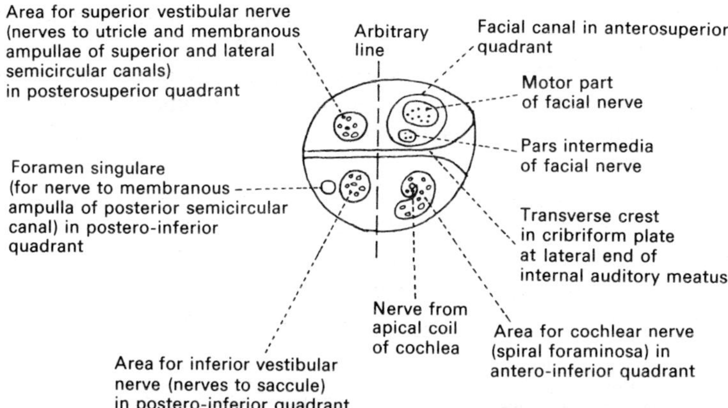

Fig. 1.39. The bony cribriform plate at the lateral end of the left internal auditory meatus (viewed from inside the meatus). The transverse crest and the arbitrary vertical line divide the bony plate into four quadrants.

and the rods, prevent any communication with the endolymph. Like the perilymph it is low in potassium and high in sodium so does not inhibit the passage of nerve impulses. It is probably derived from the perilymph of the scala tympani through small holes in the basilar membrane.

The detailed anatomy of the cochlea is described in Chapter 2, and the details of the cochlear afferent and efferent fibres are described in Chapter 3.

INTERNAL AUDITORY MEATUS

This is a short canal leading from the inner surface of the bony labyrinth to the posterior surface of the petrous where it opens into the posterior cranial fossa. The anterior wall measures 8 mm and the posterior wall 5 mm; the opening (the porus) of the meatus therefore lies obliquely (Figs. 1.32 and 1.38).

The contents of the meatus are the cochlear nerve, the vestibular nerve, the VII nerve and its pars intermedia part, and the internal auditory artery and vein. These nerves leave the brain at the groove between the pons and

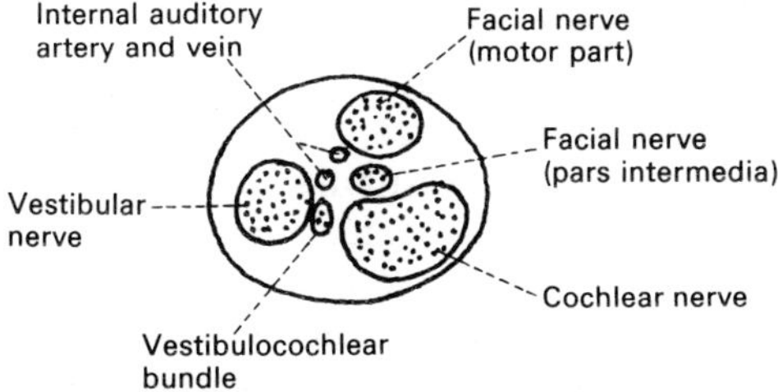

Fig. 1.40. Transverse section near the middle of the left internal auditory meatus.

medulla superolateral to the olive, and they first lie in the cerebellopontine angle before entering the meatus. The outer end of the meatus is closed by a plate of bone called the cribriform plate through which the nerves pass to their destination; it is convenient to divide it into four quadrants. The nerves passing through the quadrants are shown in Fig. 1.39.

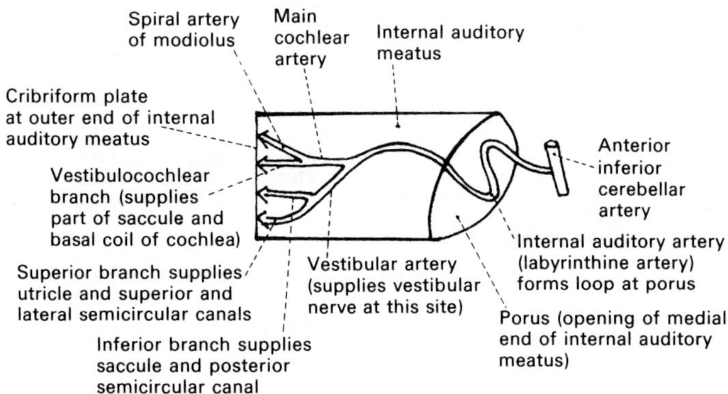

Fig. 1.41. Plan of the left internal auditory artery in the internal auditory meatus.

Each nerve carries around it as far as the cribriform plate an extension of the subarachnoid space containing cerebrospinal fluid. The dura lines the whole meatus being carried in from the porus by the nerves; it also forms a common sheath around them. The nerve supply of the dural sheath is probably by a small branch from nerve cells in the sensory root of N. V belonging to the mandibular part of N. V since pain from an acoustic neuroma at the porus is usually referred to the temporal region anterior to the auricle in the distribution of the auriculotemporal nerve (from mandibular part of N. V).

The arrangement of the contents halfway along the meatus is shown in Fig. 1.40.

The cochlear afferent fibres receive their Schwann sheath and myelin sheath on entering the bony spiral lamina (lamina spiralis). They lose their Schwann sheath at the inner end (the porus) of the internal meatus which is the site where an acoustic neuroma may develop. The myelin sheath, however, remains and is continued into the brainstem, being necessary for the conduction of the nerve impulses.

The vestibular afferent fibres acquire their Schwann sheath and myelin sheath on leaving the vestibular receptors (the cristae and the maculae). Like the cochlear afferents the vestibular fibres also lose their Schwann sheath at the porus of the internal meatus but the myelin sheath is continued into the brainstem. Many of the vestibular fibres are unmyelinated; in contrast most of the cochlear afferents are myelinated and this is probably due to the more precise information carried. The course of the vestibulocochlear efferent fibres has been described on page 39.

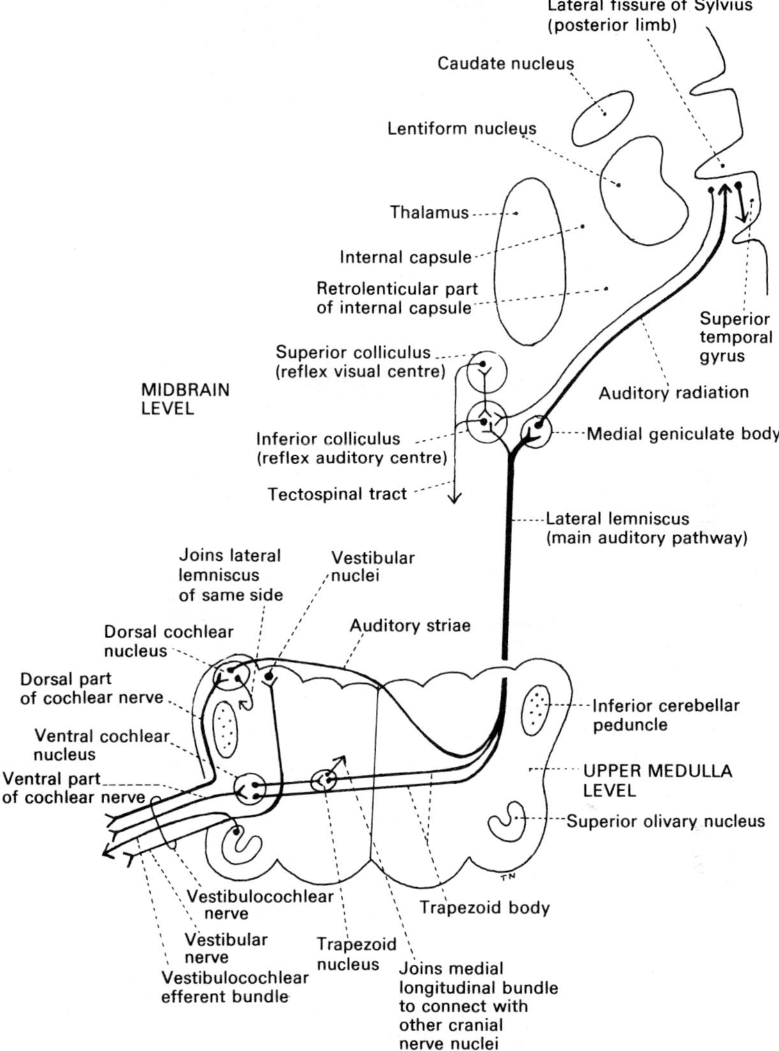

Fig. 1.42. Diagram of the central connections of the left cochlear nerve.

BLOOD VESSELS IN INTERNAL AUDITORY MEATUS

The internal auditory artery arises from the anterior inferior cerebellar or basilar artery. It commonly forms a loop at the porus, then near the outer end of the meatus it divides into a main cochlear and a main vestibular branch (Fig. 1.41). The internal auditory vein drains to the sigmoid sinus or inferior petrosal sinus.

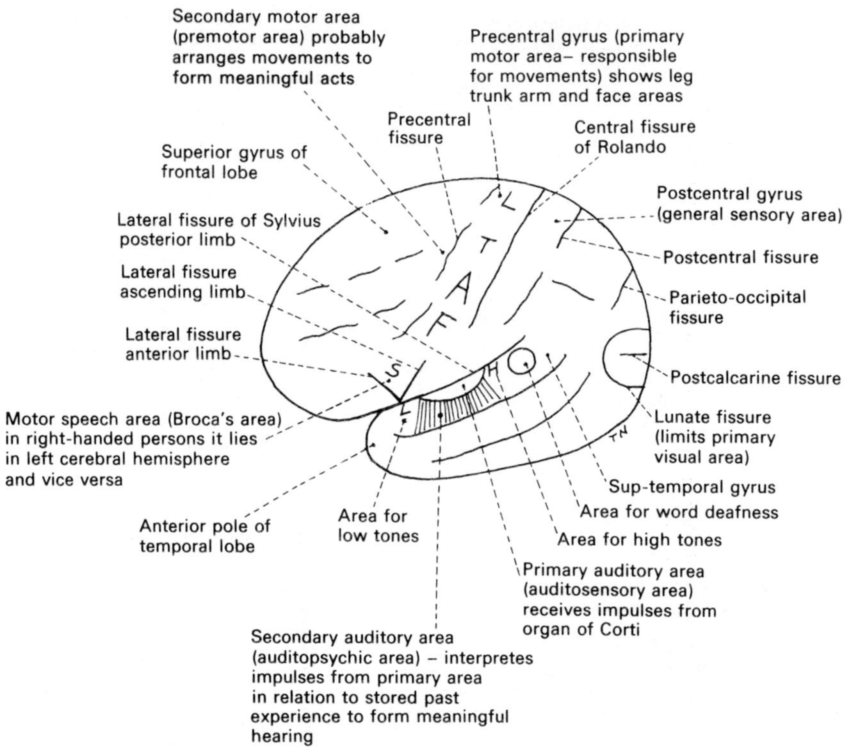

Fig. 1.43. Plan of the fissures and gyri of the left cerebral hemisphere: lateral surface. The arm and face areas in the precentral gyrus are larger than the other areas because the movements are more complicated.

The facial nerve (N. VII)

This runs an important part of its course in the ear. It consists of two parts, the main motor part and a pars intermedia part. Its nuclei lie in the floor of the fourth ventricle in the region of the colliculus facialis. The nuclear arrangements are shown in Fig. 1.44.

The main motor nucleus and the parasympathetic (sup. salivatory) nucleus lie deeply. The motor fibres then wind dorsally around the nucleus of N. VI producing the colliculus. They now run ventrally to emerge from the brainstem at the lower border of the pons. The fibres from the main motor nucleus form the main part of the facial nerve. The parasympathetic fibres together with taste fibres form the pars intermedia part.

The nuclei have higher connections—the main motor nucleus is connected to the lower part of the precentral gyrus, chiefly of the opposite side but fibres also ascend to the precentral gyrus of the same side especially in the part of the facial nerve which supplies the upper half of the face. If one facial nerve is damaged above the main motor nucleus the upper half of the face therefore escapes paralysis because its fibres are connected to both

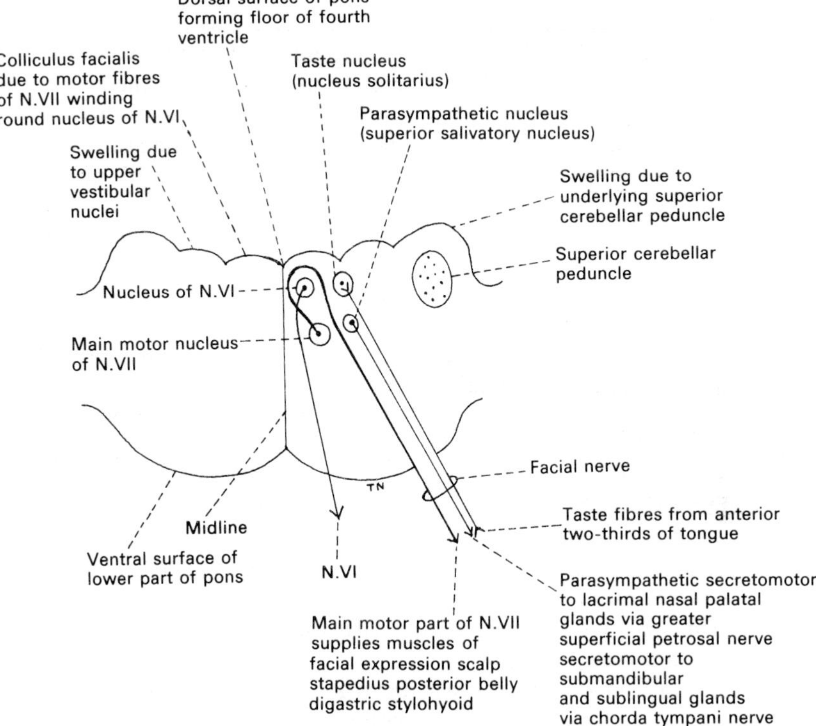

Fig. 1.44. Section of the brainstem through the lower part of the pons at the level of the colliculus facialis in the floor of the fourth ventricle, showing the nuclear arrangements of N. VII. The parasympathetic and the taste fibres form the pars intermedia of N. VII.

cerebral hemispheres. The parasympathetic nucleus is connected by fibres which cross the midline and ascend to the hypothalamic region which is the headquarters of the autonomic nervous system. The taste fibres relay in the taste nucleus; the pathway is then continued across the midline and ascends to relay in the thalamus then passes to the taste cortical area which is at the lower end of the postcentral gyrus. In this area the impulses are received and then interpreted.

On leaving the lower border of the pons the main part of the facial nerve and its pars intermedia part first cross the cerebellopontine angle then run in the internal auditory meatus (Fig. 1.38). They enter the facial canal at the upper anterior quadrant of the cribriform plate at the outer end of the meatus (Fig. 1.39). The facial canal then crosses the bony vestibule immediately behind the bony cochlea to reach the medial wall of the middle ear. At this point it bends at right-angles and at the bend is the geniculate ganglion (facial ganglion) and the hiatus of the canal (Fig. 1.21). The facial canal now runs backwards and slightly downwards above the oval window and lies in the medial wall of the attic. On reaching the aditus it forms a swelling below the lateral semi-circular canal and partly in the floor of the aditus. It now bends sharply downwards and descends in the posterior wall of the middle ear (Fig. 1.19); this is called the vertical part of the canal. The nerve then emerges from the stylomastoid foramen and passes through the parotid gland to supply the muscles of facial expression. The afferent fibres (proprioceptive) from the facial muscles probably run with the three divisions of N. V.

The branches of the facial nerve given off in the facial canal are five in number:

1. The greater superficial petrosal nerve. This is given off from the geniculate ganglion then passes through the hiatus into the middle cranial fossa. It consists of parasympathetic and taste fibres. The parasympathetic fibres pass through the geniculate ganglion without relay and finally relay in the sphenopalatine ganglion, then supply secretomotor fibres to the lacrimal gland, the glands of the nose, nasopharynx and palate. The taste fibres come chiefly from the palate. They have their nerve cells in the geniculate ganglion but there is no relay; thereafter they join the pars intermedia to reach the taste nucleus in the pons.
2. A branch from the geniculate ganglion also passes to the tympanic plexus on the promontory and is probably parasympathetic.
3. A branch is given off in the vertical part of the facial canal to supply the stapedius muscle.
4. The chorda tympani nerve is given off 6 mm above the stylomastoid foramen. It consists of parasympathetic and taste fibres. The parasympathetic fibres relay in the submandibular ganglion then supply secretomotor fibres to the submandibular and sublingual salivary glands. The taste fibres come from the anterior two-thirds of the tongue. They have their nerve cells in the geniculate ganglion then pass without relay to join the pars intermedia nerve.
5. A branch passes out of the facial canal about 4 mm above the stylomastoid foramen and joins the auricular branch of N. X. It is said to carry sensory fibres from a small area of the outer part of the posterior wall of the external meatus. Their nerve cells are in the geniculate ganglion from which they pass without relay to join the pars intermedia nerve. In the brain stem they are said to join N. V. These fibres are believed to explain the occurrence of a vesicular eruption on the posterior wall of the external meatus in cases of herpes of the geniculate ganglion. This is usually associated with lower motor neuron paralysis of N. VII.

THE TEMPORAL BONE

This contains the bony part of the external meatus, the bony part of the Eustachian tube, the middle ear, the mastoid antrum and air cells, the whole of the inner ear, and the internal auditory meatus. It consists of four morphological parts named the petromastoid part, the squamous part, the tympanic part, and the styloid process. Figs. 1.45–1.49 show the special features.

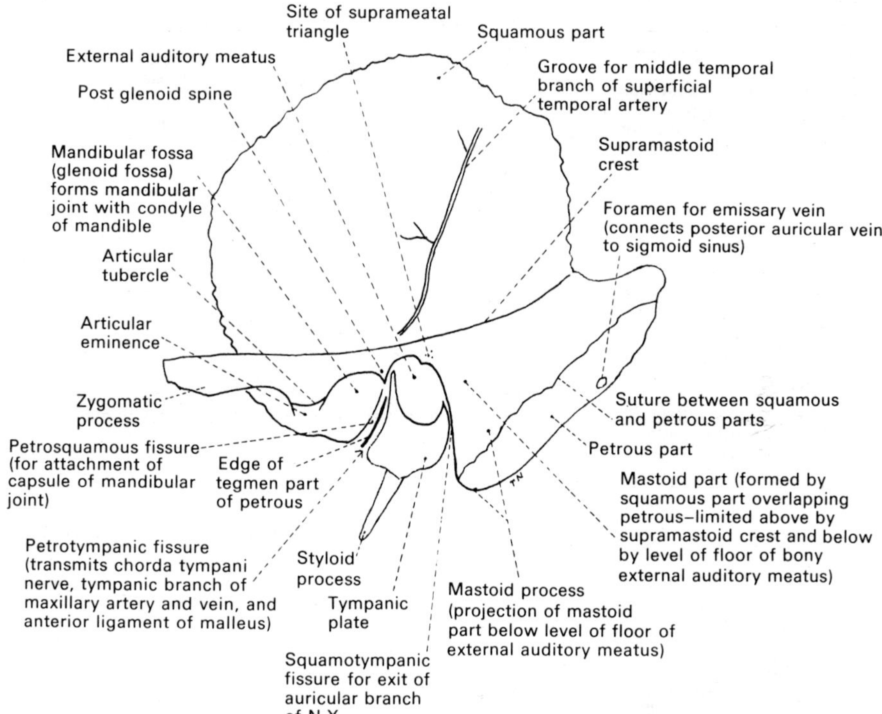

Fig. 1.45. Lateral aspect of the left temporal bone. Only small parts of the petrous are visible in a lateral view, namely the lower part of the mastoid process and the edge of the tegmen in the squamotympanic fissure.

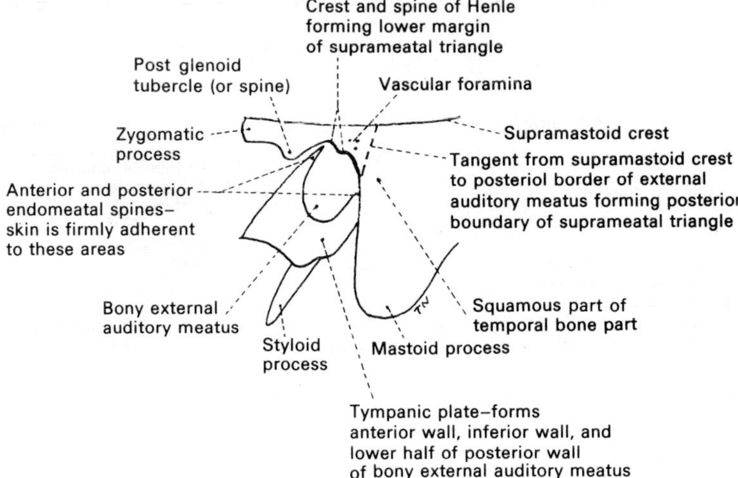

Fig. 1.46. Diagram showing the margins of the left bony external auditory meatus and the suprameatal triangle (Macewen's triangle).

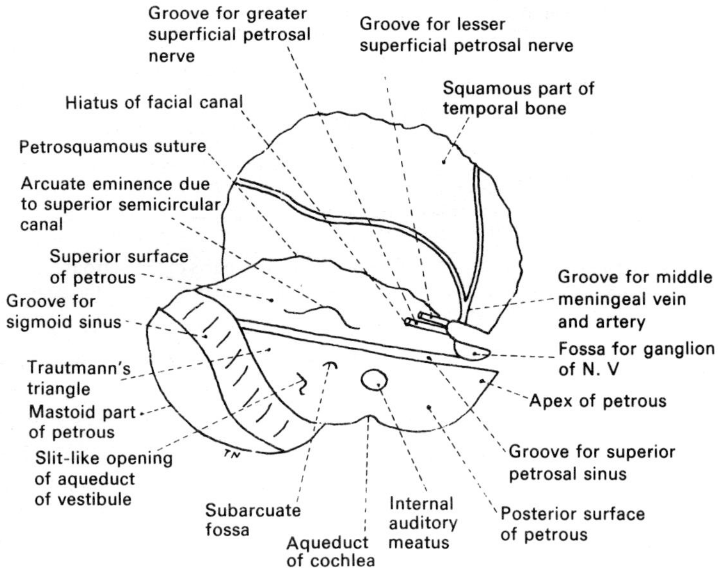

Fig. 1.47. Medial view of the left temporal bone. This also shows the superior and posterior surfaces of the petrous.

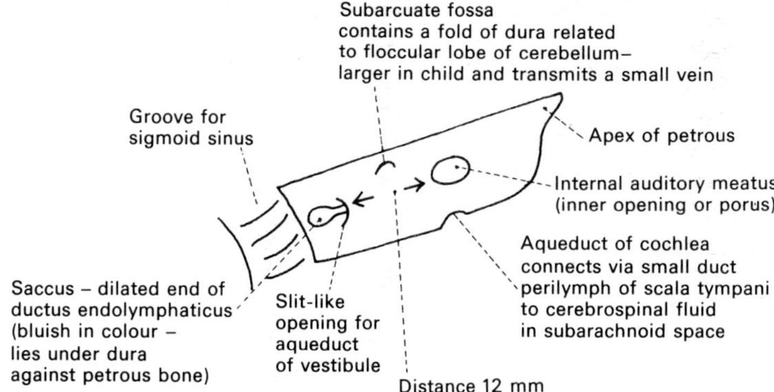

Fig. 1.48. Details of the posterior surface of the left petrous.

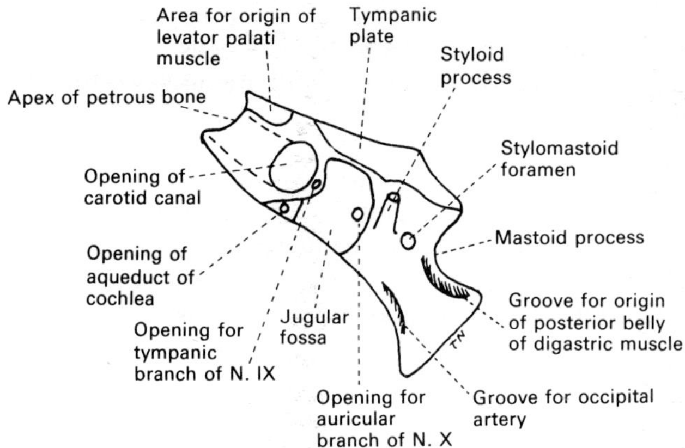

Fig. 1.49. Inferior surface of the left petrous.

2 Structure of the cochlear duct

CATHERINE A. SMITH

INTRODUCTION

Some basic knowledge of the structure of the cochlear duct is important in order to understand how the ear functions in health and disease. The cochlea is both a simple and a complex organ; simple in that although the human cochlea is approximately 35 mm long, the *histological* organization is rather similar from the basal to the apical end. It is complex in that at any one point along the basilar membrane there is a remarkable *cellular* variation; the cells in the organ of Corti and the stria vascularis have become specialized in many different ways, but the cells within each group are arranged in a very orderly manner. There are also two highly developed *extra*cellular fibrous structures, the tectorial membrane and the basilar membrane. This becomes even more remarkable when one remembers that all these cells originated in the embryo from the same layer of simple, cuboidal epithelial cells. This chapter will begin with a brief survey of the embryological development of the membranous labyrinth and continue by describing the morphology of the various cell groups of the cochlear duct, with consideration of their functional implications.

EMBRYOLOGY

The primordia of the two major sensory organs of the head (the eye and ear) appear quite early in foetal life. At the end of the third or the beginning of the fourth week in the human foetus, the auditory placodes are visible as thickenings of the ectoderm on both sides of the head. Each placode soon takes the form of a pit which very quickly sinks beneath the level of the ectodermal surface to become the auditory vesicle. Both the vestibular and the cochlear labyrinth develop from the epithelial cells of which the vesicle is composed.

The vestibular structures bud-off first. The semicircular canals begin to acquire their half-moon tubular forms during the sixth foetal week. Shortly afterwards a pseudostratified mass of cells is formed in each ampulla as well as in the utricle and saccule, from which the sensory structures of the cristae and maculae will differentiate.

The cochlea buds from the labyrinth near the saccule and elongates during the sixth foetal week, but it is not until some time later (the 22nd week according to Pearson (1967)) that the hair cells differentiate in the basal turn and changes take place in the epithelium on the lateral wall which will become the stria vascularis. Differentiation proceeds from the basal to the apical end. The last developmental phase to occur is the opening of the tunnel and the formation of the spaces of Nuel in the organ of Corti and, on the lateral wall, the vascularization and organization of the stria vascularis. Differentiation is generally believed to be complete in the seventh foetal month.

The embryological state of the inner ear at any particular time is of special interest in attempting to interpret the defects present in congenital deafnesses which may be the result of a prenatal insult. For example it has been frequently stated that prenatal rubella infections interfere with the differentiation of the cochlea, yet in more than one case (Friedmann and Wright 1966; Bordley, Brookhauser, Hardy, and Hardy 1967) it is obvious that development has continued to a normal structural differentiation. It is possible that the virus multiplies and has its toxic effect at a later period or that undiagnosed metabolic defects have been created at an early stage which are not critical for morphological differentiation up to a certain point.

THE MEMBRANOUS LABYRINTH

The adult membranous labyrinth is a closed epithelial tubular structure which has developed from the original ectodermal vesicle by the formation of elongated tubes and restricted dilations (Fig. 2.1). The human cochlea has $2\frac{1}{2}$ coils, and the basilar membrane is approximately 35 mm in length. The saccule is attached to the basal end of the cochlear duct (just above the caecum vestibulare) by a small thin epithelial tube called the ductus re-

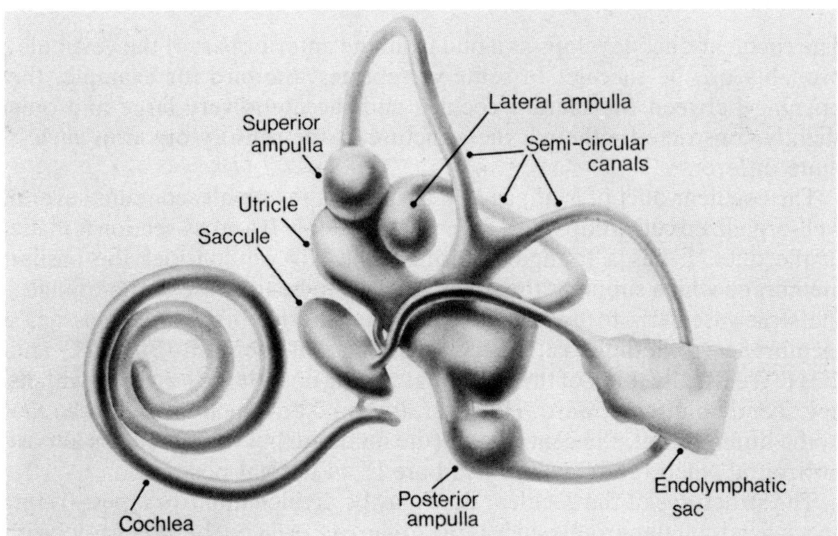

Fig. 2.1. Drawing of the human membranous labyrinth (premature infant). The endolymphatic sac has been cut off. (Redrawn from Bast and Anson (1949).) (Drawing by Suzanne Moody.)

uniens. The saccule and the utricle are joined by the two upper arms of a Y-shaped tube, the saccular duct and the utricular duct. The single base-arm of the Y forms the beginning of the endolymphatic duct which terminates in the endolymphatic sac. The sac extends into the cerebral cavity and is located beneath the dura mater of the brain.

The maculae of the utricle and saccule are compact masses of sensory and supporting cells, covered by gelatinous membranes which support the otoliths. The dilated ends of the lateral and superior semicircular canals (the ampullae) are located on the anterolateral end of the utricle, and the ampulla of the posterior canal on the posteromedial end. They contain the sensory structures of the semicircular canals, the cristae, and their gelatinous covers, the cupulae.

The membranous labyrinth, then, is a continuous epithelial structure. It is not as large as the bony labyrinth, and the fluid perilymph fills the space between the two (Fig. 2.2). The membranous labyrinth is filled with the endolymph, a fluid which has a high concentration of potassium, approximately 144 meq/l (Smith, Lowry, and Wu 1954). This is quite different from the potassium concentration of perilymph (5 meq/l) and most other tissue fluids. The fact that a fluid with a potassium concentration so different from that of tissue fluid or perilymph can be maintained indicates that potassium is concentrated by some special mechanism within the inner ear, and that the epithelial cells are probably joined together tightly, so that rapid ion flow from endolymph to perilymph and the converse is impeded.

THE COCHLEAR DUCT

The cochlear duct develops as a bud from the anterior part of the vestibule, probably off the saccule. In some vertebrates, the bird for example, the opening between the mature cochlea and saccule is very large and only slightly constricted although the structure of the sensory organ in each is quite different.

The cochlear duct of Man, as well as of other mammals, contains several well-organized cell groups with different functions. If a cross-section is made of the duct, it has a triangular form. Generally we consider the basilar membrane which supports the organ of Corti to be the base of the triangle, the stria vascularis to be the side, and that the hypotenuse is Reissner's membrane (sometimes called the 'vestibular membrane' (Figs. 2.2 and 2.3)). We usually think of the cochlea as resting on its large basal end with its apical end pointing upward. However, it should be remembered that *in situ* in the human skull, the central axis (the modiolus) of the cochlea is almost horizontal when the body and head are in an upright position.

The structures of the cochlear duct may be divided into two types: (i) the specialized cellular groups such as the organ of Corti and the stria vascularis, and (ii) the extracellular membranes which are the tectorial membrane and the basilar membrane (Fig. 2.4). All of these are continuous elements that reach from the basal caecum to the apical end (Fig. 2.5).

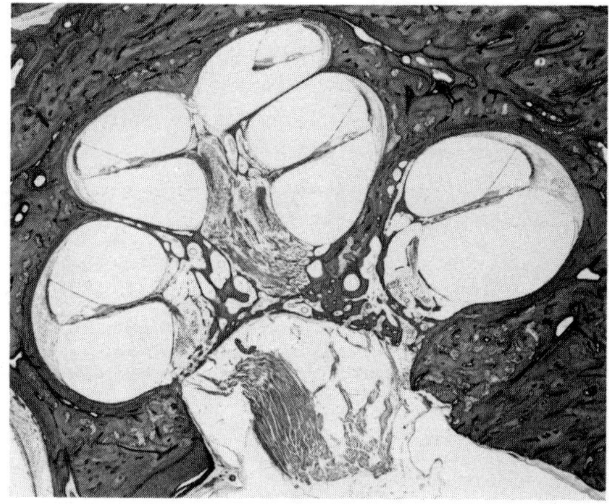

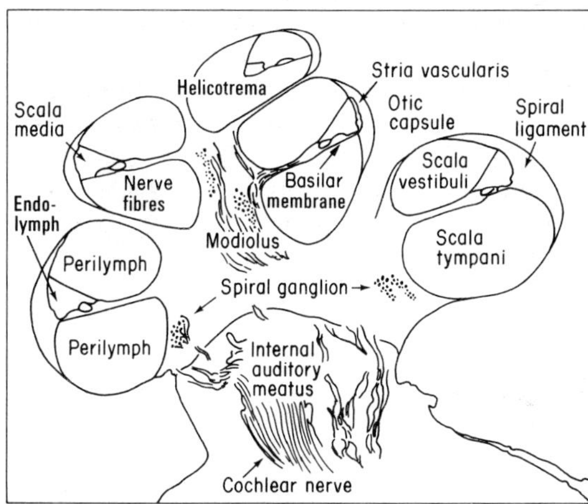

Fig. 2.2. Cross-section of the cochlea (human). Notice the 'cartilagenous rests' which are typical of the otic capsule at lower left and right, between scala tympani of the basal coil and the internal auditory meatus. A corner of the saccule is visible at the extreme lower left. × 19. (Reproduced with permission from Smith (1973).)

BASILAR MEMBRANE AND SPIRAL LIGAMENT

The basilar membrane is a fibrous structure (Figs. 2.2, 2.3, and 2.4) which spans the distance between the bony shelf of the modiolus (the bony spiral lamina through which the nerve fibres enter the cochlear duct) and the spiral ligament (which is attached to the bone of the otic capsule). Medially (near the modiolus) the fibres of the basilar membrane are attached to the bony spiral lamina, and some of the fibres extend beneath the limbus and up into it. Laterally, the fibres spread out into the spiral ligament and intermingle with the fibres of that structure. The basilar membrane is thus firmly attached both medially and laterally and resists extreme stress. For example

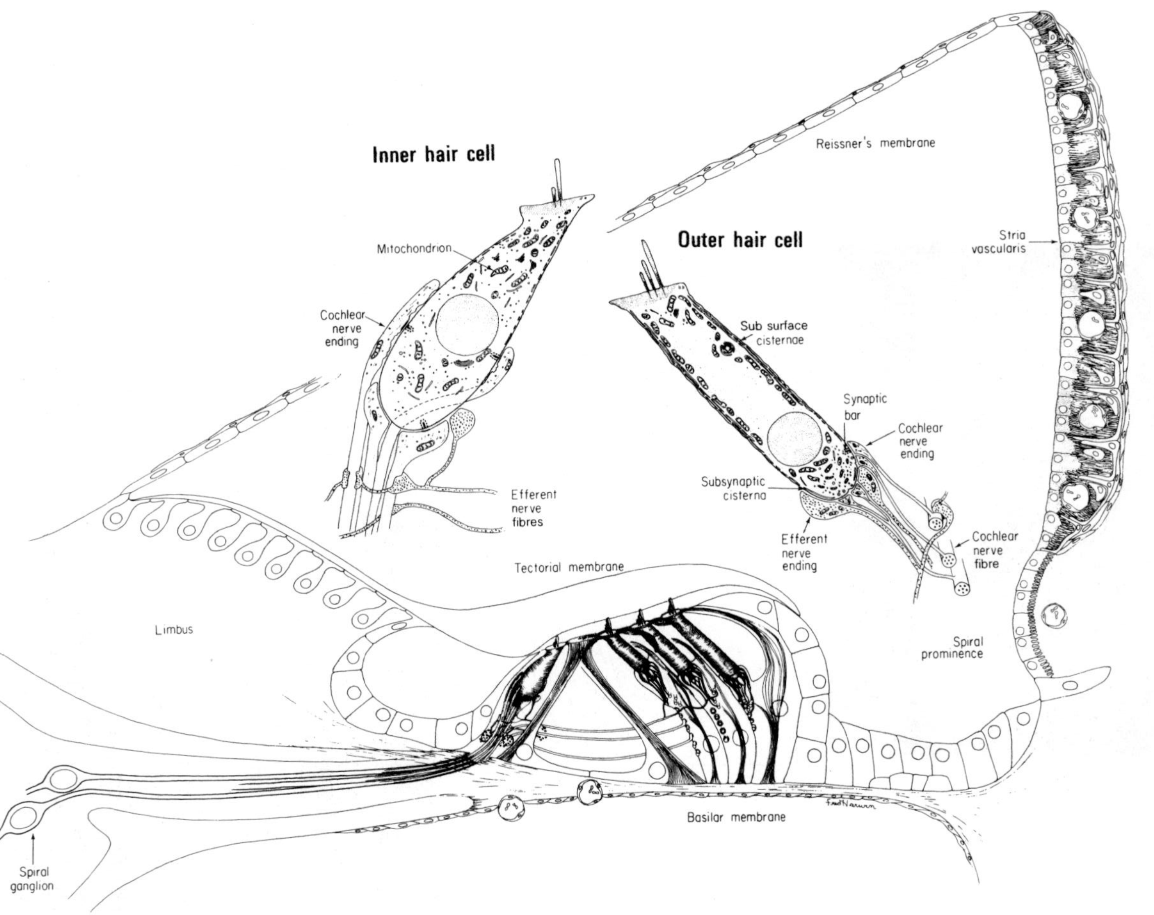

Fig. 2.3. Cross-section of the cochlear duct of the guinea pig. (Reproduced with permission from Smith (1975).) (Drawing by Fred Harwin.)

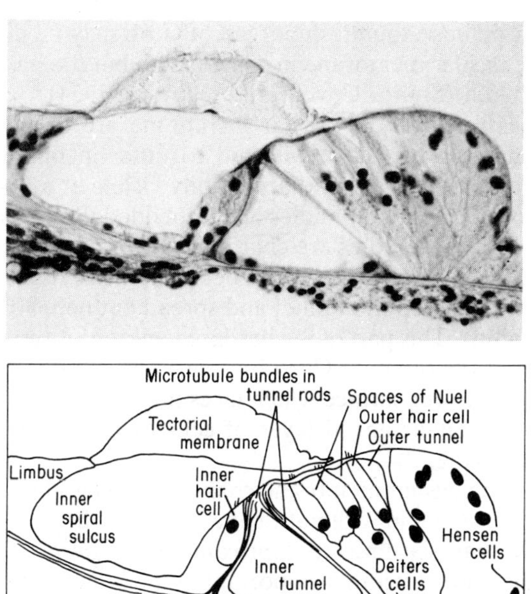

Fig. 2.4. The organ of Corti from the upper half of the squirrel monkey's cochlea. × 412.

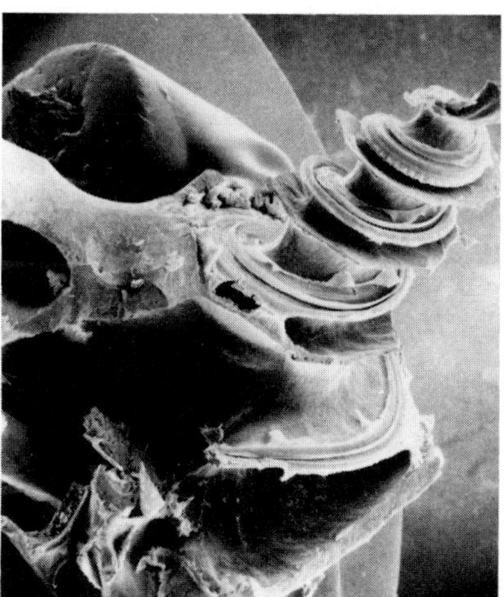

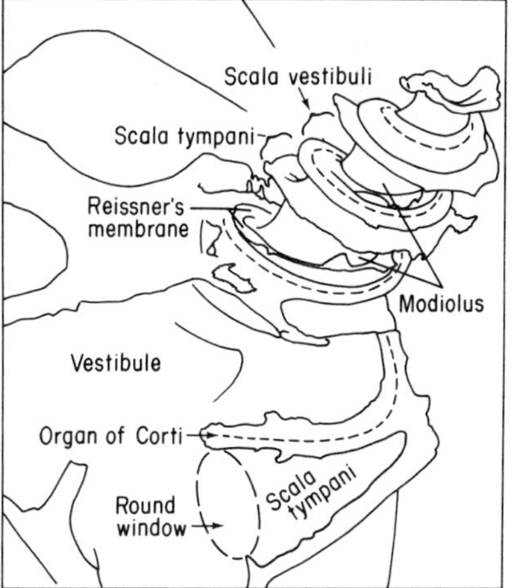

Fig. 2.5. Scanning electron micrograph (SEM) of the guinea-pig cochlea. The otic capsule has been dissected away. Reissner's membrane has been mostly removed and only some fragments of it remain attached to the inner border of the limbus. The tectorial membrane is no longer in place. The organ of Corti from basal to apical end is '*in situ*', and can be visualized as it coils around the modiolar bone. × 20.

in exposures to intense sound, the organ of Corti may be dislodged completely from the basilar membrane in some places but the basilar membrane itself is not broken (Smith, Covell, and Eldredge 1954).

Some of the fibres of the basilar membrane are organized into long filamentous strands which are collected together in bundles. These are disposed in a radial direction and are readily visible at a light microscopic level. These coarse rounded bundles are embedded in a dense mass of very short fibres. The fibre bundles are characteristic of the more lateral part of the membrane which is called the 'pars pectinata'. The fibres in the bundles tend to separate beneath the tunnel and spread out beneath the inner hair cells and the limbus. This part of the basilar membrane is separated from the epithelial cells of the organ of Corti by a very thin fibrogranular layer, the basal lamina. The lower surface which faces the perilymph of scala tympani is covered by loosely-arranged layer of cells of mesenchymal origin, the mesothelial cells (Fig. 2.4).

The width of the basilar membrane changes from basal to apical end. It is approximately 0.08 mm in width at the basal end of the human cochlea and increases more than six times to approximately 0.5 mm at the apical end. This regular increase in width is important in the fulfilment of one property that von Bekesy (1960) found to be essential for propagation of the travelling wave: a system with continuously changing mechanical properties.

The spiral ligament is not really a ligament, but is a loosely-arranged mass of connective tissue fibres and cells to which the lateral epithelial wall of the cochlear duct is attached (Fig. 2.2). It houses the blood vessels on the lateral wall of the cochlea. The tissue fluid which surrounds the spiral ligament cells, fibres, and blood vessels is freely diffusable with the perilymph in scala tympani and scala vestibuli.

THE ORGAN OF CORTI

The organ of Corti is composed of the sensory cells and their supporting cells. The afferent and efferent nerve fibres pass between the supporting cells to terminate on the sensory cells; the efferent axons also make axodendritic synapses on the cochlear nerve fibres (Fig. 2.3).

Supporting cells

The supporting cells include the centrally located tunnel rod cells, the inner and outer phalangeal cells, the (inner) border cell, and Hensen's cells. The basal parts of the cells except some of the last are situated on the basilar membrane and their apical ends reach to the surface of Corti's organ (Figs. 2.6–2.8). The reticular lamina is composed of the apical ends of the sensory cells and only those supporting cells which actually touch the hair cells, so that Hensen's cells are excluded (Fig. 2.7). The apical ends of all the cells are bound together by 'tight' junctions; at their basal ends, the supporting cells are packed together on the basilar membrane but they are not joined by occluding junctions. Ions or small molecules which penetrate the basilar

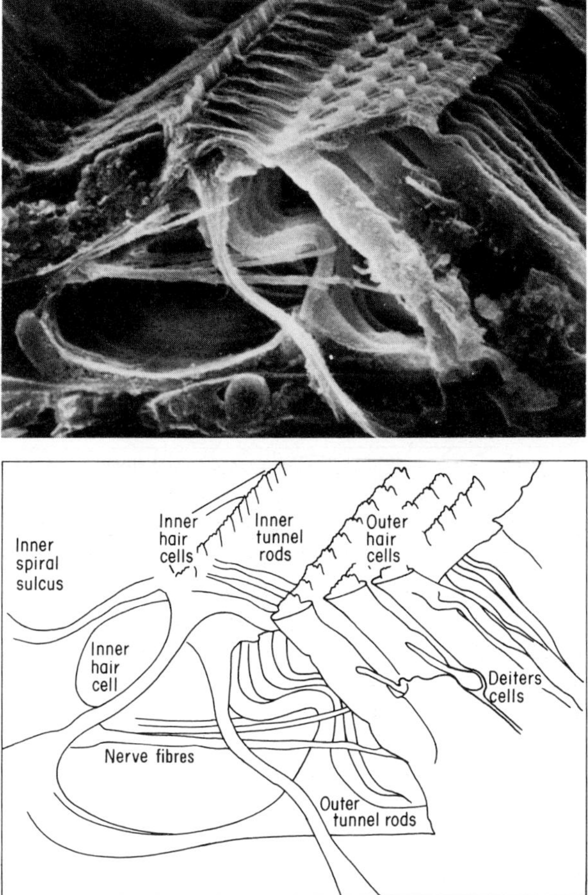

Fig. 2.6. SEM of the guinea-pig organ of Corti. × 2900. (Reproduced with permission from Engstrom (1974).)

membrane can readily diffuse between the cells and up in between the hair cells. On the other hand, the occluding junctions at the reticular lamina inhibit diffusion of ions *between* the cells; it is well known that diffusion of ions *across* cell membranes is subject to certain restrictions. The barrier between endolymph and perilymph at the organ of Corti is placed at the reticular lamina rather than at the basilar membrane.

The supporting cells about the inner hair cells (the inner phalangeal and the border cells) do not have any remarkable cytoplasmic structure (Fig. 2.9). They probably aid in maintaining the position of the inner hair cells and their related nerve fibre bundles and separate the sensory cells from each other. The flat apical ends of the sensory cells and the protruding hairs (or stereocilia) are bathed in endolymph.

The tunnel rod cells and the outer phalangeal (or Deiters) cells have

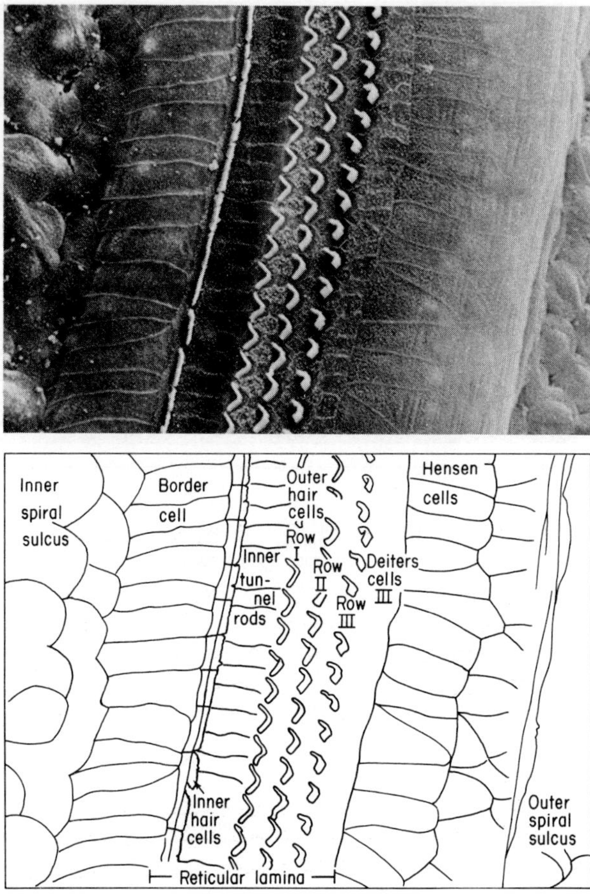

Fig. 2.7. SEM of the surface of the organ of Corti of the guinea pig. × 825. (Reproduced with permission from Smith (1975).)

become differentiated in a more unusual way. The basal parts of both types of cell are situated on the basilar membrane and the nerve fibres pass between them. The basal end of each of the outer hair cells is supported in a cup formed by a Deiters cell (Figs. 2.3 and 2.6). The upper half of each tunnel rod and each Deiters cell is constricted with the result that spaces are formed between them (Figs. 2.3, 2.6, and 2.10). These are called the inner and outer tunnel and the spaces of Nuel and they are filled with fluid. Quite obviously if the slender columns of the tunnel rods and Deiters cells are to support and hold upright the hair cells, especially in an organ that is constantly vibrating, some special cytoplasmic adaptation is necessary. It was observed many years ago that these cells contained bundles of filaments which were called 'tonofilaments'. It is now known that these are bundles of microtubules, cytoplasmic structures found in all cells. Unusual aggregates

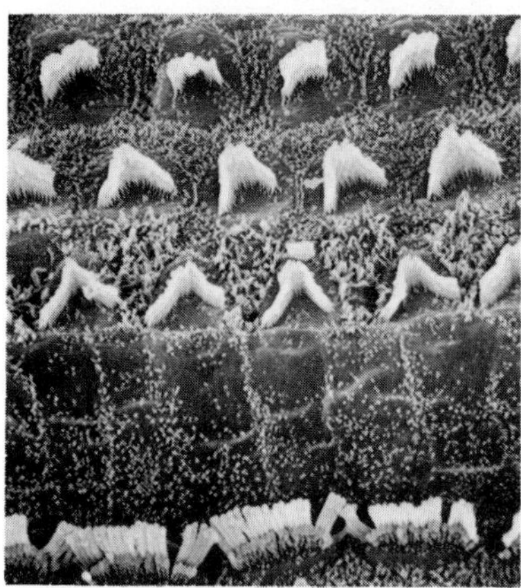

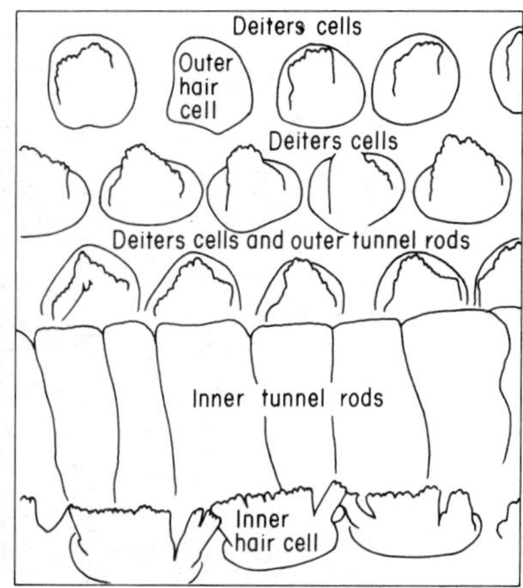

Fig. 2.8. Higher magnification of the reticular lamina, guinea pig. × 2000.

of microtubules in cells usually have the function of transport or skeletal support. In the organ of Corti, they undoubtedly give skeletal support to the structure. The bundles of microtubules extend from the base of each of the tunnel rods and Deiters cells up into the constricted processes and then turn about 45 degrees and spread out in the reticular lamina (Figs. 2.3, 2.4, and 2.10). The organ of Corti is thereby supported by the microtubular bundles, but in addition the tubules provide stiffness for the reticular lamina, a feature which is important for the detection of small movements of the basilar membrane (Smith 1978).

The other cells which are considered to be a part of the organ of Corti are the Hensen cells. All of these cells do not touch the basilar membrane but they cover the last Deiters cells as a layer. Hensen's cells in the basal coil are low and cuboidal in form. In the apical coils, they are much larger and contain numerous lipid granules.

One interesting question that has been asked frequently and has aroused considerable controversy is: What is the nature of the fluid that fills the tunnel and bathes the outer hair cells? Is it perilymph, endolymph, or another fluid? It was first indicated by Tasaki, Davis, and Eldredge (1954), who used electrophysiological measurements, that the boundary of the endolymph space was at the reticular lamina and not at the basilar membrane. More recently, electron-dense tracers have shown that materials of small molecular weight such as horseradish peroxidase pass freely from scala tympani across the basilar membrane into the tunnel and spaces of Nuel (Duvall, Quick, and Sutherland 1971). It is possible that the concentration of some substances such as protein may not be the same in the fluid within the organ of Corti (which is avascular) as in scala tympani, but most certainly it is not endolymph, and without doubt is similar to perilymph (and other tissue fluid) in its ionic composition.

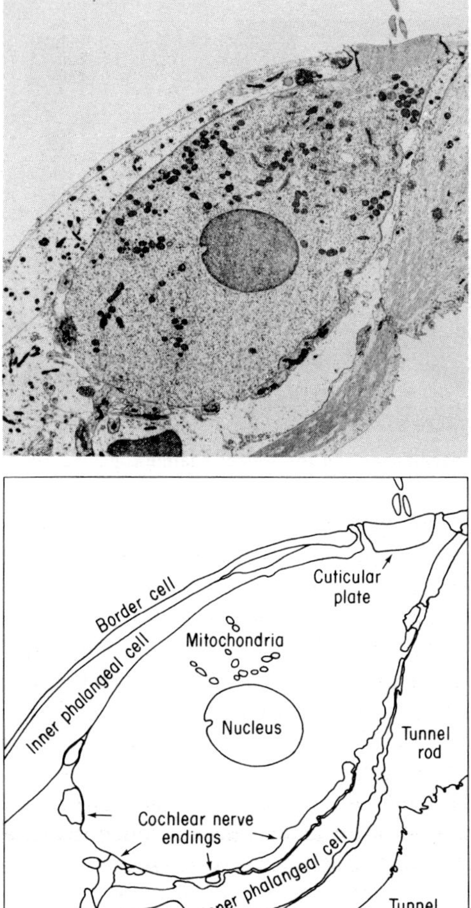

Fig. 2.9. Transmission electron micrograph (TEM) of inner hair cell of the guinea pig. × 4300. (Reproduced with permission from Smith (2978).)

Sensory cells

All the hair cells in the cochlea and the vestibule are characterized by certain features. They are all columnar cells which are separated from the fibrous base (basilar membrane or connective tissue) of the organ by supporting cells. The nerve fibres course between the supporting cells and terminate on the sides and the basal ends of the hair cells. The apical ends of the sensory cells contain a compact fibrogranular material (called the cuticular plate) a material which also fills the protruding stereocilia (Figs. 2.9 and 2.10). With only a few exceptions (some reptilian hair cells (Wever 1967)), the hairs are inserted into fibrogelatinous membranes. In the cochlea this is the tectorial membrane.

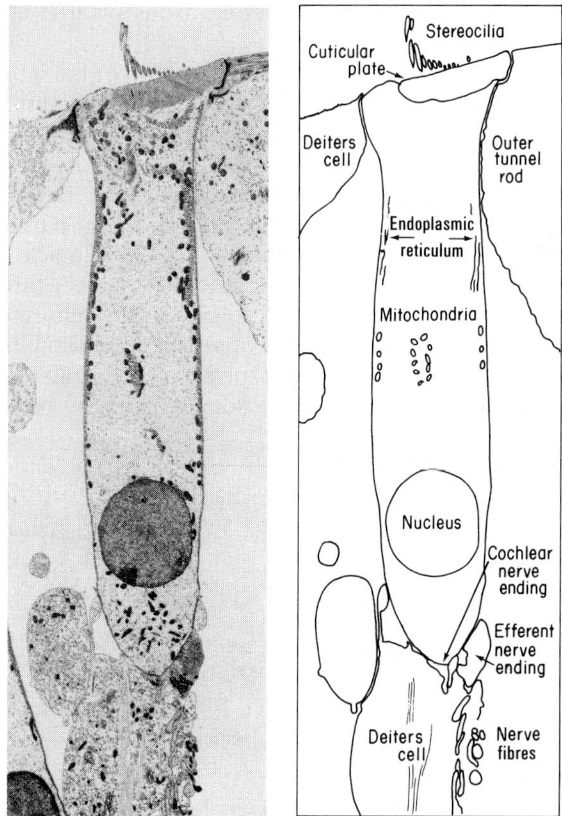

Fig. 2.10. TEM of outer hair cell of the guinea pig. × 4200. (Reproduced with permission from Smith (1978).)

INNER HAIR CELLS

The inner hair cells in the mammalian cochlea represent a widely-distributed form of hair cell; most other hair cells found in the vestibules, cochleae, and lateral line organs of lower vertebrates are similar in structure. It is a flask-shaped cell with a slightly enlarged and rounded bottom (Figs. 2.3, 2.4, and 2.9). Cochlear nerve endings in the shape of small or large knobs terminate on the base of the cell; some of the nerve fibres continue up along the side of the cell, with intermittent synapses, for distances up to ten micrometres. Membrane thickenings are present on both pre- and postsynaptic membranes and synaptic bar structures are often found within the hair cell cytoplasm adjacent to the presynaptic membrane thickenings. The synaptic bar structures are bars or balls composed of a dense fibrogranular material surrounded by a row of vesicles. It is believed they may represent a transmitter substance storage site. Efferent nerve endings have been found on inner hair cells in guinea pigs but they are infrequent and it is not known if the efferent axons synapse on inner hair cells in the human ear.

Organelles are scattered throughout the cytoplasm of the inner hair cells (Fig. 2.9). Clusters of mitochondria, endoplasmic reticulum, or Golgi apparatus may be found at the apical or basal ends and a single row of vesicles lines the apical plasma membrane but there is no morphological evidence, such as is present in the outer hair cell, that there may be any remarkable restriction of metabolic activities to different parts of the cell.

The hairs which are packed closely together on the apical end are all stereocilia (Figs. 2.6, 2.8, and 2.11). The innermost two or three rows are short and stubby and almost vestigial. The cilia in the outermost row are more than twice as long as the others. The tips of all the cilia on the inner hair cell are definitely flattened (Fig. 2.11) in contrast to the rounded tips of outer hair cell cilia (Figs. 2.10 and 2.12). The long axis of the bundle is fairly

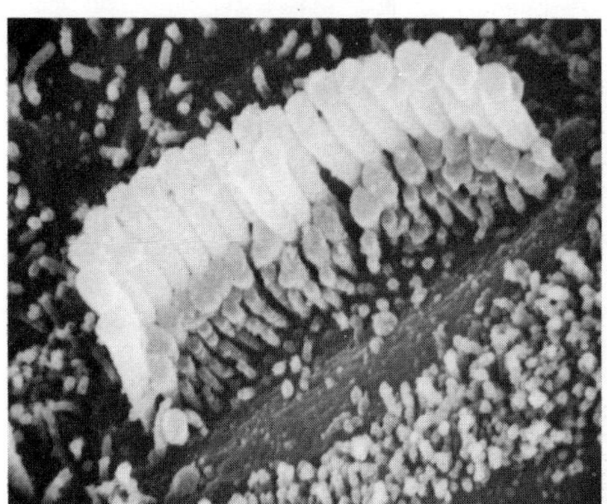

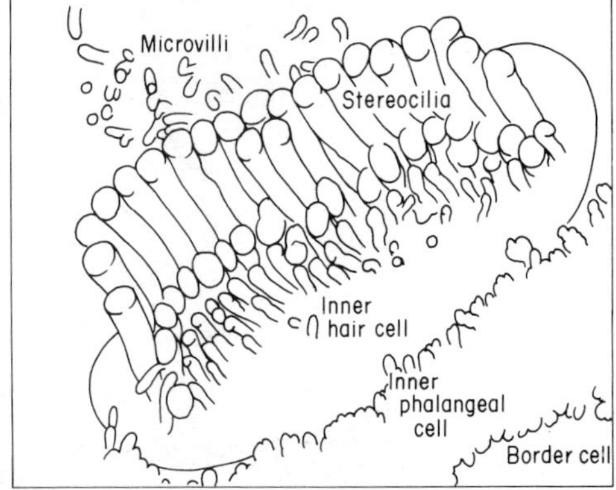

Fig. 2.11. SEM of the inner hair cell surface, guinea pig. × 12 000.

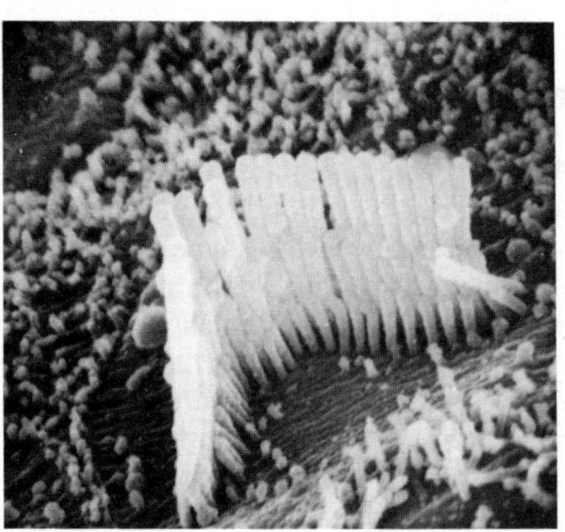

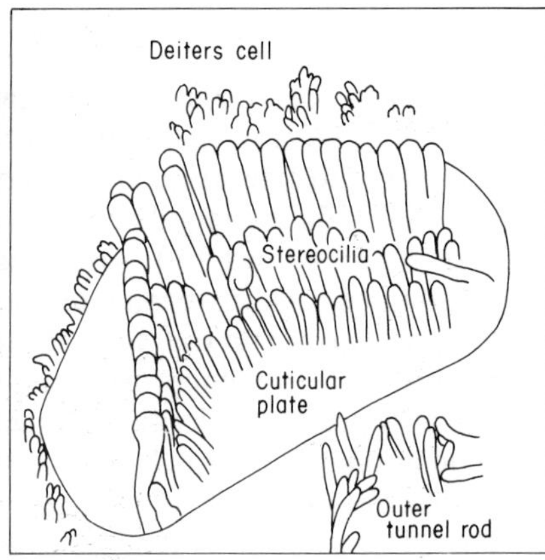

Fig. 2.12. SEM of the outer hair cell surface, guinea pig. × 12 000. (Reproduced with permission from Smith (1975).)

straight and parallel to the spiral axis of the cochlea. For many years there has been a question regarding the precise relationship between the tips of the hairs and the tectorial membrane in the mammalian cochlea. Although it seems quite clear now that the tallest of the *outer* hair cell stereocilia are inserted into the tectorial membrane (Fig. 2.13), it is still unclear if this is also true of *inner* hair cell cilia. It is probable that the tallest row of inner hair cell cilia are in contact with the tectorial membrane but not inserted.

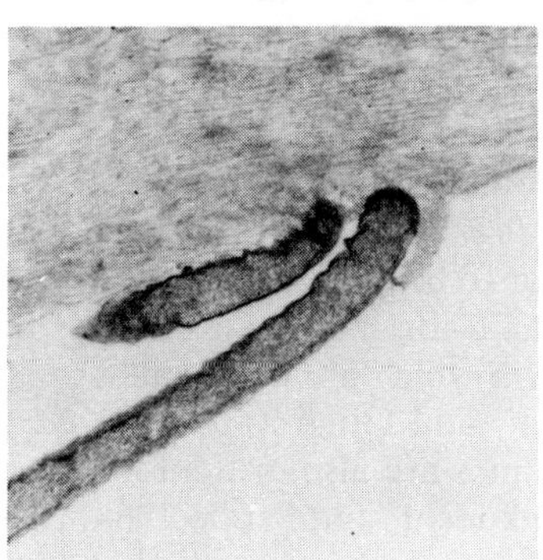

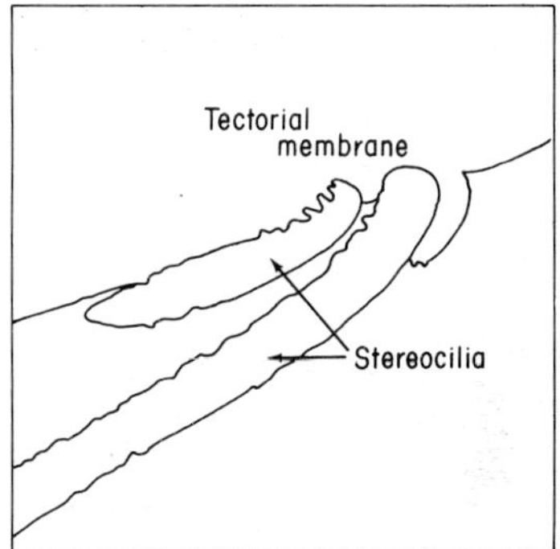

Fig. 2.13. TEM showing the tips of two stereocilia from an outer hair cell inserted into the tectorial membrane, chinchilla cochlea. × 26 000. (Reproduced with permission from Smith (1968).)

OUTER HAIR CELLS

The outer hair cells are arranged in three spiral rows external to the tunnel (Figs. 2.6–2.8). Bredberg (1968) counted an average of 13 400 outer hair cells and 3400 inner hair cells in late-foetal human cochleae. It is a tall columnar cell, 14 μm in height in the basal coil and 44 μm tall near the apex in the squirrel monkey's cochlea. Its basal end is supported in a shallow cup formed by the Deiters cell and its apical end is inserted into the reticular lamina (Figs. 2.4, 2.10, and 2.12). The remainder of the cell is surrounded by the fluid in the tunnels and/or the spaces of Nuel.

The outer hair cells are more highly differentiated than the inner hair cells (Fig. 2.10). When the cells are cut in longitudinal section, the large nucleus is visible in the lower one-third of the cell. It almost fills the cross-sectional diameter of the cell and divides it into a large supranuclear and a smaller infranuclear part each of which has a quite different cytoplasmic organization. The infranuclear part of the cell contains many mitochondria and membranes of endoplasmic reticulum as well as the synaptic bar structures adjacent to the nerve endings. At least half of the cell membrane of this portion of the cell is covered by afferent and efferent nerve endings and it seems reasonable to assume that the basal part of the outer hair cell is closely related to the process of neural stimulation.

It is not difficult to distinguish the sensory nerve endings from the efferent terminals because they are different in size and in cytological organization.

The cochlear nerve endings are small, (approximately one μm in diameter) and contain only a few vesicles plus an occasional mitochondrion. Synaptic bar structures are often present adjacent to the presynaptic membrane within the hair cell. The efferent nerve endings, which are the terminals of the olivocochlear axons, are much larger and are packed with small vesicles and mitochondria. A sub-synpatic cisterna is invariably present within the hair cell adjacent to each efferent terminal.

The supranuclear part of the cytoplasm except for that part just beneath the cuticular plate has few cytoplasmic membrane profiles or other organelles. The endoplasmic reticulum is organized into flat cisternae or vesicles adjacent to the plasma membrane (Fig. 2.10). The cisternae are laminated into honeycombed layers in some rodents such as guinea pigs and chinchillas but form only a single layer in many other mammals, including Man. These sub-surface cisternae appear to be closely bound to the plasma membrane and we assume there is a rapid ion interchange across the cell membrane powered by the mitochondria which are adjacent.

Mitochondria, endoplasmic reticulum, and Golgi apparatus are found just beneath the cuticular plate. Lysosomes are also present in this region and it has been reported (Kimura, Schuknecht, and Sando 1964) that they are numerous in human hair cells which have been studied in temporal bones of older individuals.

The hairs (or stereocilia) on the outer hair cells (Figs. 2.7, 2.8, and 2.12) have some features that are different from those on the inner hair cells. They are more numerous and have a different shape and arrangement. The cilia on the first and second rows of outer hair cells have a marked V shape whereas in the third row the form may be more crescentic (Fig. 2.7). The hairs are arranged in rows of step-like lengths with an orderly progression in height. The cilia themselves are more slender than the inner hair cell cilia and rounded rather than flat on top. The tallest outer hair cell cilia make shallow indentations into the tectorial membrane (Fig. 2.13) and even leave faint imprints in tectorial membranes as observed by scanning or transmission electron microscopy.

STRIA VASCULARIS

The stria vascularis forms the lateral wall of the cochlear duct (Figs. 2.2 and 2.3). It is held in place by the spiral ligament and in some degree by its connection to the radiating arterioles and the draining venules which are continuous with the capillary networks of the stria. The marginal cell layer is the only cell group in the structure which is definitely formed by the ectoderm from the auditory vesicle; the source of the intermediate cells and the basal cell layer is questionable at present but the basal cells may be mesodermal in origin.

There are three cell types in the stria vascularis which are distinctive both in location and in cytological structure (Fig. 2.14). The marginal cells are so-named because they face the endolymph and form the endolymphatic

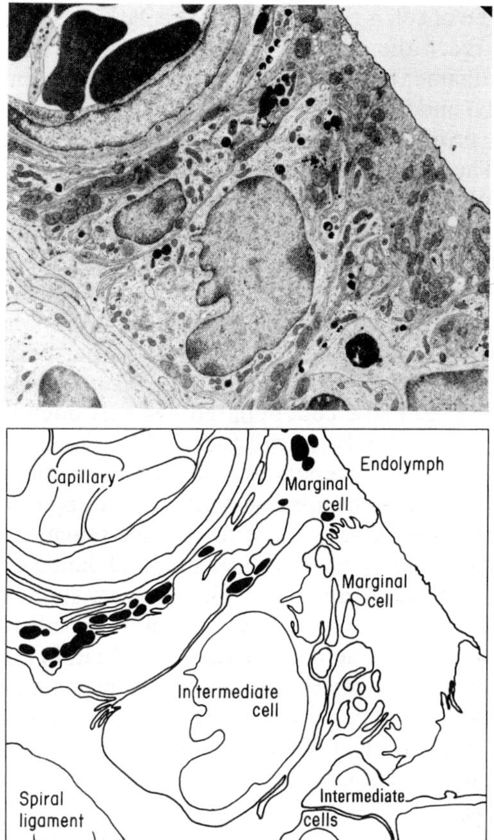

Fig. 2.14. TEM of stria vascularis from the guinea pig. The mitochondria are featured in the marginal cell at upper left in the drawing in order to emphasize the basal extensions of the cell. × 5700.

margin of the structure. They are joined together by occluding junctions at their apical ends. The basal cell membrane of each marginal cell is tremendously enlarged by the presence of innumerable finger-like cell processes which are closely packed together, are applied to the endothelial cells of the capillaries and interdigitate with the intermediate cell processes. The marginal cells have a dense cytoplasm which is packed with vesicles, rough endoplasmic reticulum, Golgi apparatus, large mitochondria, and RNA granules. These cells are the only ones of the stria which are in contact with the endolymph; they are the major cells in which the extensive capillary bed is embedded; the stria vascularis has the highest ATPase activity in the cochlea (Kuijpers and Bonting 1969). For these reasons, among others, one can assume that the marginal cells play a major role in the concentration of potassium in the endolymph. In all probability the high d.c. potential that can be measured in cochlear endolymph is associated with this process.

The second type of cell is the intermediate cell (Fig. 2.14). The intermediate cells do not reach the endolymph surface. Neither are they in contact with the spiral ligament, but are interposed in an intermediate position between marginal and basal cells. Their cell membranes have a small number of finger-like protrusions which interdigitate with some of those from the marginal cells. They have been called 'light cells' in the past, because their cytoplasm has only a moderate number of small mitochondria and few other organelles. Pinocytic vesicles are often visible within the cytoplasm. If there is any particulate matter in the extracellular space, material of a similar appearance is also present within small and large vesicles within the intermediate cells. Duvall *et al.* (1971) found that when horseradish peroxidase (an electron-dense tracer substance) was injected intravenously, it rapidly entered the extracellular space of the stria and was then taken up by the intermediate cells. These cells apparently act as scavengers in the stria.

The third cell type is the basal cell (Fig. 2.14). These flattened cells are usually several layers in thickness and separate the stria from the spiral ligament. Cellular extensions are also sent up between groups of marginal and intermediate cells (Hinojosa and Rodriquez-Echandia 1966). The flat surfaces of the basal cells are very closely apposed and are bound together by many small occluding junctions. These would impede ion and fluid movements and thus prevent ready diffusion of substances from the perilymph in the spiral ligament to the tissue fluid within the stria vascularis and vice versa. Investigators (Hinojosa 1972; Duval *et al.* 1971) who have used tracer substances have shown that this is indeed the case in experimental animals. The stria vascularis seems to be a small discrete organ with its own capillary bed, closed off from the neighbouring tissue by the basal cell layers.

LIMBUS AND TECTORIAL MEMBRANE

The limbus spiralis is a mass of connective tissue located at the medial angle of the cochlear duct (Figs. 2.2 and 2.3). It is a solid structure composed of columns of fibrillar material with interspersed cells and capillaries. A layer of epithelium overlays it. The lateral edge of the limbus is cavitated to form the inner spiral sulcus, and the upper edge forms a definite lip which overhangs the sulcus (Fig. 2.4).

The epithelial cells are bottle-shaped, with enlarged, rounded basal bulbs. The apical ends of the cells spread out into large flat plates which cover the limbic surface. The basal bulbs are arranged in radial rows, a feature which is quite obvious if one views the limbus from above. The epithelial layer is continuous with Reissner's membrane at its medial edge.

The tectorial membrane covers the epithelial plates of the limbus and seems firmly attached to the epithelial cells. It is an extracellular fibrous structure, and similar to the basilar membrane in that it is not enclosed in a membrane (Figs. 2.4 and 2.13). Unlike the basilar membrane it is not covered by a cellular layer. It is freely exposed to endolymph on its upper (or vestibular surface) as well as on its lower surface which spans the inner spiral sulcus and extends over the organ of Corti. The tectorial membrane is often curled up or under in certain pathological conditions including extreme hyperstimulation. It may even be detached at the lip of the limbus but it is usually still attached to the major part of the limbic surface. It is assumed that the epithelial cells play some role in the maintainence of the tectorial membrane substance.

REISSNER'S MEMBRANE

Reissner's membrane is a thin, flat, cellular membrane which extends from the medial edge of the limbus to the upper (or vestibular) edge of the stria vascularis. It is composed of two sheets of cells (Fig. 2.3). The cells that face the endolymph are epithelial in origin and are low cuboidal, almost squamous, in form. They are joined together by occluding junctions. A second layer of cells, which is mesenchymal in origin, faces the perilymph. These cells are very flat and are only loosely joined together.

Questions about the permeability, and the functional properties of Reissner's membrane have been raised many times. Kuipers and Bonting (1969) have shown it is rather low in adenosine triphosphatase activity so it seems unlikely that it has any remarkable ion transport activity. Hinojosa (1971) found that ferritin readily crossed from perilymph to endolymph across Reissner's membrane. It appeared that the ferritin did not penetrate the occluding junctions between the cells but was carried through the cells in pinocytic vesicles. Ferritin injected into the endolymph space was not found in Reissner's membrane cells. It appears that some molecules of small molecular weight can pass from perilymph to endolymph but not in the opposite direction.

VASCULAR SUPPLY

The labyrinthine artery is usually a branch of the anterior inferior cerebellar artery in man. However, there are variations in its derivation: sometimes it is derived from the basilar artery (Nabeya 1923). Smith (1951) found that, in guinea pigs, the anterior vestibular artery was often derived directly from the anterior inferior cerebellar artery instead of being a branch of the labyrinthine artery. In general, the labyrinthine artery is the sole source of blood for the membranous labyrinth. There are no collateral arteries.

The artery divides into the anterior vestibular artery and the common cochlear artery in the internal acoustic meatus. A vestibulocochlear branch is given off the common cochlear artery which supplies part of the lowermost basal coil of the cochlea as well as the vestibule. This branch was first described by Seibenmann (1894), but is not always present (Axelsson 1968). In short, although there seems to be some variability in the pattern of supply to the lower part of the basal coil in man, the remainder of the cochlea is invariably supplied by branches from the cochlear artery. The main importance of this branching pattern resides in the fact that an embolism in the vestibulocochlear branch could produce sudden high frequency hearing loss (plus vestibular symptoms) without affecting the rest of the cochlea.

The cochlear artery ramifies considerably within the modiolus and sends separate arteriolar branches to the lateral cochlear wall, to the limbus and spiral lamina, to the spiral ganglion cells and their peripheral processes in Rosenthal's canal, and to the cochlear nerve in the modiolus (Fig. 2.15). The capillary beds in each of these locations (except in the modiolus) form networks which are continuous in a spiral direction.

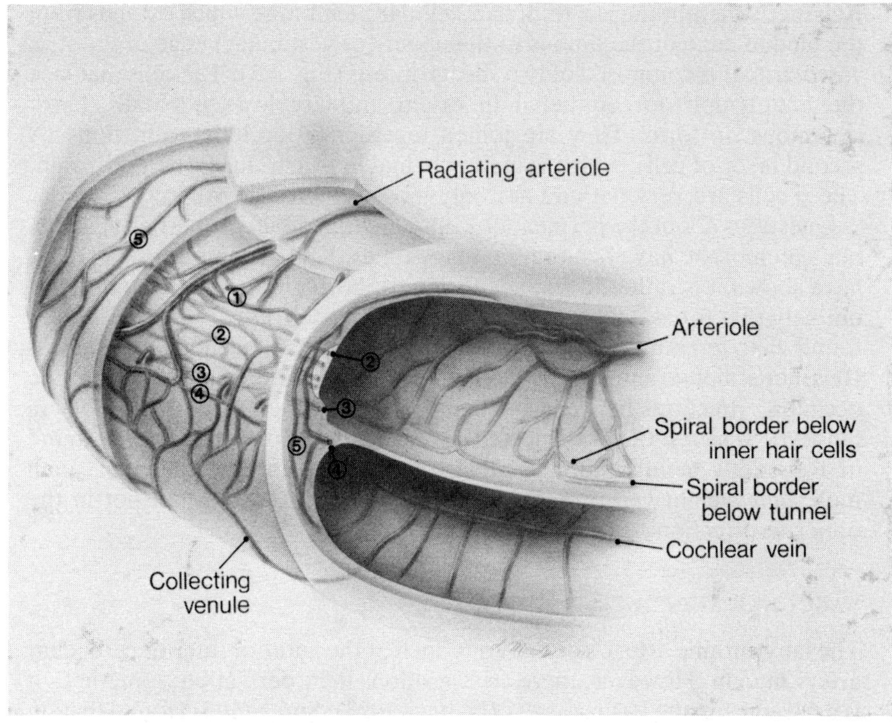

Fig. 2.15. Semi-schematic drawing showing the location of the capillary beds of the human cochlea. The capillaries in the lateral wall are numbered: (1) capillary network in the vestibular spiral ligament; (2) network in the stria vascularis; (3) network in the spiral prominence; (4) network in the tympanic spiral ligament; (5) arteriovenous arcades. (Drawing by Suzanne Moody.)

Lateral cochlear wall

Arteriolar branches radiate out through the bone over scala vestibuli and ramify in the vestibular part of the spiral ligament. Distinct and separate branches are sent to capillary beds in each of five locations: (i) a network in the upper (vestibular) part of the spiral ligament, (ii) the wide network in the stria vascularis, (iii) the narrow network in the spiral prominence, (iv) the network in the tympanic spiral ligament, and (v) the arteriovenous arcades in the depth of the spiral ligament (Smith 1951, 1954; Scuderi and del Bo 1952; Axelsson 1968). The second and the fifth capillary regions are of special interest.

The network of the stria vascularis is an intra-epithelial bed of capillaries. The marginal cells and their basal processes abut upon the endothelial cells of the capillaries and along with some intermediate cell processes completely enclose the network. The network is complete and continuous from the basal to the apical end of the human cochlea and that of other mammals. It is supplied by arteriolar branches which enter at regular intervals and by other small vessels which exit at regular intervals and empty into the venules in the tympanic spiral ligament. The cells of the stria vascularis thus have available to them a large pool of blood with innumerable sources of supply and drainage, so that a continuous fluid turnover is possible. It is separate from the network in the spiral prominence, which is close to but not within the epithelium and it has no connection with the capillaries in the spiral ligament.

The arteriolar branches to the fifth group course in the thicker part of the spiral ligament. They do not form a net, with cross-branches. These small vessels take a straight course from arteriole to venule generally without branching. These are the arteriovenous arcades.

Limbus and basilar membrane

Other arterioles branch from the cochlear artery and enter Rosenthal's canal. They form a network among the myelinated nerve fibres and radiate out with the nerve fibres towards the organ of Corti.

Some branches deviate up to the limbus and join a radial, looping network there. This is located in the neighbourhood of the epithelial cells which cover the limbus. Other branches continue outward below the inner spiral sulcus and terminate in a looped network which has two discontinuous borders, coursing in a spiral direction. The outermost border is beneath the tunnel and has been given the name of 'vas spirale' in the past; the inner border is beneath or near the inner hair cells. Both of these capillary borders are located among the mesothelial cells, outside the fibres of the basilar membrane. There are no other blood vessels close to or within the organ of Corti.

The spiral ganglion cells and the nerve fibres, both in Rosenthal's canal and within the modiolus, are well supplied with blood vessels.

The venous drainage of the cochlea is carried by the cochlear vein which is a large, thin-walled vessel located in the bony wall of the modiolus. It empties into the vein of the cochlear aqueduct which courses in a separate bony channel but follows the direction of the cochlear aqueduct. Nabeya (1923) observed that there were some collateral channels between the cochlear vein in the basal turn and the dural veins. There are no lymphatic vessels in the inner ear.

SUMMARIZING REMARKS

The membranous labyrinth is a closed epithelial tube whose cells are joined together by occluding junctions so that ion movements between endolymph and perilymph are inhibited. The cochlear division of the labyrinth has well organized cell groups which are continuous from basal to apical ends so that no single segment of the basilar membrane is favoured over another by histological organization. The large fluid spaces of the endolymph and perilymph including those within the organ of Corti allow a ready diffusion of ions and metabolites throughout the cochlea. Although the capillary areas are supplied by arterioles which course in a radial direction, the capillary networks themselves have a spiral direction and in some cases, as in the stria vascularis, there is no break in the continuity of capillary bed from basal to apical end. All of these features assure a regular and even supply of metabolites to a sensory receptor organ that is similar from one end of the cochlea to the other with the end result that, in most mammals, no one frequency region is favoured over another. Of course, there are always exceptions, one of these being bats: their remarkable high-frequency sensitivity may be aided by certain structural modifications of the organ of Corti in the lower basal turn (Pye 1966). However, the ears of Man and most other mammals do not have any such specialized features and the histological organization of the cochlear duct favours equal sensory reception over a wide frequency range.

Acknowledgement

The courtesy of Berit Engstrom who furnished the micrograph of Fig. 2.6 is greatly appreciated.

BIBLIOGRAPHY

AXELSSON, A. (1968). The vascular anatomy of the cochlea in the guinea pig and in man. *Acta oto-lar.* Suppl., 243.

BAST, T. H. and ANSON, B. J. (1949). *The temporal bone and the ear.* Thomas, Springfield, Illinois.

VON BEKESY, G. (1960). Experimental models of the cochlea, with and without nerve supply. In *Neural mechanisms of the auditory and vestibular systems*, (ed. G. Rasmussen and W. F. Windle) pp. 3–20. Thomas, Springfield.

BORDLEY, J. E., BROOKHAUSER, P. E., HARDY, J., and HARDY, W. G. (1967). Observations on the effect of prenatal rubella in hearing. In *Deafness in childhood*, (ed. F. McConnell and P. Ward) pp. 123–41. Vanderbilt University Press, Nashville.

BREDBERG, G. (1968). Cellular pattern and nerve supply of the human organ of Corti. *Acta oto-lar.* Suppl., 236.

DUVALL, A. J., QUICK, C. A., and SUTHERLAND, C. R. (1971). Horseradish peroxidase in the lateral cochlear wall. An electron microscopic study of transport. *Archs. oto-lar.* **93,** 304–16.

ENGSTROM, B. (1974). Scanning electron microscopy of the inner structure of the organ of Corti and its neural pathways. In *Inner ear studies* II (ed. H. Ades and H. Engstrom) *Acta oto-lar.* Suppl. 319, 57–66.

FRIEDMANN, I. and WRIGHT, M. I. (1966). Histopathological changes in the foetal and infantile inner ear caused by maternal rubella. *Br. med. J.* **ii,** 20–3.

HINOJOSA, R. (1971). Transport of ferritin across Reissner's membrane. *Acta oto-lar.* Suppl., 292.

—— (1972). Electron microscope studies of the stria vascularis and the spiral ligament after ferritin injection. *Acta oto-lar.* **74,** 1–14.

—— and RODRIGUEZ-ECHANDIA, E. L. (1966). The fine structure of the stria vascularis of the cat inner ear. *Am. J. Anat.* **118,** 631–64.

KIMURA, R., SCHUKNECHT, H. F. and SANDO, I. (1964). Fine morphology of the sensory cells in the organ of Corti of man. *Acta oto-lar.* **58,** 390–408.

KUIJPERS, W. and BONTING, S. L. (1969). Localization and properties of ATPase in the inner ear of the guinea pig. *Biochim. biophys. Acta* **173,** 477–85.

NABEYA, D. (1923). A study in the comparative anatomy of the blood vascular system of the internal ear in Mammalia and in Homo (Japanese). *Acta scholae med.* **6,** 1–132.

PEARSON, A. A. (1967). *The development of the ear*, American Academy of Ophthmology and Otology, Rochester, Minn.

PYE, A. (1966). The Megachiroptera and Vespertilionoidea of the Microchiroptera. *J. Morphol.* **119,** 101–20.

SCUDERI, R. and DEL BO, M. (1952). La vascolarizzazione del labirinto unamo. *Archo. ital. Otol. Rinol. Lar.* Suppl. 11.

SIEBENMANN, F. (1894). *Die Blutgefasse im Labyrinthe des menslichen Ohre.* J. Bergmann, Wiesbaden.

SMITH, C. A. (1951). Capillary areas of the cochlea in the guinea pig. *Laryngoscope, St. Louis* **61,** 1073–95.

——(1954). Capillary areas of the membranous labyrinth. *Ann. Otol. Rhinol. Lar.* **63,** 435–48.

—— (1968). Ultrastructure of the organ of Corti. *Advmt. Sci., Lond.* **122,** 419–33.

—— (1973). Anatomical correlates of deafness. *J. acoust. Soc. Am.* **54,** 576–88.

—— (1975). The inner ear, its embryological development and microstructure. In *The nervous system* (ed. D. Tower) Vol. 3, pp. 1–18. Raven Press, New York.

—— (1978). Structure of the cochlear duct. In *Evoked electrical activity in the auditory nervous system*, (ed. R. F. Naunton and C. Fernandez). Academic Press, New York.

—— COVELL, W. P., and ELDREDGE, D. H. (1954). The effects of intense sound on the cochlea. Wright Air Force Development Center Technical Report, pp. 141–53.

——LOWRY, O. H., and WU, M.-L. (1954). The electrolytes of the labyrinthine fluids. *Laryngoscope, St. Louis* **64,** 141–53.

TASAKI, I., DAVIS, H., and ELDREDGE, D. H. (1954). Exploration of cochlear potentials in guinea pig with a microelectrode. *J. acoust. Soc. Am.* **26,** 765–73.

WEVER, E. G. (1967). The tectorial membrane of the lizard ear: species variations. *J. Morph.* **123,** 355–72.

3 Neuroanatomy of the cochlea

H. SPOENDLIN

Three components of the cochlear innervation are known (Fig. 3.1): (i) the afferent innervation with the cochlear neurons, the bipolar ganglion cells of which form the spiral ganglion in Rosenthal's canal in the modiolus. These connect the cochlear receptor to the cochlear nuclei. (ii) The efferent olivocochlear neurons known as the olivocochlear bundle originating in the homo- and contralateral superior olivary complex as originally described by Rasmussen (1942). They reach the periphery together with the vestibular nerve and cross over to the cochlear nerve only within the internal acoustic meatus through the anastomosis of Oort. (iii) The third component finally consists of the autonomic innervation originating in the cervical sympathetic trunk.

For the study of the neuroanatomy of the cochlea we used a specially developed block-surface technique which allows quantitative evaluation of practically all important components of the cochlea; either in surface view

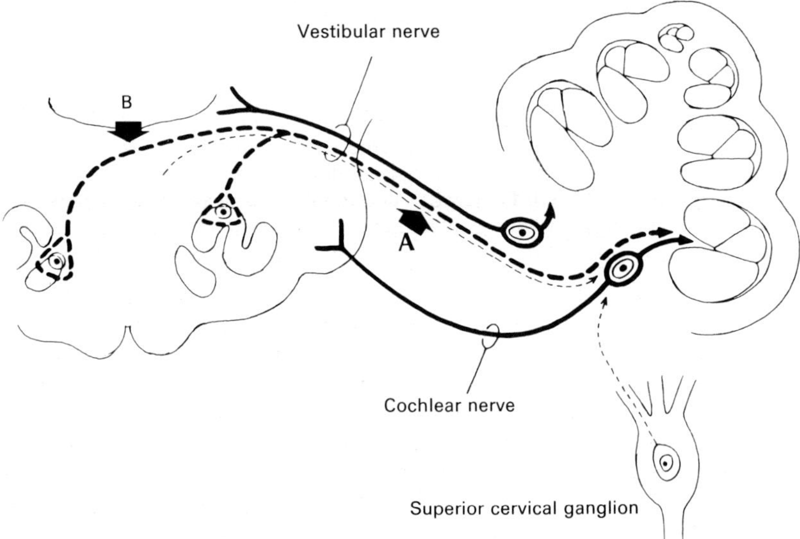

Fig. 3.1. Schematic representation of the three innervation components of the cochlea: the bipolar cochlear sensory neurons of the cochlear nerve (full heavy lines), olivocochlear efferent neurons (interrupted heavy lines), and adrenergic innervation from the superior cervical ganglion (interrupted thin lines). A gives the lesion site for selective interruption of the entire efferent nerve supply of the cochlea and B indicates the lesion site for the so called midline lesion for the interruption of the contralateral efferent nerve supply only.

with interference contrast light microscopy of semi-thin sections or ultra-thin sections of any desired portion in any desired sectional plan for electron microscopy (Fig. 3.2). The findings were photographically documented at every step (Spoendlin and Burn 1974).

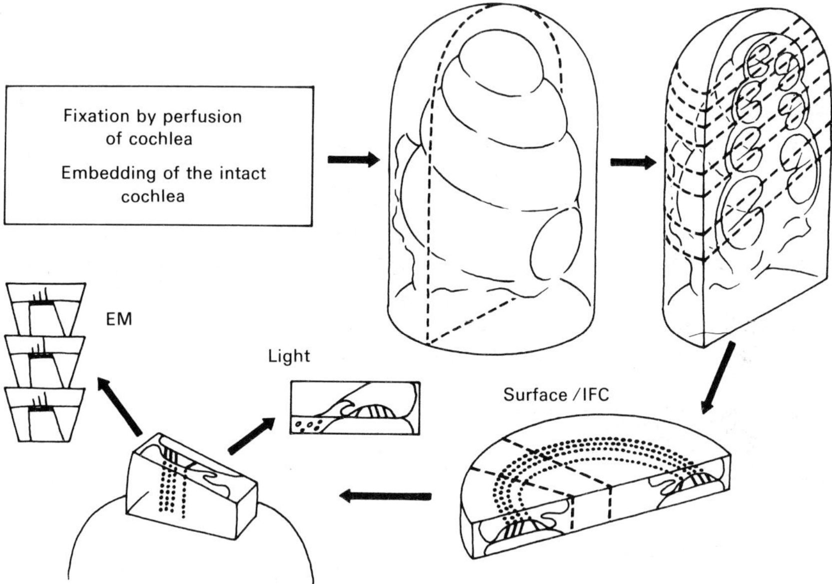

Fig. 3.2. Schematic representation of the block surface technique for the morphological evaluation of the cochlea.

To demonstrate the adrenergic innervation we used the histochemical method of Falk, Hillarp, Thieme, and Torp (1962) where, with an appropriate filter-combination, all adrenergic nerve fibres appear with a very specific green fluorescence. Using this technique in normal animals and after various lesions such as extirpation of the superior cervical or stellate ganglion or by section of the tympanic plexus we found in the cat two different independent adrenergic innervations of the inner ear (Fig. 3.3). One is strictly perivascular, originating in the stellate ganglion and reaching the inner ear through the perivascular plexus of the vertebral, basilar, and anterior inferior cerebellar and labyrinthine artery. This perivascular plexus can be followed as far as the greater arteriolar branches in the modiolus but is never found in the blood vessels of the spiral ligament of stria vascularis. The second type of adrenergic innervation is not associated with the blood vessels. It originates in the superior cervical ganglion and reaches the inner ear via the tympanic plexus. This component is most pronounced in the osseous spiral lamina where it forms a fairly rich terminal plexus just below the habenula and is especially pronounced in the apical turns of the cochlea (Fig. 3.3). This independent adrenergic innervation, however, does not enter the organ of

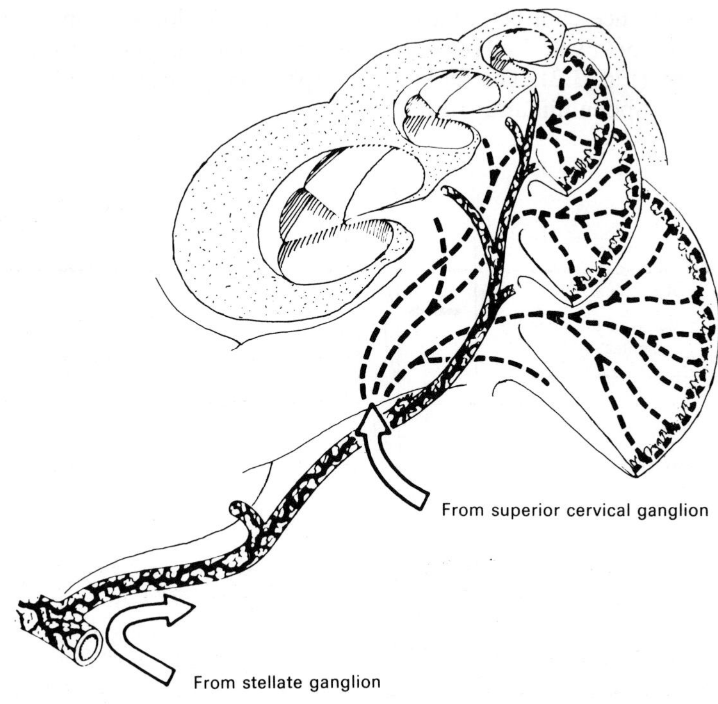

Fig. 3.3. Schematic representation of the two types of adrenergic innervation of the cochlea. One originating from the superior cervical ganglion which is independent of the blood vessels and the other originating from the stellate ganglion which follows the blood vessels.

Corti through the habenular openings and therefore does not interfere directly with the receptor process in the organ of Corti (Spoendlin and Lichtensteiger 1965, 1967; Paradisgarten and Spoendlin 1976). The two independent types of adrenergic innervation are less distinct in other species such as the rabbit (Densert 1974) and the guinea pig (Terayama, Holz and Beck 1966), but it has been confirmed in the cat.

The transformation of acoustic information into bioelectrical neural information in the acoustic nerve occurs in several steps, each of which is closely associated with certain structures of the inner ear (Fig. 3.4). The first step is the mechanical analysis of sound in the cochlea by means of travelling waves according to the tonotopical organization—low frequencies stimulating the cochlear apex and high frequencies almost exclusively the basal portions of the cochlea. This step depends entirely on the mechanical properties of the cochlea, particularly the basilar membrane. The second step is the mechano-electrical transformation in the cochlear hair cells. The functional expression of this step is the cochlear microphonic which is the exact electrical copy of the stimulating acoustic waves. The third step is the important coding of this acoustic message into neural activity. This occurs in

Cochlea	Mechanical analysis	Travelling waves
Sensory cells	Mechanical electric transduction	Microphonics
Nerve endings, terminal unmyelinated nerve branches	Coding of acoustic information	Generator potential ?
Myelinated nerve fibres	Transport to CNS	Action potential

Fig. 3.4. The four steps of information processing in the cochlea with the corresponding underlying structures (left column) and the functional expression (right column).

the nerve endings and terminal unmyelinated portions of the cochlear neurons within the organ of Corti, and is influenced by efferent activity. The functional expression of this step is a generator potential possibly measured as summating potentials. The final step is the transfer of the information from the receptor to the central nervous system through the cochlear neurons in the form of action potentials which are all or nothing responses and probably originate in the area of the habenula.

The third and fourth step depend entirely on structural characteristics, that is the distribution and the interconnections of the afferent and efferent cochlear fibres. The speed of the action potential propagation is dependent on the calibre of the nerve fibre and from the thickness of its myelin sheath. In the cochlear nerve all fibres have very similar diameter with an unimodel distribution from 4–6 micrometres and a myelin sheath of about 50 lamellae, which is the structural basis of a uniform conduction velocity, probably a very important basic functional feature. The number of cochlear neurons varies considerably in different species with about 30 000 in Man, but 50 000 in the cat (Schuknecht 1962; Spoendlin 1969) and about 250 000 in whales (Hall 1966). Very few unmyelinated fibres are found within the trunk of the cochlear nerve in contrast to the vestibular nerve where there are many. The calibre of myelinated fibres in the vestibular nerve vary considerably from 2 to 15 micrometres (Spoendlin 1972). A great number of unmyelinated fibres is also found in the olivocochlear bundle which can be selectively studied at the level of the anastomosis of Oort or within the intraganglionic spiral bundle which represents the peripheral course of the olivocochlear fibres. In contrast to the cochlear nerve trunk there are many unmyelinated fibres of varying calibres among the peripheral axons of the cochlear neurons in the osseous spiral lamina where afferent, efferent, and addrenergic fibres are intermingled (Paradisgarten and Spoendlin 1976). All fibres lose their myelin sheath before they enter the organ of Corti through the habenular openings (Fig. 3.5).

In order to study the distribution of the afferent and efferent nerve fibres within the organ of Corti, the two systems must be distinguished. The efferent system can be selectively eliminated by transsection of the olivo-cochlear fibres at the level of the vestibular nerve or vestibular root without interfering with the afferent cochlear nerve supply. After such lesions the

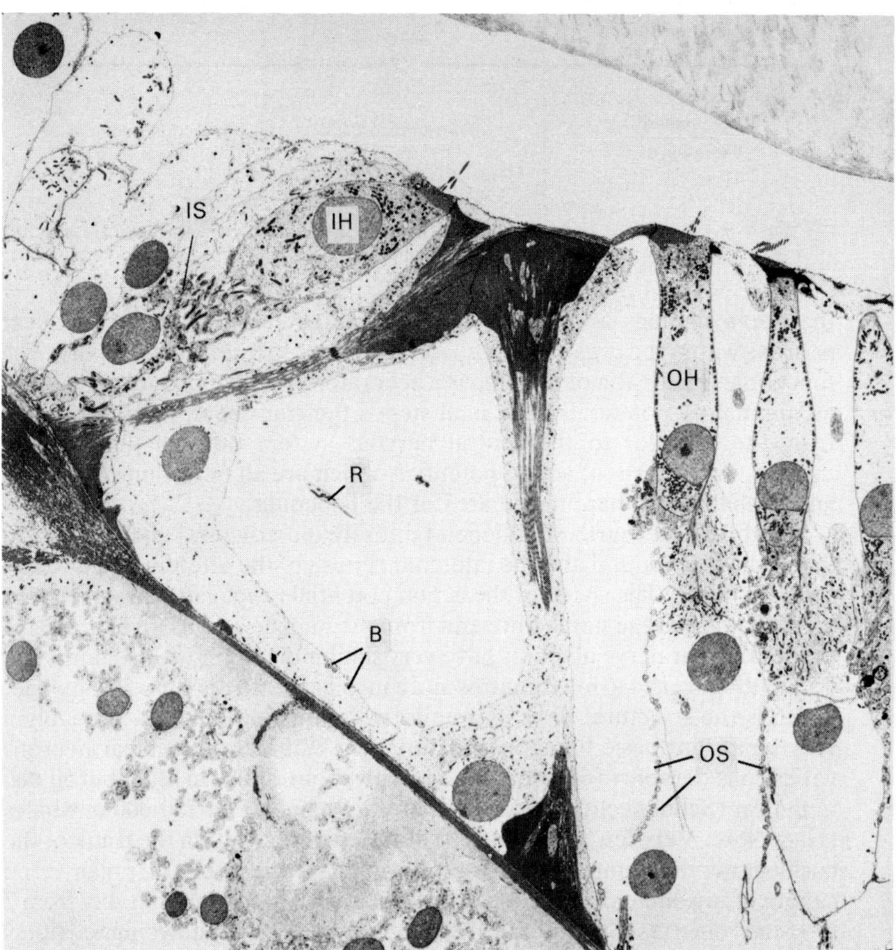

Fig. 3.5. General view of the organ of Corti with outer hair cells (OH) and inner hair cells (IH), the principal nerve fibre tracts within the organ of Corti are the inner radial and inner spiral fibres (IS), the tunnel radial fibres (R), the basilar fibres (B), and the outer spiral fibres (OS).

efferent neurons begin to degenerate within a few hours and disappear completely within a few days. This includes practically all the inner spiral fibres, the upper tunnel radial fibres, and all the very numerous large vesiculated nerve endings at the base of the outer hair cells, showing clearly that they all belong to the efferent innervation system (Spoendlin 1966, 1969) (Figs. 3.6 and 3.7). The great majority of nerve endings at the base of

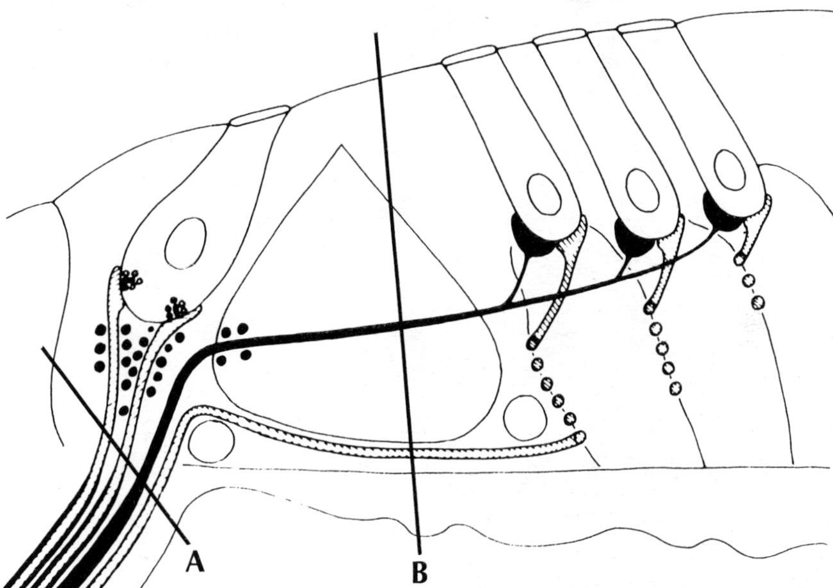

Fig. 3.6. Radial innervation schema of the organ of Corti with efferent nerve fibres (full lines) consisting of the inner spiral fibres, the tunnel radial fibres and the large nerve endings at the outer hair cells, and the afferent nerve fibres (hatched lines) consisting of inner radial fibres, basilar fibres, and outer spiral fibres with small nerve endings at the outer hair cells. A and B represent the sectional plans for the numerical evaluation of the nerve fibres as represented in the diagram of fig. 3.11.

the outer hair cells are of the large vesiculated efferent type which is very surprising as there are very few small afferent nerve endings associated with the outer hair cells (Fig. 3.7). The number of efferent terminals at the base of the outer hair cells is greatest in the basal turn and decreases gradually towards the cochlear apex, where they are restricted to the first row of outer hair cells. Using the Maillet method the efferent fibres can be stained quasi-selectively and well demonstrated in surface preparations.

There has been much discussion about the homo- and the contralateral efferents (Iurato, personal communication). According to our experiments with selective elimination of the contralateral efferents by lesions at the floor of the fourth ventricle and according to recent findings of Warr (1978) with identification of efferent neurons by uptake of horseradish peroxidase (HRP) and radioactive amino acids, the great majority of the efferents to

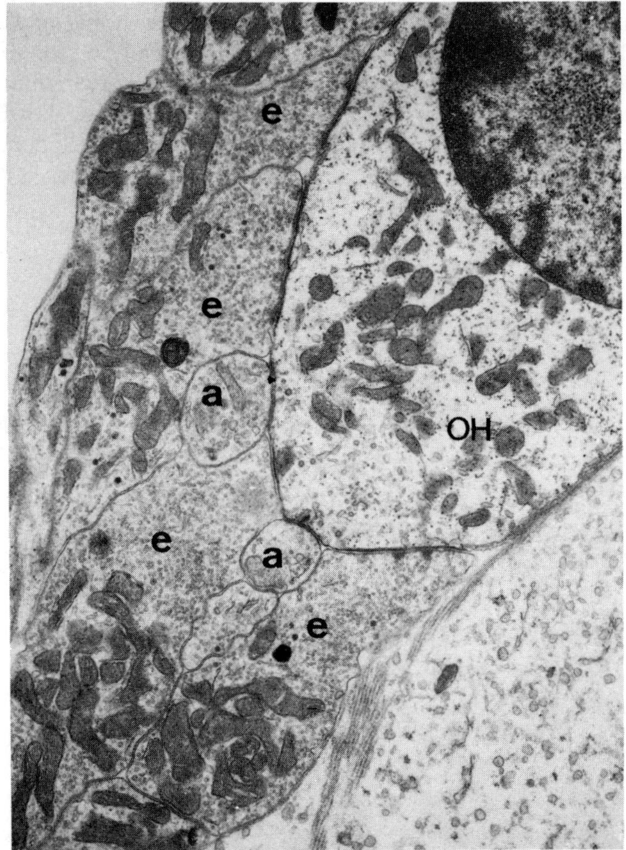

Fig. 3.7. Base of an outer hair cell (O H) of the basal turn of a guinea pig with a great number of efferent nerve terminals (e) and some afferent small nerve endings (a).

the outer hair cells originate in the large cells in the contralateral accessory olivary nucleus whereas the great majority of the efferents at the level of the inner hair cells originate in small cells in the homolateral main superior olivary nucleus (Fig. 3.8).

There is evidence that the efferents for the outer and inner hair cells represent two different types of neurons. The efferents of the outer hair cells are usually large fibres with diameters up to 1.5 μm which degenerate very rapidly after transection, whereas the efferents of the inner hair cell region are small and take several days to degenerate. In addition Warr (1978) showed that the efferent for the inner hair cells originate in small ganglion cells, whereas the efferents of the outer hair cells originate in large ganglion cells. Furthermore the inner spiral fibres have a tendency to increase from the base to the apex whereas the efferent endings at the outer hair cells decrease from base to apex. Finally, there is a basic difference in the synaptic connections of the efferents to the outer and inner hair cells. At the

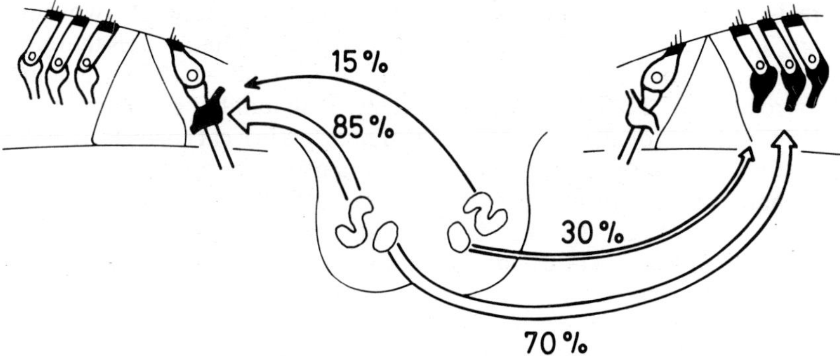

Fig. 3.8. Schematic representation of the homolateral and contralateral efferent nerve supply from the superior olivary nucleus and the accessory olivary nucleus. (Adapted from Warr (1978).)

level of the outer hair cells the efferent synapse almost exclusively with the receptor cell as such but at the level of the inner hair cells they almost exclusively synapse with the afferent nerve fibres associated to the inner hair cells. They are presynaptic in respect of the afferent synapse at the level of the outer hair cells and postsynaptic at the level of the inner hair cells (Fig. 3.9).

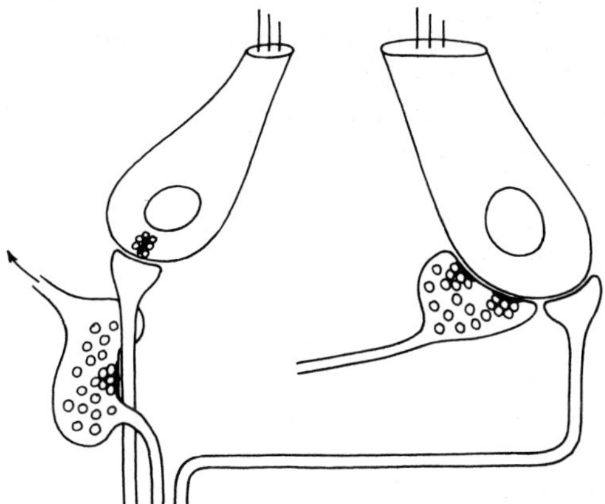

Fig. 3.9. Schematic representation of the synaptic contacts of the efferent fibres at the base of the outer hair cells (right) and at the afferent nerve fibres below the inner hair cells (left).

The only fibres left after elimination of the efferents are the inner radial fibres, the basilar fibres, and the outer spiral fibres. These represent the afferent innervation of the organ of Corti. The few basilar fibres are the only afferent fibres reaching the area of the outer hair cells. They can be counted as they pass between the base of the outer pillar cells in tangential sections through this area (Fig. 3.6). Evaluated over long distances of the cochlea there is an average of one basilar fibre penetrating between two outer pillars. The number of afferent fibres going to the outer hair cells is therefore about equal to the number of outer pillars, which in the cat cochlea amounts to approximately 2500. This is an extremely small number compared to the entire population of about 50 000 cochlear neurons in a cat cochlea. It means that only 5 per cent of all afferent cochlear neurons are associated with the outer hair cell system which represents more than three-quarters of the receptor cells of the cochlea. More evidence can be provided for this surprising 20:1 ratio of afferent innervation of inner and outer hair cells. If we reconstruct the area of some inner hair cells on the basis of serial sections after elimination of the efferent innervation we find that the great majority of all nerve fibres entering the organ of Corti through the habenular openings lead directly, unbranching, to the base of the nearest inner hair cell and only about one fibre in twenty turns outwards to the outer hair cells (Fig. 3.10). Finally, we can compare the total number of afferent and efferent nerve fibres entering the organ of Corti at the level of the habenula with the number of all fibres crossing the tunnel towards the outer hair cells in corresponding tangential sections in normal animals (Fig. 3.11). The numbers show that only about 15 per cent of all fibres entering the organ of Corti cross the tunnel towards the outer hair cells. Since two-thirds of the tunnel-crossing fibres are the efferent upper tunnel radial fibres, the basilar fibres represent only about 5 per cent of the total afferent neuron population, the same small percentage as we found on the basis of the other evaluation. There is little doubt that in fact the outer hair cell system is only associated to a small minority of afferent neurons whereas the great majority of all afferent neurons is associated to the inner hair cell system. After the demonstration of this surprising situation in the cat, similar ratios between neurons associated to the outer and inner hair cells have been found in the guinea pig (Spoendlin 1969; Morrison, Schindler and Wersäll 1975) and in Man (Nomura 1976).

Within the habenula the fibres associated with the outer hair cells cannot be distinguished from the other fibres but they are usually situated in the most distal portion of the habenular opening. In contrast to the fibres for the inner hair cells they take an independent spiral course immediately after the habenula for about five pillars before they penetrate between the inner pillars to cross the bottom of the tunnel as basilar fibres and reach the area of the outer hair cells where they form the outer spiral fibres between the Deiter cells. These outer spiral fibres gradually climb up towards the base of the outer hair cells where each fibre in its terminal portion gives off collaterals which end as afferent nerve ending at the base of outer hair cells. Each fibre sends collaterals to about ten outer hair cells and each outer hair cell receives collaterals from several outer spiral fibres according to the principal of multiple innervation (Spoendlin 1970, 1973).

The length of the basalward spiral course of outer spiral fibres can be estimated from the number of the basilar fibres reaching the outer hair cell area (1 fibre per pillar cell) and the number of the outer spiral fibres (about

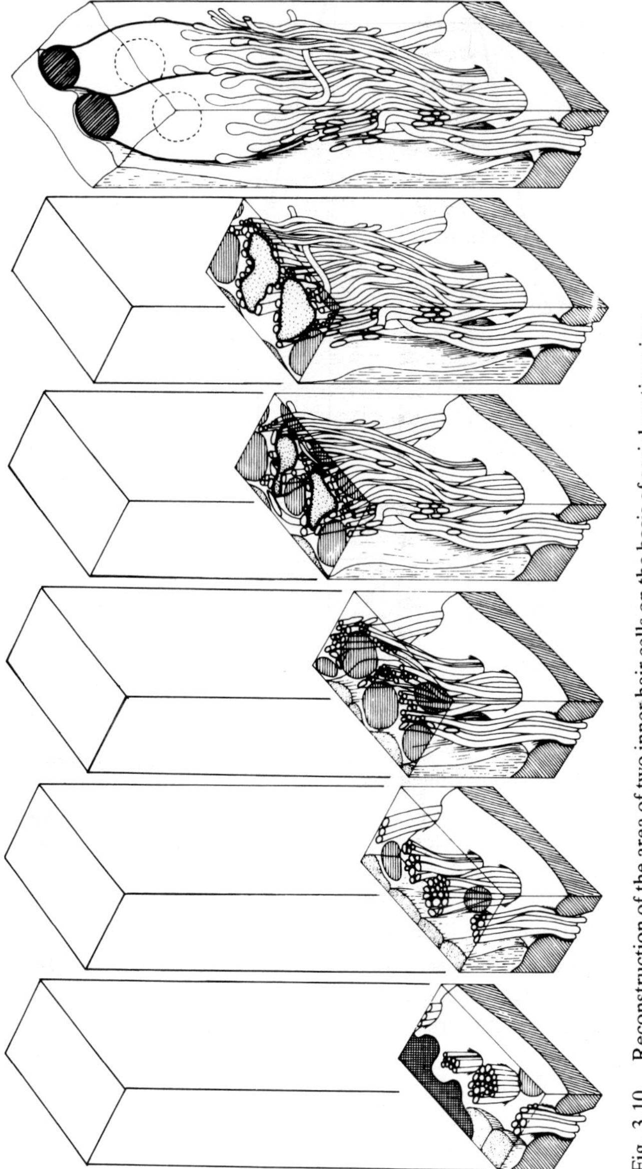

Fig. 3.10. Reconstruction of the area of two inner hair cells on the basis of serial sections in a cat where the efferent nerve fibres have been eliminated previously by section of the vestibular nerve. The great majority of all afferent nerve fibres leads directly unbranched to the nearest inner hair cell.

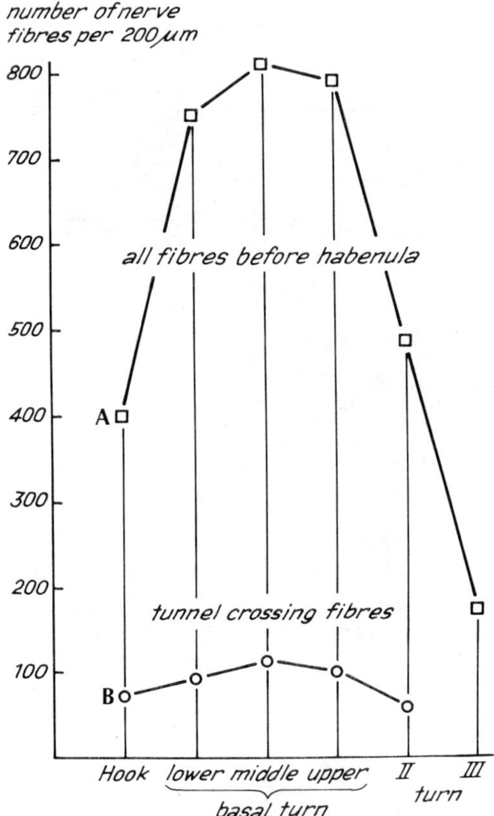

Fig. 3.11. Diagram comparing the number of nerve fibres entering the organ of Corti at the level of the habenula (A) and the nerve fibres crossing the tunnel of Corti (B).

100 at any one place). The average length is thus 0.5 mm (Spoendlin 1969). This agrees with that measured directly in stained silver preparations by Smith and Haglan (1973).

There is no morphological evidence for direct functional interaction between the afferent fibres from inner and outer hair cells at any level. In no place are there direct contacts or even synapses between the axons of the two fibre systems. Within the habenular openings all fibres are individually surrounded by the processes of a special habenular satellite cell, which seems to take the role of the individual Schwann cells proximal to the habenula (Fig. 3.12).

The calibre of the fibres varies considerably along their course through the organ of Corti. Where the fibres pass mechanically important supporting structures such as the basilar membrane at the habenular region or the pillars their diameter is especially reduced and the axoplasm is rather empty (Fig. 3.13). The ultrastructural organization of the axoplasm varies to a

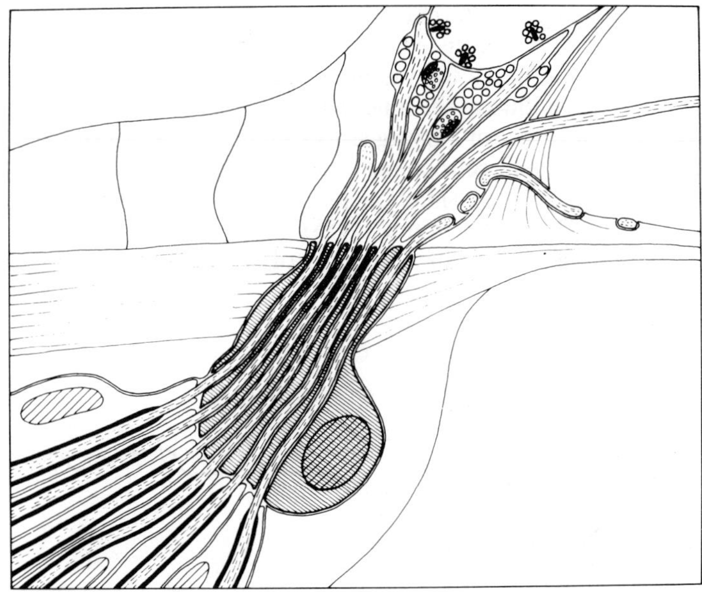

Fig. 3.12. Schematic representation of one habenular opening with the satellite cell which surrounds all nerve fibres penetrating the habenula without their myelin sheath. The nerve fibres destined for the outer hair cells tend to take an independent course immediately after the habenula.

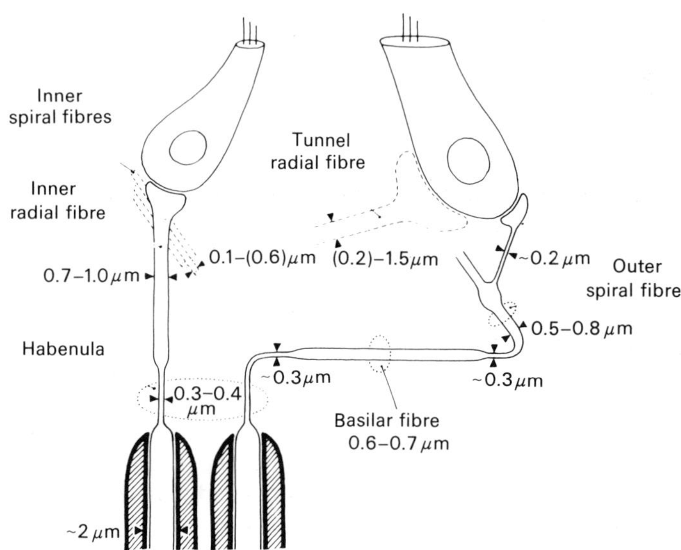

Fig. 3.13. Diameters of the nerve fibres in the organ of Corti of the cat.

certain extent between afferent fibres to outer and inner hair cells. The fibres for the outer hair cells contain mainly neurocanaliculi in their axoplasma whereas the fibres for the inner hair cells contain predominantly neurofibrils. The endings at the inner hair cells usually form synaptic complexes with synaptic bars of varying sizes (Smith and Shöstrand 1961). The endings of the outer hair cells on the other hand have no synaptic ribbons in the cat and only relatively small ones in the guinea pig (Rodriguez 1967; Spoendlin 1970; Dunn and Morest 1975).

The innervation pattern of the organ of Corti can be summarized as follows (Fig. 3.14).

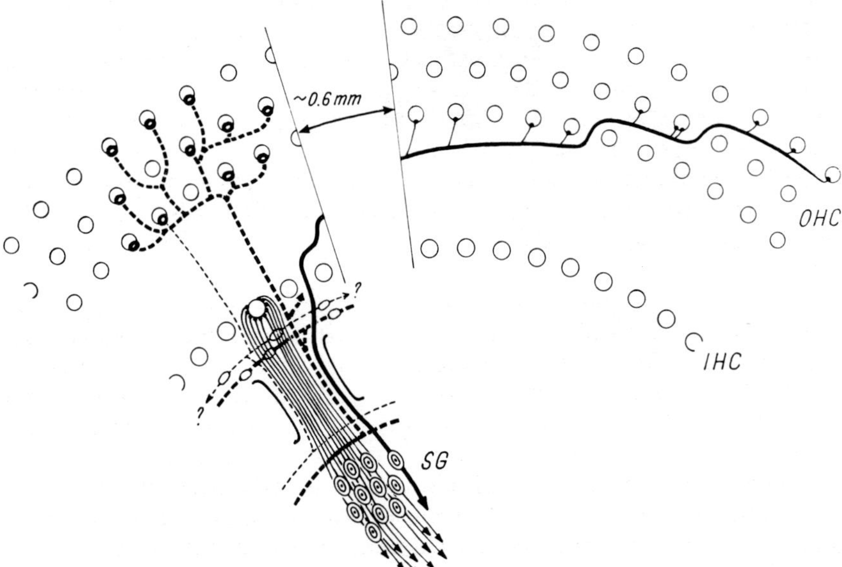

Fig. 3.14. Horizontal innervation schema of the organ of Corti of the cat. The afferent nerve fibres are represented by full lines, the efferent by interrupted lines. The afferent neurons associated with the inner hair cells are shown by thin lines, the afferents destined for the outer hair cells by heavy lines. The mainly contralateral efferent fibres are represented by heavy interrupted lines and the homolateral efferent fibres by thin interrupted lines.

THE AFFERENT INNERVATION

(i) The great majority of afferent neurons of the cochlear nerve (95 per cent in the cat and 90 per cent in the guinea pig (Spoendlin 1972; Morrison *et al.* 1975) and in Man (Nomura 1976) are associated with the inner hair cells and only a small minority (5 per cent in the cat and 10 per cent in the guinea pig) with the outer hair cells. (ii) The fibres associated with the inner hair cells are strictly radial where as the fibres for the outer hair have a considerable spiral distribution. (iii) Each inner hair cell is innervated by about 20 unbranched individual afferent neurons and each outer hair cell is innervated by branches from several neurons, each of which participates in the innervation of about ten outer hair cells. (iv) The innervation modus is therefore basically different for the inner hair cell system with its great divergence (1:20) and for the outer hair cell system with its considerably convergence (10:1). (v) The ultrastructural difference mainly of the synaptic contact with the hair cells indicate different functional mechanisms in the neurons of the outer and of the inner hair cell system.

THE EFFERENT INNERVATION

(i) The efferents of the outer hair cell system consists of large nerve fibres showing a basically radial distribution. The great majority of these fibres originate from large cells in the accessory superior olivary complex of the contralateral side and they degenerate very promptly after transection of the axon. (ii) The efferents for the inner hair cell system consist of small fibres, the majority of which originate in small cells of the homolateral main superior olivary nucleus. They have a considerable spiral distribution and synapse only with the afferent dendrites but not directly with the hair cells. They present a delayed degeneration after transection of the axons in the vestibular nerve.

The afferent neurons for the outer and inner hair cells differ not only in their anatomical distribution and structure but also in their biological behaviour. The afferent fibres at the inner hair cells are very sensitive to metabolic disturbance such as anoxia or osmotic changes and react with a pronounced swelling of the axon, whereas the afferent fibres for the outer hair cells are rather resistant to such influences (Spoendlin 1975).

The degeneration behaviour is also different. After section of the cochlear nerve in the inner acoustic meatus without disturbance of the cochlear blood supply in the cat, most cochlear neurons degenerate within two months; however, the organ of Corti remains intact (Fig. 3.15). This retrograde degeneration is a peculiar phenomenon in sensory bipolar neurons after amputation of one axon and is also well known in the spinal ganglion (Ranson 1905; Andres 1961). The normal spiral ganglion of the cat consists of about 95 per cent myelinated, large, bipolar ganglion cells (type I) and about 5 per cent of essentially unmyelinated small predominantly pseudomonopolar ganglion cells (type II) (Figs. 3.16 and 3.17). Not all ganglion cells react to the same extent to section of their axons. Some cells survive and respond only by loss of the myelin sheath and reduction of the endoplasmic reticulum, whereas others undergo complete degeneration and disappear and again others are not affected at all. In the cochlea 90–95 per cent of the spiral ganglion cells will disappear within six months following the section of the cochlear nerve. The surviving ganglion cells are the type II cells which seem not to be affected by the retrograde degeneration after section of the cochlear nerve (Fig. 3.18(a)) and a small number of altered type I cells which have lost their myelin sheath and which are referred to as type III cells. However, most axons of the bipolar type III cells remain

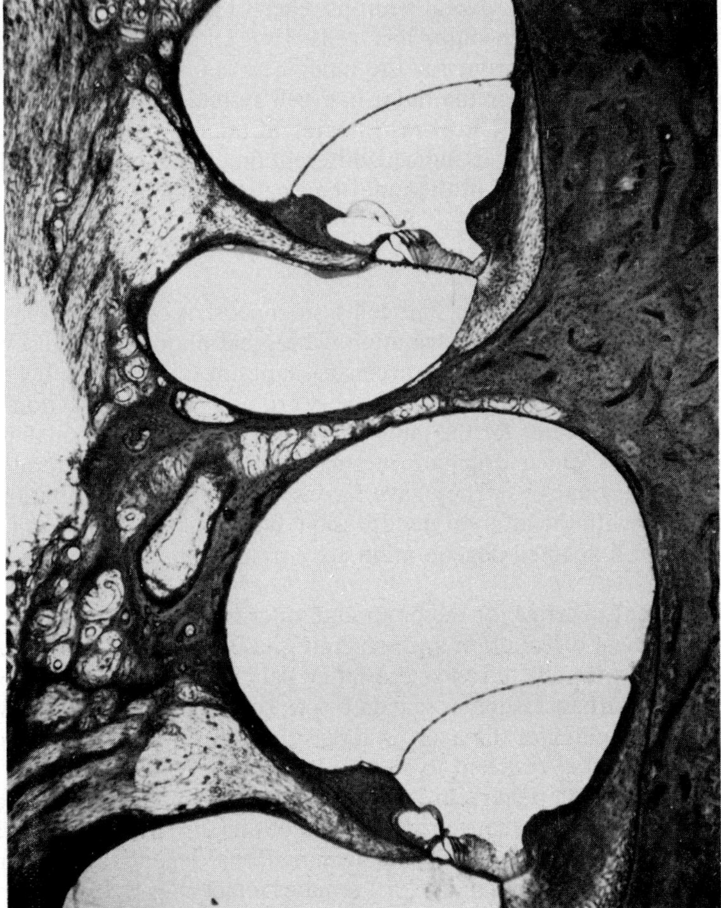

Fig. 3.15. Two cochlear turns of a cat one year after transection of the VIIIth nerve. The organ of Corti remains intact but there is a great loss of ganglion cells within the spiral ganglion where only a few cells remain.

myelinated (Fig. 3.16). With longer survival times these type III cells have a tendency to be more and more reduced in number, so that after two years only few remain beside a normal population of type II cells (Spoendlin and Suter 1976) (Fig. 3.19).

In the organ of Corti most inner radial fibres associated with the inner hair cells disappear at the same time at which the type I ganglion cells in the spiral ganglion degenerate. The afferent nerve supply of the outer hair cells consisting of the basilar and outer spiral fibres with their endings at the base of the outer hair cells on the other hand remains numerically and morphologically unchanged irrespective of the length of the survival time (Figs. 3.21 and 3.22). These surviving afferent neurons to the outer hair cells must therefore be related to the few surviving ganglion cells, particularly the type

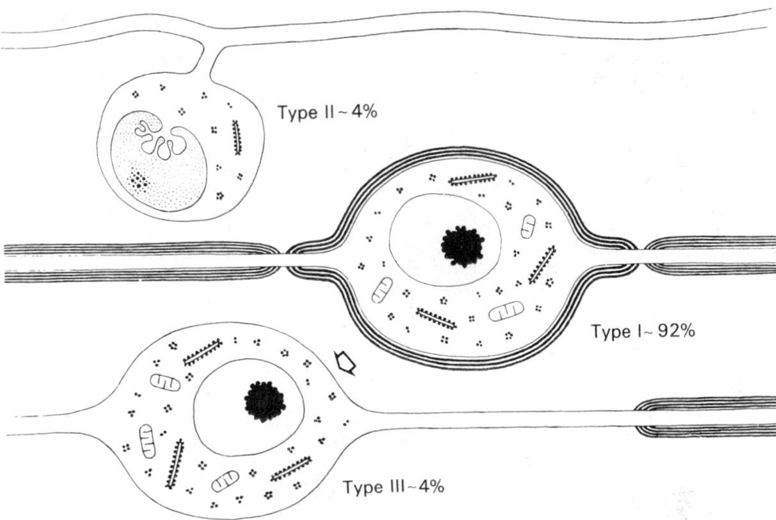

Fig. 3.16. Schematic representation of the different types of ganglion cells found in the spiral ganglion of the cat.

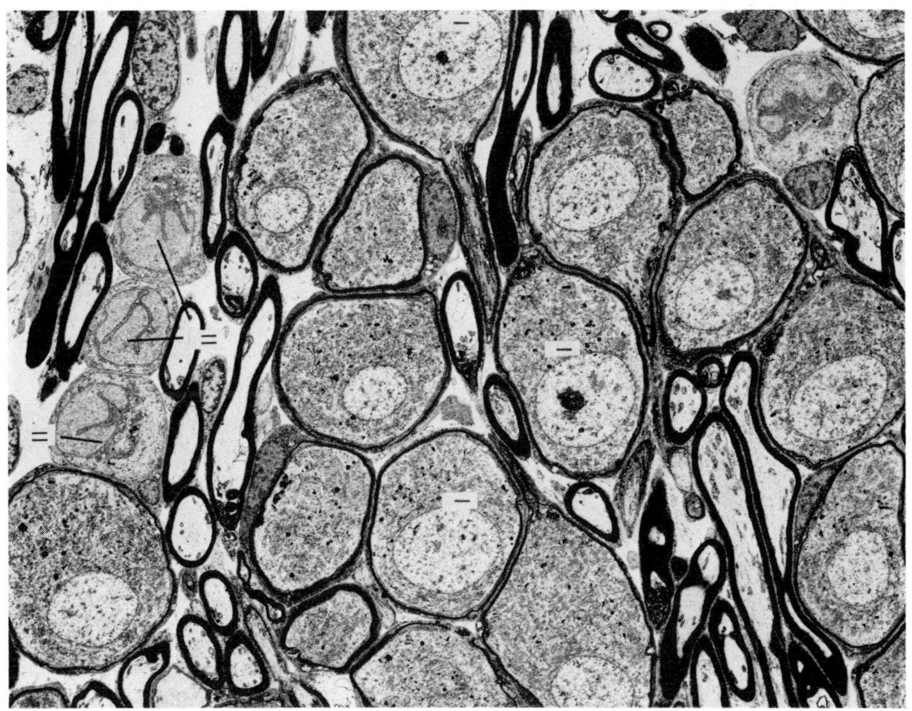

Fig. 3.17. Low magnification picture of a normal spiral ganglion of a cat with the majority of type I ganglion cells and a few type II ganglion cells.

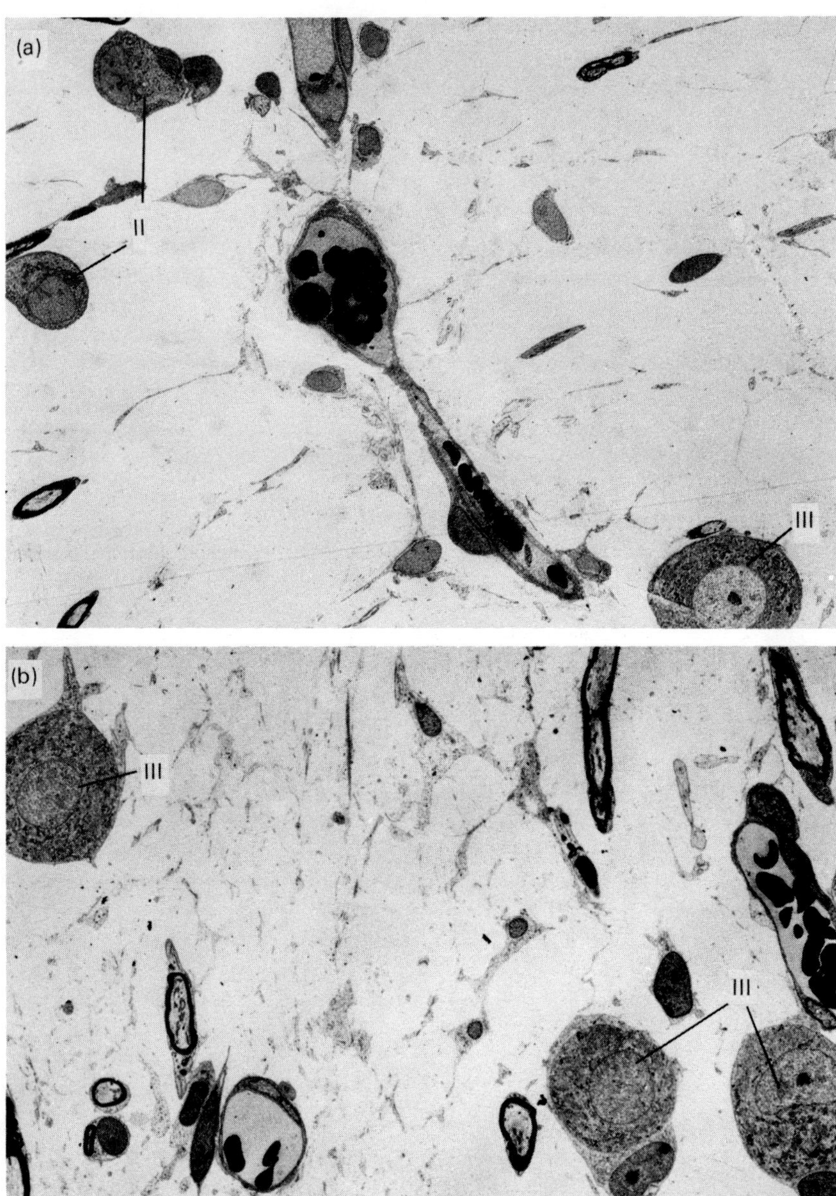

Fig. 3.18. Part of a spiral ganglion of a cat: (A) Eight months after transsection of the VIIIth nerve. The majority of the surviving ganglion cells are of type II and only a few are of type III. (B) One year after retrograde degeneration following destruction of the organ of Corti, most surviving ganglion cells are of type III.

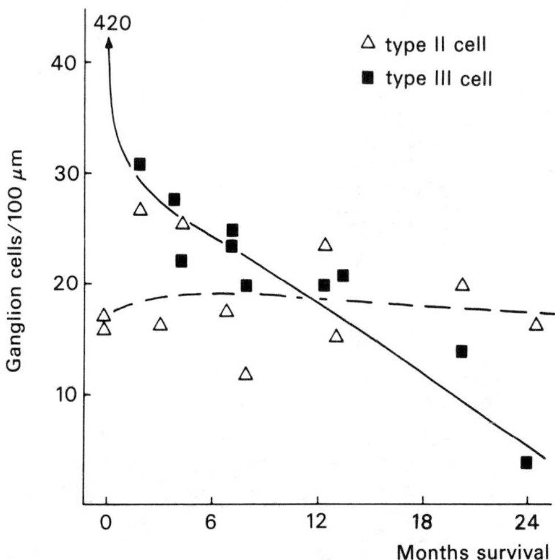

Fig. 3.19. Schematic representation of the degeneration time course of type II and type III ganglion cells in the spiral ganglion of the cat. The number of type II cells remains more or less constant with increasing surviving times, whereas the type III cells continue to be reduced with increasing survival time.

II cells whose numbers are not reduced with increasing survival times. (Fig. 3.20).

The area of the inner hair cells, however, is not completely deprived of all nerve fibres after section of the VIIIth nerve. A small number of unusually large fibres are found instead of the normal radial fibres (Spoendlin 1971). These giant fibres take their origin in the few surviving myelinated nerve fibres in the osseous spiral lamina (Fig. 3.25) and therefore probably belong to the surviving type III ganglion cells, which are the only remaining cells to have myelinated axons (Spoendlin and Suter 1976). The fibres penetrate the organ of Corti through every fifth to tenth habenular opening and divide into spirally expanding branches making synaptic contacts with several inner hair cells (Fig. 3.20). When the efferent nerve supply is preserved in cases with selective section of the cochlear nerve there are synaptic contacts between inner spiral efferent fibres and these giant fibres.

Three to eight months after section of the cochlear or VIIIth nerve few of these giant fibres remain, but with the longer survival times, their number increases to become surprisingly large. Two years after the lesion the area between the habenula and the inner hair cells is usually completely filled with spirally running nerve fibres of varying calibres in spite of the fact that only very few ganglion cells and myelinated nerve fibres are left in the spiral ganglion and the osseous spiral lamina (Fig. 3.23) (Spoendlin and Suter

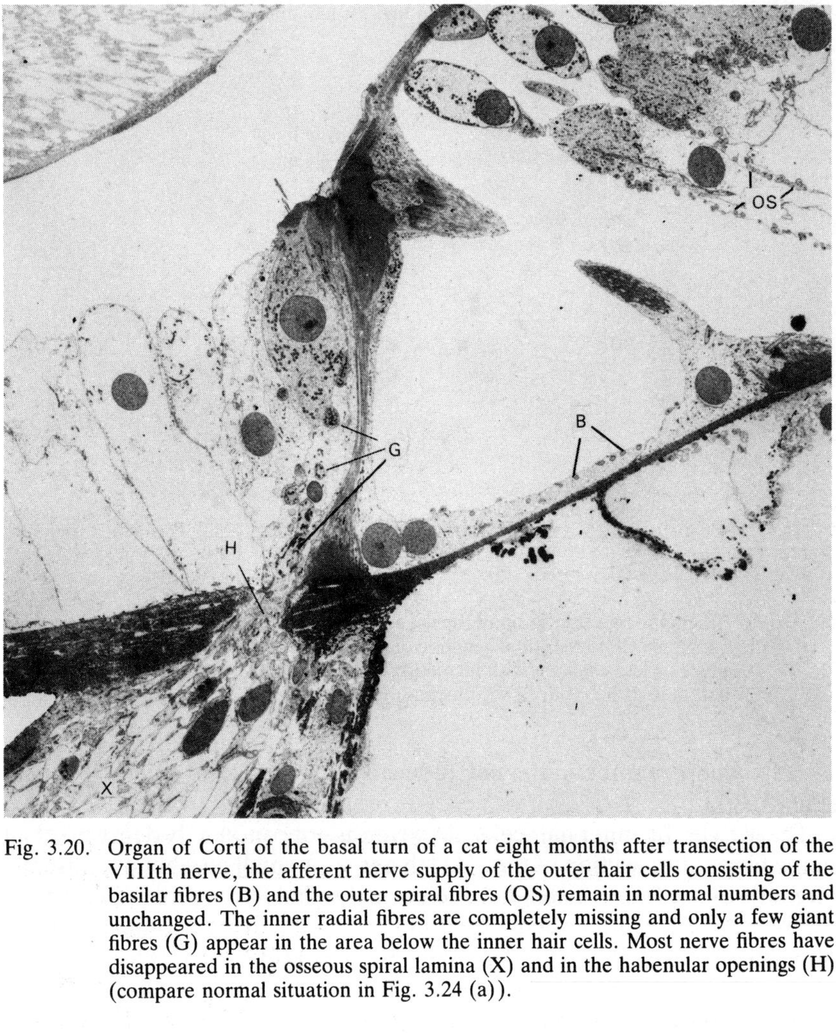

Fig. 3.20. Organ of Corti of the basal turn of a cat eight months after transection of the VIIIth nerve, the afferent nerve supply of the outer hair cells consisting of the basilar fibres (B) and the outer spiral fibres (OS) remain in normal numbers and unchanged. The inner radial fibres are completely missing and only a few giant fibres (G) appear in the area below the inner hair cells. Most nerve fibres have disappeared in the osseous spiral lamina (X) and in the habenular openings (H) (compare normal situation in Fig. 3.24 (a)).

1976). It must be assumed that the few remaining neurons left after degeneration of the cochlear nerve undergo enormous ramification and proliferation to produce these neuroma-like agglomerations of spiral fibres in the area of the inner hair cells along the entire cochlea (Fig. 3.25).

A similar retrograde degeneration occurs after damage to the peripheral axons of the cochlear neurons by destruction of the organ of Corti. This type of retrograde generation has been known for a long time, but there have been discussions on what type of alterations in the organ of Corti produce it (Bredberg 1968; Schuknecht 1953). Selective loss of outer hair cells has little effect on the cochlear neurons whereas loss of inner hair cells, even when the supporting structures of the organ of Corti of the outer hair cells remain, is followed by massive retrograde degeneration of the cochlear neurons

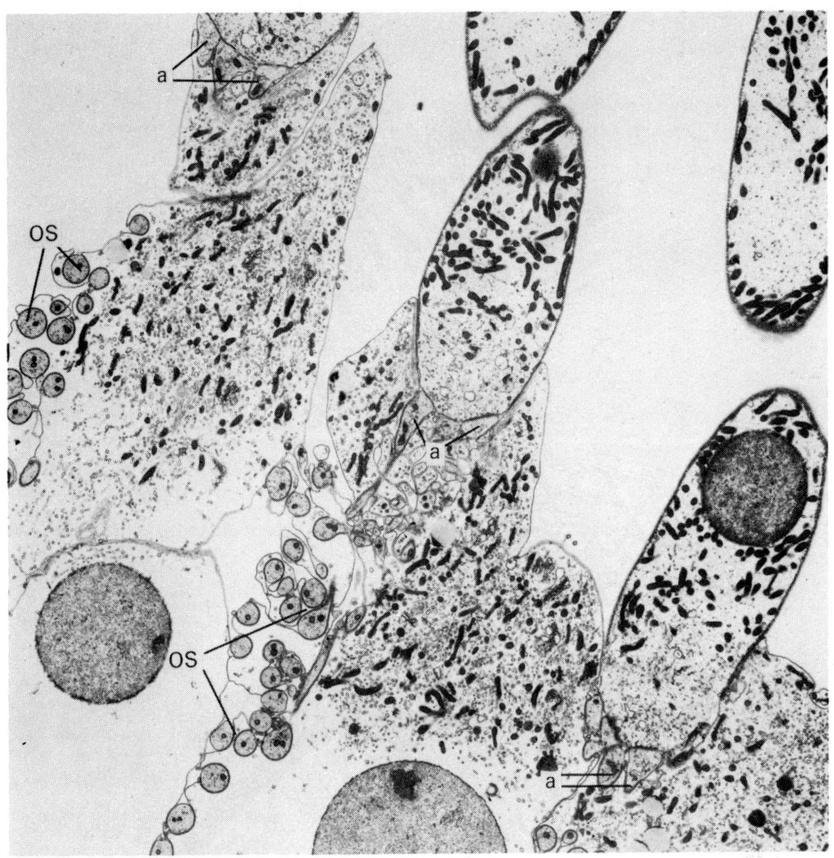

Fig. 3.21. Area of the base of some outer hair cells in a cat several months after transection of the VIIIth nerve showing the afferent nerve terminals with normal appearance and normal numbers (a) and a normal population of outer spiral fibres (OS).

(Spoendlin 1975). Although there is in general a good correlation between the number of destroyed inner hair cells and the degree of retrograde degeneration (Johnsson 1974), we have observed degeneration in areas with inner hair cells present or no degeneration in areas with extensive loss of inner hair cells (Figs. 3.26 and 3.27). The crucial factor for the initiation of retrograde degeneration is most probably the irreversible direct damage of the peripheral unmyelinated segments of the cochlear neurons associated with the inner hair cells, a situation which occurs generally, but not necessarily, in conjunction with inner hair cell destruction.

After complete destruction of the organ of Corti (by acoustic overstimulation, intoxication with ototoxic antibiotics, or direct mechanical damage) retrograde degeneration never affects all neurons (Fig. 3.28). About 10 per cent are always spared provided the cochlear blood supply is not impaired.

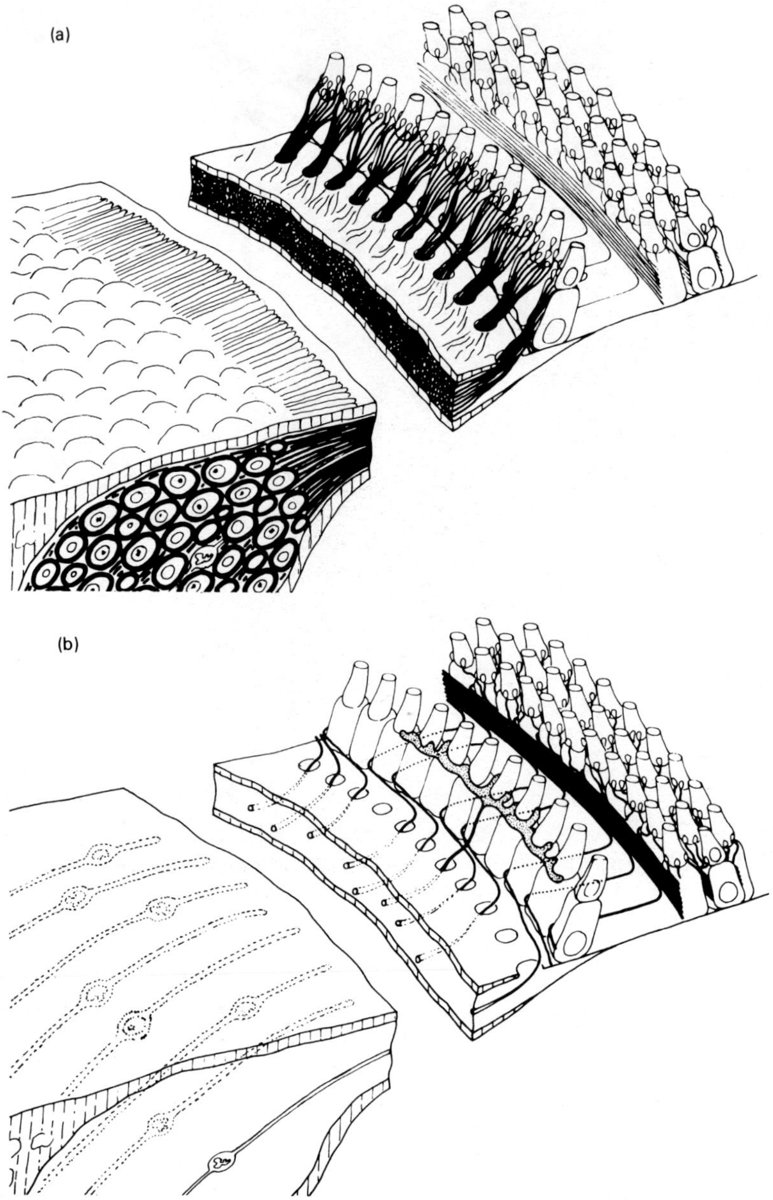

(a)

(b)

Fig. 3.22. Schematic representation of the innervation of the organ of Corti and the spiral ganglion: (A) Normal situation where the great majority of all neurons leads to the inner hair cells. (B) Several months after transection of the VIIIth nerve. The afferent nerve fibres for the outer hair cells as well as the type II ganglion cells in spiral ganglion remain unaffected in normal numbers, whereas the inner radial afferent nerve fibres for the inner hair cells have completely disappeared and only a few giant fibres which normally do not exist appear in this situation.

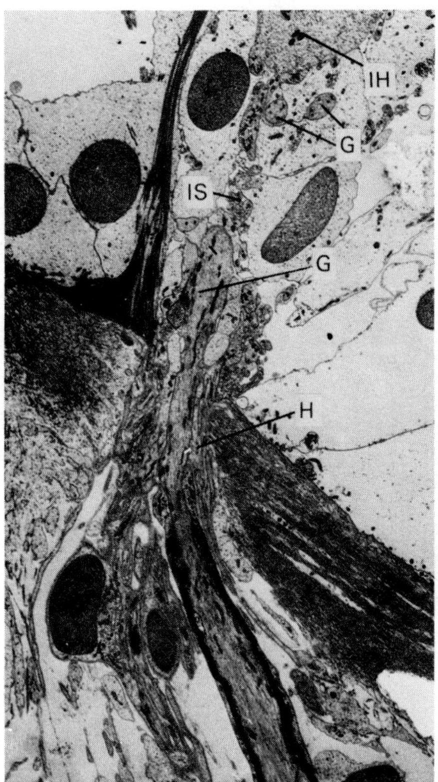

Fig. 3.23. Area of the habenula in a cat where the cochlear nerve has been transected eight months previously. The efferent inner spiral fibres (IS) are still present, whereas the normal afferent inner radial fibres are lacking and are replaced by a few giant fibres (G) which originate in the few remaining myelinated nerve fibres in the osseous spiral lamina. Habenula opening (H), inner hair cell (IH).

A higher percentage, up to 97 per cent, however, degenerates when the axons in the osseous spiral lamina are damaged closer to the spiral ganglion. The degree of retrograde degeneration seems to be related to the distance of the axon damage from the ganglion cell bodies. The closer to the cell bodies the damage occurs the more completely the neurons degenerate. Degeneration is always more pronounced in the basal turn and a greater percentage of neurons survive in the apical turns (Fig. 3.29). The process of retrograde degeneration after destruction of the organ of Corti is very slow and proceeds over several months. Most cells loose their myelin sheath, the cytoplasmic organelles are reduced, and the nuclei frequently take an irregular shape so that sometimes these cells are difficult to distinguish from type II ganglion cells. After survival times of a year or more the remaining cells, at least in the cat, are usually of type III (Fig. 3.26) and ganglion cells with all the criteria of type II cells are extremely rare, unlike the situation

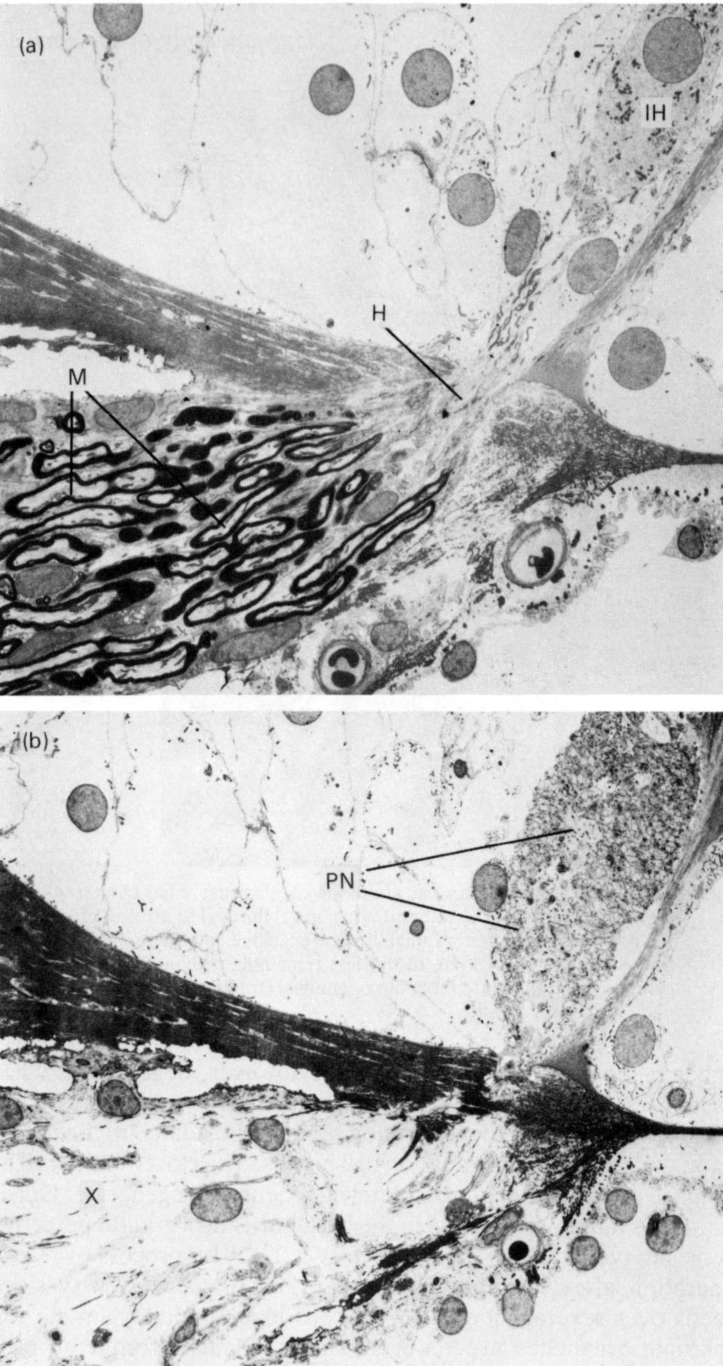

Fig. 3.24. Area of the osseous spiral lamina habenula and inner hair cells in the basal turn of cat: (A) Normal situation with many myelinated nerve fibres in the osseous spiral lamina (M), which lose their myelin sheaths before they penetrate through the habenular opening (H) and lead directly to the nearest inner hair cell (IH). (B) Same area as in (A), two years after transection of the VIIIth nerve. Most nerve fibres have disappeared from the osseous spiral lamina (X). In the area of the inner hair cell, there is a great number of unmyelinated radial nerve fibres (pN) which represent an enormous proliferation of axons in this area.

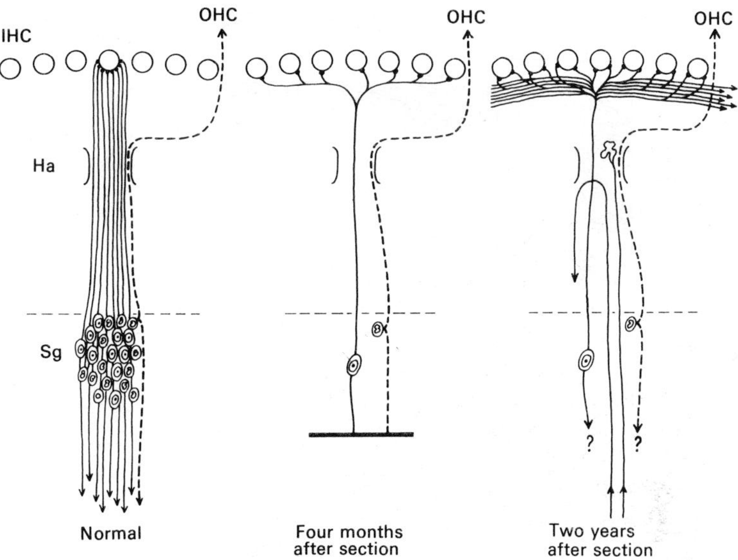

Fig. 3.25. Schematic representation of the nerve fibres in the normal cat (left), four months after section of the VIIIth nerve (centre), and two years after section of the VIIIth nerve (right).

after transection of the cochlear nerve where normal type II cells are found in the usual numbers (Fig. 3.26). The reason for this peculiar difference of retrograde degeneration after section of the cochlear nerve and after destruction of the organ of Corti is not yet clarified. It could possibly suggest that the type II neurons send their axons only to the organ of Corti and are not connected to the central nervous system, so that lesions of the cochlear nerve in the internal acoustic meatus would not reach and affect them at all in contrast to the destruction of the organ of Corti which would affect them extensively being intimately connected to the outer hair cells. The fact that we find practically no unmyelinated nerve fibres in the cochlear nerve trunk could support this view, since the axons of type II cells are essentially unmyelinated. It also could explain why it has so far proved impossible to find two distinct populations of neurons by single nerve recordings in the cochlear nerve trunk (Kiang 1965). On the other hand it would not be clear at all how the outer hair cell system which is associated to the type II neurons could participate in the cochlear function, when there is practically no morphological evidence for synaptic contacts to the majority of cochlear neurons of type I. Thus the question of the central connections of the type II neurons still remains open.

According to the innervation pattern the outer hair cell system can work on the basis of spatial summation not possible for the inner hair cell system, which, however, is quantitatively much more important and much better suited for tono-topical frequency perception and a greater dynamic range.

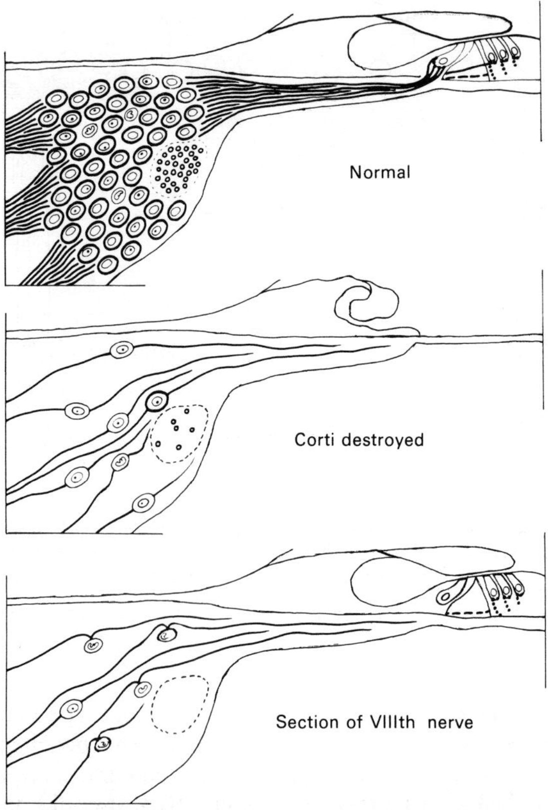

Fig. 3.26. Schematic representation of the degeneration pattern after destruction of the organ of Corti and after section of the VIIIth nerve as compared to the normal neuron population in the spiral ganglion and the organ of Corti.

Accordingly one would assume that the outer hair cell system has a higher sensitivity but a small dynamic range which would be in agreement with some electrocochleographic findings.

Other concepts of the outer hair cell system have been brought forward such as a monitoring action on the inner hair cell system (Lynn and Sayers 1970). This however would presume a functional interaction between the fibres of the outer and inner hair cells which again has been a domain of many postulates and speculations (Evans 1974; Zwislocki and Sokolich 1974) but for which unfortunately so far there is no clear structural evidence nor direct functional evidence (Rohman and Boerger 1977) to be found. The only place where the fibres are close enough for a possible functional interaction is in the habenular area, where they are surrounded by a common satellite cell. Whether such a satellite cell could mediate functional interaction between the different nerve fibres remains an open question.

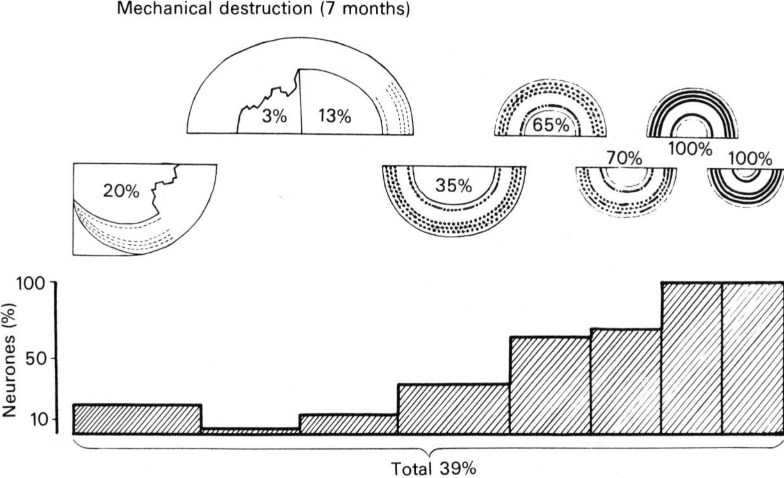

Fig. 3.27. Schematic representation of the retrograde degeneration in a cat cochlea seven months after mechanical destruction of a part of the basal turn. The percentages in the cochleogram give the amount of surviving neurons in the spiral ganglion and the osseous spiral lamina.

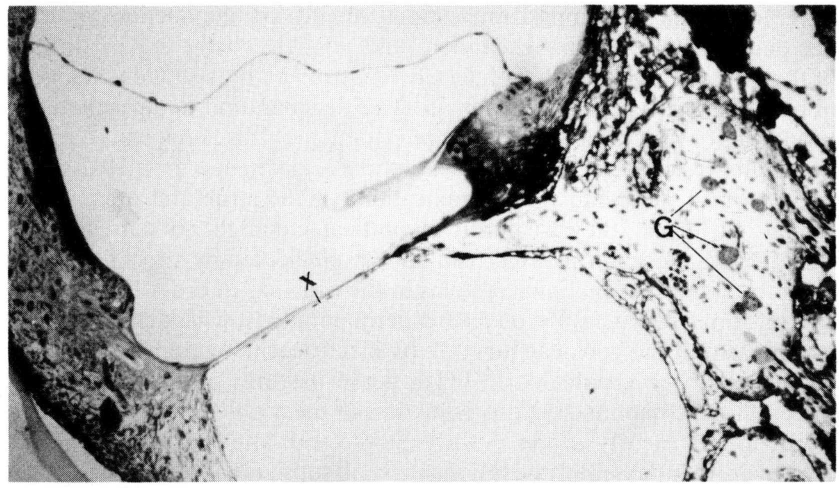

Fig. 3.28. Histological section through the basal cochlea turn of a guinea pig one year after destruction of the organ of Corti by acoustic trauma. The organ of Corti has completely disappeared (X) and only a few ganglion cells (G) remain in the spiral ganglion.

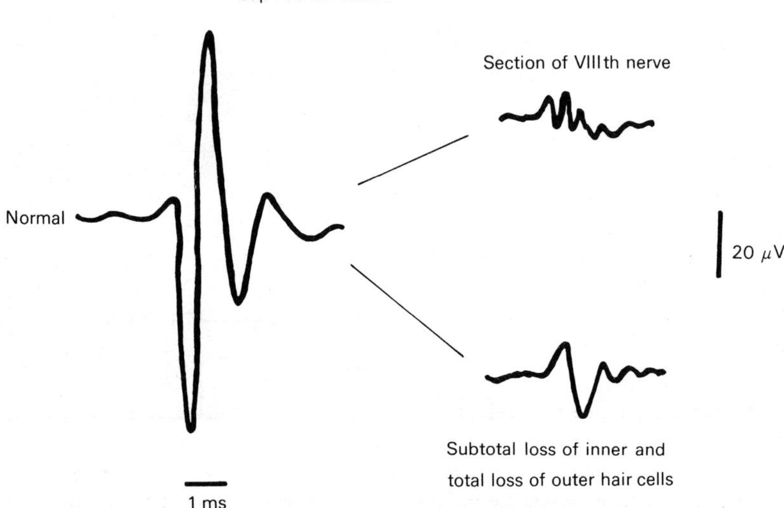

Fig. 3.29. Compound action potentials recorded from the round window of the normal cat after section of the VIIIth nerve and after heavy damage to the organ of Corti.

There is no structural evidence for synaptic contacts between satellite cell and the fibres, so that the functional interaction, if it occurs at all, could only occur as an electrical field effect. Also the diameters of the nerve fibres might have important functional implications mainly on conduction velocity, decrement of electrotonic excitation, and possibly on the spike initiation at the initial segments, which might be determined by a sudden change of fibre diameter, e.g. at the habenula. The degeneration and regeneration properties of the cochlear neurons are evidently of basic importance for the possibility of successful electric stimulation of deaf ears.

Even if all these functional implications of the structural organization seem to be logical, they are purely theoretical and might not correspond to the effective mechanisms which can only be elucidated by direct recordings from the different functional systems in the cochlea. In order to get objective information we have produced experimentally typical damage patterns and measured the cochlear function by electrocochleography.

Section of the cochlear or VIIIth nerve has only a minor immediate effect on the compound actions potentials of the cochlear nerve by the loss of the usually clearly visible P_1 waves in the high-intensity stimulus range. However, four days after the lesion and in all subsequent recordings normal action potentials have completely disappeared, whereas cochlear microphonics where unchanged, showing that the cochlear blood supply was not impaired. Instead of normal action potentials very strange stimulus-related electrical responses were recorded in all these animals. Latencies were very short and did not change very much with stimulus intensities. They had maximum amplitudes between 10 and 20 μV and they were usually maintained over several milliseconds (Spoendlin and Baumgartner 1977) (Fig. 3.29).

This functional status must be correlated to the anatomical situation after section of the VIIIth nerve with nearly complete loss of afferent neurons associated to the inner hair cells but an intact afferent nerve supply of the outer hair cells and mainly the 5 per cent type II neurons left in the spiral ganglion. If the small unusual potentials prove not to be artefacts they are most likely related to the afferent nerve supply of the outer hair cells. We must assume that the numerous nerve fibres in the organ of Corti, which represent the afferent nerve supply to the outer hair cells, produce some electrical activity upon stimulation. The complex and changing form of these recorded responses probably expresses highy dissociated and poorly synchronized activity, and the short latencies indicate a very peripheral origin (peripheral to the initial segment of the neurons).

An entirely different picture results if secondary nerve degeneration is the consequence of the destruction of the organ of Corti by locally applied ototoxic antibiotics or direct mechanical damage. A single dose of 500 mg Neomycin injected into the bulla of a cat leads to complete loss of inner and outer hair cells except for a few remaining abnormal inner hair cells. After one year 80–90 per cent of the cochlear neurons have degenerated and disappeared. Most of the surviving neurons are of the type III and a corresponding number of myelinated nerve fibres is found in the osseous spiral lamina. In contrast to the degeneration following transection of the VIIIth nerve the afferent nerve supply of the outer hair cell disappears or is severely impaired.

In the electrocochleographic recordings the cochlear microphonics are entirely missing but weak yet typical compound action potentials can still be recorded (Fig. 3.29) in spite of the total loss of outer hair cells and subtotal loss of inner hair cells. Circumscribed mechanical destruction of the organ of Corti in the basal turn usually produces an almost complete loss of outer hair cells throughout the cochlea with a relatively good preservation of the inner hair cells. The functional consequence is a complete lack of cochlear-microphonic which illustrates that the outer hair cells are the main source of the cochlear-microphonic and that they do not reflect activity of the inner hair cell. On the other hand still relatively strong and typical compound cochlear action potentials (CAP) can be recorded. The reduction of the CAP is proportional to the reduction of myelinated cochlear nerve fibres (type I and III neurons) which frequently does not correspond to the loss of hair cells.

There is a principal difference between secondary nerve degeneration following sectioning of the VIIIth nerve and following damage to the organ of Corti. After section of the VIIIth nerve only an extremely few myelinated nerve fibres but an intact afferent nerve supply to the outer hair cells remains and no normal CAPs can be recorded, whereas after destruction of the organ of Corti a greater number of myelinated nerve fibres remains but the afferent nerve supply of the outer hair cells has disappeared or is highly impaired and some typical CAPs can still be recorded proportional to the remaining nerve fibres (Fig. 3.29).

REFERENCES

ANDRES, K. H. (1961). Untersuchungen über morphologische Veränderungen in Spinalganglien während der retrograden Degeneration. *Zellforsch. mikrosk. Anat.* **55,** 49–79.

BREDBERG, G. (1968). Cellular pattern and nerve supply of the human organ of Corti. *Acta oto-lar.* Suppl. **236,** 1.

DENSERT, O. (1974). Adrenergic innervation in the rabbit cochlea. *Acta oto-lar.* **78,** 1.

DUNN, R. A. and MOREST, D. K. (1975). Receptor synapses without synaptic ribbons in the cochlea of the cat. *Proc. nat. Acad. Sci. USA* **72,** 3599–603.

EVANS, E. F. (1974). Auditory frequency selectivity and the cochlear nerve. In *Facts and models in hearing* (ed. E. Zwicker and E. Terrhardt), pp. 118–29. Springer Verlag, Berlin.

FALK, B., HILLARP, N. A., THIEME, G. and TORP, A. (1962). Fluorescence of catecholamines and related compounds condensed with formaldehyde. *J. Histochem. Cytochem.* **10,** 348.

HALL, J. G. (1966). Hearing and primary auditory centres of the whales. *Acta oto-lar.* Suppl. **224,** 244–50.

—— (1974). An electron microscopical analysis of the square areas and diameters of the cochlear nerve fibres in the cat. *Acta oto-lar.* **77,** 305–10.

JOHNSSON, L. G. (1974). Sequence of degeneration of Corti's organ and its first-order neurons. *Ann. Otol. Rhinol. Lar.* **83,** 294–303.

KIANG, N. Y. S. (1965). *Discharge patterns of single fibres in the cat's auditory nerve,* Research Monograph No. 35, pp. 84–92. MIT Press, Cambridge, Mass.

LORENTE DE NO (1933). Anatomy of the VIIIth nerve. *Laryngoscope, St. Louis* **43,** 1–38.

—— (1937). Symposium: neural mechanisms of hearing, sensory endings in the cochlea. *Laryngoscope, St. Louis.* **47,** 373–7.

—— (1976). Some unresolved problems concerning the cochlear nerve. *Ann. Otol. Rhinol. Lar.* Suppl. **34,** 85.

LYNN, P. A. and SAYERS, B. MC. A. (1970). Cochlear innervation signal processing and their relation to auditory time intensity effects. *J. acoust. Soc. Am.* **47,** 525–32.

MORRISON, D., SCHINDLER, R. A., and WERSÄLL, J. (1975). A quantitative analysis of the afferent innervation of the organ of Corti in guinea pigs. *Acta oto-lar.* **79,** 11–23.

NOMURA, Y. (1976). Nerve fibres in the human organ of Corti. *Acta oto-lar.* **82,** 157–64.

PARADISGARTEN, A. and SPOENDLIN, H. (1976). The unmyelinated nerve fibres of the cochlea. *Acta oto-lar.* **82,** 157–64.

RANSON, S. W. (1905). Retrograde degeneration in the spinal nerve. *J. comp. Neurol.* **16,** 1.

RASMUSSEN, G. L. (1942). An efferent cochlear bundle. *Anat. Rec.* **82,** 440.

RODRIGUEZ, E. E. L. (1967). An electron microscopic study on the cochlear innervation I. The recepto-neural junctions at the outer hair cells. *Z. Zellforsch. Mikrosk. Anat.* **78,** 30–46.

ROHMANN, G. and BOERGER, G. (1977). Filter function of the guinea pig cochlea after degeneration of outer hair cells. *Archs. Oto-rhin.-lar.* **215,** 223–9.

SANDO, I. (1964). The anatomical interrelationship of the cochlear nerve fibres. *Acta oto-lar.* **59,** 417–36.

SCHUKNECHT, H. F. (1953). Lesions of the organ of Corti. *Trans. Am. Acad. Opthal. Oto-lar.* **57,** 366.

—— (1962). Neuroanatomical correlates of auditory sensitivity and pitch discrimination in the cat. In *Neural mechanisms of the auditory and vestibular systems.* Rasmussen and Windle, Springfield, Illinois.

—— IGARASHI, M., and GACEK, R. R. (1965). The pathological types of cochleosaccular degeneration. *Acta oto-lar.* **59,** 154.

SMITH, C. A. (1975). Innervation of the cochlea of the guinea pig by use of the Golgi stain. *Ann. Otol. Rhinol. Lar.* **84,** 443

—— and HAGLAN, B. J. (1973). Golgi stains on the guinea pig organ of Corti. *Acta oto-lar.* **75,** 203–10.

—— and SHÖSTRAND, F. (1961). A synaptic structure in the hair cells of the guinea pig cochlea. *J. Ultrastruct. Res.* **5,** 184–92.

SPOENDLIN, H. H. (1966). *The organization of the cochlear receptor.* Karger, Basel.

—— (1968). Ultrastructure and peripheral innervation pattern of the receptor in relation to the first coding of the acoustic message. In *Hearing mechanisms in vertebrates* (ed. A. V. S. deReuck and J. Knight) pp. 89–119. Churchill, London.

—— (1969). Innervation pattern in the organ of Corti of the cat. *Acta oto-lar.* **67,** 239–54.

—— (1970). Structural basis of peripheral frequency analysis. In *Frequency analysis and periodicity detection in hearing.* (ed. R. Plomp and F. G. Smoorenburg) pp. 2–36. Sijthoff, Leiden, The Netherlands.

—— (1971). Degeneration behaviour of the cochlear nerve. *Arch. klin. exp. Ohr. Nas. Kehlk. Heilk.* **200,** 275–91.

—— (1972a). Innervation densities of the cochlea. *Acta oto-lar.* **73,** 235–48.

—— (1972b). Autonomic nerve supply to the inner ear. *Proceedings of vascular disorders and hearing defects workshop.* John Hopkins University.

—— (1973). The innervation of the cochlear receptor. In *Basic mechanisms in hearing* (ed. A. R. Møller) pp. 185–234. Academic Press, New York.

—— (1974). Neuroanatomy of the cochlea. In *Facts and models in hearing* (ed. E. Zwicker and E. Terhardt) pp. 18–32. Springer Verlag, Berlin.

—— (1975a). Neuroanatomical basis of cochlear coding mechanisms. *Audiology* **14,** 383–407.

—— (1975b). Retrograde degeneration of the cochlear nerve. *Acta oto-lar.* **79,** 266–75.

—— and BAUMGARTNER, H. (1977). Electrocochleography and cochlear pathology. *Acta oto-lar.* **83,** 130–5.

—— and BRUN, J. P. (1974). The block-surface technique for evaluation of cochlear pathology. *Archs. Otolar.* **208,** 137–45.

—— and LICHTENSTEIGER, W. (1965). Die adrenergene Innervation des Labyrinthes. *Pract. Oto-rhino-lar.* **27,** 371–2.

—— and —— (1976). The sympathetic nerve supply to the inner ear. *Arch. klin. exp. Ohr. Nas. Kehlk. Heilk.* **189,** 346–59.

—— and SUTER, R. (1976). Regeneration in the VIIIth nerve. *Acta oto-lar.* **81,** 228–36.

TERAYAMA, Y., HOLZ, E., and BECK, CH. (1966). Adrenergic innervation of the cochlea. *Ann. Otol. Rhinol. Lar.* **75,** 1–18.

WARR, B. (1978). The olivocochlear bundle: its origins and terminations in the cat.

In *Evoked electrical activity in the auditory nervous system* (ed. R. F. Naunton and C. Fernández) Academic Press, New York.

ZWISLOCKI, J. J. and SOKOLICH, W. G. (1974). Neuro-mechanical frequency analysis in the cochlea. In *Facts and Models in Hearing* (ed. E. Zwicker and E. Terhardt) pp. 107–17. Springer Verlag, Berlin.

4 Physiology of the ear

A. R. D. THORNTON

INTRODUCTION

Hearing is the perception and recognition of sound waves received by the ear. Sound waves are longitudinal pressure waves transmitted through a medium. They are generally received by the hearing system as an airborne signal and, less commonly, by contact with vibrating structures (bone conduction). This chapter will deal with the more common air conduction signals and the stages that they pass through to produce auditory perception within the peripheral auditory mechanism.

The peripheral system, like Caesar's Gaul, is divided into three parts. These are represented in the block diagram shown in Fig. 4.1. The outer ear

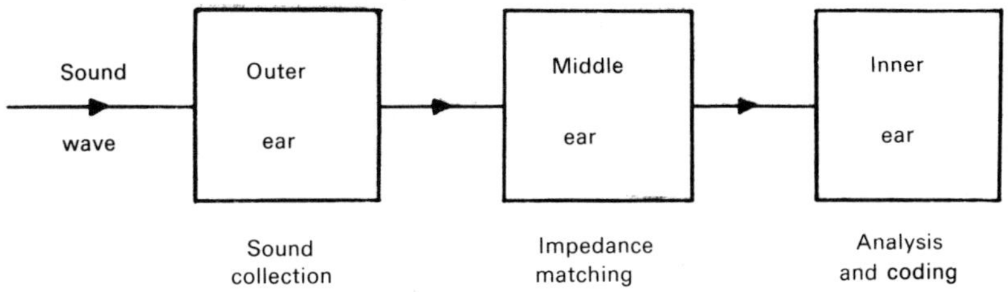

Fig. 4.1. Block diagram outlining the functions of the three parts of the peripheral hearing system.

collects the sound, passing it down the acoustic meatus to the tympanum. The vibrations of the tympanum are transmitted mechanically through the middle ear which provides an impedance match for the fluid of the cochlea or inner ear. The middle ear also contains muscles that are activated as part of a feedback system within the auditory pathway. The cochlea or inner ear is filled with fluid and the vibrations from the middle ear are passed into this fluid. Here the vibrations deform the membraneous portions of the inner ear and this mechanical deformation is transformed, by the sensory cells, into electrical and chemical events which initiate nerve impulses in the auditory nerve.

The anatomy and innervation of these structures has been dealt with elsewhere in this book. This chapter will summarize the biophysics and physiology of each of the three parts of the peripheral system. For more detailed information, the reader is referred to von Békésy's original treatise, *Experiments in hearing* (1960); Littler's book, *The physics of the ear* (1965); and, of more recent origin, a detailed account of the peripheral auditory system by Dallos, *The Auditory Periphery* (1973) and Section VI of *Scientific foundations of otolaryngology*, edited by Hinchcliffe and Harrison (1976).

THE OUTER EAR

The outer ear comprises the auricle or pinna and the external acoustic meatus. In some animals, the auricle is large and moveable and aids sounds localization. In Man, only weak vestigial musculature to the auricle is present and the whole structure adds only a little to man's ability to localize sounds. The defraction of sound waves around the head and the auricle does slightly increase the pressure at the entrance of the ear canal. However, the complex structure of the auricle means that the pressure changes vary markedly with the direction of the sound source.

The external acoustic meatus is oval in cross-section and forms a slight S shape as it proceeds medially towards the tympanum. The lateral third of the meatus is cartilaginous and, in this region, there are sebaceous and ceruminous glands, which secrete wax, and small hairs. The shape of the meatus, the hairs, and the wax all combine to protect against the entry of foreign bodies and to form a safe, thermally stable environment for the more delicate structures of the middle and inner ears.

The structure of the outer ear modifies the sound field that it receives. Various estimates of its resonant frequency have been made and these range from about 3000 to 4000 Hz. The resonant peak can produce an amplification of up to 20 dB but, because of the complex, asymmetrical structures involved, the gain varies a great deal with frequency and with direction of the sound.

THE MIDDLE EAR

The middle ear is an air filled cavity within the temporal bone of the skull. It extends from the tympanum medially to the bony cochlear wall. The oval and round windows provide the two openings, through this bony wall, by which the middle ear communicates with the cochlea. Above, the attic is connected with the mastoid air cells by the tympanic antrum which increases the effective volume of the middle ear. The inferior tympanic cavity communicates with the nasopharynx by means of the auditory (Eustachian) tube. The entire cavity is covered with a smooth mucous membrane lining.

The tympanum is a cone-shaped structure comprised of three layers. The outermost layer is continuous with the lining of the ear canal and the innermost layer is continuous with the lining of the middle ear. It is the central fibrous layer, comprised of radially and concentrically oriented fibres, which provides structural stability for the tympanum. The three ossicles, the malleus, incus, and stapes, connect the tympanum to the round window cavity. A simplified, diagrammatic representation of the middle ear structures is shown in Fig. 4.2.

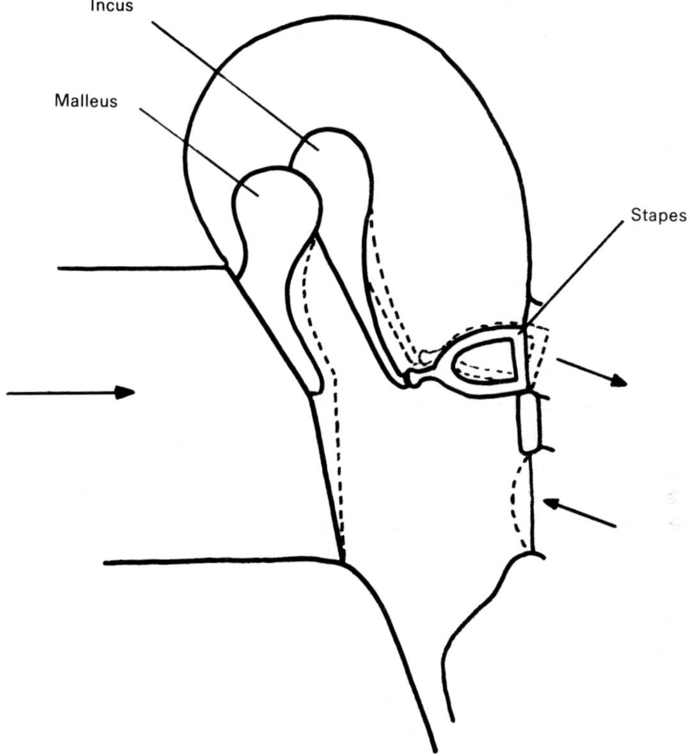

Fig. 4.2. Diagrammatic representation of the response of the middle ear to a positive pressure wave. The dashed lines represent the position to which the tympanum, ossicles, and round window move.

In the transmission of sound waves, one of the most important properties of the medium, in which the sound wave is travelling, is its impedance. In relation to the cochlear fluids, air has a relatively low impedance. A sound wave, passing from a low impedance medium to a high impedance medium, would have much of its energy reflected from the junction between the two media. To avoid this loss in sound transmission, the middle ear system provides a match between the impedance of air and the impedance of the cochlear fluids. The way in which this impedance match is achieved will be considered in greater detail later.

The auditory tube is not normally patent and is opened by swallowing or by Valsalva's manoeuvre. It provides drainage for the middle-ear space and, more importantly, equalizes the air pressure on each side of the tympanic membrane. The mucosal lining of the middle ear space absorbs air and this, together with atmospheric pressure changes, is why an intermittent air exchange through the auditory tube is required.

The reduction of volume flow, required to match the air–cochlear fluids impedance difference, may be achieved by the ossicles acting as a system of levers to reduce the motion of the tympanic membrane and by the reduction in surface areas of the tympanic membrane and the oval window. The movement of the ossicular chain, in response to a positive pressure increase, is illustrated in Fig. 4.2. The ossicular chain is suspended from various ligaments so that it can rotate about an axis formed by the short process of the incus and the anterior process of the malleus. Thus, as the tympanic membrane moves inwards the attached manubrium causes a rotary motion of the head of the malleus. This rotary motion is passed on to the incus which engages with the malleus to form a relatively rigid joint. This produces a lever action on the long process of the incus which is reduced in displacement owing to the shorter length of the long process of the incus compared to the length of the manubrium. Finally, this lever action is coupled to the head of the stapes and is transmitted to the stapes footplate and to the cochlear fluid via the oval window. The stapes footplate is held in place by an annular ligament which attaches it more firmly at its lower periphery than elsewhere. Thus the stapes does not move like a piston but, as shown in Fig. 4.2, has a rocking action reducing still further the effective displacement. However, measurements of ossicular action have shown that this lever ratio reduction is very small, reducing the displacement at the tympanic membrane by a factor of about 1.3 or possibly even less than 1 (Tonndorf and Khanna 1976).

The major component, that provides the impedance match, is the reduction in area between the tympanic membrane and the oval window. However, with the complex movement of both the tympanic membrane and the stapes footplate, the areas which are effective in obtaining the impedance match are difficult to assess. Békésy (1960) considered that the tympanic membrane vibrated as a stiff plate which rotated about the axis of ossicular rotation formed by the short process of the incus and the anterior process of the malleus. If the tympanic membrane vibrated in this way, not all of its area would contribute to ossicular displacement and the concept of an 'effective area ratio' originated. This was estimated as approximately two-thirds of the total area ratio between the tympanum and the stapes footplate. More recently, holographic studies have shown that the vibration of the tympanic membrane is not of this form. At low frequencies, the vibration pattern is uniform but above approximately 3 kHz the vibration pattern increases in complexity and different modes are introduced (Tonndorf and Khanna 1976). Again, at frequencies above 3 kHz, the displacement of the malleus becomes smaller relative to that of the tympanic membrane and, above 4 kHz, only the manubrium of the malleus and the area immediately around it forms the effective part of the transmission system. Thus, at frequencies below 3 kHz, the whole area of the tympanic membrane should be taken into account when calculating the area ratio. For Man, based on the data given by Littler (1965), this area ratio has a value of approximately 21 or 26 dB. This, combined with the ossicular lever ratio, gives a total transformer ratio of about 28 dB. This figure is comparable to the loss, found in human ears, after fenestration operations in which the middle-ear transformer action no longer occurs.

Békésy (1960) carried out a quantitative assessment of the middle-ear transformer ratio in Man using cadaver ear material. A sound wave was applied to the ear canal and, through an opening in the vestibule, a second sound wave was applied to the stapes footplate. The amplitudes and phases of these two waves were adjusted until the ossicles no longer moved, then the pressure ratio was measured. The results of this experiment gave values for the middle ear transformer ratio of about 20 dB at low frequencies rising to a maximum of 26 dB between 2 and 3 kHz and then falling fairly steeply. Calculations of the acoustic power transferred by the middle ear have shown good agreement with the normal threshold curve. This implies that the middle ear is largely responsible for the shape of this threshold curve rather than any properties of the cochlea itself.

Another function of the middle ear is to provide protection for the delicate structures of the cochlea. Various mechanisms exist to provide this protection which is most effective at low frequencies. Firstly, the middle-ear muscles provide some protection. The tendon of the tensor tympani muscle attaches to the manubrium of the malleus and the tendon of the stapedius muscle connects to the neck of the stapes. These are striated, pennate muscles which can produce high tension with very little displacement and are the effectors of the middle ear muscle reflex. The stapedius contracts to pull the head of the stapes in a posterior direction at right angles to the plane of rotation of the chain whereas the tensor tympani pulls the manubrium of the malleus in an anteriomedial direction. Thus, these two muscles pull in opposing directions and produce a stiffening of the ossicular chain. Loud sound will cause the reflex contraction of these muscles thus attenuating the transmission of energy through the middle ear. Secondly, there is slippage of the joints between the ossicles. At very low frequencies, of the order of 60 Hz and below, the incudomalleolar joint will slip and reduce the energy transmission to the cochlea (Tonndorf and Khanna 1976). Finally, there is some experimental evidence which suggests that the impedance of the internal ear may be increased for high sound pressure levels. Such an increase would reduce the effective power transfer across the middle ear as there would be an impedance mismatch.

Summarizing the data for the outer and middle ears, it is found that they function to produce a system of matching the low impedance of the air to the higher impedance of the cochlea. This transformer action occurs because of the resonance of the ear canal, the ossicular lever action and the area ratio of the tympanic membrane to the stapes footplate. This matching system enables the maximum energy to be delivered to the cochlea but optimal transformer matching is achieved only over the frequency range between 1 to 3 kHz. The sensitivity of the hearing system, as measured by the threshold–frequency curve, matches closely the power transfer function of the middle ear and is most probably determined by the middle-ear transfer function. Finally, the action of the middle ear musculature and the partial decoupling of the ossicular chain provides protection of the cochlea against high sound level signals. This protection is greatest at low frequencies.

THE INNER EAR

The inner ear may be divided into two main components. Firstly, there is a system of interconnecting ducts and cavities within the temporal bone, lined with periosteum, which forms the bony labyrinth. This is filled with perilymph and has two membraneous openings at the oval and round windows. Secondly, contained within these bony labyrinths is the membraneous labyrinth. The part of the labyrinth which is of relevance here is the cochlea. The bony cochlea forms a snail-shaped structure coiled around a central core, the modiolus. From the modiolus protrudes a thin shelf, the ossius spiral lamina, which partly divides the cochlear spiral into two areas. These are illustrated diagrammatically in Fig. 4.3. The vibrations from the

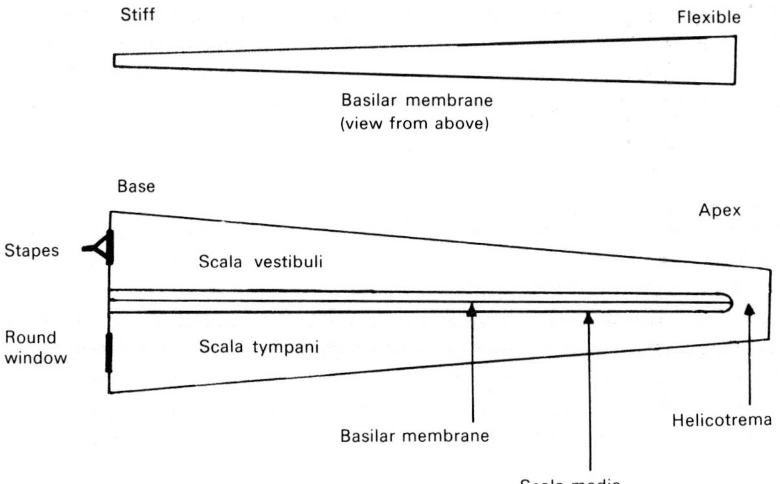

Fig. 4.3. Diagrammatic representation of the basilar membrane and a section through the inner ear.

stapes footplate pass into the fluid of the upper area, scala vestibuli, to initiate the hearing processes of the cochlea. The scala vestibuli connects to the lower area, the scala tympani, at the helicotrema. The scala tympani also communicates with the middle-ear space at the round window membrane. Between these two areas, is the membraneous cochlea or scala media. This is formed by two membranes, the basilar membrane which forms the floor of the cochlear duct and Reissner's (or vestibular) membrane. The scala media terminates before the end of the bony cochlear duct, at the helicotrema, to form a closed duct which is filled with endolymph. Endolymph is similar to intracellular fluid and has a high potassium concentration and a low sodium concentration. In contrast, perilymph is like interstitial fluid having a high sodium and a low potassium content. This difference in ionic concentrations of the cochlear fluids would be expected to lead to a difference in steady state (d.c.) potentials and, within the cochlea, there are several d.c. potentials which are independent of any stimulation and are maintained metabolically. Taking the potential of the scala tympani as zero, the scala vestibuli is slightly more positive but is approximately the same potential. The scala media has a potential of about + 100 mV and this is known as the endocochlear potential. It results from specific metabolic activity of the stria vascularis and the net potential is a balance between this and the potassium ion diffusion potential. Within the organ of Corti, there is a negative potential of between 70 to 100 mV. At present it is not clear whether this potential is the normal intracellular potential or whether there is sustained extracellular negativity. There is a further polarization of the hair cell interior, which is maintained at about − 80 mV relative to the extracellular space.

The cochlea carries out the functions of transducing, coding, and analysing the vibratory signal which arrives from the stapes footplate. The vibratory signal is first transduced to various electrical potentials; these are then coded, producing impulses in the cochlear nerve, and, during this process, a basic analysis of the incoming signal is performed. These three aspects will be considered separately.

Transduction

The vibrations, coming from the stapes footplate, cause deformations in the scala media and, in particular, produce vibrations of the basilar membrane. The details of the wave motion produced will be discussed later. It is generally accepted that the hair cells, and their cilia, provide the main link in the transduction chain. Fig. 4.4 shows, in diagrammatic form, an outer hair cell with its cilia. At least the tallest cilia of the outer hair cells are in contact with the bottom surface of the tectorial membrane (Spoendlin 1966). The connection between the cilia and the tectorial membrane, together with the relative motion of the reticular lamina and tectorial membrane, means that a vertical displacement of the basilar membrane is translated into a lateral displacement of the cilia. This is illustrated diagrammatically in Fig. 4.5. The basilar membrane, tunnel of Corti, and reticular lamina form a single mechanical entity which rotates around a flexible connection at the osseous spiral lamina. The tectorial membrane appears to rotate about a different point, located at the edge of the spiral limbus. This difference between the points of rotation of the two surfaces results in the relative lateral displacement of the cilia. This displacement produces a radial shear relative to the orientation of the cochlear spiral. Tonndorf (1960), using a theoretical model in which the basilar membrane was restrained along both of its edges, was able to show that, in the region proximal to the maximum of the wave motion the dominant curvature runs in the radial direction, whereas the region distal to the maximum has maximum curvature in a longitudinal direction. Because shearing force is proportional to the underlying curva-

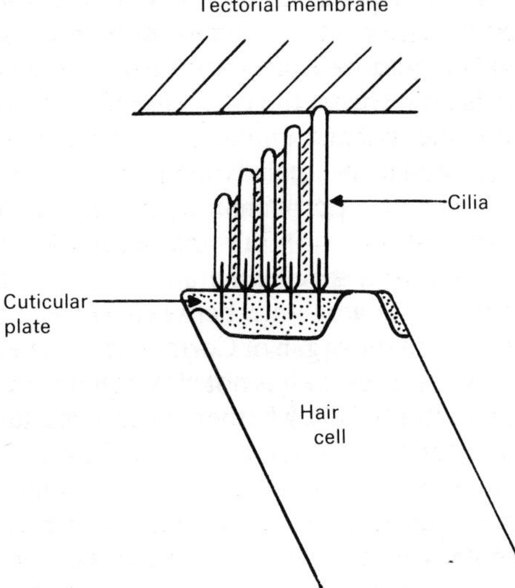

Fig. 4.4. Diagramatic representation of an outer hair cell. The tallest of the cilia is embedded in the tectorial membrane.

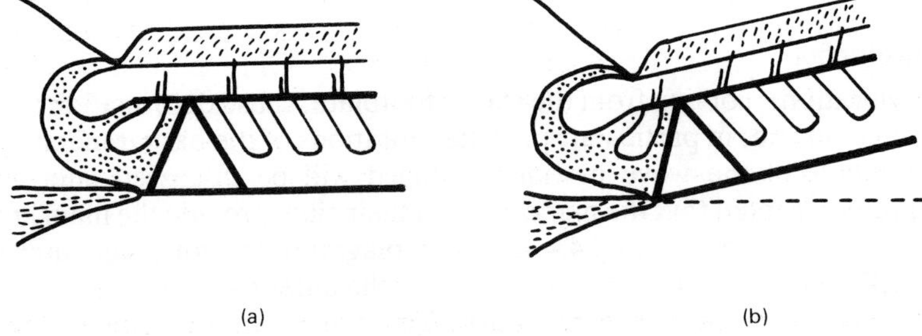

Fig. 4.5. Illustration of how the displacement of the basilar membrane is transformed into a shearing action on the cilia of the hair cells. In (a) the basilar membrane is at its normal resting position. In (b) the basilar membrane has been displaced upwards. The basilar membrane, tunnel of corti, and reticular lamina have rotated about their connection at the osseous spiral lamina whereas the tectorial membrane has rotated about the edge of the spiral limbus. This results in a lateral displacement of the cilia relative to the surface of the hair cell.

ture of the membrane, these two different shear modes, radial and longitudinal, are predominant in different regions of the basilar membrane. Generally, work has been concentrated on the radial bending of the cilia and the effects of the longitudinal shear have not been well studied.

Nevertheless, the vibratory motion of the basilar membrane is translated into a shearing force on the outer hair cells. The cilia of the inner hair cells make no apparent contact with the tectorial membrane and it would appear that the relative movement between the reticular lamina and tectorial membrane produces movement of the endolymph and the viscous drag this creates on the cilia of the outer hair cells results in their displacement. The viscous drag is proportional to the velocity in the endolymphatic fluid. Therefore, whilst the force acting on the cilia which are attached to the tectorial membrane is proportional to the relative displacement of the basilar membrane, the viscous force acting on the unconnected cilia is proportional to the velocity of the basilar membrane. This suggests distinct functional roles for the two sets of hair cells and, because of the attached cilia, the outer hair cells can be stimulated at smaller displacements than those required for the inner hair cells.

The exact manner of the next stage in the transduction process is not well understood. The deformation of the cilia leads to a change in the electrical resistance of some part of the hair cell structure. Whether this occurs at the cilia themselves, by a transmitted deformation of the hair cell boundary or from changes brought about by the cilia transmitting a deformation to the cuticular plate is not clear. Nevertheless, a resistance change within some part of the hair cell structure does occur and this results in a change in the current flow through the hair cells. The endolymphatic potentials create a voltage difference of about 170 mV across the cuticular surface of the hair cell and this maintains the receptor current which is the first electrical event following acoustic stimulation. This current is considered to be responsible for the release of chemical transmitters within the hair cell which initiate a permeability change in the postsynaptic membrane of the first order neuron. This produces a local depolarization which is conducted electrotonically in the dendritic section of the nerve. This potential change then initiates the all-or-none nerve impulses in the axons of the cochlear nerve. It is by this complex and incompletely understood mechanism that the acoustic signal is transduced into a nerve impulse.

Coding

The coding of the acoustic signal gives rise to various stimulus-related bioelectric potentials. The first of these are the receptor potentials, the cochlear microphonic (CM) and the summating potential (SP).

Wever and Bray (1930), in recording electrical potentials from the auditory nerve of the cat, noted that if their signals were fed to a loudspeaker then sounds presented to the cat's ear could be reproduced by the loudspeaker. Adrian (1931) suggested that these electrical changes were generated in the cochlea and were due to some form of microphonic action. Saul and Davis (1932) and Davis, Derbyshire, Lurie, and Saul (1934) came to similar conclusions and suggested that the CM arises from the hair cells of the cochlea as part of the process of mechanical deformation. Whilst a number of alternative hypotheses have been suggested, the hair cell hypothesis of Davis has been most widely accepted. As its name implies, the CM reproduces, to a reasonable degree of fidelity, the pressure wave form of the sound presented to the ear. The reproduction is not perfect because the frequency dependent amplitude and phase characteristics of the middle- and inner-ear systems alter the waveform. Thus, it is perhaps more accurate to describe the CM as reproducing the vibratory pattern of the basilar membrane. The amplitude of the recorded CM is proportional to the intensity of the stimulus for low and moderate intensity levels but at higher intensities the CM generators saturate and the response amplitude first limits and then decreases with further increase in stimulus intensity. The departure from linearity at high stimulus intensities is accompanied by the production of harmonic distortion components. These data reflect the properties of the gross CM where the recording electrode is sited outside the hair cell and the signal it receives is the vectorial sum of the output of several hundred generators. Whitfield and Ross (1965) showed that, if the hair cells are regarded as independent generators, the weighted sum of their individual responses will produce a spatial filtering effect on the gross CM. This argument was able to explain why the CM input–output function turned over and decreased at high intensities and why the recorded waveform did not show large amounts of distortion products.

At the lower end of the stimulus intensity range, the CM is proportional to the stimulus intensity and the limit at which the CM is measured depends only on the experimental techniques used. There appears to be no intrinsic threshold limit for the CM. The gross CM, and the summating potential which will be discussed later, is produced predominantly by the outer hair cells. The inner hair cells do produce receptor potentials but of a much smaller amplitude. Studies of receptor potentials following the destruction of outer hair cells show responses which are reduced by a factor of 30 to 40 dB. However, although the recorded CM is produced mainly by the outer hair cells, approximately 90 per cent of the cochlear nerve fibres connect with the inner hair cells. This emphasizes the difficulties involved in trying to obtain correlations between the gross receptor potentials and the responses of the cochlear nerve.

Davis, Fernández, and McAuliffe (1950) noted that a tonal stimulus can elicit a d.c. potential change within the cochlea. This is the summating potential (SP) which to some degree reflects the envelope of the stimulus. The SP persists for the whole of the stimulus duration and, like the CM, it can be measured from any location in the vicinity of the cochlea but with maximum amplitude in the scala media. The amplitude and the polarity of the SP depend upon complex interactions of stimulus intensity, stimulus frequency and electrode location. Dependent upon the combination of these parameters, the SP may be of the same polarity or of opposite polarity in the two scalae. The SP does not show any refractoriness nor does it appear to adapt to high stimulation rates. As the stimulus intensity is increased the SP amplitude also increases and shows no evidence of reaching a saturation limit. Whilst the SP is the sum of several positive and negative components (see Dallos 1973) the gross SP, recorded in the normal human, is a negative deflection when recorded at the round window or from the bony promentory. Various hypotheses have been put forward to explain the generation of the SP. As early as 1952, Davis, Tasaki, and Goldstein suggested that the SP could be the result of asymetrical distortion in the CM generating process. Later, Whitfield and Ross (1965) also produced evidence that the SP results from the non-linearity of the CM generators and their concept of phase cancellation, to produce the spatial filtering referred to earlier, was able to explain the relatively large size of the SP compared to the size of the fundamental CM component. This is because the phase cancellation procedure does not affect the SP which could then be larger than the distorted CM from which the SP is derived.

Whilst it is recognized that the gross receptor potentials, both CM and SP, do not necessarily reflect the essential steps in coding the acoustic information at the cochlear level, it is most probably that the intracellular CM and SP are necessary steps in the processing chain. Thus, the receptor potentials within the individual cell provides a mechanism directly responsible for the liberation of chemical transmitter which in turn stimulates the neural connections to the hair cell. These ideas have recently been strengthened by the work of Sellick and Russell (1978) who obtained recordings of CM and SP from an intracellular electrode. Within the afferent section of the auditory nerve, the fibres show a resting discharge and respond to sound stimulation by increasing firing rate or better synchronization of activity. For low frequency periodic waveforms, the neural spikes occur in synchrony with the stimulus waveform. At higher frequencies, above approximately 5000 Hz, such time-locking can no longer be achieved. In addition, the primary fibres have some degree of frequency selectivity and have a characteristic frequency at which the fibre responds with maximum sensitivity.

Analysis

The cochlea carries out a basic analysis of the stimulus and encodes the analysis in a form suited to the central nervous system. The first of the analysis mechanisms is known as the place principle or travelling wave concept. Békésy (1960) received his experimental measurements which showed that the stiffness of the basilar membrane was high in the basal turn and decreased as the membrane extended to the apical region. Studies on cadaver ears and on mechanical models of the cochlea led to an understanding of the travelling wave phenomenon. Fig. 4.6 shows the travelling wave pattern set up in the basilar membrane by a low-frequency tone. It was found that the envelope of the membrane displacement rises slowly to a maximum value and then decreases with a steeper slope. The position of this maximum value varies with frequency in accordance with the place principle. That is the location of the maxima are different for different frequencies; high frequencies have their maxima located in the basal turn and lower frequencies have their maxima located apically. Békésy's measurements were limited by the techniques available at that time but more recent measurements (Johnstone and Boyle 1967) have confirmed Békésy's findings although altering somewhat the numerical values involved. The travelling wave obtains its particular characteristics from the dimensions and properties of the cochlear partition. The change in basilar membrane width and in its stiffness as it progresses from base to apex are the main

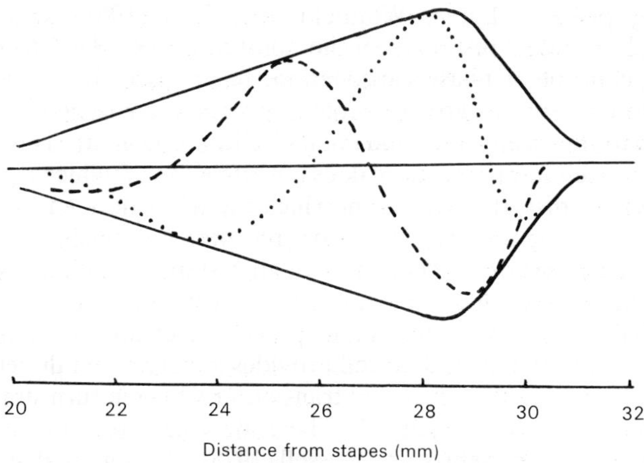

Fig. 4.6. Travelling wave motion along the basilar membrane in response to a 200 Hz tonal stimulus. The solid line represents the envelope of the travelling wave motion. Two examples of the travelling wave itself are illustrated by the broken lines. (After Békésy (1960).)

factors involved. Thus, a basic analysis of the frequency components in the stimulus can be carried out by this place mechanism. However, at low frequencies, below 100 Hz, the travelling wave extends over virtually the entire length of the basilar membrane and there is no clear maximum in the wave envelope. Clearly, the place principle cannot provide an analysis of the frequency component in these low-frequency signals.

However, if the frequency is low enough, an individual nerve fibre can produce impulses which are time-locked to the period of the signal. Thus the frequency of the stimulus may be identified as the time interval between nerve impulses will correspond to the signal period. Such a mechanism can work up to frequencies of approximately 1000 Hz. In practice, time-locked neural responses can be observed up to 3000 or 4000 Hz and, as nerve fibres cannot sustain discharge rates more than about 200 per second, the question arose as to how the cochlear nerve could be time-locked at these frequencies. Wever (1949) proposed his 'volley' theory to explain this. Single auditory neurons would still be phase-locked to a sinusoidal stimulus but as the frequency of the stimulus increased the impulse in that neuron would still occur at a particular phase of the cycle but would not occur on every cycle. Thus the interspike interval would be an integral multiple of the signal period. If a large number of individual fibres respond to a sinusoidal signal, there will always be some fibres that respond on any particular cycle and so, between all the fibres, volleys of nerve impulses will occur which are time-locked to higher frequency stimuli. Experimental evidence places the limit of this mechanism as somewhere between 4000 and 5000 Hz. Hence, using a combination of the travelling wave and volley mechanisms, a frequency analysis of the entire audible range of frequencies can be carried out.

If recordings are taken from a single fibre in the cochlear nerve for a range of stimulus frequencies, the stimulus intensity may be adjusted until the nerve responds at a predetermined firing rate. This produces the 'tuning-curve' of the nerve fibre. It has been known for many years that the tuning properties of the cochlear nerve fibres were much better than the equivalent tuning curve provided by the travelling wave envelope along the basilar membrane. This led to a consideration that there was a 'second filter' which would improve the frequency selectivity properties of the basilar membrane to match those measured within the cochlear nerve fibres. The work of Sellick and Russell (1978) has shown that the intracellular CM and SP exhibit tuning curves which match those found in cochlear nerve fibres. Thus, at the level of the hair cell, the frequency resolution of the peripheral auditory system has already been improved. The mechanism of this process is not understood but may involve the basic hydrodynamic processes that stimulate the hair cells or the two types of shear mechanism that have been described earlier.

It can be seen that, even at the level of the cochlear nerve, the auditory system has already provided a sophisticated time-frequency analysis of the input signal. Further analyses occur within the auditory brainstem and much of the auditory processing which is based on simple, physical characteristics of the signal seem to occur before cortical levels are reached.

REFERENCES

ADRIAN, E. D. (1931). The microphonic action of the cochlea in relation to theories of hearing. In *Report of a discussion on audition*, pp. 5–9. Physics Society, London.

BÉKÉSY, G. VON (1960). *Experiments in hearing*. McGraw-Hill, New York.

DALLOS, P. (1973). *The auditory periphery biophysics and physiology*. Academic Press, New York.

DAVIS, H., FERNÁNDEZ, C., and MCAULIFFE, D. R. (1950). The excitatory process in the cochlea. *Proc. nat. Acad. Sci. USA* **36**, 580–7.

—— TASAKI, T., and GOLDSTEIN, R. (1952). The peripheral origin of activity, with reference to the ear. *Cold Spring Harb. Symp. quant. Biol.* **17**, 143–54.

—— DERBYSHIRE, A., LURIE, M., and SAUL. L. (1934). The electric response of the cochlea. *Am. J. Physiol.* **107**, 317–32.

HINCHCLIFFE, R. and HARRISON, D. (1976). *Scientific foundations of otolaryngology*. Heinnman, London.

JOHNSTONE, B. M. and BOYLE, A. J. T. (1967). Basilar membrane vibrations examined with the Mössbauer technique. *Science, N.Y.* **158**, 389–90.

LITTLER, T. S. (1965). *The physics of the ear*. Pergamon Press, London,

SAUL, L. and DAVIS, H. (1932). Action currents in the central nervous system: I. Action currents of the auditory tract. *Archs Neurol. Psychiat., Chicago* **28**, 1104–16.

SELLICK, P. M. and RUSSELL, I. J. (1978). Intracellular studies of cochlear hair cells. In *Evoked electrical activity in the auditory nervous system* (ed. R. F. Naunton and C. Fernández) Academic Press, New York.

SPOENDLIN, H. (1966). *The organisation of the cochlear receptor.* Karger, Basel.

TONNDORF, J. (1960). Shearing motion in scala media in cochlear model. *J. acoust. Soc. Am.* **32**, 238–44.

TONNDORF, J. and KHANNA, S. M. (1976). Mechanics of the auditory system. In *Scientific foundations of otolaryngology* (ed. R. Hinchcliffe and D. Harrison) pp. 237–52. Heinemann, London.

WEVER, E. G. (1949). *Theory of hearing.* Wiley, New York.

—— and BRAY, C. (1930). Action currents in the auditory nerve in response to acoustic stimulation. *Proc. nat. Acad. Sci. USA* **16**, 344–50.

WHITFIELD, I. C. and ROSS, H. F. (1965). Cochlear microphonic and summating potentials and the outputs of individual hair cells generators. *J. acoust. Soc. Am.* **38**, 126–31.

5 Psychophysics of hearing pertaining to clinical audiology

LOIS L. ELLIOTT

This chapter is written primarily for readers who are not acquainted with the field of psychoacoustics and who need to gain basic understanding of those aspects of hearing science that underlie frequently used clinical audiology tests. Since it is not possible in a single chapter to do justice to the details of present knowledge about human hearing and since many important questions remain unresolved, this account will touch only on some basic fundamentals. The interested reader is referred to texts by Hirsh (1952) and Green (1976) for further information on this subject.

The psychophysics of hearing may be described as dealing with relations between the physical stimulus (sound) and the subjective experience of the listener. Although the experience of hearing is subjective, it may be evaluated from the listener's responses. In general, one may say that clinical audiology tests are based on comparisons between the behaviour, or performance, of the patient being tested and performances typically observed in a group of normal listeners.

Audiologists have two main reasons for administering hearing tests to patients. One is to determine how well the individual can function in the normal, hearing world. This world involves understanding the speech of others as well as detecting and identifying environmental sounds such as door-bells, telephones, and traffic noises. A subsidiary aspect of this first purpose concerns the use of hearing tests in selecting the 'best' hearing aid (when an aid is considered appropriate) to improve the auditory functioning of an individual with impaired hearing. A second purpose of clinical audiology tests is to provide information that can assist in diagnosing the nature of the hearing problem and in identifying other health problems, such as neurological disorders, that may be detectable via auditory tests at an earlier stage in the course of the disease than is possible by other diagnostic procedures.

Psychoacousticians, or scientists who study hearing, have additional reasons for administering hearing tests since their primary goal is to explain the principles of normal hearing (that is, 'how people hear'). Many psychoacousticians assume that increased knowledge of normal hearing will provide a basis for designing improved sensory aids for people with impaired hearing. There is also increasing recognition of the idea that psychoacoustic study of hearing-impaired listeners, and comparisons with normal listeners, facilitates understanding of both normal and impaired hearing.

In summary, the goals of the clinical audiologist as well as the goals of the psychoacoustician involve measurement of listeners' behaviour and, often indirectly, measurement of the listeners' subjective auditory experiences.

MEASUREMENT CONSIDERATIONS

Characteristics of the measurement situation can range from loose to tight control. An example of a loosely controlled test is the tuning fork procedure, where a tuning fork is struck, held to the patient's ear, and then moved away as the patient indicates when the sound is no longer perceived. Precise measurement of the sound intensity at which the patient can no longer hear the tone is not possible and, if the tuning fork has been dropped or bent, its frequency characteristics may diverge from those intended. The extreme opposite of the tuning fork procedure might be a computer-controlled test that incorporates precise specification of the stimulus frequency and intensity and that records every stimulus presented and every response. In this situation the patient, wearing headphones, might be seated in front of a panel holding two, three, or four lights, each of which is illuminated sequentially to mark an 'observation interval'. The test stimulus is presented to the patient in one of the observation intervals (over many trials, the stimulus is presented randomly in all possible intervals) and, on each trial, the patient pushes a button to indicate the observation interval during which the stimulus was heard. It is possible in the computer-controlled task for the patient to be informed, after each trial, whether the response was correct (i.e. to give the patient 'feedback'). Often such feedback helps the patient learn the task more quickly and produces less variable test results.

Whether one uses a loosely controlled hearing test, a carefully controlled test, or one of the many audiological procedures that fall along the intervening continuum there are many sources of potential variability in the test results. These include variability of the patient, variability in the test stimuli, and variability in the procedures that are used to obtain, record, and interpret the patient's responses.

A patient may give variable test results for a number of reasons. Instructions may not have been clear and the patient may not understand what is expected. The patient's criterion for reporting presence of a tone may be very conservative one day (for example, the patient waits until absolutely certain that the tone is clearly perceived) and may be lenient another time. The patient's attention may wander, particularly if there are distracting sights or sounds in the nearby environment. The patient's general health, state of alertness, and interest in the test procedures may change from day to day. Generally, it may be said that test procedures that allow the examiner to assess possible sources of patient variability will provide more interpretable test results than would otherwise be possible.

Test variability may occur because of changes in the stimuli presented. It has been mentioned that the frequency of a tuning fork may change and both the frequency and intensity of audiometers can deviate from the dial settings. (Calibration procedures and standards discussed in Chapter 8 are designed to prevent inaccuracies in clinical audiometers.) It should also be noted that a noisy environment (e.g. a test room that does not meet specifications for quiet—see Chapter 6) can introduce apparent variability into the test results.

The examiner's potential contribution to test variability is not always acknowledged. When the examiner controls the timing of stimulus presentations, it is imperative that no extra cues signal the patient to respond. Furthermore, if the examiner does not follow a predetermined protocol for determining the *intensities* of stimuli as well as the order of frequencies, the outcome of the hearing test may be different from that where a specific protocol is used. A final example of potential examiner-introduced variability concerns the testing of speech understanding. Typically, the patient is instructed to repeat back words, sentences, or nonsense syllables that are presented at controlled intensity levels. If the patient's response is not tape-recorded, thus allowing verification of the responses, there is always the possibility that the examiner will misunderstand the words as the patient pronounces them. (Of course, speech understanding tests that require written responses, or pointing to pictures, eliminate this possible source of variability.)

The implications of these potential sources of variability in hearing testing should emphasize the necessity for careful and precise control of the test situation. Even when control is maximized, patient responses will exhibit variability; less usually occurs within a single test session and more across different test days. While this is true of normal listeners, it has also been found that hearing-impaired listeners often exhibit greater-than-normal variability.

Psychoacousticians require *very* precise measurements of patient or subject response since, frequently, their purpose for collecting a set of data is to decide between two or more different models of auditory system functioning and small differences in test results may have major, theoretical significance. Increasingly, however, clinicians require and obtain equally precise measurements of patients' auditory responses. To date, this has been most true of those situations where the purpose of the clinical audiology test 'battery' is to facilitate diagnosis of special medical problems. Of course, even the most routine clinical testing requires a considerable degree of precision since erroneous results could impinge undesirably upon the prospect of ameliorating the patient's hearing problem.

UNITS OF MEASUREMENT

Since the above discussion has emphasized that clinical audiology is dependent upon rather precise measurement procedures, one may ask in what units these measurements are most frequently made. The three physical dimensions that form the cornerstones of traditional audiological tests are intensity, frequency, and time.

Intensity is usually measured in decibels (dB) and must be stated relative to a reference value. Frequently, intensity is measured in pressure units (sound pressure level—SPL) with the reference of 0.0002 dyn/cm^2 or, more recently 2×10^{-5} N/m^2 or 2×10^{-5} pascal (Pa). Decibel measurements represent the ratio between the sound intensity being measured and the reference level. Although, as a rough rule of thumb, one may think of intensity as most directly related to the subjective experience of loudness, there is not a one-to-one relationship between the subjective experience and the physical quantity, as will be discussed shortly.

We speak of the physical basis of sound as being a 'sound wave', that is, a rapid change in pressure. One group of sound waves is characterized by sinusoidal pressure changes and may be described by *frequency* or the number of times the sinusoidal cycle recurs in a unit of time (usually a second). These are called 'pure tones'. The formerly used terminology for frequency of 'cycles per second' (c.p.s.) has been replaced by 'hertz' (Hz) which has exactly the same meaning. The subjective experience that is most closely related to sound frequency is pitch, with high-pitched sounds being those having higher frequencies, and vice versa.

Pure tones are sometimes referred to as *simple* acoustic stimuli to differentiate them from *complex* stimuli which cannot be described by a relatively simple mathematical formula. Many environmental sounds have complex acoustic waveforms but one might say that the complex stimuli to which most of us accord greatest attention are those of human speech.

The third cornerstone dimension, time, has often not been given as much attention as either frequency or intensity. However, recent investigations are indicating that its role may be more important than previously thought. Duration of the auditory stimulus and the amount of time between stimuli are usually measured in seconds, milliseconds (ms—thousandths of a second), or microseconds (μs—millionths of a second). For some time it has been known that the ease with which an auditory stimulus of low intensity can be detected is, in part, a function of its duration ('temporal integration'). In the last several decades it has been learned that some speech sounds are distinguished by discriminating certain temporal differences that are measured in milliseconds (Studdert-Kennedy 1976). There are also some special tests used for identifying special auditory and other problems that depend on the ability of the listener to continue to perceive an auditory stimulus over a period of time (e.g. tests for auditory adaptation, Chapter 15).

SENSITIVITY

The measurement of auditory sensitivity involves determining the least intense stimulus that the patient can just detect (that is, just say 'I hear it' as opposed to 'I do not hear it'). Human listeners hear acoustic stimuli in the frequency range from about 20 to 20 000 Hz. At sound frequencies below 20 Hz, the subjective experience is one of feeling vibrations; at frequencies higher than 20 000 Hz, humans usually experience no subjective response at the time of stimulation. (It is well known, of course, that animals such as dogs and cats, and especially bats, are able to hear sound frequencies that are above the range of human hearing.) Fig. 5.1 shows responses of young,

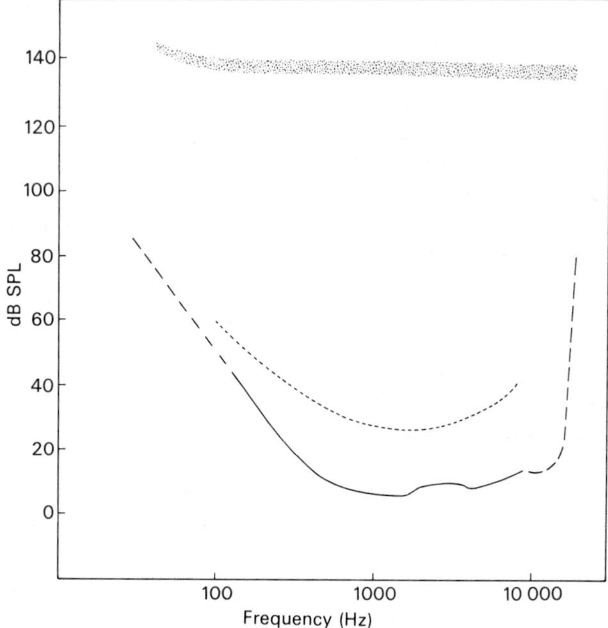

Fig. 5.1. Normal auditory sensitivity in sound pressure level (SPL) re 0.0002 dyn cm^2 or 2×10^{-5}Pa, as a function of frequency for young listeners. The solid line connects the points of the ANSI 1969 standard and is extrapolated (dashed lines) to other frequencies using the averages of several psychoacoustic studies. The dotted line represents an 'equal loudness contour'. The stippled line, at the top, is the region of discomfort and pain.

normal human listeners who have no history of ear disease or noise exposure and expresses these responses in SPL units. The lowest curve of this figure represents the normal 'threshold' of auditory sensitivity and indicates that human listeners are most sensitive to sounds with frequencies between 1000 and 4000 Hz.

Psychoacousticians have devoted considerable attention during the 1950s and 1960s to the theory of signal detection (Green and Swets 1966) which was developed, in part, to take account of the observer's criterion in judging the presence or absence of a signal. Formerly, the psychoacoustic testing methods that were frequently used were the method of adjustment and the single-interval, 'yes–no' procedure. In the former, the experimenter or the subject varied one characteristic of the signal, such as intensity, until the listener judged it as having some specified value—such as the intensity at which the signal could be 'just detected'. In the 'yes–no' procedure, the listener was required on each trial to indicate whether or not the signal occurred. Both methods reflected the listener's criterion, which was not directly assessed.

Signal-detection theory (Swets 1964) assumes that noise in the stimulus may be considered as resulting in two partially overlapping response probability distributions—one to noise alone and the other to signal-plus-noise. The difference between the means of these two probability distributions is defined as d' and may be considered a measure of sensitivity.

Empirically, d' may be measured either by encouraging the listener to change his response criterion on different sets of trials by actually changing the proportion of times the signal is presented. Another measurement procedure requires the listener to assign a confidence rating to each judgment; these responses are then statistically manipulated to obtain a Receiver Operating Characteristic (ROC) curve.

By emphasizing the importance of the listener's response criterion, signal detection theory has revolutionized thinking concerning 'thresholds'. It is also interesting to note that Swets (1961) commented prophetically, 'We can forego estimating the response criterion in a forced-choice experiment. Under the forced-choice procedure, few observers show a bias in their responses large enough to affect the sensitivity index d' appreciably.' This is precisely what has happpened; today almost all research investigators and many clinical specialists use a two-, three, or four-alternative forced-choice procedure.

In clinical audiological measurement, it is usually sufficient to keep in mind that 'threshold' is the intensity at which a signal can be detected 50 per cent of the time. This implies, of course, that some of the time, signals with intensities greater than the 'threshold' level may not be detected and that the listener will sometimes detect signals with intensities lower than the 'threshold'.

The measurement of pure-tone sensitivity, both for stimuli presented through headphones (via 'air conduction') and for stimuli transmitted via a vibrator placed on the mastoid process behind the pinna or (occasionally) on the centre of the forehead (i.e. via 'bone conduction') constitutes the most basic clinical test used by audiologists. The frequencies at which sensitivity is usually measured (125, 250, 500, 1000, 2000, 4000, and 8000 Hz) are an octave apart. A typical audiogram form contains these signal frequencies printed across the horizontal axis. The intensity measures that are printed along the left, vertical axis of the form are not in sound pressure level units but are labelled dB HL, where HL stands for 'hearing level'. One may think of the lower, curved line in Fig. 5.1, which represents normal auditory sensitivity of the 'threshold' of young, normal listeners, as being pulled taut and relabelled 0 dB HL on the standard audiometric form (Fig. 5.2). Decibel values on the audiometric form that are below the 0 dB HL line represent greater intensities than normal threshold levels (i.e. than 0 dB HL); negative HLs, which appear above the 0 dB HL line, represent sounds that are less intense than the average, normal threshold level. Thus, conversion from sound pressure level to hearing level and expression of the patient's auditory sensitivity or 'threshold' in dB HL on a standard clinical, audiogram form: (i) focuses attention on the comparison between the patient's sensitivity and normal sensitivity; (ii) effectively subtracts out the differential sensitivity across sound frequencies that characterizes the res-

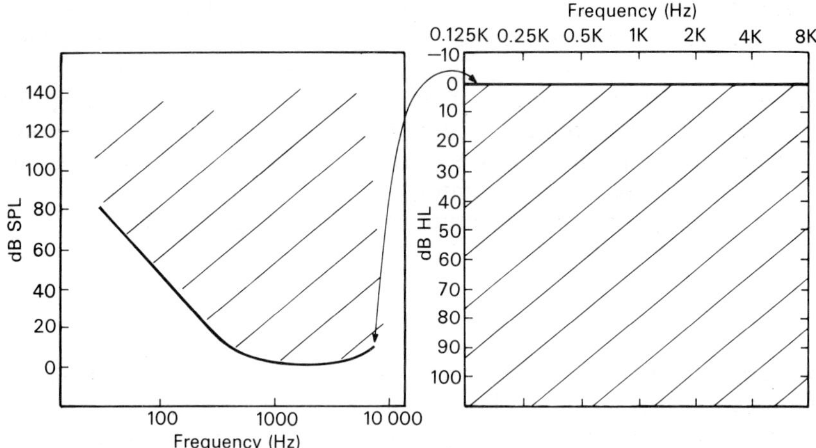

Fig. 5.2. Diagram illustrating conversion from the sound pressure level (SPL) scale to the hearing level (HL) scale. The arrow connecting the two parts of the figure points, in each case, to the line representing normal 'threshold'. The cross-hatched areas represent the regions of sound pressures that are more intense than normal 'thresholds'.

ponses of all normal listeners; and (iii) reverses the up–down directionality of intensity change from that usually used in psychoacoustic reports.

LOUDNESS

It was stated earlier that the subjective experience of loudness is primarily related to sound intensity. Psychoacousticians have studied the manner in which loudness changes as a function of intensity change; data show that the increase in loudness as a function of increased intensity differs somewhat across signal frequencies.* The dotted line in Fig. 5.1 represents an 'equal loudness contour' that was determined by having normal listeners equate the loudness of one pure-tone signal with the loudness of another. Notice that this line is neither perfectly parallel with the abscissa nor equally distant from the threshold line.

Audiologists have two major reasons for evaluating a patient's subjective experience of loudness. The first derives from the fact that some disorders of the peripheral auditory system are characterized by 'recruitment' which is an abnormal increase in loudness (as a function of intensity increase—see also Chapter 15). Thus, clinicians are able to use data about a patient's loudness experience to assist in determining the nature of the hearing problem. The second reason concerns the fact that there is a point at which a

* S. S. Stevens conducted many experiments on the growth of loudness as a power function of sound pressure. In Stevens' 1966 paper, cross-modality matches of loudness with other perceptual continua (e.g. warmth, pressure on the palm, etc.) are described and certain consistencies across the 'families' of power functions are derived.

sufficiently intense sound produces discomfort and pain for normal listeners (see Fig. 5.1). For most hearing-impaired listeners, the discomfort level occurs at an intensity about equal to or slightly lower than that where normal listeners experience discomfort. If the clinician contemplates the fitting of a hearing aid or if the clinician is attempting to determine an appropriate intensity level for administering a suprathreshold test, it is often important to determine the patient's discomfort level or the maximum intensity that can be tolerated. Another measure that is frequently obtained is 'most comfortable loudness' (MCL).

PITCH

The subjective experience that is most closely associated with the dimension of frequency is that of pitch. Clinical audiologists typically test the sensitivity of patients at differing frequencies but there are few routinely used clinical procedures that involve measuring the patient's ability to perceive pitch. If a patient reports that a suprathreshold pure tone does not sound 'tone-like', this observation has potential diagnostic significance. The examiner may also learn that the same signal frequency produces two different tonal sensations in the two ears; this condition is called *diplacusis* and is of potential clinical importance. Although psychoacousticians have devoted considerable energy to determining how well normal and hearing-impaired listeners can discriminate between two stimuli having different frequencies, this type of task has not typically been used when testing a patient in the clinical context. However, an evaluation of patients with implanted cochlear prostheses employed a pitch discrimination task and obtained useful results (Bilger 1977). Since many speech sounds are distinguished by the frequencies and change in frequency of component concentrations of sound energy or *formants* (see Pickett 1980), and since hearing-impaired listeners may have reduced frequency-analysing abilities (Danaher, Osberger, and Pickett 1973), it is likely that clinical tests of the future will address the question of how well a patient is able to discriminate small changes in sound frequency (see following discussion of frequency selectivity). Synthesized speech stimuli may be used in some of these procedures. Such tests may provide useful diagnostic information and they also may be helpful in evaluating different sensory aids.

MASKING

The term masking refers to the situation where one sound stimulus interferes with perception of another. Masking occurs in many everyday situations—for example, in noisy subways; in crowded restaurants; and in homes where voices, the television set, and other electrical appliances may produce sounds at a level to 'drown out', or mask, conversations.

Masking used in audiologic tests is usually a wide band of noise, a narrow band of noise, or a 'babble' or several talkers. In this context, 'noise' refers to a random mixture of many different frequencies. For example, a wide-band noise should contain all frequencies between 20 and 20 000 Hz at approximately equal intensities while a narrow-band noise can be produced by filtering out frequencies above and below the end points of the band. In actual practice, the width of a narrow (or indeed any other) band of noise is defined as the frequency difference between the two points at which the sound intensity is 3 dB less than at the centre of the band. Frequencies just beyond both end-points are present in the narrow band masker at reduced intensities and the extent to which outlying frequencies are present is determined by the steepness of the filter.

The psychoacoustic literature on masking is large and growing. It is possible to state some basic fundamentals but it must be remembered that these are gross oversimplifications: (i) A more intense sound will mask a less intense sound more than the reverse. (ii) A pure tone will mask another pure tone having a higher frequency more than it will mask a pure tone having a lower frequency. (iii) A narrow band of noise will mask pure-tone signals having frequencies located within the frequency limits of the band more than it will mask signal frequencies outside the band. (iv) If a wide band noise is used to mask a pure-tone signal, only those frequencies within the wideband noise that are relatively close to the signal frequency (i.e. that are within the 'critical band') will exert a masking effect on the signal. (v) A sound presented simultaneously with another sound will have a greater masking effect on it than it will have on a sound that precedes it or follows it. Nevertheless, a sound has some masking effect on stimuli that occur just before it ('backward masking') or just after it ('forward masking'), where 'before' and 'after' are of the magnitude of 0, 10, 20, and 30 ms for normal listeners and somewhat longer for hearing-impaired subjects (Elliott 1975).

The concept of the 'critical band' was originally based on the assumption that the narrow band of noise frequencies that surround a pure tone and that are *equal to it in power* are responsible for masking the tone. This type of 'critical band' is calculated from the signal-to-noise ratio at the threshold of the tone in the noise and is called a 'critical ratio'. Later investigators studied the 'critical band' directly by modifying the width of a noise band and determining the bandwidth at which psychoacoustic responses (such as detection of a signal or loudness of the noise) begin to change. Different bandwidths are obtained for critical bands measured in these two ways, with the latter being about 2.5 times the width of the critical ratio. It should also be noted that critical bands are wider for higher frequencies, being almost 160 Hz wide at 1000 Hz, and 700 Hz wide at 4000 Hz.

Interest in critical bands was stimulated by theoretic considerations of the auditory system as a 'bank' of band pass filters (Scharf 1970). Investigators have attempted to determine the relations between critical bandwidths on the one hand, and masker intensity (Scharf and Meiselman 1977) or masker duration, on the other. There has also been interest in the question of whether critical bands in cochlear-impaired ears are the same width as in normal-hearing listeners, but a conclusive answer is not available (Scharf

1978). The general interest now is in relating the construct of critical bands to frequency analysing capabilities of the auditory system via psychological and physiological tuning curves (Wightman, McGee, and Kramer 1977; Dallos, Ryan, Harris, McGee, and Özdamar 1977). This approach is also likely to be modified in order to develop new clinical tests for evaluating *frequency selectivity* in hearing-impaired listeners.

Psychoacousticians have many reasons for studying masking phenomena; most relate to testing models of auditory system function. In the past, the audiologist has had primarily two reasons for using masking. The first was to isolate the ear being tested from the non-test ear. For example, if the sensitivity of one ear is considerably better than the sensitivity of the other ear, then when one intends to test the poorer ear it is possible for stimuli to travel around or through the head to the better ear and to be detected there. A wide variety of clinical situations, including the testing of speech understanding, require masking to isolate the test ear.

Interaural attenuation, or the amount of sound energy that is lost by sounds travelling around or through the head, varies as a function of signal frequency, head configuration, and earphone coupling to the head. A conservative procedure for air conduction testing is to apply masking to the non-test ear whenever it is necessary to present a signal to the test ear that is 40 dB or more higher than the air- or bone-conduction threshold in the non-test ear (Sanders 1972). For bone-conduction testing, a conservative procedure is to assume no cross-cranial attenuation and always to mask the non-test ear (see also Chapter 15). It has also been shown that a relatively intense sound presented to one ear can mask signals presented to the other ear, even when direct transmission of acoustic energy around or through the head can be ruled out—a phenomenon that is termed 'central masking'.

With the exception of some special tests for functional hearing impairment (see Chapter 15), the second typical reason for the clinical audiologist to employ masking concerned procedures for testing a patient's understanding of speech. It is well accepted that some people who can understand a spoken message when it is presented in quiet have considerable difficulty understanding speech when it occurs in noise. When testing a patient with speech in noise, the clinician controls the signal level (i.e. the intensity of the speech) and the signal-to-noise (S/N) ratio. This latter quantity is expressed in decibels and represents the number of decibels by which signal intensity exceeds (for a +S/N) or is less than (−S/N) the noise intensity.

It has been established that the ability of normal listeners to understand speech presented in noise or babble is a function of: the signal level and the S/N ratio; the acoustic frequencies present in the noise; the familiarity of the test materials to the listener and their frequency of usage; the number of syllables in the stimulus words; the redundancy and predictability of the test materials, if sentences are used; and, the listener's level of language competence. The clinician's purpose for administering speech tests under conditions of masking is to compare performance with that expected of normal listeners. Sometimes the terminology used by clinicians for this use of masking is 'competing noise' or 'competing speech' to distinguish it from the ear-isolation purpose.

BINAURAL HEARING

The terms 'monaural' and 'binaural' are frequently used to describe stimulation of one or of two ears. 'Monaural', or its synonym 'monotic', refers to the situation in which a stimulus is presented to only one ear. This occurs, usually, only in an artificially contrived situation where the listener wears one active headphone or a 'receiver' in one ear. Of course, if a listener has a profound unilateral hearing loss, or a 'dead ear', he is effectively receiving monotic stimulation. The word 'binaural' is not sufficient for many audiologic purposes. 'Binaural' means stimulation of the two ears, but does not make clear whether the same or different stimuli are delivered. The term 'diotic' refers to the condition in which *exactly* identical stimuli are presented to both ears. This usually occurs only when headphones transmit the same stimulus or when the listener is postioned immediately in front of the sound source (and the environment on both sides of the listener is equally reverberant). The term 'dichotic' refers to the condition where different stimuli are delivered to two ears. In most everyday situations, one ear is closer to the sound source than the other or the reverberation qualities of the environment differ on the right and left sides of the listener. Head shadow effects, which occur when the sound source is on one side and the acoustic stimulus must bend around the head to reach the more distant ear, also produce dichotic stimulation. And, finally, when the pinnae and the ear canals are of unequal size or shape, the resonant effects they exert on the sound stimulus (that is, the extent to which they cause some frequencies to be differentially amplified) will differ at the two ears and dichotic stimulation may result. Hence, dichotic listening is the general rule in daily life.

The term 'dichotic' is also used to refer to carefully controlled laboratory situations where the experimenter deliberately presents differing stimuli to the two ears. Note that this may refer to differences in frequency, intensity, duration, time of arrival of the stimulation at the ears, or to all of these.

The stimulus cue of difference in time of arrival (or of phase difference between two otherwise identical sinusoids) is a primary cue for localizing the source of the sound. Localization refers to the subjective experience that a sound originates at a particular physical place. This term is reserved for situations that are sometimes called 'field listening'—that is, for times when the listener does not wear headphones and when there is a speaker or other sound source from which the stimulus emanates. Data on normal listeners indicate that the ability to discriminate different sound source positions varies as a function of the frequency of the stimulus and the position of the source relative to the listener. For sound sources located in front of the listener, positions that differ by one to three degrees can usually be distinguished as being different.

Localization is an important parameter in daily living situations since it is the process whereby we determine which way to look when someone calls us across a large space or whereby we decide on which side to take aim at a buzzing mosquito. Generally, the clinician does not test the ability of a patient to localize sounds; however, the mechanism of localization can serve as a convenient vehicle for determining whether or not a difficult-to-test patient can *hear* sounds. For example, in testing young children, it is common to have two speakers or sound sources in the test suite and to associate each speaker with an object or toy that can provide positive reinforcement if the child turns toward the source. A tone or speech signal is presented through one of the speakers and, when the child turns to face that speaker, the eyes of the teddy bear sitting on top of it light up. It has been demonstrated that children having normal motor skill and normal intelligence and who are between the ages of about six months to one year readily learn the head-turning task (which is sometimes called an orienting response) and enjoy the test procedure. Were they not able to localize the source of the sound stimulation, it would not be possible to test their auditory sensitivity in this manner.

The process by which the listener is able to localize the sound source concerns the different times of arrival of the signals reaching the two ears. When headphones are used to transmit the two signals that differ in time of arrival, the process is usually termed lateralization. Experimental data demonstrate that, depending upon the frequency of the stimuli, differences in interaural times of arrival on the order of 20–30 microseconds (μs) can be detected by normal listeners; some can detect interaural time differences as small as 10 μs. There is also evidence that, to some extent, differences in time of arrival of the two stimuli can be offset by intensity differences. That is, within limits, when one stimulus arrives at one ear later than the stimulus to the other ear, it can still be perceived as arriving simultaneously if it is more intense than the other.

Stimuli presented via headphones are usually perceived as 'localized' either within the head or at one or the other of the ears. Thus, in the previous paragraph, when we referred to perceiving two stimuli as occurring simultaneously, the actual judgment the listener would usually make would be that the percept appeared to be located in the centre of the head. This is sometimes referred to as 'localization in the medial sagittal plane'. Recently, it has been learned that a patient's ability to lateralize sounds or to centre two dichotic stimuli may provide useful diagnostic information concerning certain types of auditory pathology (Hawkins and Wightman 1978).

One especially important dichotic phenomenon has been given the name 'masking level difference' (MLD). This refers to the situation where the listener is presented both with a signal and with masking noise and where one of these (either signal or masker) is identical at both ears (that is, diotic) and the other is not identical in a very special way. When MLDs are studied in the laboratory, the phase of either the signal or the masker is identical at both ears (0° phase difference) while the phase of the other component differs. The measure obtained is the intensity at which the signal can be just detected or the percentage of words correctly reported *in comparison to the situation when the special MLD conditions are not present.* For example, if a low-frequency tone, which is presented in wide-band noise that is perfectly correlated in phase at both ears (i.e. has a 0° phase difference), is varied in phase from 0° to + or −180°, the signal intensity that is necessary to detect the presence of the tone may be decreased as much as 10, 12, or 15 dB. It is this change in sensitivity as a function of the change in interaural phase of signal or masker (but not both) that is referred to as the MLD. It is well known that the largest MLDs are obtained using low-frequency, pure-tone signals and that the size of the MLD decreases as signal frequency increases.

The MLD phenomenon can assist a normally hearing listener who attempts to understand the speech of a conversationalist in a noisy environment. In this case, the background noise usually is transmitted from a distance greater than the distance that separates the two talkers and, thus, is relatively highly correlated with respect to phase whereas the speech of a talker standing to one side or another will arrive at the listener's ears relatively uncorrelated. The MLD effect allows the listener to understand the talker's speech at a lower intensity level than if the talker's speech arrived at the listener's ears in a perfectly correlated manner. This is sometimes called the 'cocktail party effect'.

Most studies of MLDs have been accomplished by psychoacousticians who have been interested in studying binaural auditory processing. This procedure is not part of the typical clinical test 'battery'. However, relatively recent data have demonstrated that patients having certain auditory pathologies of the central nervous system demonstrate diminished or absent MLDs (Olsen and Noffsinger 1976); hence, this procedure may gain increased popularity for clinical purposes in the future.

One final type of binaural test procedure deserves brief mention. In the last decade there has been interest in the patient's performance when two different speech stimuli are presented simultaneously to the two ears and the patient is asked to repeat both of them (Berlin and McNeil 1976). Performance on this task is sometimes used as a measurement of lateralization and integrity of the central auditory system and there are suggestions in the literature that, properly administered, this type of test can provide information that is useful for diagnostic purposes.

OTHER CONSIDERATIONS

This chapter has focused on measuring a listener's performance in response to particular stimulus variables. A critical aspect of this situation is that the investigator knows *with certainty* to what dimension of the stimulus the listener is responding. This may appear a simple requirement, but we have already seen that in the case of a patient with asymmetrical hearing loss, failure to apply masking to the non-test ear may produce erroneous results. Are there other, potentially misleading situations where data collected by psychoacousticians and clinicians can lead to incorrect conclusions? The answer is 'yes'.

The physical characteristcs of sound and the fact that many listeners have hearing losses that affect their sensitivity to some frequencies but not to others (e.g. a high-frequency hearing loss) conspire to create special challenges. For example, a rapidly turned on pure tone that continues for, say 3 seconds, and that is then rapidly turned off, will have a sinusoidal wave form for the centre portion of the stimulus, but will have a wave form that includes a broad band of frequencies at the beginning and end of the stimulus. A listener with a hearing loss at the target frequency but with better sensitivity at other frequencies may respond to the stimulus by detecting the splatter of acoustic energy that is produced by the abrupt stimulus onset. This situation may be largely curtailed by shaping the 'rise' and 'fall' times of the stimulus—that is, by having the pure tone attain its maximum amplitude gradually. Standards of audiometers specify appropriate rise/fall times for pure tone stimuli and authors of scientific publications are expected to provide this information when the listener's performance could be affected by this experimental parameter.

The above example of a 3 second tone was selected to allow the stimulus to achieve a 'steady-state' condition after 'onset' and before 'offset'. The spectrum of a short tone does not achieve a steady state condition (where its spectrum is characterized by a sinusoid); indeed, Fourier analysis shows that as tones become increasingly short, their spectra contain an increasingly large number of different frequencies. Thus, very short tonal stimuli are not used in audiological testing since a patient with a sharply-sloping hearing loss *could* detect the signal on the basis of a frequency other than the target stimulus.

A related situation, where the patient responds to frequencies other than the intended signal, can occur in the case of distortion. Most typical is harmonic distortion, where frequencies at some octave intervals above the signal frequency are inadvertently introduced by the equipment used in testing. Audiometer calibration procedures are designed, in part, to maintain distortion within low and tolerable limits.

It is recognized that the auditory system, itself, is non-linear. Investigations of auditory non-linearities have, in the past, often concerned the perception of pitch associated with temporal characteristics of the stimulus (as contrasted with pitch associated with energy at a particular frequency) or saturation of the neural (physiological) response as the intensity of stimulation increases (Goldstein 1967; Green 1976). Non-linearities within the auditory system that are associated with the simultaneity of two or more stimulus frequencies ('two-tone suppression') have been identified and this information is now being incorporated into sophisticated models of auditory processing of complex stimuli such as speech (Sachs and Young 1980).

CONCLUDING STATEMENT

This chapter has demonstrated that many standard audiologic tests are based on principles of psychoacoustic performance. As stated at the outset, it has only touched on fundamentals of hearing that pertain to clinical audiologic procedures. Until recently, there has usually been a wide gulf between test procedures and topics considered important by clinicians and psychoacousticians, but in some settings, the distance is narrowing. As more sophisticated sensory aids for the hearing impaired are developed and as diagnostic tests for special auditory and neurological disorders become more elegant and more illuminating it is likely that the interests of clinicians and psychoacousticians will move somewhat closer.

REFERENCES

BERLIN, C. I and MCNEIL, M. R. (1976). Dichotic listening. In *Contemporary issues in experimental phonetics* (ed. N. J. Lass) pp. 327–87. Academic Press, New York.

BILGER, R. C. (1977). Evaluation of subjects presently fitted with implanted auditory prostheses. *Ann. Otol. Rhinol. Lar.* Suppl. 38, **86**, 1–176.

DALLOS, P., RYAN, A., HARRIS, D., MC GEE, T., and ÖZDAMAR, Ö. (1977). Cochlear frequency selectivity in the presence of hair cell damage. In *Psychophysics and physiology of hearing* (ed. E. F. Evans and J. P. Wilson) pp. 249–58. Academic Press, London.

DANAHER, E. M., OSBERGER, M. J., and PICKETT, J. M. (1973). Discrimination of formant frequency transitions in synthetic vowels. *J. Speech Hearing Res.* **16,** 439–51.

ELLIOTT, L. L. (1975). Temporal and masking phenomena in persons with sensorineural hearing loss. *Audiology* **14,** 336–53.

GOLDSTEIN, J. L. (1967). Auditory non-linearity. *J. acoust. Soc. Am.* **41,** 676–89.

GREEN, D. M. (1976). *An introduction to hearing.* Lawrence Erlbaum, Hillsdale, New Jersey.

—— and SWETS, J. A. (1966). *Signal detection theory and psychophysics.* Wiley, New York.

HAWKINS, D. B. and WIGHTMAN, F. L. (1978). Interaural time discrimination in cochlear-impaired listeners. *J. acoust. Soc. Am.* **63** S1–S52.

HIRSH, I. J. (1952). *The measurement of hearing.* McGraw Hill, New York.

OLSEN, W. and NOFFSINGER, P. D. (1976). Masking level differences for cochlear and brainstem lesions. *Ann. Otol. Rhinol. Lar.* **85**, 820–5.

PICKETT, J. M. (1980). *The sounds of speech communication.* University Park Press, Baltimore.

SACHS, M. B. and YOUNG, E. D. (1980). Effects of non-linearities on speech encoding in the auditory nerve. *J. acoust. Soc. Am.* **68,** 858–75.

SANDERS, J. W. (1972). Masking. In *Handbook of clinical audiology* (ed. J. Katz) pp. 111–42. Williams and Wilkins, Baltimore.

SCHARF, B. (1970). Critical bands. In *Foundations of modern auditory theory* (ed. J. V. Tobias) Vol. I, pp. 157–202. Academic Press, New York.

—— (1978). Comparison of normal and impaired hearing II. Frequency analysis, speech perception. *Scand. Audiol.* Suppl. 6, 49–106.

—— and MEISELMAN, C. H. (1977). Critical bandwidth at high intensities. In

Psychophysics and physiology of hearing (ed. E. F. Evans and J. P. Wilson) pp. 221–32. Academic Press, London.
STEVENS, S. S.. (1966). Matching functions between loudness and ten other continua. *Percept. Psychophys.* **1**, 5–8.
STUDDERT-KENNEDY, M. (1976). Speech perception. in *Contemporary issues in experimental phonetics* (ed. N. J. Lass) pp. 243–93. Academic Press, New York.
SWETS, J. A. (1961). Is there a sensory threshold? *Science,* **134**, 168–77.
—— (1964). *Signal detection and recognition by human observers.* Wiley, New York.
WIGHTMAN, F. L., MCGEE, T., and KRAMER, M. (1977). Factors influencing frequency-selectivity in normal and hearing impaired listeners. In *Psychophysics and physiology of hearing* (ed. E. F. Evans and J. P. Wilson) pp. 294–306. Academic Press, London.

6 Acoustics in audiology

J. J. KNIGHT

It may be claimed that in many audiological studies it is as necessary to have a basic understanding of acoustics as it is of the anatomy, physiology, and pathology of the ear. Although in the past many otologists concentrated their interest on the ear itself, it is in the past half century since active collaboration was established with physicists and electrical engineers with acoustical knowledge that rapid progress in audiology has been achieved, leading to much more accurate diagnosis and hence to better, and more appropriate, treatment than was possible previously.

Today, the total breadth of acoustical studies is enormous (Fig. 6.1.) and covers from the lowest infrasonic to the highest ultrasonic frequencies, from geophysical exploration to fish detection, and from design of concert halls to means of examining blood flow or to the specification of improved hearing aids for particularly difficult cases. While the same underlying concepts apply in all these fields, this chapter is devoted to a brief description of the more important fundamentals of acoustics that have a bearing on audiology. Even so as the breadth of coverage of acoustics necessary for audiology is wide, the treatment here must be correspondingly limited. This is not necessarily disadvantageous as none of the principles described are new and are to be found described in most acoustics textbooks from Rayleigh (1877), Wood (1940), Richardson (1947, 1953), Beranek (1949), Stephens and Bate (1966), etc. For terminology the reader is referred to British Standard 661 (1969).

PHYSICAL ACOUSTICS

Acoustics is the name for the science of sound and it is a branch of physics. Sound is a form of energy like electricity, light, and heat. Sound energy is converted eventually into heat, although the quantity of heat produced by normal sounds is very small. Sounds usually can be traced to something vibrating, such as a tuning fork, the diaphragm of an earphone, or the cone of a loudspeaker. Such vibrating surfaces impart energy to the surrounding air and waves consisting of compressions and rarefactions travel outwards as *progressive waves* from the source of sound at a speed (velocity) determined by the elasticity of the air (proportional to its pressure) and its density. In air at 20° C, the speed of sound is 344 metres per second (1127 feet per second or 768 m.p.h.); *supersonic* is the term reserved for speeds of travel greater than this. The speed of sound, c is given by the product of the frequency, f and the wavelength, λ.

$$c = f\lambda.$$

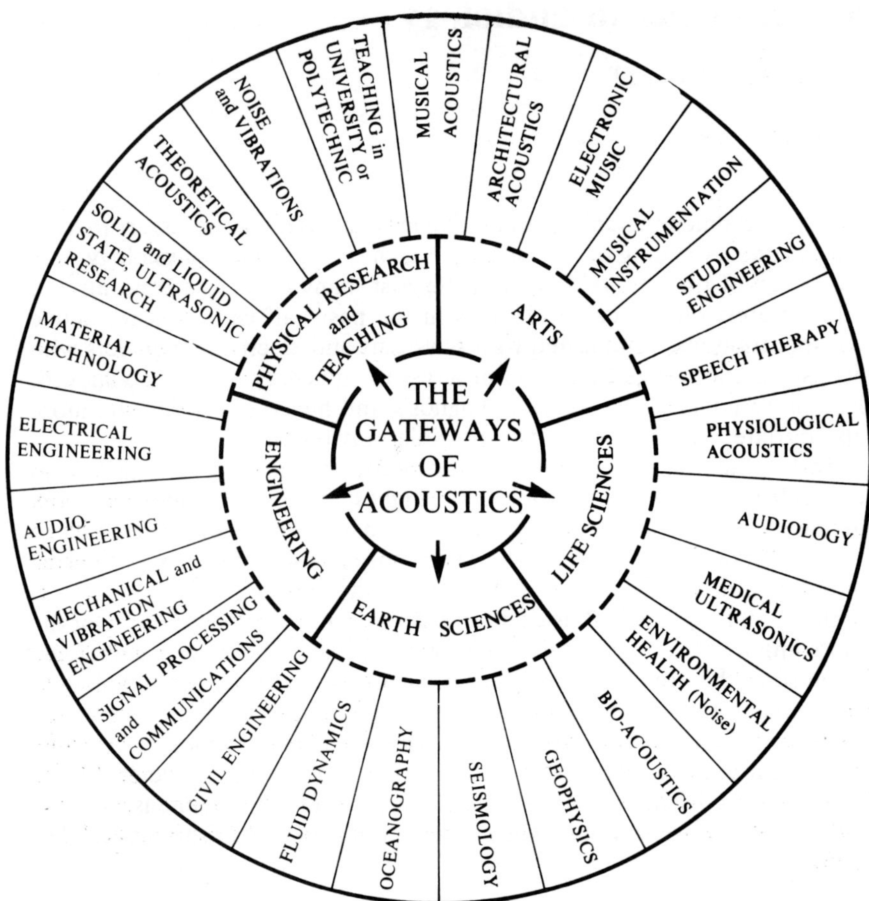

Fig. 6.1. Acoustics today. (By courtesy of the Institute of Acoustics.)

Sound can, of course, be propagated in other gases, liquids, and solids at different speeds, but it is not propagated at all in a vacuum where there are no particles to transmit the motion. Sound waves are *longitudinal* as the direction of particle vibration is in the direction of travel of the waves. Waves on the surface of water caused by a sudden disturbance give a two-dimensional picture of the situation except that they are *transverse*, i.e. the particle motion is at right angles to the direction of wave travel. It is convenient to visualize sound waves in the same way by plotting the *particle displacement* at right angles to the direction of the wave, but it must be understood that the actual sound waves are longitudinal.

Reference was made earlier to a tuning fork which has a special place in audiological assessment because it can be made to vibrate at its own characteristic single frequency to produce a *pure tone*. The waveform of the sound which results is smooth and continuous as the sine function in trigonometry (the ratio of the side opposite the particular angle, to the hypotenuse in a right-angled triangle). Hence it is known as a *sinusoidal wave*. The time of one complete vibration is called a *period*, e.g. for of a pure tone of frequency 500 vibrations per second, or hertz (Hz), the period is 1/500th of a second, or 2 milliseconds (ms). The motion of the vibrating tuning fork dies away as its energy is transferred to sound energy in the surrounding air. Sound becomes less intense the greater the distance from the source because the available energy is spread over spheres of increasingly greater radius centred on the source; *intensity* is measured by the amount of energy passing in one second through an area of one square centimetre at right angles to the direction of travel.

The familiar *Inverse Square Law* of physics applies to the decrease of sound intensity, I with distance, r when there are no reflecting surfaces as in a *free field* where:

$$\frac{I_1}{I_2} = \frac{r_2^2}{r_1^2}.$$

In terms of sound pressure, P the pressure varies inversely with distance. In audiology, it is convenient to use the logarithmic decibel (dB) scale in these measurements as such a scale represents the behaviour of the ear better than a linear one. Then the two intensities, I_1 and I_2 are said to be separated by an interval of x decibels when

$$x = 10 \log_{10} \frac{I_1}{I_2} = 10 \log_{10} \frac{p_1^2}{p_2^2}$$

$$= 20 \log_{10} \frac{p_1}{p_2}$$

where p_1 and p_2 represent the corresponding sound pressures. One decibel change in sound is a pressure change of approximately 12 per cent, corresponding to a change in intensity of 26 per cent.

In air, p_2 the reference sound pressure is taken as 2×10^{-5}Pa and the resulting calculation gives the *sound pressure level* (SPL).

In terms of decibels, application of the Inverse Square Law means a reduction of 6 dB on doubling the distance from the source, or 10 dB when distance is trebled—a useful rule which is applicable to free-field tests of hearing, say, at distances of up to 5 m from the source in a large room well treated with sound absorbent.

In its application to the use of tuning forks in hearing tests, the decibel unit enables otological tuning forks to be calibrated with regard to their decay characteristics so that a particular fork may be found to have a decay of 5 dB/s in air, and 7 dB/s when pressed in a standard way to the mastoid process. Hence, with the aid of a stop watch, an examiner with normal hearing can assess the difference in thresholds of a subject with impaired hearing, frequency by frequency with a series of calibrated forks.

In sound propagation, the wavelength is important for, when the wavelength is much larger than an obstacle the sound bends round it. This is the case with audible sound obstructed by a barrier such as a picket fence, where the sound bends round the individual obstacles, illustrating the so-called *diffraction* of sound. However, with higher frequencies (i.e. with shorter wavelengths), sound is reflected or scattered in many directions and a shadow is formed. Thus walls can be used as barriers against high-frequency noises.

Sound is reflected wherever there is a change in the *characteristic impedance,* Z (the product of the density, ϱ and the speed of sound, c) of the medium in which it travels.

$$Z = \varrho c$$

The term *specific acoustic impedance* refers to the characteristic impedance of a medium at a point in a progressive plane wave propagated in a free field. Almost complete reflection takes place at a gas–liquid interface whereas transmission from liquids to solids is easier because there is less difference in the characteristic impedances. An *echo* is heard when the reflected sound returns to the listener's ear after approximately 1/15 s. With propagation in air, this involves a total path length of about 23 m or a distance to the reflecting object of 11.5 m.

With acoustic impedance measurements of the ear for diagnostic use as described in subsequent chapters, the quantity that is measured, Z_A is the ratio of sound pressure, p to *volume velocity, V*.

$$Z_A = \frac{p}{V}.$$

Volume velocity is the product of particle velocity and effective area.

As in the analogous electrical case, acoustic impedance consists of *acoustic resistance,* R_A and *acoustic reactance,* X_A where

$$Z_A = \sqrt{(R_A{}^2 + X_A{}^2)}$$

and the phase angle, θ between the two components of impedance is given by

$$\theta = \tan^{-1}\frac{X_A}{R_A}.$$

Modern acoustic impedance instruments used for diagnostic measurement of the middle ear often measure in terms of the reciprocal of impedance which is termed *admittance*, Y_A. The corresponding components of admittance are *conductance*, G_A and *susceptance*, B_A where

$$Y_A = \sqrt{(G_A{}^2 + B_A{}^2)}.$$

A violin string when bowed emits a particular frequency, as does a tuning fork when struck on a resilient pad, and an organ pipe when air is blown across its mouth to produce a wide band of frequencies of which one is accentuated by the pipe. These are examples of *resonant frequencies*. In the organ pipe the phenomenon can be shown to be caused by the interaction of two progressive sound waves of equal intensity and the same frequency, travelling in opposite directions to produce a *stationary* wave. The incident progressive wave originating from the mouth is almost totally reflected at the far end and travels back along the tube causing the interaction. Special conditions occur at points separated by distances separated by one quarter of a wavelength where positions of maximum air particle movement alternate with points of almost no movement. The effect is an undesirable one if it occurs in rooms where it can cause regions of reduced sound intensity alternating with others of high intensity.

ROOM ACOUSTICS

In ordinary rooms, much of the sound energy is reflected from the walls, floor, and ceiling. The consequence is that sound heard at any point in the room consists of a sound that has travelled by the direct path from the source, together with many other reflections from different surfaces that arrive later after corresponding intervals of time. The Inverse Square Law no longer applies to this situation where there are significant reflections. In the ultimate situation, sound waves can travel equally in all directions with the result that the sound pressure is the same everywhere in the room. A perfectly *diffuse* sound field is then said to exist. Special reverberation-rooms create these conditions with reflective wall surfaces which are deliberately made non-parallel to prevent formation of stationary waves.

If a sound is generated in a room with perfectly reflecting walls, there will be hardly any dissipation of energy and the intensity will continue to build up as long as the source is maintained. In the opposite case of a room with completely absorbent walls (an *anechoic* room), there will be no reflections and the Inverse Square Law will apply.

In most situations in ordinary rooms, there will be considerable wall reflections but also some absorption in the carpets and furnishings. The reflections from the boundaries will cause the sound to persist after the source has stopped until the energy is dissipated. This persistence of sound is known as *reverberation*. It is measured by the *reverberation time*, T, which is the time taken for the intensity to fall to one millionth of its original value, i.e. to fall by 60 decibels.

In simple terms:

$$T = \frac{k \times \text{Volume}}{\text{Total Absorption}} \quad \text{seconds}$$

where k = 0.16 for measurements in metres
0.05 for measurements in feet.

Absorption is specified in terms of an *absorption coefficient*, A which is the ratio of the absorbed energy to the incident energy. The relation to the *reflection coefficient*, R is

$$A = 1 - R.$$

Whereas the absorption coefficient of an open window is unity at all frequencies, special acoustic tiles mounted on wooden battens will absorb only 85 per cent of the energy of sound (i.e. $A = 0.85$) at frequencies of 1 kHz and above, and only 50 per cent at 250 Hz. An unpainted brick wall will only absorb 5 per cent of the sound at 1 kHz and 3 per cent at 250 Hz.

The design of concert halls and auditoria requires detailed consideration of the above acoustical principles but a number of uncertain factors are also involved as illustrated by some expensive constructions of recent times which have not been eminently satisfactory. The basic acoustical requirements in auditoria include adequate loudness with no perceptible echoes and no undue reverberation for speech, but with a suitable amount of reverberation for music; good sound exclusion is required to keep out external noise. The critical distance of just less than 12 m is important in relation to ceiling height and absorbents are often applied to the back of the hall and to the upper parts of the walls to suppress echoes.

In London, St Paul's Cathedral is notable for its reverberation time of 11 s when empty, which is reduced to 6 s with a full congregation. Here also, the Albert Hall echoes challenged generations of acousticians for almost a century until the recent installation of suspended diffusers provided a solution. On the other hand, the Royal Festival Hall, sited alongside a main railway line crossing the river Thames in 1951, was well received by the critics, but it has been improved lately by the installation of many electro-acoustic channels of *assisted resonance* to control the reverberation time at a corresponding number of frequencies.

Optimum reverberation times for concert halls for speech and music vary between 1 and 2 s according to size. For music alone, the reverberation time should be less. In broadcasting studios for speech 0.75 s is a suitable reverberation time. It was half a century ago when Knudsen (1929) showed that speech intelligibility decreased by roughly 6 per cent for every increase of one second in the reverberation time at 500 Hz, but this and other basic acoustical facts are still occasionally overlooked by those responsible for constructing new buildings, particularly those for specialized use. The following section deals with the design of audiometric rooms while for the design of educational facilities for deaf children the reader is referred to Fourcin, Joy, Kennedy, Knight, Knowles, Knox, Martin, Mort, Penton, Poole, Powell, and Watson (1980).

AUDIOMETRIC ROOMS

Extremely quiet conditions have to be created in order to determine normal hearing thresholds and usually the ideal environment is found only in research centres such as the National Physical Laboratory, the Building Research Establishment, etc. The cost of a single anechoic test facility is very high today. When hearing tests are to be performed on patients with impairment of hearing, often less perfect acoustic conditions can be tolerated and a reasonable compromise is to ensure that the overall sound level inside audiometric test rooms does not exceed 30 dB(A). However, it should be mentioned that such a level is insufficiently quiet for determination of air conduction thresholds of a normal ear for the lowest test frequencies even using earphones (as in tests of the better ear in cases of unilateral hearing impairment). If the tests are conducted not with earphones but in a free field, the ambient noise must be much less, as it also must be for measurement of low-frequency bone-conduction thresholds. Financial considerations demand this compromise, but even 30 dB(A) is difficult to achieve and calls for special constructional techniques.

It is the lower frequencies of general ambient noise that are the most difficult to exclude but, if sufficient care is taken to reduce the octave-band sound pressure levels below 250 Hz, the levels in the higher frequency bands will tend to look after themselves. The contributions from the 63 and 125 Hz octave bands should be reduced to less than 35 dB SPL. To achieve these levels requires the employment of fully-isolated rooms, or double-box structures, in which an inner room is supported on resilient mountings to attenuate structure-borne noise; the walls being supported on the floating floor, and the ceiling by walls. A suitable size of inner room for general audiometric use is at least 2.4 × 2.4 m with a height of 2.1 m. For testing young children, the room should be at least 6.3 × 4.8 m with a height of 2.1 m.

The inner room is protected at all parts by a double structure, made as separate and as massive as possible. Access is provided by massive air-tight doors in each of the two leaves. If reveals are constructed between the door frames, they must not provide a rigid connection between the leaves. This also applies to window reveals. Lining the walls and ceiling of the inner room with sound-absorbent material and carpeting the floors helps to attenuate any sound which enters the room, but only to the extent of about 5 dB; it also reduces sounds created in the room and simplifies speech communication with hearing-impaired patients, particularly with those using hearing aids. To meet these requirements the reverberation time of the inner room should be less than 0.5 s at 500 Hz.

The most difficult task is to provide ventilation without loss of insulation, but ventilation is essential because the patient, at least one audiology technician and a quantity of electronic apparatus will be enclosed in the heat—as well as sound—insulated, room. In the course of an average test session of duration, say 30 minutes, conditions can otherwise become extremely hot and unpleasant, and so cause erroneous results to be obtained. Ducted mechanical ventilation will be required with an air flow of approximately 2700 l/min for the inner room of minimum size designated for general use, but the ducts must not form a solid bridge between the two leaves of the structure. Moreover, the duct system and its construction must not permit the passage of air-borne sound from the outside to the inner room to a significantly greater extent than can occur through the general double structure. This often entails the use of heavy-wall ducting and of sound-absorbent duct linings. The possibility of noise passing along the ducts must be borne in mind, either from outside the building, or from the mechanical ventilation equipment, or from another room connected to the system. The only form of protection is sound-absorbent lining of the ducts and/or the introduction of suitably designed splitters. Noise caused by air turbulence in passing through grilles must be minimized. The design of duct systems is an expert task and specialist advice should be obtained.

Prefabricated acoustic booths suitable for audiometry are available commercially from several manufacturers. Locally constructed booths are not recommended as commercial products have the advantage of a guaranteed performance. Typical noise reductions obtained from prefabricated booths are from 20 dB in the 31.5 and 63 Hz octave bands to 50 dB or more in the 500 and 1000 Hz octave bands, with still greater reduction at higher frequencies. Because of the limited attenuation for low frequencies it is necessary to site audiometric booths in areas of low ambient noise, preferably where the noise is less than 40 dB(A). Weight of the booth is another consideration from the point of view of the strength of floor on which it is placed. A booth of internal floor area 1.8 m × 1.8 m can weigh up to 2000 kg. Although booths are available with floor areas as small as 0.9 × 1.1 m, they are not recommended for normal use.

Adequate illumination must be provided within the test room or booth. Filament lamps cause less electrical interference with high gain amplifiers, used for amplifying electrophysiological signals in audiological tests, than do fluorescent tubes, but filament lamps have the disadvantage of generating more heat. On the other hand, if fluorescent light sources are employed, the ballast or starting choke should be mounted remotely from the inner test room.

Pure-tone audiometry is normally required to be operated by an audiology technician within the test room with the patient and the apparatus. However, with the increasing employment of recorded speech audiometry and self-recording (Békésy) audiometry, a certain amount of mechanical noise is generated by apparatus which consequently must be operated from a lobby outside the test room. An ample ventilated space, for apparatus and a technician, of at least 3.5 × 1.8 m must be provided for the lobby with multiple electrical screened cable connections as dictated by the equipment to carry various forms of communication, transmission of signals from lobby to test room and vice versa. Observation is often desirable either through a double-glazed plate-glass window of appropriate acoustic design (which may be one-way) or by a closed-circuit television link; the latter will require extra suitably screened connections to avoid electrical interference with the audiometric channels.

Additional points needing special consideration are provision of an electrical mains supply of at least six thirteen-ampere socket outlets in each test room and lobby, the decoration—particularly where young children are to be tested in larger facilities of this type, and alarms for warning the occupants in case of fire.

There exist relatively few adequately-designed test rooms in hospitals at the present time, reference is made to those designed for children's tests at the Audiology Centre, Heston, Middlesex (Fisch 1963) and at the Royal National Throat, Nose and Ear Hospital and its Nuffield Hearing and Speech Centre, London. These are sufficiently quiet and are ventilated.

At the Nuffield Centre, the outer rooms are constructed with 178 mm solid concrete floor and roof, 229 mm brick internal walls, and 356 mm external walls. The rooms inside these are formed with a 152 mm concrete slab and stand on a resilient studded rubber mat mounting (Metalastic Ltd) and have 229 mm brick walls with a 152 mm concrete roof. There is a 203 mm space between the inner (test) rooms and the outer rooms which are draped with a fibreglass quilt. The test rooms, and the lobby in the outer rooms from the corridor are both lined on walls and ceiling with 19 mm acoustic tiles on wooden battens, and the floors are covered with carpet and a foam underlay. From the corridor to the lobby in the outer room there are two special doors 54 mm thick. These doors are of sandwich construction having sheets of 1 mm thick lead incorporated in the laminations and the edges of the doors are closed against the frames with magnetic plastic seals. From the lobby in the outer room to the test room, a similar pair of doors is fitted. Care was taken to ensure that there was no solid connection between the inner and outer rooms, and all electrical connections are flexible.

Measurements by the Building Research Establishment gave values of attenuation from corridor to test room of 48, 54, 52, 55.5, 58,5, 63.0, and 71.5 dB in the seven one-third octave bands centred on the frequencies 63–250 Hz. The fact that some noise originates from other regions than the corridor is indicated by measured octave band sound pressure levels in the test room of 32, 38, 18, and 12 dB in the bands centred on 31.5, 63, 125, and 250 Hz with normal quiet conditions in the corridor.

In the main building of the Royal National Throat, Nose and Ear Hospital (See Fig. 6.2.) a suite of six ventilated audiometric rooms using an inner prefabricated construction within a brick shell, gives an ambient level of 20 dB(A), with octave band levels of 44, 31, 31, and 29 dB in the bands centred on 31.5, 63, 125, and 250 Hz.

ACOUSTIC MEASUREMENTS

It would be out of place here to attempt to reproduce the wealth of information contained in the classic works on measurement of sound such as Beranek (1949) or Fletcher (1953) where most requirements for measurements of an audiological nature are included. As space is also a limiting factor, the reader is referred to the above treatises in the first instance, the information to be updated and supplemented by reference to relevant Standards and helpful literature available from the instrument manufacturers, e.g. Broch (1979) and Peterson and Gross (1974).

The basic measure of sound pressure level was defined earlier in this chapter. It is obtained using a combination of a high-quality microphone, a

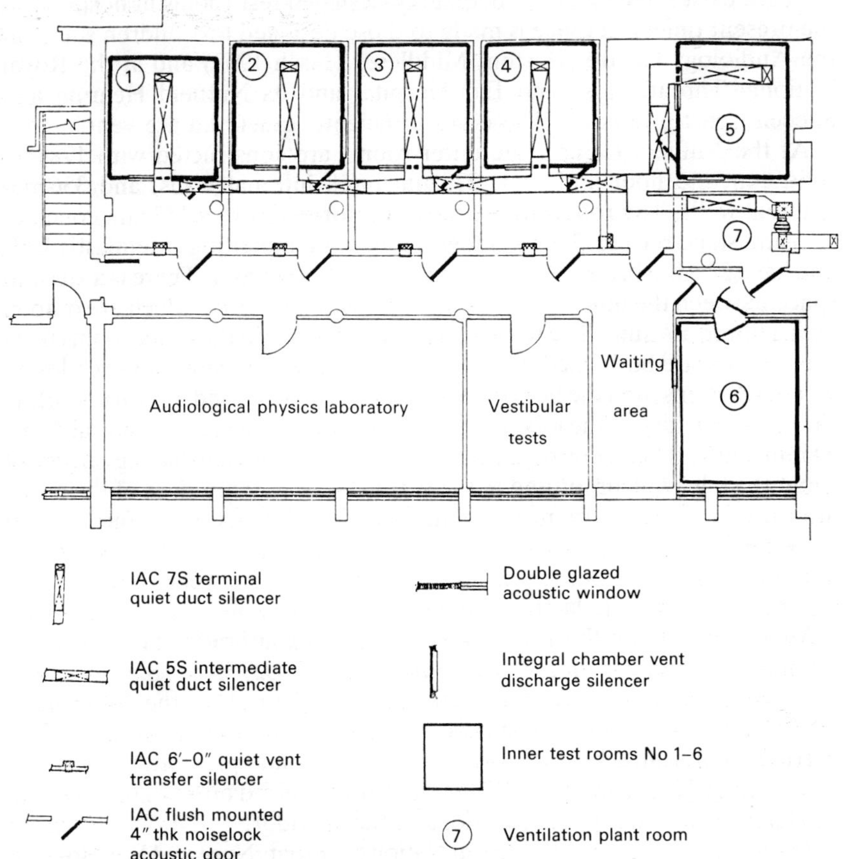

Fig. 6.2. Modular acoustic audiometric facility at the Royal National Throat, Nose and Ear Hospital, London. (Industrial Acoustics Co. Ltd.)

special amplifier, and a meter which is read visually, or a level recorder to give a permanent record. The entire apparatus must be able to deal with all frequencies in the same way, i.e. it must have a *flat frequency response*. In the laboratory there needs to be little restriction as to size of the apparatus and many comprehensive facilities are possible. For many purposes, however, a hand-held portable sound level meter is preferable. As well as measuring sound pressure level, by introduction of certain *frequency and time-weighted networks,* corresponding *sound levels* can be obtained. The frequency-weighting networks are designated A, B, C, D, and Flat while the time-weighting characteristics are Slow S, Fast F, Impulse I, and Peak. A new International Electrotechnical Commission (IEC) Publication No. 651 (1980) is a consolidated revision of the earlier Publications No. 123 (1961), 179 (1973), and 179A (1973) relating to sound level meters, precision sound level meters, and impulse sound level meters respectively. These are now superseded and the new Standard designates sound level meters in four grades of precision according to the allowed tolerances. Type O is intended as a laboratory reference standard, Type 1 is comparable to the previous precision grade, Type 2 is suitable for general field applications, while Type 3 is intended primarily for field noise survey applications.

Many acoustic measurements needed in audiology are in relation to the various effects of noise. For example, the hearing of workers exposed in the course of their occupation to industrial noise is at risk if the continuous noise level is as much as 90 dB(A) during an eight hour daily exposure, five days per week for a matter of years. In Britain, and in many other countries, an *equivalent continuous noise level*, L_{eq} of 90 dB(A) is accepted as equal to an exposure of 93 dB(A) for four hours, 96 dB(A) for two hours, etc. on the basis of equal damage being caused by the same amount of energy spread over different times. However, in the USA a 5 dB(A) allowance is made for doubling the exposure time instead of the British 3 dB(A). The different ways of calculating L_{eq} that result are given in the International Organization for Standardization (ISO) Recommendation 1999 and in the US Occupational Safety and Health Act. Personal sound exposure meters (also called noise dosemeters) are small devices that can be worn and which can integrate a function of A-weighted sound level to give the *sound exposure*. In a forthcoming IEC publication to deal with these meters, it is likely that two types will be specified to correspond with Types 2 and 3 of IEC 651. The meter is expected to be calibrated in the physical unit of pascal-squared-hours (Pa^2.h) rather than to read a percentage of a legal limit of exposure as at present. Work is also proceeding within IEC to draft a standard for integrating sound level meters.

With noises such as road traffic noise, the peak noise levels are important and an index called the *ten per cent level*, L_{10} is used. It is the level of noise in dB(A) exceeded for just 10 per cent of the time. The average L_{10} value for each hour from 06.00 hr to 24.00 hr correlates well with dissatisfaction and is referred to as L_{10} (18 hours).

When the public complain about noise from nearby factories, it is found that the annoyance depends on factors such as the loudness of the noise, in tonal components, intermittency, and duration. These are taken into account in a *corrected noise level*, CNL, based on measurements in dB(A) to which corrections are applied according to the character of the noise. A British Standard, BS 4142 (1967) describes the method of rating such noise.

Conditions for audiometric rooms were discussed earlier at length. Measurement of the resulting low ambient noise levels in the quietest rooms presents difficulty. Whittle and Evans (1972) have applied the principle of energy addition to measure the total noise from the measuring system integrated over a few minutes, first with the microphone shielded from the noise, and then with it exposed. Noise signals of up to 15 dB below the system noise level can be determined in this way.

The modern acoustics laboratory is equipped with a range of sophisticated real-time narrow-band spectrum analysers and digital frequency analysers that give real-time analysis in octave and one-third octave bands of continuous and transient sounds. In the audiological context, it is of over-riding importance to ensure that periodic checks are made on the calibration and performance of all acoustic measuring equipment. Simple checks should be performed locally at frequent intervals. Six-monthly, or at least annual, objective checks of calibration should be available at regional centres equipped with secondary standard devices such as a pistonphone or a sound-level calibrator, with traceability to national standards.

REFERENCES

BERANEK, L. L. (1949). *Acoustic measurement.* Chapman and Hall, London.

BRITISH STANDARDS INSTITUTION (1967). BS 4142. Method of rating industrial noise affecting mixed residential and industrial areas. London.

—— (1969). BS 661. Glossary of acoustical terms. London.

BROCH, J. T. (1979). *Acoustical noise measurement.* Bruel and Kjaer, Naerum, Denmark.

FISCH, L. (1963). Building an audiology centre. *J. Laryng.* **77**, 234.

FLETCHER, H. (1953). *Speech and hearing in communication.* Van Nostrand, New York.

FOURCIN, A., JOY, D., KENNEDY, M., KNIGHT, J. J., KNOWLES, S., KNOX, E. C., MARTIN, M. C., MORT, J., PENTON, J., POOLE, D., POWELL, C. A., and WATSON, T. J. (1980). Educational facilities for deaf children. *Br. J. Audiol.* Suppl. 3.

INTERNATIONAL ELECTROTECHNICAL COMMISSION (1980). IEC Recommendation. Publication 651. Instruments for the measurement of sound level (sound level meters). Geneva.

INTERNATIONAL ORGANIZATION FOR STANDARIZATION (1971). ISO Recommendation 1999. Assessment of occupational noise exposure for hearing conservation purposes. Geneva.

KNUDSEN, V. O. (1929). Hearing of speech in auditoriums. *J. acoust. Soc. Am.* **1**, 57.

PETERSEN, A. P. G. and GROSS, E. E. (1974). *Handbook of noise measurement*, 7th edn. General Radio, Concord, Mass.

RAYLEIGH, LORD (1877). *Textbook of sound*, Vols. 1 and 2. Macmillan, London.

RICHARDSON, E. G. (1947). *Textbook of sound*, 4th edn. Arnold, London.

—— (1953). *Technical aspects of sound*, Vols. 1–3. Elsevier, London.

STEPHENS, R. W. B. and BATE, A. E. (1966). *Acoustics and vibrational physics*, 2nd edn. Arnold, London.

WHITTLE, L. S. and EVANS, D. H. (1972). A new approach to the measurement of very low acoustic noise levels. *J. Sound Vibrat.* **23**, 63.

WOOD, A. (1940). *Acoustics.* Blackie, London.

7 Acoustics of normal and pathological ears

J. J. ZWISLOCKI

INTRODUCTION

The third quarter of the twentieth century witnessed the acceptance of acoustic measurements in the ear canal as a clinical method which has since become a routine part of the audiological tests. Fundamentally, the method relies on changes of acoustic characteristics produced at the tympanic membrane by middle-ear pathology and by contractions of middle-ear muscles. The potential clinical usefulness of such changes, especially with respect to the acoustic stapedius reflex, was first demonstrated by Metz (1946). Later, systematic laboratory studies allowed us to associate specific changes with specific pathologies (Zwislocki 1957b; for review see Zwislocki and Feldman 1970). The rapid growth of what may be called 'acoustic method' was made possible by acquisition of a sufficient understanding of the acoustic properties of normal and pathological ears (Békésy 1941, 1960; Zwislocki 1957b, 1962; Onchi 1961; Møller 1961), by the introduction of sufficiently simple physical principles to acoustic measurements in the ear canal (Zwislocki 1957a, 1961, 1963), and by clever exploitation of the findings of Békésy (1941), and Thomsen (1958) that the acoustic properties of the middle ear depend critically on the static pressure differential across the tympanic membrane (Terkildsen and Thomsen 1959; Terkildsen and Scott Nielsen 1960). Since intelligent diagnostic interpretation of acoustic measurements in the ear depends on an at least rudimentary knowledge of relevant mechanical and acoustical relationships and on some understanding of the acoustic middle-ear function, this chapter is devoted to these topics.

The next section concerns some of the most relevant mechanical and acoustical relationships, especially the impedance and admittance concepts, and rudiments of electromechanical and electroacoustic analogies. Readers familiar with these topics may want to omit it; however, those who are not, are encouraged to make a serious effort to master it.

THE CONCEPTS OF ACOUSTIC IMPEDANCE AND ADMITTANCE

Current measurements of acoustic middle-ear characteristics are usually made in terms of either acoustic impedance or admittance. Both measures have been borrowed from the theory of electrical networks. There, the electrical impedance measured at the input terminals of a network and called input impedance is defined as the ratio between the voltage applied to the terminals and the current flowing through them. The situation is schematized in Fig. 7.1, in which Z_E denotes the input impedance, E the input

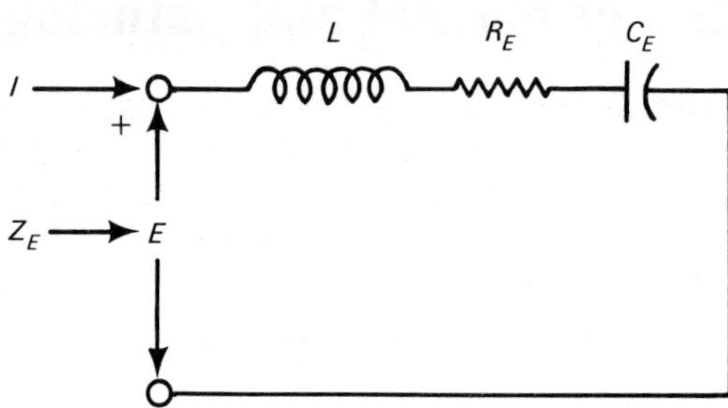

Fig. 7.1. An electrical series resonant circuit. Z_E is the input impedance; I is the input current; E is the input voltage; L is the inductance; R_E is the resistance; and C_E is the capacitance.

voltage, and I the input current. In mathematical shorthand the input impedance is defined as $Z_E = E/I$. Admittance is nothing more than reciprocal impedance: $Y_E = I/Z_E = I/E$.

Both concepts, impedance and admittance, apply only to sinusoidal currents, and their values usually change when the frequency of the current is changed. Perhaps the main difficulty in using them arises from the fact that they cannot be completely expressed in terms of real numbers we are used to in everyday life but require so-called complex numbers. This requirement may be gleaned from Fig. 7.2 in which the relationship between sinusoidal and circular motions is illustrated. In Fig. 7.2(a), E denotes the radius of a circle, which is drawn at an angle θ_E relative to the horizontal axis. Such a radius is called 'phasor' in the parlance of the electrical network theory, and the horizontal axis is called the real axis. The projection of the phasor on the vertical axis, called imaginary axis, is obtained by drawing a horizontal line between the tip of the phasor and the axis. The magnitude of the projection may be denoted by $E_\mathrm{j}(\theta_E)$, where the subscript j means that the projection is made on the imaginary axis, and (θ_E) signifies that the magnitude of the projection depends on the angle θ_E, called 'phase'. The projection $E_\mathrm{j}(\theta_E)$ on the imaginary axis is called the imaginary part of the phasor $E(\theta_E)$. The projection of this phasor on the real axis, $E_\mathrm{R}(\theta)$, is called its real part. We should remember from trigonometry that the projection of the phasor $E(\theta_E)$ on the vertical axis is equal to the product of the length of the phasor $E(\theta_E)$ and the sine of the angle θ_E:

$$E_\mathrm{j}(\theta_E) = \mathrm{j}|E| \sin \theta_E.$$

The symbol j indicates that the projection is on the imaginary axis, and $|E|$ denotes the length of the phasor $E(\theta_E)$, which is independent of the angle. Similarly, the horizontal projection of the phasor is

$$E_\mathrm{R}(\theta_E) = |E| \cos \theta_E.$$

In the symbolic phasor notation the phasor E can be expressed as the sum of its real and imaginary parts: $E = E_\mathrm{R} + E_\mathrm{j}$. In the trigonometric notation, we obtain

$$E(\theta_E) = |E| \cos \theta_E + \mathrm{j}|E| \sin \theta_E.$$

The j symbol associated with the imaginary part alerts us to the fact that the real and imaginary components of the phasor E stand at right angles to each other and cannot be added arithmetically. From trigonometry we know that the length of the phasor E squared is equal to the sum of the squares of its horizontal and vertical components

$$|E|^2 = (|E|^2 \cos^2\theta_E + |E|^2 \sin^2\theta_E).$$

Because the phasor E is composed of a real and an imaginary part, which are at right angles to each other and cannot be added arithmetically, it is not described by a real number but by a number called 'complex'.

Imagine now that the phasor E rotates around its point of origin anticlockwise with an angular velocity ω. Under these conditions, the angle θ_E is given by the relationship $\theta_E = \omega t + \theta_{E0}$, where θ_{E0} means the angle from which the rotation begins. For a starting angle of 0, $\theta_E = \omega t$, or $\omega = \theta_E/t$, which means that ω is measured in angular units per second. Traditionally,

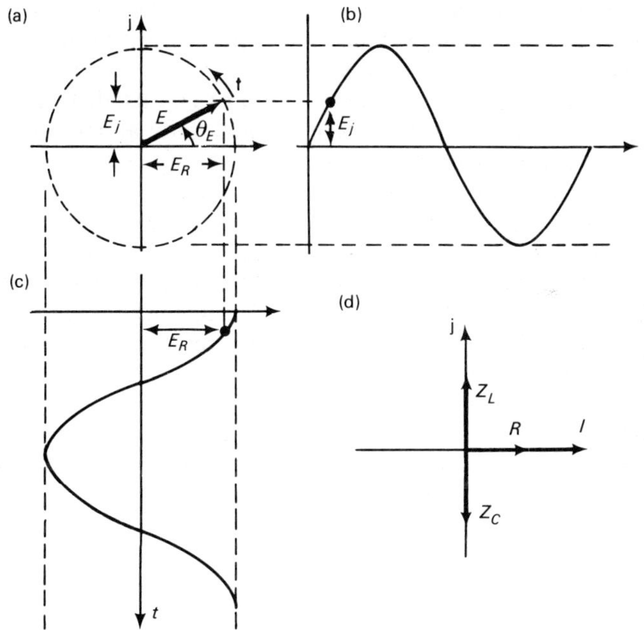

Fig. 7.2. The relationship between circular and sinusoidal motions. (a) Circular motion: E = *phasor;* θ_E is the angle between the phasor and the real axis; E_R is the projection of the phasor on the real axis; E_j is the projection of the phasor on the imaginary axis; arrow labelled with the letter t is the direction of circular motion with a uniform angular velocity $\omega = 2\pi f$, where $\pi \simeq 3.14$; and f is the frequency of rotation in cycles per second, or Hertz. (b) Projection of phasor E on the imaginary axis as a function of time of rotation. (c) Projection of phasor E on the real axis as a function of time of rotation. (d) Phasor diagram showing the angular relationships among the impedances of a resistance (R), an inductance (Z_L), and a capacitance (Z_C); I indicates the current phasor which serves as a reference for the impedance phasors.

radians rather than degrees are used as the angular units. An angle of 360° is equal to 2π or about 6.28 radians. When we take for $t = T$ the time required for a full rotation of 360°, or 2π radians, $\omega = 2\pi/T$. The time T required for a full rotation is called a period. The inverse value of the period gives the number of full rotations per second, or frequency f. Consequently, $\omega = 2\pi f$. It should be clear that, for an assumed rotating phasor E, its vertical and horizontal projections are $E_j = j|E| \sin (\omega t + \theta_{E0})$ and $E_R = |E| \cos (\omega t + \theta_{E0})$. When these projections are plotted as functions of time, as this is done in Figs. 7.2(b) and 7.2(c), sinusoidal curves result. Such curves can be seen when a sinusoidal voltage is projected on the screen of an oscilloscope.

To understand the concept of impedance and of its reciprocal, admittance, sufficiently well for meaningful acoustic measurements in the ear, one additional theoretical step is necessary. We may assume that phasor $E(\theta_E)$ in Fig. 7.2(a) symbolizes a voltage amplitude associated with a phase that is determined by the initial condition (θ_{E0}), an angular velocity ω, and time t: $\theta_E = \omega t + \theta_{E0}$. Projection of $E(\theta)$ on the horizontal axis gives us the instantaneous value of the voltage. Similarly, current amplitude associated with a time dependent phase may be indicated by a phasor I with a phase $\theta_I = \omega t + \theta_{I0}$. Since the electrical impedance is defined as the ratio of voltage to current, we must have $Z_E = E(\theta_E)/I(\theta_I)$. But what is the ratio of two phasors? The phasor algebra tells us that it is a phasor itself. Its magnitude is equal to the ratio of the magnitudes of the numerator and the denominator, $|Z| = |E|/|I|$, and its phase to the difference between the numerator and denominator phases, $\theta_Z = \theta_E - \theta_I = \omega t + \theta_{E0} - \omega t - \theta_{I0}$. Since the ωt terms cancel each other, we have $\theta_Z = \theta_{E0} - \theta_{I0}$. This means that the angle, or phase, of an impedance phasor is independent of time.

Measurements on electrical networks show that a voltage applied to an electrical resistance produces a current that is in phase with the voltage ($\theta_{I0} = \theta_{E0}$). Accordingly, the impedance of a resistance is a phasor with a phase 0. Such a phasor coincides with the real axis and can be described by a real number, $Z_R = R = |E|/|I|$. On the other hand, voltage applied to an inductance generates a current that is delayed by a quarter period (90°, $\pi/2$) relative to the voltage. As a consequence, the impedance of an inductance is a phasor with a phase $\pi/2$, $Z_L = j\omega L = E/I$. The symbol L indicates the magnitude of the inductance. The inclusion of $\omega = 2\pi f$ means that the impedance is directly proportional to current frequency; the inclusion of j signifies that the impedance has a phase, or angle, $+\pi/2$. Voltage applied to a capacitance produces a current that precedes the voltage by a quarter period. Accordingly, Z_C, the impedance of the capacitance is described by the phasor $Z_C = -j/wC_E$. It is inversely proportional to the current frequency and has a phase of $-\pi/2$. The positions of the three impedance phasors together with the position of the reference current phasor are indicated in Fig. 7.2(d).

In Fig. 7.1 an electrical circuit is shown in which an inductance, L, a resistance, R_E, and a capacitance, C_E, are shown connected in series. The input impedance, Z_i, of such a circuit is equal to the sum of the impedances of its elements — $Z_i = Z_L + Z_C + Z_R$. Introducing the expressions for the component impedances defined above, we obtain

$$Z_i = j\omega L - \frac{j}{\omega C_E} + R_E.$$

This can be simplified to

$$Z_i = \underbrace{j(\omega L - \frac{1}{\omega C_E})}_{\text{Reactance}} + \underbrace{R_E}_{\text{Resistance}}$$

since the impedances of the inductance and capacitance are on the same imaginary axis and can be arithmetically subtracted from each other. Note that, when $\omega L = 1/\omega C_E$, the imaginary part of the impedance disappears, the impedance becomes real and goes through a minimum. This is the point at which the current through the circuit is maximum. Of course, when the impedance is minimum, its reciprocal value, the admittance, is maximum.

When the network elements are connected in parallel, as shown in Fig. 7.3, the admittances rather than impedances sum

$$Y_i = \underbrace{j(\omega C - \frac{1}{\omega L})}_{\text{Susceptance}} + \underbrace{\frac{1}{R_E}}_{\text{Conductance}}.$$

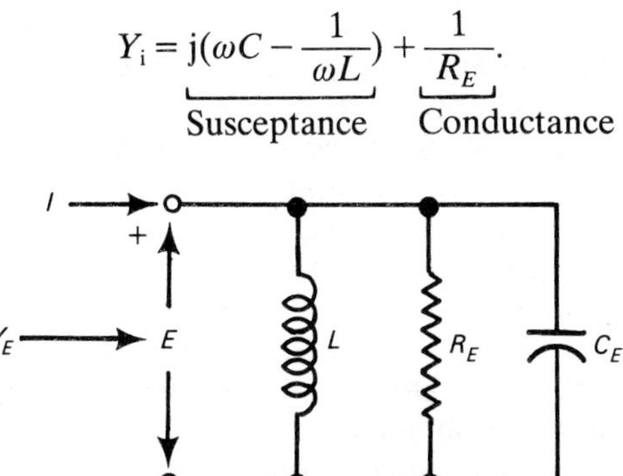

Fig. 7.3. An electrical parallel (antiresonance) circuit. Y_E is the input admittance; I is the input current; E is the input voltage; L is the inductance; R_E is the resistance; and C_E is the capacitance.

Again, the admittances of the capacitance and inductance can be subtracted from each other arithmetically. When they are equal, they cancel each other completely and the admittance becomes equal to the conductance, $1/R_E$, which is equal to the reciprocal value of the resistance. Under these conditions, the admittance is minimum and its reciprocal, the impedance, is maximum. Note the reciprocal effects of the series and parallel connections of the network elements. When the inductive and capacitive components are equal in a series network and cancel each other, the impedance becomes minimum. This effect is called resonance. When the two components cancel each other in a parallel network, the impedance becomes maximum—an effect often called antiresonance.

Physical measurements have shown that fricative resistance, inertance of a mechanical mass, and compliance of a spring have analogous effects to the electrical resistance, inductance, and capacitance, when mechanical force is regarded as an analogue of electrical voltage and mechanical velocity as a analogue of electrical current. By the same token, mechanical impedance, defined as a ratio between mechanical force and velocity, becomes an analogue of the electrical impedance — $Z_M = F/U$. Of course, mechanical admittance is the reciprocal of mechanical impedance — $Y_M = 1/Z_M$. Remember that, by analogy to electrical networks, a mechanical impedance, or admittance, is composed of an imaginary and a real part and cannot be described by a real number, except at the point of resonance or antiresonance.

Similarly to a mechanical impedance, we can define an acoustic impedance. The difference is that, in acoustics, the impedance is defined as a ratio between sound pressure and volume velocity rather than between force and velocity. The relationships between the acoustic and mechanical impedances and between velocity and volume velocity are illustrated in Fig. 7.4(a). The mechanical force acting on the diaphragm with the effective surface area A is equal to sound pressure, P, multiplied by the effective area. In Fig. 7.4(a) the effective area A is equal to the projection of the geometric area of the curved diaphragm on a plane perpendicular to the direction of motion. We have for the force $F = P \cdot A$. The volume velocity is equal to the volume displacement of the diaphragm per second. If the whole diaphragm, with the exception of its suspension, moves with the same velocity U, the volume velocity of the diaphragm is equal to the product of this velocity and the effective area — $\hat{V} = AU$. We can express the mechanical impedance measured at the diaphragm as $Z_M = F/U = P \cdot A/U$. When we divide the rightmost fraction by the effective surface area A, we obtain $Z_S = P/U$. This is called specific impedance. Dividing the specific impedance in turn by the effective surface area, we obtain the acoustic impedance $Z_A = P/U \cdot A = P/\hat{V}$. In words, the acoustic impedance is defined as the ratio between sound pressure and volume velocity. It is the impedance measured in the ear canal by the currently available instrumentation.

Whereas mechanical impedance elements are determined by fricative resistance, mass inertance, and spring compliance, the elements of acoustic impedance result from geometric configurations through which acoustic gas oscillations are transmitted. When air flows through a porous material or a narrow passage, the flow is opposed by a fricative resistance. A narrow passage or tube has, in addition, an inertance effect. Dilation in a conduit acts as a compliance. It is well known that air enclosed in a container acts like a spring. The arrangement of Fig. 7.4(a) represents a mechano-acoustic system. The mechanical part consists of the mass (mechanical inertance) of the diaphragm and of the compliance and resistance of its suspension. The acoustic part is made up of the compliance of the cavity behind the diaphragm, the inertance and resistance of a narrow passage between this cavity and a second cavity, and the compliance of the second cavity. The

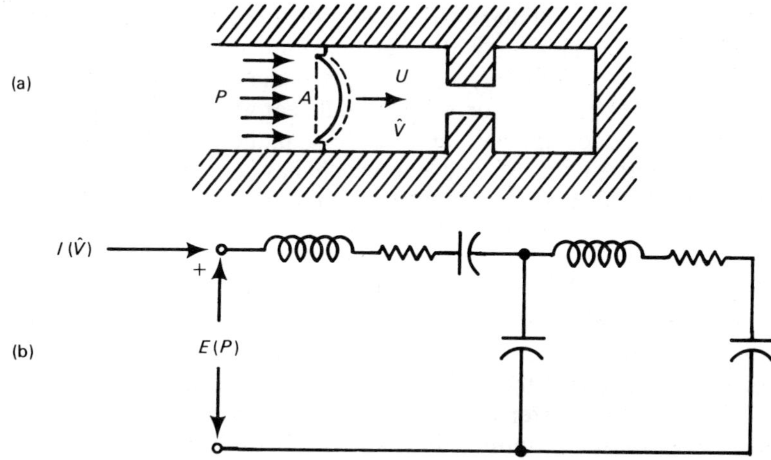

Fig. 7.4. A mechano-acoustic system and its electrical analogue. (a) The mechano-acoustic system. P is the sound pressure at the diaphragm indicated by the heavy curved line (the dashed curved line indicates the mode of diaphragm displacement); A is the effective area of the diaphragm (projection of the diaphragm on a plane perpendicular to the direction of motion of the diaphragm); U is the velocity of motion of the diaphragm; $\hat{V}$ is the volume velocity of the diaphragm ($U \cdot A$). (b) The electrical analogue. I is the input current which is the analogue of volume velocity; E is the input voltage which is the analogue of sound pressure. The first three series elements (inductance, resistance, and capacitance) are the analogues of the acoustic inertance, resistance, and compliance of the diaphragm. The numerical values of the acoustic impedance elements are obtained by measuring the mechanical mass, resistance, and compliance of the diaphragm and dividing the obtained values by the effective area of the diaphragm squared (A^2). The first shunt capacitance from the left is the analogue of the acoustic compliance of the volume of air behind the diaphragm. The acoustic compliance is numerically equal to $C_A = V/\varrho.c^2$, where V is the volume of air; ϱ is the density of air; and c is the speed of sound propagation in the air. The series inductance and resistance following the shunt capacitance are the analogues of the acoustic inertance and resistance of the constriction separating the two volumes of air. The inertance is equal to $M_A = \varrho l'/A_c$, where A_c is the cross-sectional area of the constriction and l' is the effective length of the constriction ($l' \simeq l + 0.85\, d$, where d is the diameter of the constriction). The resistance, $R_A = 128\, \mu l'/\pi d^4$, where μ is the viscosity of air. The second shunt capacitance is the analogue of the acoustic compliance of the second volume of air.

electrical analogue of this mechano-acoustical system is shown in Fig. 7.4(b). Note that it consists of two series-resonance circuits separated by a shunt capacitance. The shunt capacitance, together with the second resonance circuit, has the effect of producing an antiresonance. More generally, as the current frequency is increased gradually, the input impedance of such a network is first determined predominantly by the capacitances and is strongly negative imaginary. Then, as the effects of the inductances increase, it goes through a first minimum coinciding with the first resonance of the network. This resonance, by the way, is not the same as that of the first series circuit of the network. As the frequency is further increased, the impedance increases to a maximum coinciding with the antiresonance of the network. Finally, at a still higher frequency, the impedance will go through another minimum coinciding with a second resonance.

At this place, it should be pointed out that the system of Fig. 7.4 is a reasonably good approximation of the middle ear with a missing incus or a disarticulated incudostapedial joint. Such a pathological middle ear is simple compared to the normal ear which has several resonances and antiresonances. This is discussed in the next section.

THE MIDDLE EAR AS AN ACOUSTIC TRANSFORMER

For a satisfactory interpretation of acoustic measurements in the ear canal, such as impedance or admittance measurements or tympanometry, it is necessary to realize that the main acoustic function of the middle ear is to provide maximum transfer of acoustic energy from the ear canal to the cochlea. Such transfer requires a tight coupling between the cochlea and the tympanic membrane. As a consequence, the acoustic input impedance of the cochlea is reflected in the acoustic impedance measured at the tympanic membrane. Theory and more recent measurements agree that the cochlear input impedance is high and resistive (for review see Zwislocki 1975). It provides most of the resistive component of the tympanic membrane impedance. When the cochlea is disconnected from the tympanic membrane through an ossicular disarticulation, the acoustic resistance measured at the tympanic membrane drops dramatically.

The transmission of acoustic energy from the ear canal to the tympanic membrane strongly depends on the difference between the tympanic membrane impedance and the acoustic impedance of air in the ear canal. The greater the difference, the less energy is transmitted. More specifically, the ratio of transmitted to incident energy obeys the formula $E_t/E_i = 4Z_d \cdot Z_{air}/(Z_d + Z_{air})^2$, where E_t — transmitted energy, E_i — incident energy, Z_d — impedance at the tympanic membrane, Z_{air} — impedance of air in the ear canal. In an average ear canal of 0.44 cm^2 cross-sectional area, the acoustic impedance, Z_{air}, amounts to 92 acoustic ohms. The acoustic input impedance of the human cochlea has been estimated to be 3.5×10^5 acoustic ohms (Zwislocki 1975). It is much larger than the air impedance, and the transmission formula tells us that, if the cochlear impedance were reflected directly at the tympanic membrane, only 0.1 per cent of the incident acoustic energy would be transmitted to the tympanic membrane. The situation is improved considerably by the transformer action of the middle ear. The action is provided mainly by the lever ratio between the malleus and incus and by the ratio of the effective surface areas of the tympanic membrane and the stapes footplate (Békésy 1960). An idealized transformer system of the middle ear is shown in Fig. 7.5. The lever system rotates around the axis 0 which is identical with the axis of rotation of the ossicular chain. The symbols l_m and l_i indicate the effective levers of the malleus and incus. According to Békésy, their ratio amounts to 1.3. The symbols A_d and A_{st} stand for the effective areas of the tympanic membrane and stapes footplate

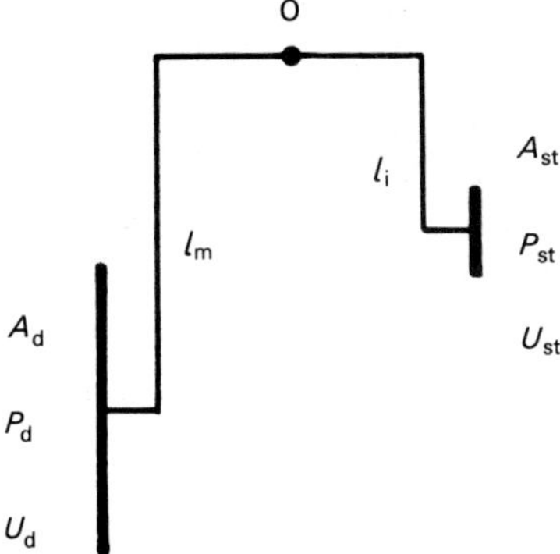

Fig. 7.5. Schematic of the idealized transformer system of the middle ear. A_d, U_d are the effective area and velocity of the tympanic membrane, P_d is the sound pressure at the membrane; l_m, l_i are the effective levers of the malleus and incus; A_{st}, U_{st} are the effective area and velocity of the stapes footplate; P_{st} is the sound pressure in the cochlea at the oval window; and 0 is the axis of rotation.

and have according to Békésy the numerical values of 0.55 and 0.032 cm^2. The sound pressures at the tympanic membrane and stapes are denoted by P_d and P_{st}, and the corresponding average velocities by U_d and U_{st}. From mechanics we know that the system is in equilibrium when the moments, that is the products of forces and lever lengths, are equal, $l_m A_d P_d = l_i A_{st} P_{st}$. In this relationship the forces are equal, of course, to the products of pressures and effective areas. Rearranging the terms of the equation a little bit, we obtain $P_{st}/P_d = l_m A_d / l_i A_{st}$. If we introduce the numerical values for l_m, l_i, A_d, and A_{st}, we obtain a pressure ratio of about 22.4, equivalent to a gain of about 27 dB. This means that, for a given sound pressure in the ear canal, the sound pressure in the cochlea is 27 dB higher. In reality the pressure transformation is somewhat smaller because of energy losses in the middle ear.

The geometry of the lever system of Fig. 7.5 tells us that the ratio of velocities U_d, U_{st} must be equal to the ratio of the levers l_m, l_{st} — $U_d/U_{st} = l_m/l_{st}$. As we have seen, volume velocity is equal to the product of average velocity and effective area. Accordingly, $\hat{V}_d/\hat{V}_{st} = A_d U_d / A_{st} U_{st} = l_m A_d / l_i A_{st}$. Multiplying the pressure ratio by the ratio of the volume velocities, we obtain $P_{st}\hat{V}_d / P_d \hat{V}_{st} = (l_m A_d / l_i A_{st})^2$. Since $P_{st}/\hat{V}_{st} = Z_{st}$ and $\hat{V}_d/P_d = 1/Z_d$, we also have $Z_{st}/Z_d = (l_m A_d / l_i A_{st})^2$. This is the impedance transformation between the cochlea and the tympanic membrane. From this transformation we can calculate the magnitude of cochlear impedance measured at the tympanic membrane — $Z_d = (l_i A_{st} / l_m A_d)^2 \cdot Z_{st}$. With the numerical values we already introduced, we obtain approximately $Z_d \simeq 700$ acoustic ohms. With the value of cochlear impedance so reduced, about 40 per cent of acoustic energy would be transferred from the ear canal to the tympanic membrane. In fact, the impedance is even further reduced by a certain amount of decoupling between the tympanic membrane and the stapes, as is discussed in the next section.

NORMAL AND PATHOLOGICAL MIDDLE-EAR SYSTEMS

Whether explictly or implicitly, current diagnostic interpretations of acoustic measurements in the ear canal are based on the following analysis of the middle-ear system (Zwislocki 1962, 1963). Grossly, the acoustic function of the normal human middle ear may be represented by the block diagram of Fig. 7.6. The diagram essentially follows the flow of acoustic energy from the

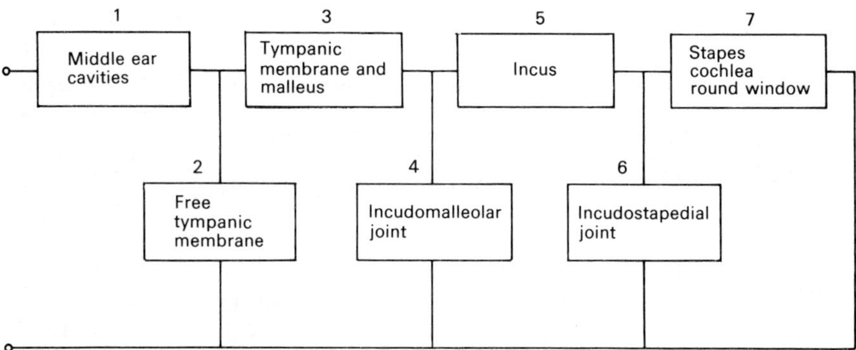

Fig. 7.6. Functional block diagram of the middle ear.

tympanic membrane to the cochlea. Although, coming from the ear canal, the acoustic waves first encounter the tympanic membrane, the first block of the diagram represents the system of the middle-ear cavities located behind the tympanic membrane. This reversal emphasizes the fact that the entire volume displacement of the membrane is transmitted to the air of the cavities, irrespective of whether the motion is imparted to the malleus or not. Block number 2 stands for those parts of the tympanic membrane that can move reasonably freely even when the malleus is fixed. Block 3 comprises the malleus with its ligamental attachments and the tensor tympani, as well as the part of the tympanic membrane that is closely coupled to the malleus. The next block, number 4, indicates a possible relative motion between the malleus and the incus in the incudomalleolar joint. To the best of our knowledge, the joint is practically rigid, and in a normal ear, the malleus and incus rotate as one rigid body around their axis of gravity (e.g. Békésy 1960). However, under pathological conditions, a partial or complete disarticulation between these two ossicles can take place. Block 5 comprises the incus and its ligaments; block 6 indicates relative motion between the incus and the stapes in the incudostapedial joint. To the best of our knowledge, such motion takes place even in a normal human ear, in contradistinction to the ears of some other mammals where the joint may be regarded as practically rigid up to reasonably high sound frequencies. The flexibility of the joint in the human ear decouples to a certain extent the stapes from the tympanic membrane and weakens the effect of stapedial ankylosis on the acoustic impedance or admittance measured in the ear canal. Finally, block 7 stands for what may be called the cochlear complex that includes the stapes with its elastic attachments—the stapedius muscle and the annular ligament, the resistive cochlear input impedance, and the elastic round-window membrane. All the blocks connected in series are associated with acoustic energy flow from the tympanic membrane to the cochlea. The shunt blocks indicate where the energy is diverted from the cochlea and provide varying amounts of decoupling between the tympanic membrane and the middle-ear parts located medially to the shunt. Because of this decoupling they limit the diagnostic usefulness of the acoustic impedance measurements. For instance, incudostapedial disarticulation completely prevents detection of stapedial ankylosis in such measurements. Perforation of the tympanic membrane makes it impossible to detect acoustically any additional pathology in the middle ear. In general, the shunts suggest that pathological changes in the vicinity of the tympanic membrane have a stronger effect on the acoustic impedance measured at the membrane than do more medial changes.

At very low sound frequencies, the inertance (mass) effects of the ossicles and of air columns in the narrow passages of the cavity system of the middle ear are insignificant, since they are proportional to sound frequency. Under these conditions the system is controlled mainly by compliances or their reciprocals, the stiffnesses of its various parts. However, it should be pointed out that, already in the vicinity of 500 Hz, the narrow passage between the tympanic cavity and the antrum produces a resonance effect. As a result, above 500 Hz and up to about 2000 Hz the cavity system of the middle ear acts as an inertance rather than a compliance (Onchi 1961)! When the frequency is low enough, probably below about 200 Hz in a normal ear, all the blocks of Fig. 7.6 may be approximated by mechanical compliances or their analogue electrical capacitances. Such an approxima-

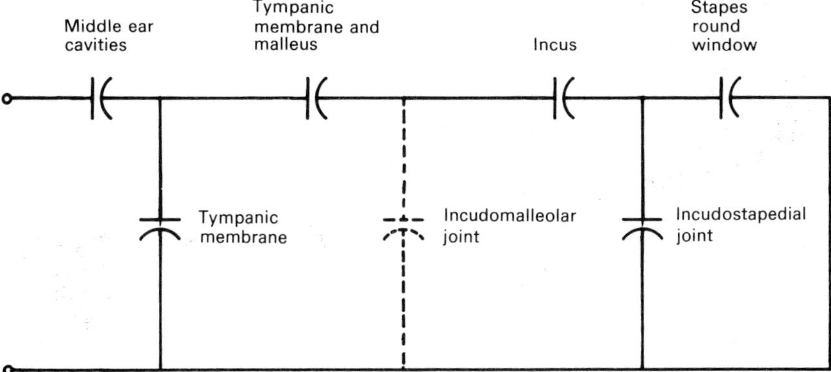

Fig. 7.7. Electrical network analogue of the middle ear at low sound frequencies.

tion is shown in Fig. 7.7. It makes it relatively easy to predict changes in acoustic impedance or admittance at the tympanic membrane, which result from pathological changes in the middle ear, if we remember that capacitances (compliances) sum when they are in parallel. For instance, the capacitances associated with the incudostapedial joint and with the stapes–round-window complex add. When the stapes capacitance is eliminated by ankylosis, the joint capacitance remains. Since the latter is almost as large as that of the stapes and round window combined, the total capacitance is decreased by little more than 50 per cent. The effect of this reduction on the impedance at the tympanic membrane is further diminished by the other capacitances of the middle-ear system. This is why the compliance measured at the tympanic membrane in the presence of stapedial ankylosis is reduced on the average by less than one half when compared to normal. On the other hand, Fig. 7.7 suggests that fixation of the malleus by adhesions must have a dramatic effect on the compliance at the tympanic membrane. This is so because all the compliances of the system are effectively disconnected from the tympanic membrane except that of the middle-ear cavities. The effect of the latter is negligible at low frequencies, especially in the presence of partial fixation of the tympanic membrane through the immobilized malleus. Under these conditions the entire compliance is due to the still moveable portion of the tympanic membrane. The compliance of this portion is only about one-fourth of the normal compliance measured at the membrane.

We can best understand the effect of ossicular disarticulation when we realize that the reciprocal values of compliances, that is the stiffnesses, add when they are connected in series. In an ear without an incus, all the stiffnesses beyond the mallear complex are eliminated and the total stiffness is determined only by the mallear complex, the tympanic membrane, and the middle-ear cavities. This stiffness is only about half the normal stiffness. In compliance terms, the absence of the incus increases the compliance measured at the tympanic membrane on the average by a factor of about 2.

Impedance measurements performed at very low sound frequencies which reflect almost exclusively stiffness or compliance contributions of various parts of the middle ear miss a considerable amount of diagnostic information inherent in inertia and resistance contributions of these parts, which manifest themselves at higher frequencies. For instance, in a normal ear, the main resonance point at which the reactance part of the impedance disappears is located near 1000 Hz. Incudostapedial disarticulation brings it down to about 500 Hz. Above this frequency the reactance is positive, whereas it is negative in normal ears. Incudostapedial disarticulation also lowers considerably the resistance measured at the tympanic membrane by eliminating its main source—the cochlea. Because impedance contributions of different middle-ear components are maximum in different frequency ranges, it must be expected that the greatest amount of diagnostic information can be obtained by measuring the impedance as a function of sound frequency. Resulting average reactance and resistance curves are shown in Fig. 7.8 for normal and otosclerotic ears and ears with ossicular

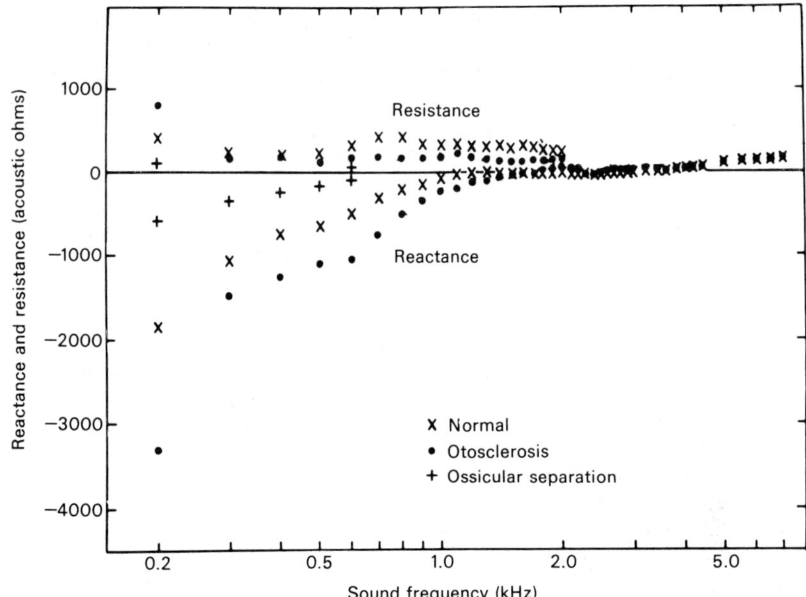

Fig. 7.8. Average reactance and resistance at the tympanic membrane measured as a function of sound frequency.

separation. Note the very low resistance and the low resonance point in the presence of the separation. Note also that, on the average, otosclerosis increases the reactance maximally around 200 and 700 Hz, but minimally around 300 Hz. Note finally that the reactance is hardly affected by otosclerosis above 1000 Hz.

In conclusion of this section a word should be added with respect to tympanometry based on static pressure variation in the ear canal. This simple method has proved itself clinically in several ways, even though the mechanisms underlying the observed stiffening of the middle-ear system in the presence of a pressure differential across the tympanic membrane are not well understood. More detailed measurements of the stiffening effect as a function of sound frequency, which would lead to impedance curves of the type shown in Fig. 7.8, would probably contribute materially to a better understanding of the effect and further increase the efficiency of the method. This could be expected in particular if the results of the measurements were interpreted in terms of the block diagram of Fig. 7.6 and the network analysis of Section 2.

REFERENCES

Békésy, G. von (1941). Über die Messung der Schwingungsamplitude der Gehörknöchelchen Mittels einer Kapazitiven sonde. *Akust. Z.* **6,** 1–16.

—— (1960). *Experiments in hearing*. McGraw-Hill, New York.

Metz, O. (1946). The acoustic impedance measured on normal and pathological ears. *Acta oto-lar.* Suppl. 63.

Møller, A. R. (1961). Network model of the middle ear. *J. acoust. Soc. Am.* **33,** 168–76.

Onchi, Y. (1961). Mechanism of the middle ear. *J. acoust. Soc. Am.* **33,** 794–805.

Terkildsen, K. and Scott Nielsen, S. (1960). An electroacoustic impedance measuring bridge for clinical use. *Archs Otolar.* **72**, 339–46.

—— and Thomsen, K. A. (1959). The influence of pressure variations on the impedance of the human eardrum. *J. Lar. Otol.* **73,** 409–18.

Thomsen, K. A. (1958). Investigations on the tubal function and measurement of the middle-ear pressure in pressure chamber. *Acta oto-lar.* Suppl. **140,** 269–78.

Zwislocki, J. (1957a). Some measurements of the impedance at the eardrum. *J. acoust. Soc. Am.* **29,** 349–56.

—— (1957b). Some impedance measurements on normal and pathological ears. *J. acoust. Soc. Am.* **29,** 1312–17.

—— (1961). Acoustic measurement of the middle ear function. *Ann. Otol. Rhinol. Lar.* **70,** 599–606.

—— (1962). Analysis of the middle-ear function. Part I: Input impedance. *J. acoust. Soc. Am.* **34,** 1514–23.

—— (1963). An acoustic method for clinical examination of the ear. *J. Speech Hearing Res.* **6,** 303–14.

—— (1975). The role of the external and middle ear in sound transmission. In *The nervous system* (ed. E. L. Eagles and D. B. Tower) Vol. 3. Raven Press, New York.

—— and Feldman, A. S. (1970). Acoustic impedance of pathological ears. *ASHA Monogr.* No. 15.

Section 2
Instrumentation

8 Audiometers

M. C. MARTIN

An audiometer is described by the International Electrotechnical commission (IEC) Vocabulary (IEC 1976) as: An instrument for the measurement of hearing acuity and, specifically, the threshold of audibility. Audiometers may be divided into two main categories (i) those that require a subjective response on the part of the listener and (ii) those that make an objective measurement of some physiological or electrophysiological response of the listener to the stimulus, and requires no response from the listener. This chapter will only deal with the former although many aspects of this will be applicable to the latter category.

PURE-TONE AUDIOMETER

Audiometers can be considered in terms of their main functional parts which are signal source, signal level control, and transducers. These parts can then be broken down further in order to specify performance in detail. Fig. 8.1 shows a functional block diagram whose performance requirements will be considered in the light of a new IEC standard (IEC 645 1979) on audiometric equipment which revises the current standards IEC 177 (1965) Pure-Tone Screening Audiometers and IEC 178 (1965) Diagnostic Audiometers.

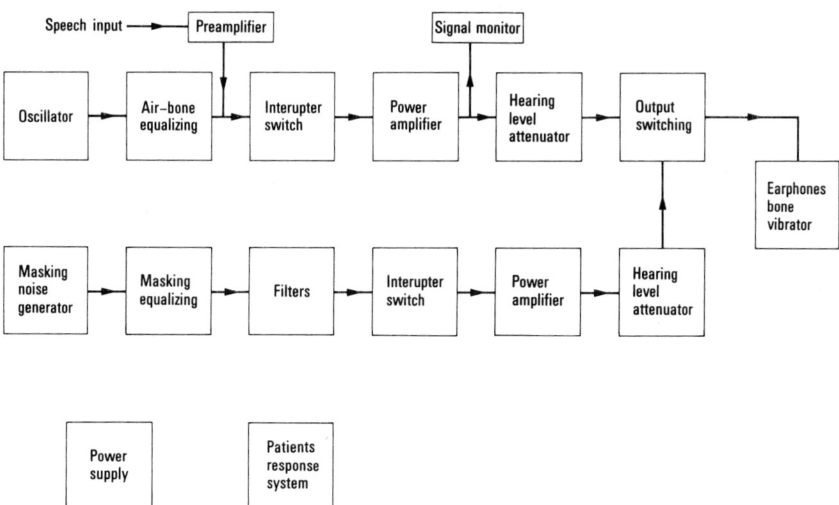

Fig. 8.1. Functional block diagram of general purpose diagnostic audiometer.

In order to get away from descriptive terms such as diagnostic and screening, the new IEC standard describes audiometers as Types 1 to 5 with Type 1 being the most sophisticated and Type 5 the very simplest. This terminology will be used throughout the chapter.

FUNCTIONAL PARTS OF AUDIOMETER

Oscillator

Pure tones are generated electronically and for audiometers the standardized frequencies are 125, 250, 500, 750, 1000, 1500, 2000, 3000, 4000, 6000, and 8000 Hz. These frequencies are required to be within ± 3 per cent of their nominal value and have a harmonic distortion content that is at least 30 dB below the fundamental. Continually variable frequency audiometers are also available and their performance specification is the same.

The method of generating the electrical oscillation has altered quite considerably over the last few years with the introduction of integrated circuits, which are inherently very stable. A factor that influences the choice of electronic circuit to be used is whether or not the oscillator is to be fixed or variable and also the type of interrupter switch circuitry.

Interrupter switch

The presentation of tones to a patient usually requires that the tone is switched on and off. This may appear to be a trivial requirement, however the interrupter switch presents some difficult problems because it has two important characteristics (i) the amount of signal attenuation provided by the switch when it is at its off position and (ii) the rise and decay characteristic of the tone when switched on and off.

IEC 645 specifies that the signal shall be attenuated by at least 70 dB for signals above 70 dB hearing level (HL) attenuator settings and be at least 10 dB below the reference equivalent threshold level for settings below this. This specification is not particularly difficult to meet and two approaches to the problem may be found. The most effective method of control is to switch the oscillator off by means of the interrupter switch thereby having no possibility of signal breaking through. However, this does raise problems in causing an oscillator to come on and go off with no audible change in frequency, or without excessive distortion during the on/off period. Oscillators of the LC type were particularly suitable and widely used in older instruments, but involved precisely wound coils which tended to be bulky.

The alternative approach is to have the oscillator running continuously and to electronically gate the signal. This method appears to be currently favoured largely due to the recent availability of efficient electronic attenuator circuits. In this case there will always be some breakthrough of signal which can be heard by a person with normal hearing at high signal output settings but obviously not heard by the deaf patient.

The rise and decay characteristics of the signal are important in order to avoid giving the persons being tested clues to the presence of the test signal while not hearing the signal itself, and thus producing misleading information on the threshold. Such clues may come about by clicks at the beginning or end of the tone caused by electrical switch contact noise, or by a very rapid rise and fall in the signal. Furthermore, any mechanical noise from the movement of the switch may give clues.

In order to minimize the problems due to the rise and decay of the tone this parameter is standardized and is detailed in Fig. 8.2. Doubts have been expressed as to how well audiometers meet this or any other requirement for rise and decay times, which in certain types of hearing loss may have a considerable effect.

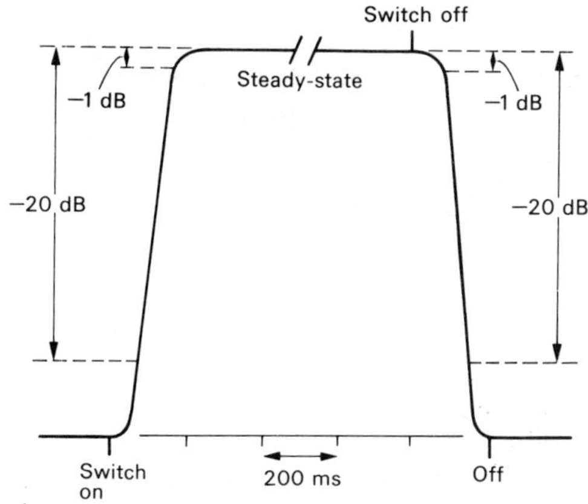

Fig. 8.2. Diagrammatic representation of rise and decay of test tone.

For self-recording audiometers the tone is very frequently a pulsed tone, the repetition rate being about two pulses per second, the rise and decay characteristic being the same as for manual audiometers.

Equalization circuit

The threshold in Man is not uniform, the ear is most sensitive at frequencies around 2 kHz and particularly insensitive at low and very high frequencies. Fig. 8.3 shows the threshold of hearing for earphone listening. This variation in the sensitivity of the ear, as well as the variability in the sensitivity of transducers used to present the signal to the listener, requires that at each frequency and ideally for each transducer used an individual adjustment should be made of the signal level. In most audiometers therefore there will be a set of variable resistors that can be adjusted to give the required output signal. The resistors are the means of calibrating the audiometer to the required standards as described in the section entitled 'Calibration of audiometric equipment'. As the calibration resistors are different for each frequency and transducer the switch arrangement is often very complex and gives rise to the major part of the wiring in an audiometer.

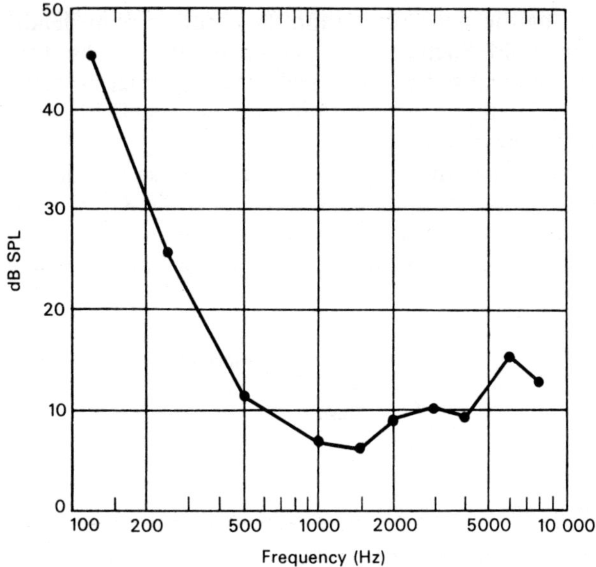

Fig. 8.3. Threshold of hearing for earphone listening using TDH39 earphones with an MX41/AR earcap. Sound pressure measured on 9A acoustic coupler. From ISO R389 (1970).

Output power amplifier

The output transducers on the audiometer require audio frequency power to operate them, the signals produced by the oscillator may have relatively high voltages but lack power. The output power amplifier provides the power to operate the transducers and basically is a good quality audio frequency power amplifier. The important characteristics of the amplifier are that it produces little distortion and has a good signal-to-noise ratio. In many audiometers the power amplifer is run at almost constant high-signal output levels with the signal being controlled by an attenuator on the output, this arrangement giving the best signal-to-noise ratio hence minimizing problems with background internal electrical noise from the audiometer.

Hearing level attenuator

The attenuator that controls the level of the signal from the audiometer is usually adjustable over a range of 110 or 130 dB. The attenuator is normally variable in steps of 5 dB and will have a reference position marked 'O' and often two steps below this marked −5 and −10. Above 'O' the attenuator will switch in 5 dB steps up to the maximum of 100, 110, or 120 dB. The expected maximum values are tabulated in Table 8.1 for different types of audiometer.

It has been previously stated that the threshold of hearing curve is not flat and therefore the 'O' position on the attenuator represents a different value of output signal at each frequency. The 'O' position is the standardized value

TABLE 8.1. *Maximum output expected from audiometers of various types (dB HL)*

Frequency (Hz)	125	250	500	1000	1500	2000	3000	4000	6000	8000
Type 1 (advanced diagnostic)										
AIR	70	90	120	120	120	120	120	120	110	100
BONE		45	60	70	70	70	70	60		
Type 2 (diagnostic)										
AIR	70	90	110	110	110	110	110	110	100	90
BONE		40	60	70	70	70	70	60		
Type 3 (simple diagnostic)										
AIR		90	100	100		100	100	100	90	80
BONE		30	50	50		50	50	50		
Type 4 (screening)										
AIR			70	70		70	70	70	70	

of the threshold of hearing and as this varies by some 40 dB over the audiometer range it means that at the end of the frequency range the output is very high compared with say 1 kHz. While this does not affect matters at low intensities it seriously affects the high output levels. If it is possible to obtain an output of 120 dB at 1 kHz and this was required at 125 Hz, 40 dB more signal is required to compensate for the fall in sensitivity of the ear, this means an increase in power of 10 000 times which very clearly the audiometer cannot give and the transducers cannot handle. Therefore on all audiometers there is a maximum signal level which varies at different frequencies. These values are tabulated in Table 8.1. It should be noted that on some audiometers the dial can be turned to a high value and the tone is still present, it will not however increase with increased dial readings above the maximum point and may well reduce in level. The best arrangement for audiometers is where the dial cannot be turned beyond the maximum point or where the signal goes off above that point.

The attenuator steps have to be accurate and their required performance is that between any two successive steps the output shall not differ from the indicated dial difference by more than three-tenths of the dial interval or 1 dB whichever is smaller IEC 645 (1980).

Output transducers

Output transducers may be of three main types: earphones, bone vibrator, or loudspeaker output. In general loudspeaker outputs are not normally available on audiometers with sufficient power at the output socket to drive a large loudspeaker. Very often there are output sockets which allow an external power amplifier and loudspeaker to be connected, see section on Free Field Audiometers.

Earphones for audiometers are very specific and cannot be replaced or changed without affecting the whole calibration of the instrument. Audio-

TABLE 8.2. *Standardized acoustic couplers*

IEC type	Cavity size	Type of earphone to be measured
303 Provisional reference coupler	6 cm³	Supra-aural for audiometer calibration
318 Wideband artificial ear for the calibration of earphones used in audiometry	Acoustic load to simulate normal ear impedance	Supra-aural for audiometer and general purposes
126 IEC reference coupler for the measurement of hearing aids using earphones coupled to the ear by means of ear inserts	2 cm³	Hearing aid both button and acoustic tube connected types

metric earphones are selected on the basis of good long-term stability and a flat frequency response as well as being able to deliver high output sounds. The earphone and the earcap that goes with it are specific to the individual audiometer they are supplied with. Calibration of earphones is described in the following section. Earphones are reasonably robust but can alter sensitivity if dropped or misused. The most commonly used types are listed in Tables 8.3 and 8.4.

Bone vibrators by comparison with earphones have a very limited dynamic range and frequency response. Fig. 8.4 shows the frequency response of a typical bone vibrator used with audiometers. At low frequencies, e.g. 250

TABLE 8.3. *Reference equivalent threshold sound pressure levels from American standard Z24.5 (1951). British Standard BS2497 (1954) and ISO 389 (1975)*

	dB ref 20(μ Pa)			
Frequency	BS 2497	ISO 389	ASA Z24.5	ISO 389
125	44.5	47	54.5	45.5
250	29.5	28	39.6	24.5
500	12	11.5	24.8	11
1000	6	5.5	16.7	6.5
1500	7.5	6.5		6.5
2000	9	9	17	8.5
3000	6	8		7.5
4000	9	9.5	15.1	9
6000	9	8		8
8000	9	10	20.9	9.5
Earphone	ST2C 4026-A	ST2C 4026-A	Western Electric 705A	Western Electric 705A
Acoustic coupler	BS artificial ear BS 2042 1953	BS artificial ear BS 2042 1953	9A acoustic coupler	9A acoustic coupler

TABLE 8.4. *Recommended reference equivalent threshold sound pressure levels in the 9A coupler (after BS 2497: Part 2 (1969). (For these data to be valid, the earphone is placed both on the ear and on the coupler with its earcushion, with one exception. When calibrating the Beyer DT 48 earphone on the 9A coupler, the cushion is removed and an adaptor, described by Mrass and Diestel (1959), is used. The values for the TDH-49 earphone are derived from a paper by Delany and Whittle (1967))*

Frequency (Hz)	Reference equivalent threshold sound pressure levels relative to 20 μ Pa (dB)							
125	47.5	51.0	44.0	46.5	46.5	51.0	45.0	47.5
250	28.5	30.5	25.0	26.0	26.0	28.5	25.5	26.5
500	14.5	13.5	11.5	10.5	11.0	10.0	11.5	13.5
1000	8.0	6.5	6.5	5.0	7.0	6.0	7.0	7.5
1500	7.5	7.0	5.5	5.0	7.0	6.5	6.5	7.5
2000	8.0	7.5	7.5	7.5	9.0	6.5	9.0	11.0
3000	6.0	8.0	8.0	6.5	10.0	9.0	10.0	9.5
4000	5.5	10.5	9.0	13.0	13.5	9.0	9.5	10.5
6000	8.0	13.5	17.0	11.0	8.5	18.5	15.5	13.5
8000	14.5	20.5	13.0	13.0	11.0	14.0	13.0	13.0
Pattern of earphone	Beyer DT 48 with flat cushion	STC 4026A	Permoflux PDR8 MX41/AR cushion	Permoflux PDR1 ADC case cushion	Permoflux PDR1 MX41/AR cushion	Permoflux PDR10 MX41/AR cushion	Tele-phonics TDH-39 MX41/AR cushion	Tele-phonics TDH-49 MX41/AR cushion

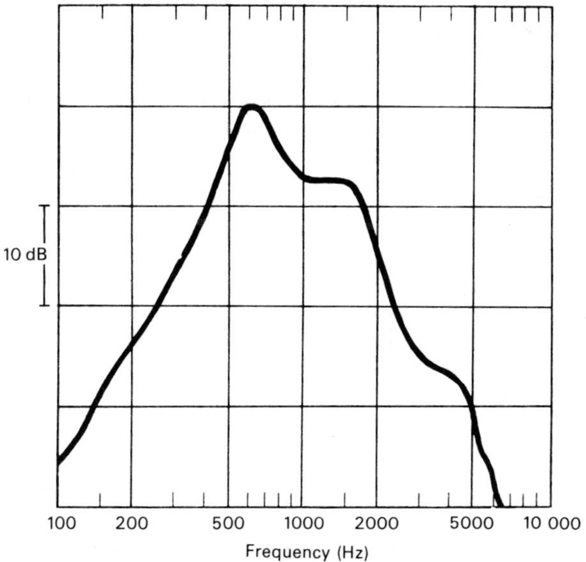

Fig. 8.4. Frequency response of typical bone vibrator used for audiometry. Output measured in terms of acceleration on an artificial mastoid.

and 500 Hz, bone vibrators have particularly poor harmonic distortion characteristics. It is for this reason that maximum measurable bone conduction hearing levels at low frequencies are extremely limited and on many audiometers the distortion content is very high at levels as low as 20 dB HL. The implication of this for the listener is that, depending upon his hearing loss, he may not hear the fundamental of the signal but may respond to a higher harmonic thus appearing to have better hearing than he really has.

CALIBRATION OF AUDIOMETERS

In order to appreciate the difficulties in audiometer calibration it is necessary to start with the standardization of the threshold of hearing for earphone listening by pure tones. With any psycho-acoustic experiment there will be an inevitable difference between the results obtained on one group of subjects and those obtained even by the same experimenter on another group. Early audiometer manufacturers each used the results of their own experiments to set the threshold of hearing for audiometers of their own make and many were very close to modern-day standards. However, differences were bound to occur and steps were taken to produce an agreed threshold of hearing.

Two different approaches were taken by the United States and the United Kingdom in arriving at national values for threshold. In the United States large scale surveys were undertaken of people attending State Fairs and a threshold arrived at for a wide range of people. In the United Kingdom two surveys under laboratory conditions using only young otological normal subjects were undertaken.

These surveys produced a set of figures very different from the USA values, Dadson and King (1952) and Wheeler and Dickson (1952). Table 8.3 gives the difference between the two standards that were finally arrived at and ISO R389 (1964) values.

The foregoing situation may have appeared not too difficult to resolve when it came to trying to get international agreement on audiometric zero. However, a further matter causes complications which has not been so far mentioned and that is the method of measuring the value of sound pressure level (SPL) that relates to audiometric zero.

There are two main methods of measuring the sound pressure for audiometric zero. The direct method is to place a probe tube microphone at a stated position under the earcap of the earphone near to the entrance to the meatus and measure the sound pressure level at this point. It is not usually possible to measure the sound pressure at the threshold of an individual due to the very low levels involved, therefore an accurately calibrated attenuator is used to relate the SPL at threshold to some higher value at which the probe tube microphone is calibrated Fig. 8.5. A disadvantage of this method is that the information obtained cannot be used to calibrate another earphone directly unless an assumption is made that the performance of other

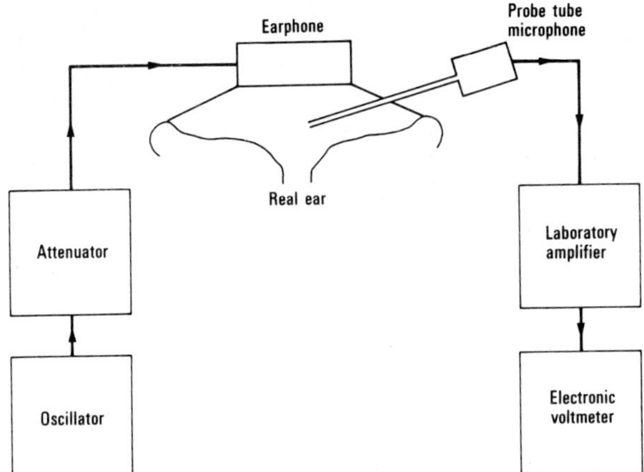

Fig. 8.5. Direct method of earphone calibration. Earphone is applied to real ear and attenuator reading noted for threshold. The sound pressure level is then increased by a known amount (x) and measured by the probe tube microphone. The threshold value for sound pressure is then that value minus (x). This procedure is repeated for a large number of otologically normal ears and the modal value of the sound pressure level for threshold at each frequency taken as being the minimum audible pressure for that earphone.

earphones of the same type are identical. Furthermore the repeatability of probe tube measurements of this type is likely to be poor.

The second method of measuring the sound pressure level for audiometric zero is an indirect method using an acoustic coupler or artificial ear: the generic term acoustic coupler, will be used in this chapter to describe all forms of acoustic coupling for the measurement of earphone performance. Acoustic couplers are devices which use a calibrated microphone to measure the sound pressure in some form of cavity. The size and shape of the cavity will obviously affect the acoustic characteristics of the device and two main types can be identified, i.e. the simple acoustic coupler and the artificial ear. An acoustic coupler such as the widely used 9A or IEC Provisional Reference Coupler IEC 303 (1970) does not attempt to reflect accurately the acoustic impedance of the real ear whereas an artificial ear such as the IEC Wide Band Artificial Ear IEC 318 (1970) does attempt to reflect accurately the average impedance of the adult ear as seen through an earphone earcap. Table 8.3 lists the standardized types of acoustic couplers and their intended use.

In order to obtain a standardized value for audiometric zero with a chosen earphone the threshold of hearing of a sufficiently large group of otologically normal subjects is measured. In this case the sound pressure level from the earphone in the real ear is not measured, but the voltage applied to the earphone in order to produce that sound pressure is measured on a laboratory-standard electronic voltmeter. From the voltage measurements for threshold thus obtained the modal value is taken for the group and applied to the earphone when placed upon an appropriate acoustic coupler (Fig. 8.6). The sound pressure developed in the acoustic coupler is then known as the reference equivalent threshold sound pressure level (RETSPL) for the modal value and the equivalent threshold sound pressure level (ETSPL) for the value of an individual ear.

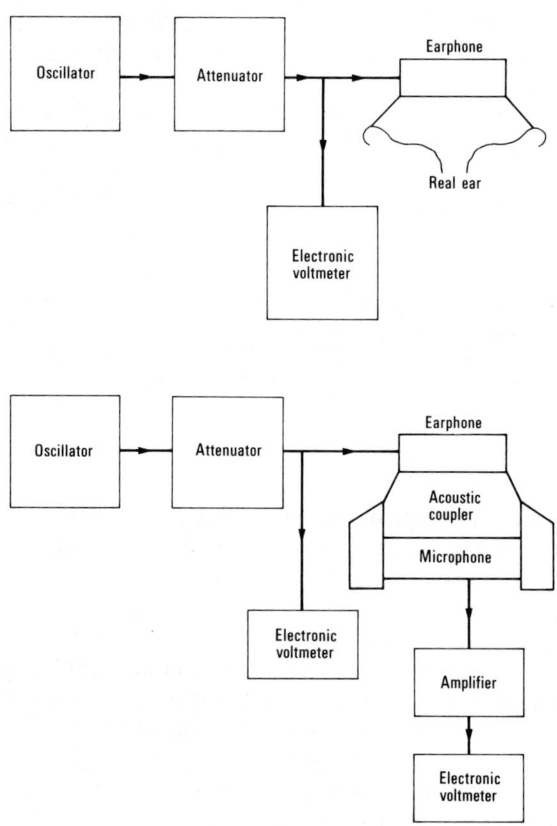

Fig. 8.6. Indirect method of earphone calibration. (1) The voltage applied to the earphone for threshold is noted at each frequency. (2) The earphone is applied to an acoustic coupler and the sound pressure measured for a known voltage to the earphone. (3) The ETSP is the sound pressure measured in (1) and (2).

The RETSPL is internationally standardized in ISO 389 (1975) which lays down the values of RETSPL for a range of earphones in a variety of acoustic couplers. The most commonly used acoustic coupler is the '9A' acoustic coupler or IEC Interim coupler. The 9A coupler is so widely used because it is very simple and RETSPL values exist for a range of earphones (Table 8.4).

It must be stressed however that if an earphone other than those listed in R389 is used a complete subjective calibration has to be undertaken by a standardizing authority. To overcome this problem a true artificial ear is necessary which would allow the user to place any form of earphone on it and to know that if a certain RETSPL is obtained that this will give audiometric zero. This situation has not been reached as yet but a wide band artificial ear, IEC 318 (1970) has been designed (Delaney, Whittle, Cook, and Scott 1967) that will allow supra-aural earphones of a wide variety to be calibrated. At present (1980) international standardization of RETSPL for this wide band ear has not been achieved although work is now going on in this area. Table 8.5 gives values standardized in the United Kingdom together with values recently produced (Robinson 1978) for the ISO working group on this subject. To date no internationally agreed method exists for the measurement of the performance of circumaural earphones although work is being undertaken into the design of a flat-plate coupler for this type of earphone.

TABLE 8.5. *Values of RETSPL for the IEC 303 wide band artificial ear. Robinson 1 and 2 refers to values suggested by Robinson (1978)*

	RETSPL values dB ref 20 μ Pa		
Frequency (kHz)	BS 2497 Part 3	Robinson 1	Robinson 2
0.125	45	43	43
0.25	27.5	26	28.5
0.5	13.5	13	13.5
1	8	8	7
1.5	7.5	7.5	7.5
2	10.5	10	8
3	11.5	10.5	8.5
4	13.5	10.5	10.5
6	13.5	20.5	22
8	16	18	20

BONE CONDUCTION CALIBRATION

The calibration of bone conduction vibrators for audiometric purposes in principle is the same as for earphones. The obvious differences are of course that some form of measuring device is needed to measure the output of the vibrator and a set of internationally agreed figures for bone conduction threshold are required.

A device called a mechanical coupler IEC 373 (1971) is specified to measure the output from bone vibrators. This device is more generally called an artificial mastoid and two main types exist, one designed in the United Kingdom (Robinson and Whittle 1967a) and the other in the United States (Weiss 1960). Fig. 8.7 shows the current commercially available device based on the NPL design.

Two main sites for the bone vibrator on the head are the mastoid and the

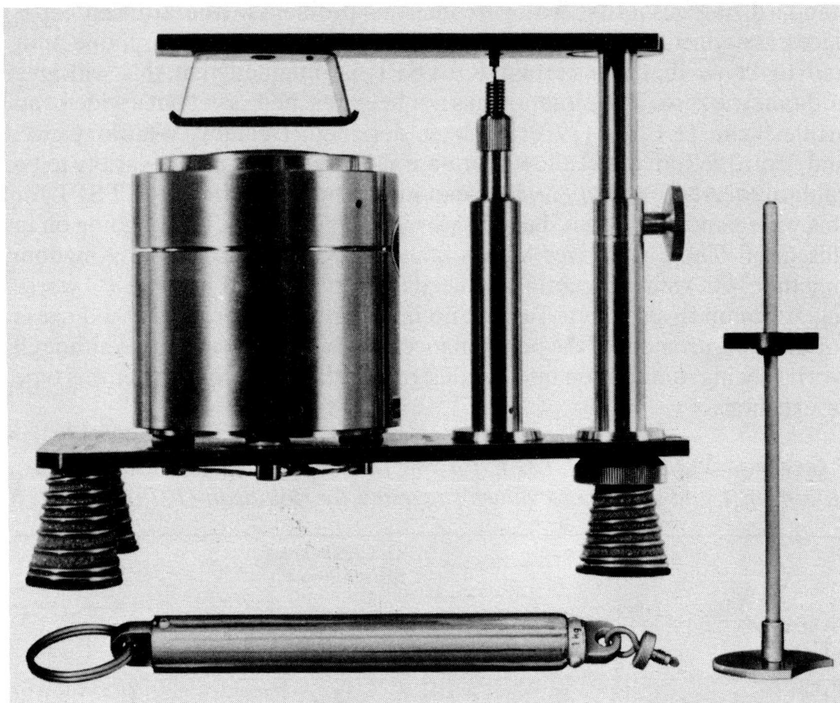

Fig. 8.7. A commercially available artificial mastoid. Courtesy B & K Ltd.

forehead. The mastoid is the most sensitive position but the forehead may be more stable. Table 8.6 gives the differences between the two positions. To date, however, no international standard exists for the threshold of hearing by bone conduction. A British Standard B S 2497 part 4 (B S I 1972) takes the view that due to the very large variance existing between the

TABLE 8.6. *Mean correction from mastoid to forehead placement of a bone conduction vibrator (Whittle 1965)*

Frequency (Hz)	Forehead sensitivity relative to mastoid position
125	− 12
250	− 14
500	− 16
1000	− 11
1500	− 9
2000	− 7
3000	− 5
4000	− 5

measurements so far made to standardize threshold (Robinson and Whittle 1966, 1967b) a single value of acceleration can be used to define threshold for practical purposes. This figure is −30 dB ref/m/s^2 measured on the IEC mechanical coupler.

A difficulty that arises in making bone conduction measurements on normal hearing people is the effect of airborne signals radiated from the bone vibrator. At frequencies above 1 kHz these can often be heard at hearing levels of 20 dB at 4 kHz thus apparently giving the person being tested a threshold 20 dB better than normal. The ear can be occluded at frequencies above 1 kHz with very little effect on threshold but of course below 1 kHz a very large increase in sensitivity occurs due to the occlusion effect (Whittle 1970).

PERFORMANCE SPECIFICATION OF AUDIOMETERS

The performance of audiometers has been specified in the past by two IEC documents, IEC 177 and 178. The former covers screening audiometers while the latter deals with diagnostic instruments. More recently IEC has consolidated all requirements for audiometers in one document IEC 645 (IEC 1980).

In outline, the general performance requirements for all audiometers will be the same but the range of frequencies, outputs, and facilities will determine the type and obviously the use of the equipment. Five types are listed and Table 8.7 gives the requirements for different types of instrument in terms of the facilities that might be found on these instruments.

The calibration of the audiometer fixes the SPL for audiometric zero which will be seen to vary by some 45 dB over the range 125 Hz to 4 kHz. At low output levels this presents no problem but it does create a difficulty at high output levels. If one wishes to measure the threshold of hearing of a patient with a 100 dB loss at 1 kHz then from Table 8.4 it may be deduced that a SPL of 107 dB will be required, i.e. (RETSPL at 1 kHz) + 100. If the same patient has a 90 dB loss at 250 Hz then 115.5 dB SPL will be required. In order to achieve the high output the earphones must be capable of handling in a linear manner the power required and the audiometer amplifier must be capable of producing the power. These requirements place a strict limit on the maximum amount of sound available from an audiometer, Table 8.1 gives the maximum levels required. Different manufacturers use varying methods to indicate when the maximum level has been exceeded. The best method is for the tone to go off above the maximum level but many instruments still have the tone available at a constant or even a reduced level above the maximum point. This may lead to misleading results with profoundly deaf patients from unwary operators.

The secondary signal source is the masking noise generator which produces random noise, four types of masking noise are specified, i.e. narrow band, broad band, weighted random noise for pure tones and weighted random noise for speech. Narrow band noise is specified as a third octave

TABLE 8.7. *Facilities to be found on various types of audiometers*

Capability	Type 1	Type 2	Type 3	Type 4	Type 5
Bone conduction	Yes	Yes	Yes		
Masking (pure-tones)					
Narrow-band noise	Yes	Yes			
Narrow-band noise or other			Yes		
Broad-band noise	Yes	Yes			
Masking (speech)					
Broad-band noise	Yes	Yes			
Speech-weighted noise	Yes	Optional			
Routing of masking					
Contralateral earphone	Yes	Yes	Yes		
Ipsilateral earphone	Yes	Optional			
Bone vibrator	Yes	Optional			
Reference tone					
Alternate	Yes	Yes†			
Simultaneous	Yes				
Alternate monaural, bifrequency	Optional				
Patient's response					
Signal system	Yes	Yes	Yes	Yes‡	
Auxiliary output (e.g. loudspeaker)	Yes	Optional	Optional		
Input for external signal source (e.g. speech)	Yes	Yes†	Optional		
Test signal indicating device	Yes	Yes			
Audible monitoring of test signal	Optional	Optional			
Operator to subject speech communication	Optional	Optional			
Noise-reducing earphones				Optional	Optional

† For automatic recording audiometers this feature is not required.
‡ For manual audiometers feature this feature is not required.

band of noise centred on the test tone, the third octave being a good approximation to the critical band.

Broad band noise is specified as having a uniform spectrum level over the range 250–6000 Hz. Weighted random noise has a spectrum such that for zero masking the sound pressure level in each one third octave band is equal to the reference equivalent threshold level for each test frequency as measured in an ear simulator. Weighted random noise for speech shall have a spectrum pressure level constant from 350–1000 Hz with a 12 dB per octave fall from 1000 to 6000 Hz.

The rise and decay times of the test tone are of prime importance in the design of any audiometer due to their influence on the detectability of the signal at threshold. If the rise or decay time is too short there is a subjective impression of a thump or click and if it is too long then there may be frequency changes and distortion in the test tone. Fig. 8.2 shows the rise and decay times for manual and self-recording audiometers. While it is of prime importance that electrical noise, i.e. clicks are not produced from the audiometer when the test signal is applied it is equally important that acoustic noise is not produced due to the mechanical movement of switches. Hence in an audiometer the movement of the hearing level dial and the tone interrupter switch are of prime importance to the designer in order to ensure a positive easy and silent movement of the switch. The audiometer must also not give any clues to the patient that the test tone is being presented by producing extraneous noise or visual clues. Some older audiometers radiated frequences above 1 kHz from the coils used in the oscillator circuits which could be easily heard by near normal hearing patients with headphones on.

The ergonomic design of the audiometer is not specified but should be a major consideration when considering the purchase of an instrument. In particular the siting of the interrupter switch and the hearing level dial. These two controls will be used tens of thousands of times in a year by an operator and therefore it should be possible to use the controls with the minimum of effort.

PRACTICAL CALIBRATION OF AUDIOMETERS

To calibrate an audiometer it is necessary to have equipment that will allow the measurement of sound pressure in an acoustic coupler, ideally over the full range of output from the audiometer. A means of measuring frequency and harmonic distortion are necessary, however measurement of rise and decay times are difficult and in most cases can be assessed by ear. Fig. 8.8 shows a block-diagram of the equipment needed for full calibration of audiometers using standard acoustic measuring equipment. Acoustic measurements can be made with little difficulty in most quiet laboratories. Electrical measurements of output are difficult to relate to the acoustic output and should not generally be used.

Appendices A–C contains procedures for the calibration and maintenance of audiometers as recommended by the Department of Health and Social Security, in the United Kingdom.

SPEECH AUDIOMETERS

A speech audiometer (Fig. 8.9) is an instrument designed specifically for delivering test material to the patient at a known intensity through earphones, bone vibrator, or from a loudspeaker. The performance of speech audiometers is detailed in ANSI S3.6 (1969) and more recently in IEC 645 audiometers IEC (1980).

The essential features of the speech audiometer are that it must have a stated frequency response characteristic and a means of monitoring the speech signal. The frequency response should be flat from 250 to 4000 Hz for acoustic input to a microphone used for live voice testing and flat from 250 to 6000 Hz for recorded material as measured in an acoustic coupler.

The monitoring meter presents difficulties as there are many ways of

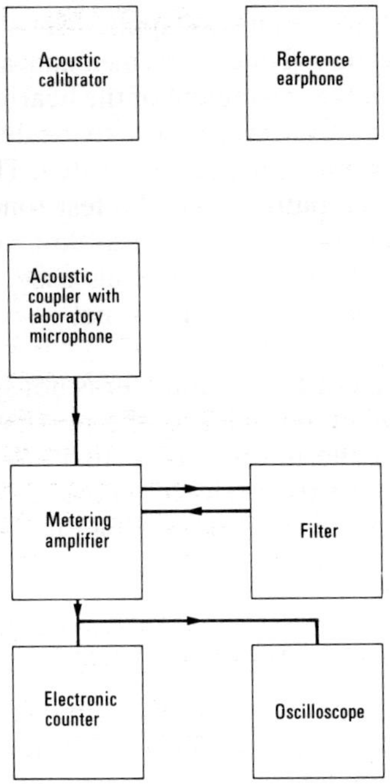

Fig. 8.8. The earphone is placed upon the acoustic coupler and the sound pressure is measured by means of the calibrated condenser microphone in the cavity. A metering amplifier with a range of at least 120 dB is necessary to measure the performance of attenuator steps. The filter can be a one-third octave type and is used to measure low acoustic levels and harmonic distortion. The electronic counter enables the frequency of the test tones to be measured quickly and accurately. The oscilloscope provides a valuable means of seeing if distortion is present if the equipment is functioning. An acoustic calibrator allows acoustic calibration at single frequencies, while a reference earphone enables a calibration at all frequencies.

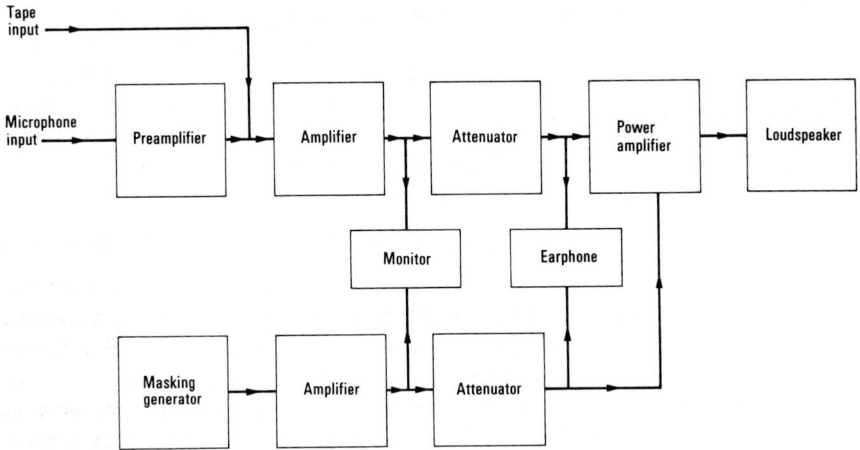

Fig. 8.9. Functional block diagram of speech audiometer.

measuring speech voltages none of which are universally acceptable (Sjogren 1973). In practice the VU meter is most widely used and is inexpensive and readily available. The output level control should meet the same audiometric standards as for pure tones. The zero point on the hearing level dial should correspond to a stated sound pressure developed in an acoustic coupler when the monitor meter is at the reference point. In the American Standard S3.6 (1969) this sound pressure is 19 dB.

Test material for speech audiometry presents further problems due to its influence on the calibration of the instrument. Fig. 8.10 shows the articulation curves for three different types of test material. On each curve three points may be readily defined:

(i) Speech detection level which is that point at which speech is just heard but not understood.

(ii) Speech reception threshold (SRT) which is the point at which 50 per cent of the test material is understood, or 50 per cent of the maximum score if 100 per cent score is not achieved.

(iii) Maximum speech discrimination score.

Speech audiometry is discussed elsewhere (Chapter 16) but for calibration purposes it may be seen from the above that a problem exists in deciding which point should be defined as the reference point. To avoid this dilemma IEC 645. Audiometers does not consider the test material but only the sound pressure for a stated signal.

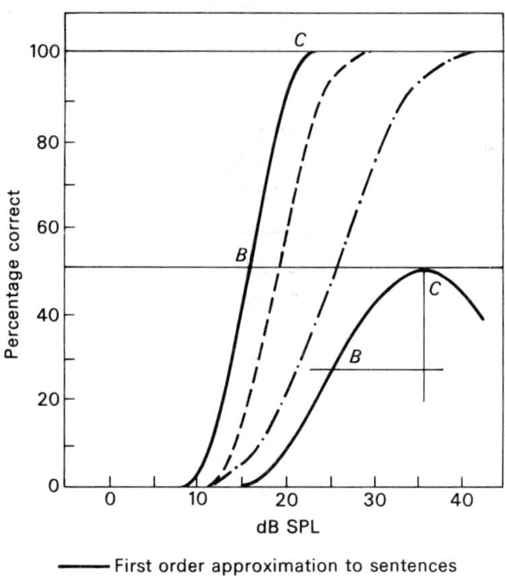

Fig. 8.10. Comparison of articulation curves for three types of speech material (from Jerger 1970). Right-hand curve shows method of measurement when 100 per cent score is not reached. *A* = Speech detection level. *B* = Speech perception level. *C* = Maximum discrimination score.

All recorded speech test material should have a calibration tone on the tape or disc. This calibration tone should be recorded at a peak level that corresponds approximately to the peak level of the speech signal. Peak values are chosen in order that the reproduction device is not overloaded when the calibration tone is set to the reference point on the monitor indicator. The calibration tone ensures, given that the audiometer is stable, that the test signals are reproduced at the correct hearing level; without the calibration tone it becomes extremely difficult to set the level of output accurately in a repeatable fashion.

While speech audiometers exist as instruments in their own right it is common practice for pure tone audiometers to contain the facility for accepting an external signal either from tape or from a microphone and preamplifier (live voice). Table 8.7 indicates that this facility should be found on Types 1, 2, and 3 audiometers.

'FREE' OR 'SOUND-FIELD' AUDIOMETERS

A free sound-field is a field whose boundaries exert a negligible effect on the sound wave. A measure of the effect of the boundaries is whether or not the signal follows the inverse square law. The term 'free field' is used in the United Kingdom while 'sound field' is used in the United States. In practice a free sound-field is only produced in an open space such as produced by a loudspeaker on a high pole or by a loudspeaker in an anechoic chamber. If a loudspeaker is placed in a room the sound-field will depend upon the size and absorption characteristics of the room. At one end of the range a good anechoic room will absorb energy over a wide wide frequency range. At the opposite end of the range a reverberant chamber will absorb very little sound. Hence rooms may vary from what may be descriptively described as very 'dead' to very 'live'.

For free field testing any room may be used providing its characteristics are borne in mind. For clinical tests a short reverberation time is preferred, 0.5 s is often suggested for good speech transmission purposes. For hearing-aid fitting, however, it may be desirable to have both long and short reverberation times. For localization purposes near anechoic conditions will be required. The free field audiometer is normally a conventional audiometer with an electrical signal taken from output socket on the audiometer and fed into a power amplifier and suitable loudspeaker. It is possible to take the signal from the headphone output of most audiometers, providing that suitable precautions are taken to load the output socket correctly and to ensure that no earth loops occurs which might affect the performace of the audiometer, particularly the hearing level attenuator. The power amplifier used will depend upon the level of output signal required but for most practical purposes a standard 20 W high-fidelity amplifier will be more than adequate.

The loudspeaker to be used should be given special consideration both for its frequency response characteristics and its power handling capabilities.

Ideally, a uniform response is required over at least 250 to 6000 Hz, the higher frequencies however may give rise to power handling problems when using pure-tones as signals. Users should examine the high-frequency power handling capability of the loudspeaker system for continuous tones, it will be seen to be very much less than the overall power handling figure for the loudspeaker system. If care is not taken over this point the high-frequency units in multiple speaker units may burn out.

A number of configurations can be used for free field audiometry but to calibrate these arrangements basically the same procedure can be used:

(i) The signal source is set to give a reference reading on the audiometer monitor meter.

(ii) The attenuator is set to some value that will give a good signal without running into any overload condition from the amplifier and loudspeaker or into background noise for the sound level meter used for measuring purposes.

(iii) A sound level meter set to a linear 'C' weighting position is placed at the position of the test subject's head. A 'fast' meter position is used to measure the sound field.

(iv) The sound field is measured for the range of stimuli to be used. This normally means making a measurement of each test frequency and recording the results in a reference book.

In making the above measurements it is essential to keep the body of the person holding the sound level meter clear of the test position. Ideally the microphone should be mounted on its own. The manner of measurement should be kept constant and not changed without noting the change.

If the test stimuli are pure tones it will be found that a small variation in position of the sound level meter will cause large changes in sound pressure. It is for this reason that warble tones and bands of noise are used for test purposes as they minimize the variations found with pure tones.

It is important to note that the sound field will not be the same value as that indicated by the audiometer hearing level dial. The gain of the amplifier may be adjusted to give the same sound pressure level as the dial reading at one frequency, say 1 kHz, but at all other frequencies the sound pressure will tend to be different. Corrections will have to be made to the results obtained from patients in response to the free-field signals.

COMPUTER-BASED AUDIOMETERS

Interactive procedures using computers has become of more interest recently and Stevenson (1975) has described a speech audiometer using two alternative forced-choice system which not only records if the response is correct or not, but the time taken to make the decision. The time for making a decision is one which conventional forms of audiometer do not take into account but which are important. A further advantage of using reaction time as a measure is that a 100 per cent correct response can be recorded by patients differentiated on the basis of the time taken to make that response.

The other use for computer-based audiometers is for obtaining threshold using strategies that can be adopted to suit the needs of the experimenter and the patients. Sakabe, Hirai, and Itami (1978). There is however little point in going to this sophistication if conventional techniques are simply implemented through a computer.

PEEP-SHOW AUDIOMETERS

The peep-show audiometer (Dix and Hallpike 1947) is a device that consists of an audiometer with the means of operating an animated figure, lighting a picture or making a toy move when a correct response is made to the test signal by a patient. The performance of such audiometers should not vary from accepted standards but the method of obtaining a response will depend upon the ingenuity of the system used.

SUMMARY

A very specific and standardized range of requirements for audiometer performance exists. Many variations are possible in the manner in which audiometers are used but very few of these require any change in performance requirements. The future development of audiometers will be with improved circuitry but it is difficult to see other changes apart from attempts to automate the system. The major difficulty is to obtain a response from the patient and the infinite variability of the individual will always make this a major problem.

APPENDIX A: ROUTINE CHECKING OF AUDIOMETRIC EQUIPMENT: RECOMMENDED PROCEDURE FOR DAILY AND WEEKLY CHECKS†

1. Introduction

Most items of audiometric equipment require to be checked on a regular basis, to ensure that items which may have become unsafe, or non-functional do not remain in service. Three levels of check procedures are defined, as under:

Stage A: Daily and weekly subjective tests
Stage B: Periodic objective tests
Stage C: Full workshop test and calibration

The frequency and scope of Stage B and Stage C procedures is covered in other recommendations; it is anticipated that Stage C procedures will be performed only on demand while Stage B procedures will be utlized at intervals of 3–12 months, depending upon the type and usage of the equipment concerned. This recommendation deals with Stage A checks only, and formalizes procedures which are already in general use in many centres.

2. Need for routine checking

In addition to the types of malfunction normally associated with electronic equip-

† Appendices A–C are reproduced by courtesy of the Department of Health and Social Security and remain subject to Crown copyright.

ment, audiometric equipment is susceptible to sudden or gradual changes in performance resulting from damage or mishandling. Such changes may not produce a complete loss of function, but may nevertheless affect the calibration of the equipment to the extent that diagnostic tests could prove misleading. The purpose of routine checking, therefore, is to ensure as far as possible that the equipment is performing in a proper manner, that its calibration has not noticeably altered and that its attachments, leads and accessories are free from any defect that might adversely affect safety.

Stage A check procedures should be performed weekly in full on all equipment in use. They may be performed more frequently if required, e.g. immediately after possible damage has been sustained or before each period of use for equipment which is not used regularly. In particular, some of the tests should be performed on each day of use to ensure that equipment is in order before commencing clinical investigations. Tests recommended for daily application are marked with asterisk in paragraph 4.

3. Subjective checking of electro-acoustic equipment

Stage A check procedures employ simple tests throughout, i.e. measuring instruments are assumed to be unavailable and are not therefore used. The most important elements of the Stage A procedure can be successfully performed only by an operator with unimpaired hearing, and this must be taken into account when determining which members of a centre's staff are to perform these tests. The ambient noise conditions under which the tests are performed must not be subtantially worse than those encountered when equipment is in use.

4. Stage A check procedure—pure-tone audiometers

(i) Clean and examine the audiometer and all accessories. Check plugs, mains leads, and accessory leads for signs of wear or damage. (Damaged or badly worn leads should be replaced.)

(ii)* Switch on equipment and leave for recommended warm-up time. (If no warm-up period is quoted by the manufacturer, allow five minutes for circuits to stabilize.) Carry out any setting-up adjustments as specified by the manufacturers. On battery-powered equipment, check battery state by the specified method. Check that earphone and bone vibrator serial numbers tally with instrument serial number

(iii)* Check calibration of both air and bone conduction by sweeping through at, for example 10 or 15 dB HL and listening for 'just audible' tones. This test must be performed at all appropriate frequencies, and for both earphones as well as the bone vibrator.

(iv)* Check through at high-level (e.g. 60 dB HL on air-conduction, 40 dB HL on bone-conduction) on all appropriate functions (and on either earphone) at all frequencies used; listen for proper functioning, absence of distortion, freedom from interrupter clicks, etc. Check all earphones (including masking insert), also the bone vibrator, for absence of distortion and intermittency; check plugs and leads for intermittency. Check that all switch knobs are secure and that lamps and indicators function correctly.

(v)* Check that patient's signal system operates correctly.

(vi) Listen at low levels for any sign of noise or hum, for unwanted sounds (break-through) arising when a signal is introduced in another channel, or for any change in tone quality as masking is introduced. Check that attenuators do attenuate the signals over their full range, and that attenuators which are intended to be operated while a tone is being delivered are free from electrical or mechanical noise. Check that interrupter keys operate silently, and that no noise radiated from the instrument is audible at the patient's position. (These tests should be performed by an operator with very good hearing.)

(vii) Check speech circuits if appropriate, applying procedures similar to those used for pure-tone functions.

(viii) Check tension of headset, headband, and bone vibrator headband. Ensure that swivel joints are free to turn without being excessively slack.

(ix) On self-recording audiometers, check mechanical operation and function of limit switches and frequency switches. Check that no extraneous instrument noise is audible at the patient's position.

NOTES

1. The check procedures described above should be carried out with the audiometer set up in its usual working situation. If a booth or separate test room is used, the equipment should be checked as installed, even if an assistant may then be required in order to carry out the procedures. The checks will then cover the interconnections between the audiometer and the equipment in the booth, but the additional connecting leads and any plug and socket connections at the junction box should be examined, as potential sources of intermittency or incorrect connection.

2. When subjective checks of bone conduction threshold levels are being performed by an operator with normal hearing, air conducted sound radiated from the back of the bone vibrator may be heard at a high enough level to invalidate this test, especially at frequencies about 1.5 kHz. Sufficient attenuation of this air-conducted sound may be achieved by wearing the air-conduction headphones (disconnected) during this test.

5. Stage A checking procedures—other equipment

Speech audiometry equipment, acoustic impedance bridges, electric response audiometry equipment etc, should also be subject to daily and weekly check procedures. These procedures should check the safety and proper operation of the equipment and should follow the general principles of the procedure for pure-tone audiometers. A check should be made of recordings used for speech audiometry. The calibration of the compliance or admittance indication on acoustic impedance bridges may be checked objectively at at least one spot value by using calibration cavities of pre-determined volume. Such cavities are usually available from the equipment manufacturer. It has been found that certain types of acoustic impedance bridge are prone to steady calibration drift; if such drifting is suspected, bridges should be checked immediately before performing tests.

6. Action on discovery of faults

Immediate action should be taken to rectify any fault discovered in applying the above procedures. Local fault reporting procedures may vary, but users should ensure that they are familiar with local arrangements for repair and maintenance of electromedical equipment. If maintenance or repair is undertaken in local workshops, a full calibration check should be performed before equipment is returned to service (this procedure should be automatic when repairs are undertaken by the manufacturer), unless the work is limited to the replacement of a mains lead or other external component that can have no effect upon calibration. (NB replacement or shortening of a headset lead, or altering the length of tubing on impedance bridges, may alter the calibration.) In many instances faulty equipment will be returned directly from the centre to the manufacturer or repairer for attention. Where this is done, the responsibility for reporting any serious defects (i.e. those capable of producing major safety hazards) to the responsible officer must not be overlooked.

When equipment is sent away for repair or calibration, it is essential that it should be sent complete with the correct earphones, bone vibrator etc. These items must not be interchanged between equipments.

APPENDIX B: CHECKLIST FOR DAILY AND WEEKLY EXAMINATION OF PURE-TONE AUDIOMETERS

Tests marked with an asterisk are recommended for daily check procedures; other checks may be performed at weekly intervals.

1. Clean equipment and examine for damage or wear.
2. * Switch on, allow warm-up, adjust according to handbook.
3. * Earphone serial numbers tally with equipment.
4. * Switch knobs are secure; switches operate freely.
5. * Lamps and indicators function correctly.
6. * Patient's signal system operates correctly.
7. * Check battery state if appropriate.
8. * Threshold levels are subjectively correct for
   (a) Air conduction.
   (b) Bone conduction.
9. * High level listening test satisfactory on:
   (a) Air conduction.
   (b) Bone conduction.
   (c) Masking (including insert).
   (d) Loudness balance.
   (e) Other functions.
10. Attenuators are silent and attenuate over proper range.
11. Noise, hum, and break-through levels are adequately low.
12. Radiated noise from instrument is inaudible at the patient's position.
13. Speech circuits (if provided) operate correctly.
14. Headbands are in good condition and tensions are correct.
15. (Self-recording audiometers). Mechanical operations, including limit switches and frequency switches, are satisfactory. Noise from instrument is inaudible at the patient's position.
16. * Reset all controls to normal operating positions for commencement of patient testing.

APPENDIX C: PREVENTIVE MAINTENANCE OF AUDIOMETRIC EQUIPMENT

Attention paid to the following suggestions will assist in maintaining equipment in good condition, thereby reducing the delay and inconvenience resulting from equipment being inoperative or under repair. These points may be especially useful to students being trained in the use of audiometers.

1. Equipment leads which are allowed to become tangled, kinked, or twisted may develop intermittent faults which can be troublesome to trace. A little time spent in keeping leads tidy will avoid more serious trouble later, as well as speeding the handling of the next patient.

2. Headphones and bone vibrators may be damaged, and their calibration affected,

by mechanical impact. These components should always be handled and stored carefully; avoid dropping them or placing them where they may be pulled off a working surface by an accidental pull on the connecting lead.

3. Do not subject equipment to dust, dampness, or large ambient temperature changes unnecessarily. While audiometric equipment should operate correctly over a wide range of temperature and humidity, large cyclic changes will tend to shorten the working life of equipment. Place dust covers over equipment which is not in use.

4. Portable audiometers are usually designed for lightness in weight rather than robustness. Larger audiometers, although often transportable, are not intended to be transported without special packing. Equipment should always be cushioned against impact when in transit.

5. Headphones and bone vibrators cannot be interchanged between audiometers (even of the same type) without affecting the calibration. If these accessory items are not permanently marked with the equipment's serial number, local markings (e.g. colour-coded tabs) may be applied in order to prevent any risk of confusion.

6. Equipment and accessories should be stored away when not in use, and adequate clean and dry storage facilities should be available. Leads and other accessories should be stored with the instrument for which they are intended, rather than in a 'communal' place. Equipment which is to be stored for long periods should have any batteries removed.

7. If a fault does occur, the equipment should be clearly labelled, indicating the nature of the fault, before anyone else attempts to use it. (Special procedures exist for reporting hazardous faults.)

REFERENCES

ASA Z24.5 (1951). American standard specification for audiometers for general diagnostic purposes. American Standards Associations.

ANSI S3.6 (1969). American national standard specifications for audiometers. American National Standards Institute.

BRITISH STANDARD 2042 (1953). An artificial ear for the calibration of earphones of the external type. British Standards Institution.

—— 2497 (1954). The normal threshold of hearing for pure tones by earphone listening. British Standards Institution.

BSI (1972). British Standard 2497 Part 4. Normal threshold of hearing by bone conduction. British Standards Institution.

DADSON, R. S. and KING, J. H. (1952). A determination of the threshold of hearing and its relation to the standardisation of audiometers. *J. Lar. Otol.* **66**, 366–78.

DELANY, M. E. and WHITTLE, L. S. (1967). Reference equivalent threshold sound pressure levels for audiometry. Acustica **18**, 227–31.

——, WHITTLE, L. S., COOK, J. P., and SCOTT, V. (1967). Performance studies on a new artificial ear. *Acoustica* **18**, 231–7.

DIX, M. R. and HALLPIKE, C. S. (1947). The peep show. *Br. med. J.* **ii**, 719.

INTERNATIONAL ELECTROTECHNICAL COMMISSION 126 (1961). IEC reference coupler for the measurement of hearing aids using earphones coupled to the ear by means of ear inserts.

—— 177 (1965a). Pure tone audiometers for general diagnostic purposes.

—— 178 (1965b). Pure tone screening audiometers.

—— 303 (1970a). IEC provisional reference coupler for the calibration of earphones used in audiometry.

—— 318 (1970b). The IEC wideband artificial ear for the calibration of earphones used in audiometry.
—— 373 (1971). An IEC mechanical coupler for the calibration of bone vibrators having a specified contact area and being applied with a specified static force.
—— (1976). International electrotechnical vocabulary, Chapter 801 Acoustics and electro acoustics, Section 08 Various apparatus.
—— 645 (1980). Specification for audiometers.
INTERNATIONAL STANDARD ORGANIZATION ISO 389 (1975), Standard reference zero for the calibration of pure tone audiometers.
JERGER, J. (1970). Development of synthetic sentence identification (SSI) as a tool for speech audiometry. *2nd Danavox Symp.,* Odense.
MRASS, H. and DIESTEL, H. G. (1959). Best immung der Normalhorschwelle fur reine Tone bei einohrigem Horen mit Hilfe eines Kopfhorers. *Acustica* **9,** 61.
ROBINSON, D. W. (1978). A proposal for audiometric zero referred to the IEC artificial ear. NPL Acoustics Report AC 85.
—— and WHITTLE, L. S. (1966). An international ring comparison of bone conduction thresholds. NPL Report AP 23.
—— —— (1967a). An artificial mastoid for the calibration of bone vibrators. *Acustica* **19**, 80–9.
—— —— (1967b). Second report on standardization of the bone conduction threshold. NPL. Aero Report AC 30.
SAKABE, N., HIRAI, Y., and ITAMI, E. (1978). Modification and application of the computerized automatic audiometer. *Scand. Audiol.* **7**, 105–9.
SJOGREN, H. (1973). Objective measurements of speech level. *Audiology* **12**, 47–54.
STEVENSON, P. W. (1975). An adaptive speech audiometer. *Int. J. Man–Mach. Stud.* **7**, 661–74.
WEISS, E. J. (1960). Air damped artificial mastoid, *J. acoust. Soc. Am.* **32**, 1582.
WHEELER, L. J. and DICKSON, E. D. D. (1952). The determination of the threshold of hearing. *J. Lar. Otol.* **66**, 379.
WHITTLE, L. S. (1965). A determination of the normal threshold of hearing by bone conduction. *J. Sound Vib.* **2**, 3.
—— (1970). Problems of calibration in bone conduction *Sound* **4**, 35–41.

9 Instrumentation for Electric Response Audiometry

A. R. D. THORNTON

INTRODUCTION

Electrophysiological tests of hearing are carried out at many centres as a routine clinical procedure. Furthermore, current research work has shown many areas, involving audiometric, audiological, and neurological applications of evoked potential (EP) measures, which provide useful data in clinical measurement and diagnosis. It seems clear that such tests will play an increasingly important role in the audiological clinic and these aspects are dealt with later in Chapters 31 and 33. As increasing diagnostic reliance is placed on evoked potential results, it becomes more important that the instrumentation used to obtain the results be well understood so that data contamination and errors of interpretation are avoided.

The recording system has to obtain from the patient an EP that is substantially free from contaminants. Contamination of the record can arise from many sources. Firstly, there is contamination from physiological noise. The EP is of a smaller amplitude than other electrical signals recorded from the same site and the recording system has to improve the signal-to-noise ratio so that a clear response may be obtained. Secondly, artifactual contamination from external electromagnetic sources can occur. These include the stimulus transducer, mains wiring, and general electromagnetic radiation. Finally, the EP may be contaminated or modified by the recording system itself. The factors involved here include sampling rate, filter settings, interstimulus intervals, electrode impedance, and the accuracy of measurement in the computer or averager.

In the sections that follow, the main requirements of electric response audiometry (ERA) instrumentation will be defined by considering the methods used to improve the response signal-to-noise ratio and to avoid or minimize contamination of the response.

BASIC TECHNIQUES

In some instances an EP of 0.1 μV will be contained in a record which has 50 μV of electrical activity due to other physiological signals, electrode contact potentials etc. The activity which is not due to the EP may be regarded as noise. Thus, the basic problem is to improve the signal-to-noise ratio (S/N) for the EP. The most powerful element in the recording system for S/N improvement is the averager and this will be considered separately. In this section other techniques which reduce the noise components will be described.

Electrodes

Electrodes in contact with the skin will generate a contact potential which can vary during the test period. The impedance of the electrode–skin junction will also determine the noise generated and the magnitude of induced electromagnetic artefacts. There are several ways in which the noise from this source may be reduced. The electrode material is a major factor in determining the contact potential. Silver has a low contact potential and further improvements can be made by using a fluid-column electrode in which the electrode itself does not touch the skin, the connection being made by a saline solution or electrode jelly (Cooper, Osselton, and Shaw 1974). Low-frequency noise may be reduced by using a reversible electrode such as silver coated with silver chloride (Ag–AgCl) (Geddes 72). Cooper *et al.* (1974) also pointed out that the distortion caused by electrode capacitance is very small for Ag–AgCl electrodes.

Traditionally preparation of the skin surface by vigorous rubbing with spirit or acetone helps to reduce the electrode–skin contact impedance. Electrode contact should be tested with an alternating current impedance meter and the impedances of each electrode pair should be both low and balanced as closely as possible. Impedances of 2000 to 3000 Ω measured at a frequency of 1 kHz give satisfactory results. Direct currenct test meters should never be used to measure electrode contact. Not only can this polarize the electrodes and add to the noise they produce but currents in excess of present safety limits can be passed through the patient.

Differential amplification

By careful selection of the electrode derivation, a situation may be achieved in which much of the noise is the same at both electrodes whilst the EP differs at each electrode of the pair. If the two electrodes are connected to a differential amplifier, the output signal is the result of subtracting the signal at one electrode from the signal at the other. Thus, noise which is common to the two electrode sites will be cancelled whilst the EP will largely be unchanged. In this way the S/N of the EP is improved. The degree to which a differential amplifier can cancel common noise is called its common mode rejection ratio (CMRR).

Much of the physiological noise is recorded as a far-field signal that is distributed widely over the scalp. In some cases the EP may be recorded as a near-field potential so that one electrode receives virtually all of the EP signal and differential amplification will improve the S/N a great deal. For other responses which are themselves recorded as a far-field signal it is more difficult to achieve this situation.

Band-pass filtering

The power spectrum of a signal represents the values of signal power at a different frequencies. Examination of the power spectra of EPs and of the noise shows that, in general, the noise spectrum extends over a much wider range of frequencies than the EP spectrum. Thus, by filtering the input signal with a band-pass filter whose frequency limits correspond to the limits of the EP spectrum, the EP will not be altered but the noise components which lie outside this filter band will be markedly reduced in amplitude. The overall noise power will be reduced and hence the EP S/N will be improved.

Limiting

Limiting or peak-clipping involves restricting the input signal within pre-set voltage limits. If these limits are set such that the signal is unaltered for most of the time that the patient is generating low levels of physiological noise, then occasional high-amplitude signals due to patient movement, swallowing, yawning, etc. will cause the limiter to operate. This ensures that the amplitude of the input signal, during these particularly noisy periods, is not as great as it could have been. This protects the recorded signal from large amplitude noise values and hence improves the S/N. The exact effects of limiting are hard to quantify but theoretical studies by Hyde (personal communication) have shown that, in high noise level records, limiting the signal to very narrow limits can give beneficial results.

TIME-DOMAIN AVERAGING

Time-domain averaging is a powerful technique for improving the S/N of periodic signals or of signals with a fixed time relationship to a detectable event.

Theory of operation

A section of the amplified signal from the electrodes is sampled using an analogue-to-digital converter (ADC). This measures the voltage of the input signal at an instant in time and this sample voltage is converted into a digital, numerical value and stored in a location in the averager memory. Such samples are taken at short time intervals until the required section of input signal has been sampled and stored. Thus, a digital representation of a section of the input signal is stored in the averager memory. This record is called a 'sweep' and the duration of the section is known as the 'window' or 'analysis time' used by the averager. It is arranged that the acoustic stimulus is delivered at the start, or perhaps more usefully, at a fixed time after the start of the window. A single sweep, stored in the memory, can be considered as containing two parts which are shown in the top half of Fig. 9. 1. The first part is the response or signal and the second is the noise. For a fixed set of stimulus parameters, it is assumed that the response is constant. Thus, when the acquisition and sampling process is repeated and the values from successive sweeps are added to the values obtained from the first sweep, the response will always occur at the same point in the sweep (it is time-locked to the stimulus) and its amplitude will increase linearly with the number of sweeps. Hence, if the original amplitude of the response is r, after m sweeps the response amplitude stored in memory will be m times greater and equal

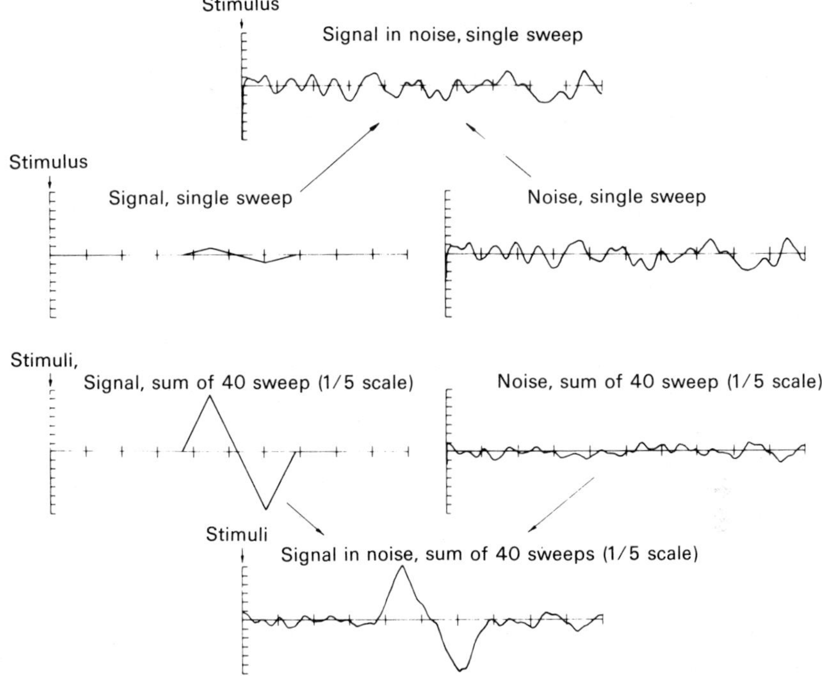

Fig. 9.1. The effects of averaging on the overall S/N, shown as the change in the response component and in the noise component.

mr. The noise processes are not time-locked to the stimulus and, at a point in the window, the noise can take any value both positive and negative for different sweeps. Clearly the noise values will not add linearly and, if it is assumed that the noise is random with a normal distribution, it can be shown that it will add according to a root-mean-square rule (e.g. see Thornton 1977a). Thus, if the original noise value is n, after m sweeps the noise will have a value equal to $\sqrt{(m)}n$. Hence, the original S/N for the response is r/n and after averaging this becomes $mr/\sqrt{(m)}\, n$ or $\sqrt{(m)}\,(r/n)$. The S/N of the EP has been improved by a factor equal to the square root of the number of sweeps. This is illustrated in the lower half of Fig. 9.1.

The enhancement of S/N by a factor of $\sqrt{m}$ will occur only if the assumptions of an invariant response and normally distributed random noise are met. If the response is variable, and this has been demonstrated (Hyde 1973), it can be shown that the degree of S/N enhancement will not be so great. Similarly, to the relief of the neurologist and others who use EEG patterns diagnostically, the EEG is not strictly normally distributed random noise. However, for EP work, where the signals are averaged, the EEG approximates adequately to this assumption (Thornton 1977b).

An aspect of averaging can also be used to eliminate fixed frequency contaminating waveforms such as mains hum. It can be shown that the process of averaging in the time domain is equivalent to comb filtering in the frequency domain and produces regularly spaced passbands whose width depends on the number of sweeps. The process is sometimes referred to as time-domain filtering. Components in the input signal which are of frequencies such that their periods are an exact multiple of the interstimulus interval (cycle time) will be time-locked and will be summated. Frequencies which have an odd number of periods in m times the cycle time, where m is the number of sweeps averaged, will be cancelled in the averaging process. The exact degree of summation or cancellation at each frequency may be calculated and a frequency domain transfer function defined. This attribute may be used to cause a particular frequency to be cancelled in the average. For example mains hum, at the line frequency of 50 Hz, has a period of 20 ms and can be cancelled, for any even number of sweeps, by having an interstimulus interval which is an odd multiple of 10 ms.

Sampling

The ADC converts the analogue voltage of the input signal into a binary number containing several binary digits or, in its more usual abbreviated form, several bits. The number of bits in the ADC determines the number of voltage levels which are used to approximate to the actual voltage of the signal. A one-bit ADC will have $2^1 = 2$ levels and the signal will be coded as having values equal to 0 or to 1. A three-bit ADC has $2^3 = 8$ levels and the signal voltage would be approximated by numbers from 0 to 7. This quantization of the signal introduces sampling errors as the fixed levels available from the ADC will not correspond exactly to the actual voltage level of the signal. This has the effect of introducing noise to the signal and the number of quantization levels will determine the precision of the digital version of the input signal. A relationship between the precision which the averaged EP can achieve, the number of sweeps required and the number of bits in the ADC can be calculated (Thornton 1979). Clearly, the greater the number of bits in the ADC the fewer the number of sweeps which are required for a given precision. Calculations for transtympanic and brainstem responses show that the eight-bit ADCs, found in some of the instruments currently on the market, give sufficient accuracy. The dynamic range, in dB, of an ADC may be calculated by multiplying the number of bits by 6. Thus, an eight-bit ADC has a dynamic range of 48 dB.

Sampling rate

The sample rate in most hard-wired averagers is determined by the number of channels selected and the window duration that is chosen. For example an averager with 1024 words of storage is set to average two channels with a window of 30 ms. This means that there are 512 sample points per channel and that 512 samples will be taken in 30 ms. Therefore the sample rate is 512/0.03 = 17 067 samples/s. The question which now arises is whether such a sample rate is an adequate one.

The sample rate which will avoid errors is related to the highest frequency present in the input signal. It should be stressed that this differs from the highest frequency of interest in the input signal. For a simple signal, such as a sine wave, it can be shown that if it is sampled at a rate greater than two samples per period then the samples will uniquely define the sine wave which can be exactly reconstructed from the sample values. Furthermore, any signal, such as an EEG, may be considered as comprising a set of sine waves of different amplitudes and frequencies. Therefore, if the EEG is sampled at a rate which is greater than two samples per period for the highest frequency present then this frequency component and all the lower frequency components will be adequately defined. This will ensure that the EEG signal itself is uniquely determined by the sample values.

If the sample rate is not high enough the signal will not be faithfully reproduced and distortion of the waveform and of the resultant averaged EP will occur. Such errors can be quite marked and are known as aliasing errors. There is no way of determining from the averaged waveform that aliasing errors have occurred. The only way to avoid the effects of such errors is to prevent their occurrence. This is done by using a low-pass filter, often referred to as an anti-aliasing filter, to limit the high frequency end of the signal spectrum. If the filter acts such that f_m is the highest frequency present in the signal then the minimum sample rate is $2f_m$ samples/s. This is known as the Nyquist rate (Nyquist 1924) after the mathematical pioneer of sampling theory. The Nyquist rate represents the *theoretical* minimum value for the sample rate. In practice higher rates have to be used for two main reasons. Firstly, the ADC produces errors in the sample values and the effect of these errors is reduced by increasing the sample rate. Secondly, and more importantly, the anti-aliasing filter does not have an infinitely steep slope and so, if it is set to a cut-off frequency of f_m, higher frequency components will be attenuated but not absent from the signal. The sample rate of $2f_m$ will not be adequate for these higher frequencies and aliasing errors will occur.

To avoid all aliasing errors the filter must have attenuated the input signal by an amount equal to the dynamic range of the ADC before a frequency equal to half the sample rate. For a filter with a 3 dB cut-off frequency set to f_c Hz with a slope of S dB per octave and using and ADC of dynamic range D, the required sample rate f_s may be calculated from $f_s = 2f_c.2^x$, where $x = (D-3)/S$.

BASIC ERA SYSTEM

A block diagram of a basic ERA system is shown in Fig. 9.2. For several of the EP measures that are in general use a two-channel system is required. Many commercial systems will provide one piece of apparatus to enable EP measures to be taken. Nevertheless, the basic elements shown in Fig. 9.2 should be included. The signal from the electrodes is amplified by a pre-amplifier and a main amplifier, which may contain the band-pass filters. The amplified signal is then passed to the limiter and to an anti-aliasing filter if

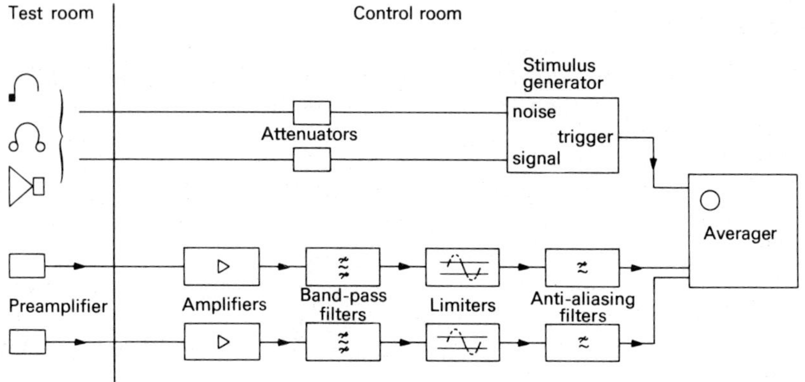

Fig. 9.2. Block diagram of a basic ERA system.

the sample rate criteria are not met by the band-pass filter. Finally, the signal is fed to the ADC of the averager. The stimulus generator provides the test signal which is passed via attenuators to the output transducers such as loudspeakers, earphones or bone-conductors. The stimulus generator should also provide masking noise and timing control for the averager.

The test environment will depend upon the type of EP to be measured, whether anaesthetic facilities are required and the type of patient population in the particular clinic. The requirements have been usefully summarized Gibson (1978). The various elements of the system will be considered separately.

Stimulus generator

The various EPs and the different applications to which they are put require a wide variety of stimuli ranging from clicks to shaped tone-bursts. These have been outlined by Gibson (1978). In addition, tone-burst stimuli should have the facility to be phase-locked and, to cancel stimulus produced electromagnetic artefacts, it is necessary to produce clicks and tone-bursts with alternating phases. Frequency-modulated stimuli may also be required as Arlinger (1976) has demonstrated useful clinical applications with such stimuli. If derived response techniques are to be used, two independent white-noise generators should be provided. One to mask the non-test ear and the second to provide the high-pass filtered noise for the derived response technique.

With click stimuli the timing control could come from the averager or from the stimulus generator but with more complex stimuli such as phase-locked tone bursts it is more convenient to use the stimulus generator to control the timing and to feed trigger pulses to the averager.

Finally, the acoustical waveform of the stimulus delivered to the patient will have been modified by the transducer. For an accurate knowledge of the stimulus the acoustical waveform should be measured and its spectrum calculated.

Amplifiers

The amplification given to the signal occurs in two stages, the preamplifier and the main amplifier. The electrode leads, which are kept as short as possible to avoid electromagnetically induced artefacts, plug into the preamplifier. The preamplifier has two main functions. Firstly, it provides the differential amplification needed to reduce the input noise. To achieve this, the common mode rejection ratio (CMRR) should be high, generally of the order of 70 to 80 dB. Normally, the CMRR is adjusted to its maximum value at a particular frequency. Often this is the line frequency which in the United Kingdom is 50 Hz. If 50 Hz is not within the recording pass-band of the system, it could improve matters by maximizing the CMRR at a different frequency.

Secondly, the preamplifier provides an impedance change, having a very high input impedance and a very low output impedance. The low output impedance minimizes electromagnetic pick-up by the long cables which lead from the preamplifier in the test room to the main amplifier in the control room.

The main amplifier then provides the major part of the amplification, the gain controls and often filter controls being included at this stage. The overall amplification system has some intrinsic noise. Perhaps the most convenient way to evaluate the amplifier noise is to take the 'referred-to-input', r.t.i., noise figure. This is the equivalent of the amplifier noise expressed as a value that would appear at the preamplifier input. This figure should be small compared to a low level EEG signal.

Filters

The filters that determine the pass-band for recording the signal play an important role in determining the waveform of the resultant averaged EP. The characteristics are often specified by the cut-off frequency, the frequency at which the filter attenuation is 3 dB below its value in the centre of the pass-band, and by the slope of the filter skirt. The full characteristics would contain the information of the filter gain by frequency characteristic and its phase by frequency characteristic. The filter will change the phase of the signal at the output relative to that at the input and this can lead to phase distortion which will alter the signal. A linear phase characteristic will preserve the correct relationships between the signal components.

The filter will also introduce a propagation delay which increases as the bandwidth gets narrower. If a stimulus marker is recorded through an appropriate filter system and used to provide response latency values then no errors will arise. However, if for example, the stimulus is presented at the same time as the sweep is triggered and the response latency is calculated from the beginning of the sweep, then the latency values will be in error by the amount of filter propagation delay.

As discussed earlier, as the filter bandwidth is narrowed, the S/N for the response is improved. However, at some point the band limits will enter the range of the response spectrum; this will eliminate components of the response distorting the waveform and reducing the response amplitude. Fig. 9. 3 shows the effects of different recording bandwidths on the PAM response and it can be seen that the response is markedly altered. Clearly, dependent upon the response being recorded and its application the band limits have to be chosen with considerable care.

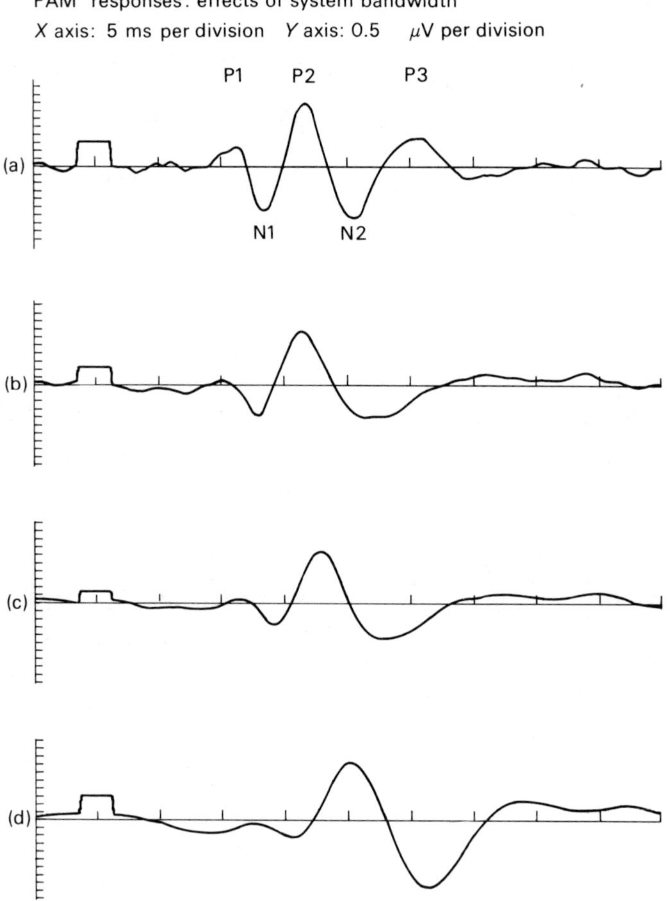

Fig. 9.3. The effects of filter bandwidth on the PAM response. The change in the waveform with various high-frequency limits is shown. The limits are (a) = 4 kHz, (b) = 500 Hz, (c) = 200 Hz, (d) = 100 Hz.

Anti-aliasing filter

The problems of phase distortion are likely to be more severe with the anti-aliasing filter than with the signal band-pass filter as the slope required is generally considerably steeper. One solution to this problem, implemented in the author's clinic, is to use an active filter which starts with a very gentle slope that gradually increases as the attenuation of the filter increases. This results in a filter which meets the anit-aliasing requirements but which has less than 1 per cent distortion in the pass-band.

Averager

The averager acquires its data from the ADC as a sample comprising a certain number of bits. This is fed to an arithmetic unit which adds the value to the value stored in the appropriate memory location. When more than one channel is used the ADC is multiplexed, in the case of four channels a sample is taken from channel 1 followed by samples from channels 2, 3 and 4 before returning to channel 1. Due to the differing requirements of different EP techniques the averager must be a flexible instrument so that the appropriate parameters may be selected for each application.

Generally, the averager includes a display which can monitor the ongoing EEG, when not averaging, and show the accumulating sum or average as it occurs. To produce a permanent record of the response a write-out device is included or the averager produces output signals to control an X–Y plotter.

Calibration

Where stimuli are the same as those used in normal audiometric practice they may be calibrated by standard procedures otherwise 'biological calibration' using a group of normally hearing subjects can be carried out. Most of the stimuli used in EP work will require biological calibration. This has been the procedure used in many centres and appears to work well. Once normal values have been set the physical parameters of the acoustic stimulus should be measured and recorded. Thereafter, at regular intervals, say six months, the objective measures of the acoustic stimulus can be measured to ensure that the system calibration is correct or to adjust the calibration if necessary.

Similarly, the recording system requires calibration. This can be carried out by using a calibration pulse, built into the system, or by measuring the system gain. In either case, the system calibration should be checked at regular intervals using external precision measuring equipment.

CLINICAL ERA SYSTEM

The basic system, described above will record clear responses under good conditions. In this section additional facilities, which are of use in obtaining results in the clinic, will be dealt with. Some of the simpler facilities, such as buffered averaging, may be found in basic averagers. Other, more complex functions such as demeaning and smoothing, are to be found in averagers with microprocessor facilities.

Buffered averaging

This technique allows sweeps that have acquired a high noise level section of EEG to be rejected and not added to the average. A sweep is acquired and temporarily stored in a reserved section of memory. The sweep values may then be examined automatically and, if one or several values exceed some preset limits, no further operations will be carried out and the system will wait for the next sweep to be acquired. If the limits are not exceeded, the sweep is then added to the values accumulating in the main memory. By eliminating the worst sweeps from the average the noise is reduced and a response with better definition is recorded.

EEG-dependent control

Buffered averaging enables the acquisition of data from quiet periods of the EEG. An alternative but somewhat less effective technique is to inhibit the control pulses, that start the averager sweep and the stimulus, until the EEG is in a quiet period. Providing that the EEG remains in a quiet state during the sweep the results will be similar to those obtained by buffered averaging. As there is no means of preventing the acquisition of a sweep during which the EEG has markedly increased in amplitude, this technique generally gives a poorer noise reduction than that given by buffered averaging. The cost of EEG dependent control may be less than that of buffered averaging as no memory space is required.

Manipulation of the averaged response

There are several basic techniques, operating on the averaged response, which are of use in the clinical situation. Perhaps the most common of these is the facility to add and subtract averaged responses stored in different sections of the averager's memory. This enables the separation of cochlear microphonic, action potential and summating potential responses (Eggermont and Odenthal 1974). An example is shown in Fig. 9.4. Trace A shows an abnormal EP recorded using the transtympanic method at a stimulation rate of 5/s. The abnormality could be due to the action potential (AP) or to the summating potential (SP). The second trace (B) shows the SP obtained by stimulating at a rate of 100/s which ensures that the AP component has been adapted. The subtraction of B from A, shown in the lowest trace, gives a normal AP and demonstrates that the abnormality was due to an abnormal SP.

Smoothing, demeaning, and detrending are also useful techniques (Bogart 1972). Smoothing the trace reduces small irregularities on the waveform. Demeaning sets the mean value of the waveform to zero and removes the effects of d.c. shifts. Detrending removes from the waveform the effects of linear trends in the record. It is of use in obtaining a better definition of a waveform but should be used circumspectly. Finally, the ability to expand the horizontal axis of the record and examine a part of the response in greater detail is most valuable.

COMPUTER SYSTEMS

These systems generally contain all of the facilities described above but use a

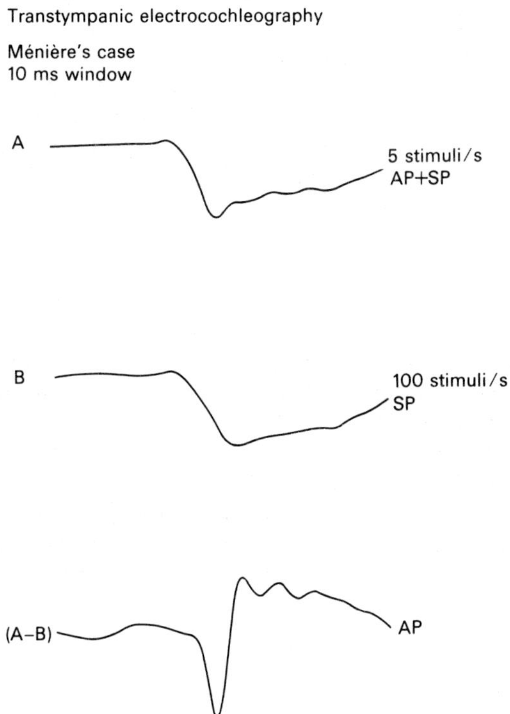

Fig. 9.4. The use of memory subtraction techniques. The top trace shows the AP and SP recorded at 5 stimuli/s. The middle trace shows a response that is predominantly SP, the AP having been adapted by the stimulus rate of 100/s. The lowest trace is the AP obtained by subtracting the middle response from the top one.

general purpose computer to carry out the averaging procedure and many additional techniques. For research work such a system provides the most flexible approach. Some of the more advanced microprocessor averagers will have some of the facilities described here and, in the future, more are likely to do so.

Backing store

Often this is provided by digital magnetic tape or by floppy disks. Once a response has been averaged, the record, together with details of the recording parameters, is written to the backing store and the next averaging run can be started. Such a facility has several advantages. As the patient is involved only for the length of time necessary to acquire the data, the test time is minimized. Once the data are obtained the patient can go and the data retrieved from the backing store for measurement and analysis at any convenient time. The data may be permanently stored and reanalysed at any time and if a new analysis technique is to be evaluated the data stored provide the means to do this.

Real-time techniques

More complex control of the averaging process is possible using a computer. Buffered averaging may be performed with asymmetrical voltage limits or the data in a sweep may be excluded from an average using both amplitude and duration criteria in which the signal must exceed the voltage limit for more than a certain minimum period. Techniques such as dynamic rejection become possible. This involves continuously evaluating the short-term r.m.s. value of the ongoing EEG. When a sweep is acquired to the buffer store, if a value in it exceeds some criterion level, which is a multiple of the EEG r.m.s. value, then the sweep is rejected. This enables the sweeps containing the largest artefacts, to be rejected. These worst sweeps will be a fixed proportion of the total number recorded but will be independent of the basic EEG level of the patient and hence avoid the problems that occur with fixed level rejection systems.

Numerical parameters values

Parameters such as peak latency and peak-to-peak amplitude can be calculated by the computer and printed on a printer to give a permanent record. This is considerably more accurate and convenient than estimating these parameter values from a screen or a plotted waveform. Automatic peak detection systems, with varying degrees of operator control involved, aid this process.

Off-line analysis

Computer systems provide the facility for complex analyses of EP data. In some cases these analyses provide a faster way to achieve a result that could be achieved in other ways. For example, to determine the optimum high-pass filter setting for recording brainstem responses, the data may be

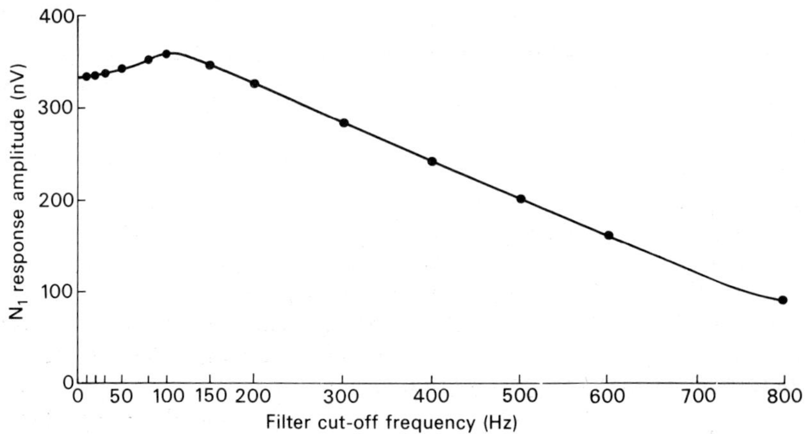

Fig. 9.5. A result from a digital filtering experiment. The amplitude of the N_1 response from the brainstem complex shows a maximum for a high-pass filter setting of 100 Hz.

obtained using a high-pass filter set to 0.2 Hz. A digital filter, which simulates the analogue filter, may then be programed in the computer and the same data then filtered at a range of higher frequencies. Fig. 9.5 shows one of the results from this experiment. The amplitude of the N_1 response is plotted against high-pass cut-off frequency and the response shows a maximum amplitude at 100 Hz.

Spectral and phase analyses (Sayers, Beagley, and Henshall 1974) or convolution techniques (Elberling 1978) have been used to elucidate the basic mechanisms underlying the EP. Statistical analyses of response parameters to provide statistical diagnostic criteria (Thornton 1976) and models of EP processes (Elberling 1976) have all used computer processing techniques. Many more examples exist and in ERA, as in many areas in science and medicine, computers are of increasing importance.

REFERENCES

ARLINGER, S. (1976). Auditory responses to frequency ramps. A psychoacoustic and electrophysiological study. *Linköping Univ. Med. Dissert.* **40**.

BOGART, B. P. (1972). Practicing digital spectrum analysis. In *Human communication: a unified view* (ed. E. E. David Jr. and P. B. Denes). McGraw-Hill, New York.

COOPER, R., OSSELTON, J. W., and SHAW, J. C. (1974). *EEG technology*. Butterworths, London.

EGGERMONT, J. J. and ODENTHAL, D. W. (1974). Action potentials and summating potentials in the normal human cochlea. *Acta oto-lar.* **316** (Suppl.), 39–61.

ELBERLING, C. (1976). Simulation of cochlear action potentials recorded from the ear canal in man. In *Proc. Symp. Electrocochleography* (ed. R. J. Ruben, C. Elberling, and G. Salomon). University Park Press, Baltimore.

—— (1978). Compound impulse response for the brainstem derived through combinations of cochlear and brainstem recordings. *Scand. Audiol.* **7**, 145–57.

GEDDES, L. A. (ed.) (1967). *Electrodes and the measurement of bioelectric events*, Chapter 1. Wiley Interscience, New York.

GIBSON, W. P. R. (1978). *Essentials of clinical electric response audiometry*. Churchill Livingstone, Edinburgh.

HYDE, M. L. (1973). Properties of the auditory evoked vertex response in man. Ph.D. Thesis, University of Southampton.

NYQUIST, H. (1924). Certain factors affecting telegraph speed. *Bell Syst. tech. J.* **3**, 324–46.

SAYERS, B. McA., BEAGLEY, H. A., and HENSHALL, W. R. (1974). The mechanism of auditory evoked EEG responses. *Nature, Lond.* **247**, 481–3.

THORNTON, A. R. D. (1977a). Computers. In *Scientific foundations of otolaryngology* (ed. R. Hinchcliffe and D. Harrison). Heinemann, London.

—— (1977b). Averaged evoked brainstem responses and their analysis for diagnostic application. In *Applications of time series analysis*. Southampton University, 23.1–23.13.

—— (1979). Considerations of analogue-to-digital converter requirements and accuracy in the measurement of averaged signals. ISVR Memorandum No. 593. University of Southampton.

10 Hearing aids

M. C. MARTIN

Today it is estimated that some two million people throughout the world are purchasing hearing aids annually, Bogeskov-Jenson (1978). It cannot be denied that the hearing aid is the one device that has been of real benefit to so many hearing impaired people. Of course the hearing aid does not meet all the needs of some people and does not give the benefit that many would like, but in spite of this it still remains the main means of maintaining communication for a very large number of people.

Hearing aids are basically simple amplifying devices, but like many simple devices there are somewhat more difficult underlying fundamental aspects that have to be understood if the best use of the device is to be made. All hearing aids can be considered as working in the same manner with variations in the way that they are packaged. The range of aids generally available can be broken into three groups: (i) body-worn aids, (ii) head-worn aids, and (iii) educational aids, which will be dealt with later in the chapter. Fig. 10.1 shows examples of body and head-worn (ear-level) types.

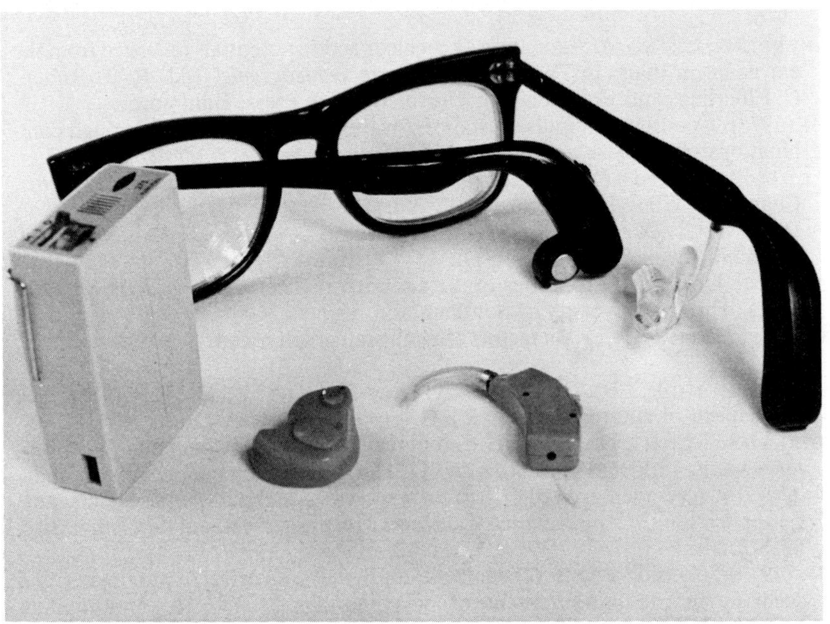

Fig. 10.1. Typical body-worn, post-aural, spectacle, and in-the-ear aids.

THE BASIC AID

Fig. 10.2 shows the basic functional parts of a hearing aid and by using this diagram it is possible to see how the overall acoustic performance of the aid is arrived at, each part will be considered in turn.

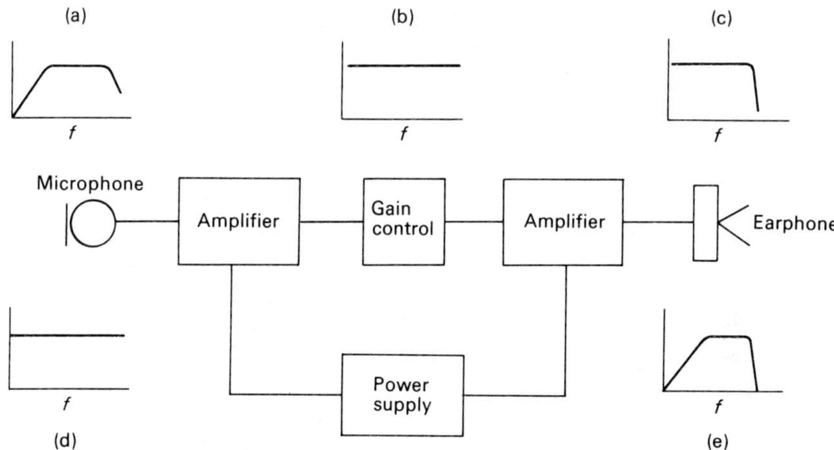

Fig. 10.2. Block diagram of functional parts of an air-conduction hearing aid. Frequency response curves (a), (b), and (c) represent responses of the microphone, amplifier, and earphone. Frequency response (d) represents a constant sound pressure input to the microphone used for testing purposes and (e) the acoustic output for the input (d). (e) therefore gives the cumulative effect of all parts of the aid on the frequency response.

Microphone

The diaphragm of the microphone responds to sound pressure presented to it producing an electrical signal that will be passed on to the amplifier. Microphones used in hearing aids today are the result of considerable development by the microphone manufacturing companies and are available in three functional types, i.e. magnetic, piezo-electric (ceramic), and electret.

Early valve hearing aids used piezo-electric (crystal) microphones because they had a high-voltage output at high impedance and were particularly suitable for feeding into valve circuits. With the advent of transistors which had a low impedance input the crystal microphones could not be used and magnetic types became prevalent. However, as semi-conductor technology advanced it became possible to obtain high-input impedances with transistors and at the same time new types of piezo-electric materials called ceramics were introduced and used in hearing aid microphones. The magnetic microphone inherently has a reduced low-frequency response and the smaller the microphone the greater this reduction; it also tends to have a 'peaky' frequency response. The ceramic microphone has a good low-frequency response which is largely dependent upon the impedance that it works into, but again it tends to have a 'peaky' high frequency response.

The electret microphone works upon the same principle as the condenser microphone except that the charge required for the condenser microphone is contained in an electret material and not provided by a polarizing voltage as in the case of the condenser microphone. Fig. 10.3 shows typical frequency responses obtained from the three types of microphone.

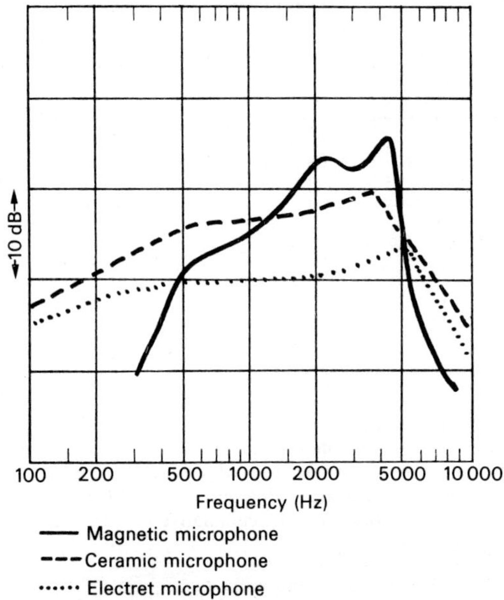

Fig. 10.3. Relative frequency response of three microphones used in post-aural hearing aids.

A further development in microphones is that of the directional microphone which makes use of a phase delay obtained from using a two-port system Fig. 10.4. The overall frequency response of the hearing aid is therefore initially determined by the microphone because the aid can only amplify the electrical signal produced by the microphone.

Amplifier

The amplifier in the hearing aid increases the electrical signal from the microphone and provides the power to operate the earphone. The frequency response of the amplifier presents little problem in that it can be flat and cover a wide frequency range as is wanted. The power output from the amplifier can be as high as is wanted, however increasing power output does increase battery current and this consideration often dictates the design. A further consideration is that of electrical noise generated in the first stages of the amplifier and this may be of prime importance with high-gain aids and those that are to be used by people with small hearing losses.

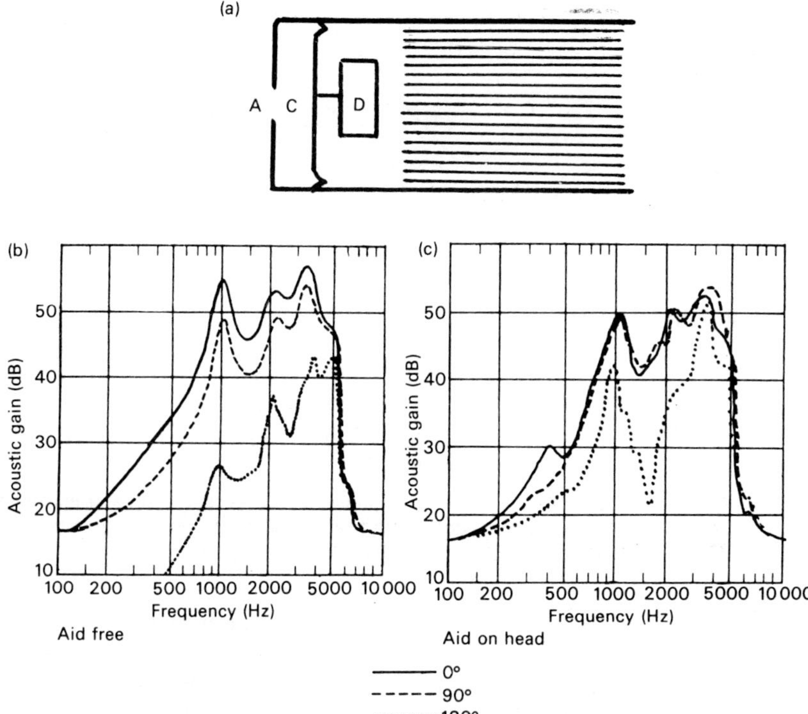

Fig. 10.4. (a). Schematic diagram of directional microphone from British Patent 1, 180, 86 (1970). Front opening A allows sound pressure to activate diaphragm C which creates electrical output from microphone element D. Rear entry B allows sound to pass through acoustic resistance in the form of narrow passages in parallel with one another. This resistance provides a phase or time delay which causes cancellation at low frequencies. The lower figures show frequency response of hearing aid with directional microphone at three different angles to the loudspeaker (b) on its own and (c) worn on the head. Sound input = 64 dB SPL, gain of aid set to maximum, output measured in IEC 2cc acoustic coupler.

The two parameters gain and output power must be clearly separated, particularly when maximum output power is considered. Gain in hearing aid amplifiers refers to voltage gain and does not require any significant battery current. Power output requires battery current and also requires that the output stage of the amplifier has a certain power handling capability. Fig. 10.5 shows the effect of increasing the input to an amplifier with various degrees of gain and maximum output. Tone control can be achieved in the amplifier circuit and normally consists of a simple bass and treble cut operating about 1 kHz.

The position of the gain control in the amplifier circuit is of importance in order to minimize the problem of over-loading the early stages. If an AGC circuit is used then the position becomes more important as it changes the nature of the input–output characteristics of the aid. If the gain control is

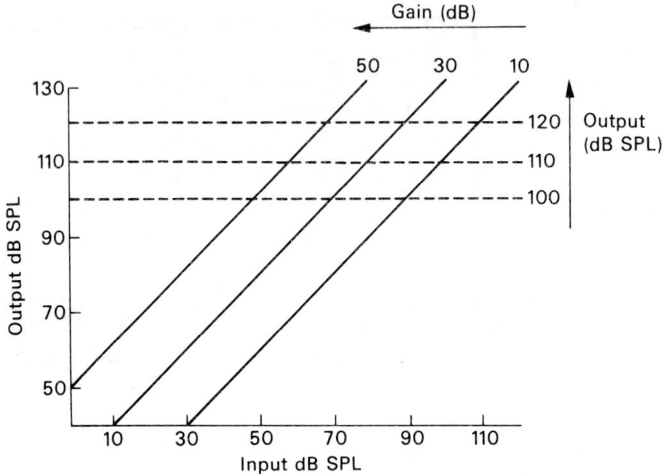

Fig. 10.5. Input–output characteristic of an amplifier. Three levels of gain and maximum output are shown. Gain and output can be adjusted independently to give in theory an infinite number of input output characteristics from two controls.

inside the feedback loop (Fig. 10.6) the control only alters gain and does not affect the maximum output. However, if the control is outside the loop then it acts as an output attenuator and alters maximum output as well as gain. Further consideration will be given to this later in the chapter.

Earphone

The earphone is the means of turning the electrical signal into an acoustic one to be delivered to the ear. The term receiver, which probably originated

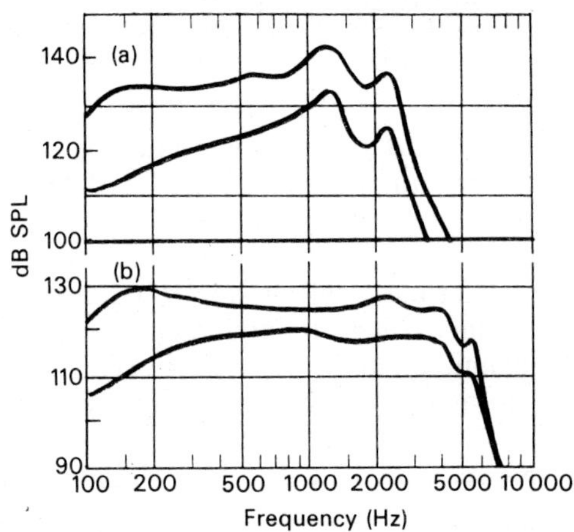

Fig. 10.6. (a). Maximum acoustic output and gain curve for high-powered earphone. (b). Output for a wide-band earphone on the same aid.

from its application in telephony, is often used to describe a hearing aid earphone but is now falling into disuse.

The hearing aid earphone is an electromagnetic device and is made in two basic shapes. The most familiar is the button type used with body-worn aids while the less familiar is that of the rectangular type used in head-worn aids. The button type earphone is designed to be fed into a closed cavity and has a good low frequency response, but a restricted high frequency. Earphones are capable of outputs up to 6 kHz or more but only at low sound pressures. Fig. 10.6 shows the frequency response of a typical high-powered earphone and a wide band earphone to emphasize this important restriction on performance. The low frequency response is normally limited by the degree of acoustic leakage from the earmould and this effect is shown in Fig. 10.7.

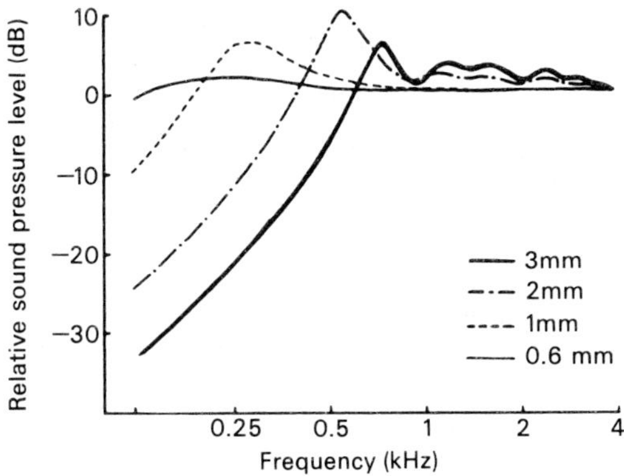

Fig. 10.7. Effect of leakage from lateral vents of different diameters in an earmould. (From Grover (1976).)

Earphones of the rectanglar type used in head-worn aids are connected to the ear by a tube, the dimensions of which will considerably affect the performance. Fig. 10.8 shows the performance of typical earphones of this type and the effect of tube configurations. The maximum output of this type of earphone is still less than that of button type earphones and they also have a poorer low-frequency response.

A bone vibrator may be used instead of a button earphone on most powerful body-worn aids. The frequency response of such vibrators is limited (see Fig. 8.4 p. 167). The earphone can therefore be seen to be the second limiting factor in determining the overall acoustic performance of the aid. The net result is that the transducers in the hearing aid limit its performance which is the case in most acoustic systems.

Power supply

The power supply in most hearing aid systems is a single primary cell often wrongly called a battery. Secondary rechargeable cells are used, often nickel–cadmium, but the main source of power is either the Leclache penlight cell for body-worn aids or the mercury cell for head-worn aids. Fig. 10.9 shows the characteristics of these different types of cell.

The size of the cell will determine its electrical capacity which is measured in milliampere hours (mA/h). Obviously the more current the amplifier

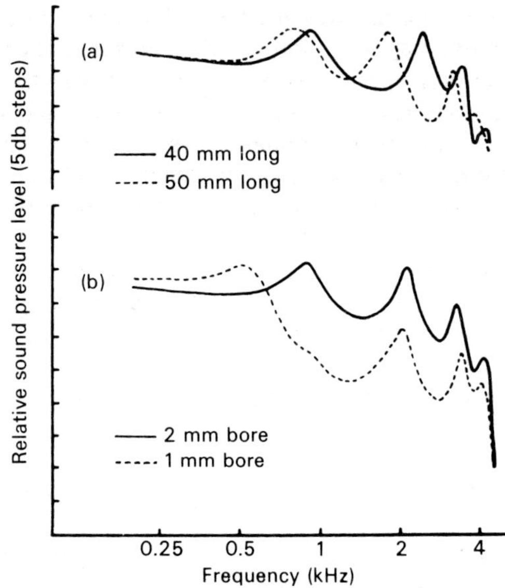

Fig. 10.8. (a). Effect of tube length on the frequency response of a post-aural receiver. (b). Effect of tube bore on the frequency response of a post-aural receiver. (From Grover (1976).)

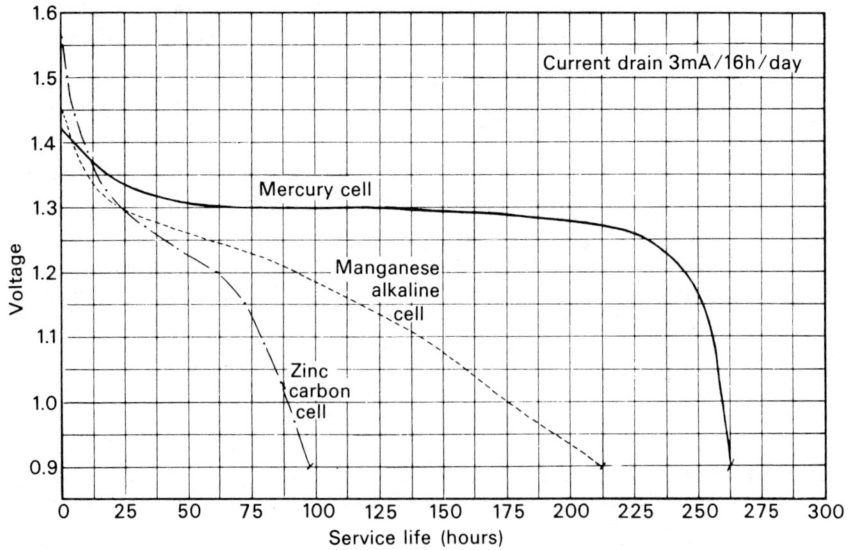

Fig. 10.9. Variation of voltage with hours of use for three types of cell. (From Martin (1970).)

takes the shorter the life of the battery, hence battery consumption is of prime consideration in the running costs of aids.

MEASUREMENT OF HEARING AID PERFORMANCE

It is vital to the understanding of hearing aids that the methods of measurement of performance, and in particular their limitations, are clearly understood. The prime factor to remember in the measurement of performance and its specification is that it does not attempt to simulate what happens on an individual, at best it represents some of the acoustic features found on an average adult human head and torso. Measurement of performance can be broken into two main types (i) standardized type testing in accordance with IEC 118 (1959) and (ii) standardized *in situ* measurements which attempt to take into account the acoustic features of a standard head and body. Burkhard and Sachs (1975) describe KEMAR (Knowles experimental mankin for acoustical research) which is becoming widely used in the United States.

Fig. 10.10 indicates the equipment required to make the basic measurements of electro-acoustic performance of hearing aids, this does not alter with the type of measurement (i) or (ii) above except for the acoustic enclosure. One of the most important features to note with the testing of hearing aids is the manner in which the acoustic output of the hearing aid is measured.

Fig. 10.11 shows the 2cc coupler described in IEC 126 (1973) and it is of prime importance to note the following warning in the scope and object of this document.

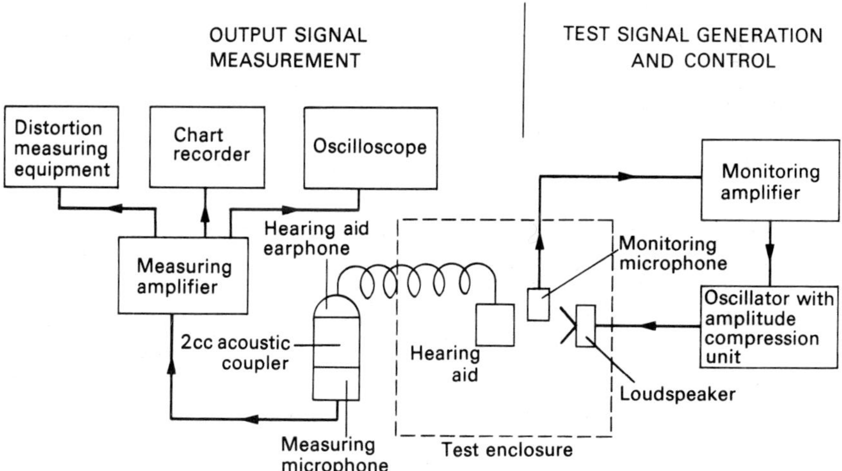

Fig. 10.10. Equipment required for measuring the acoustical performance of hearng aids. The test enclosure is often a small box which basically provides a constant sound pressure input to the aid. For use with a manikin a free-field condition is essential and hence an anechoic chamber of some size. The 2cc coupler may be replaced by an insert ear simulator such as that proposed by Zwislocki (1970).

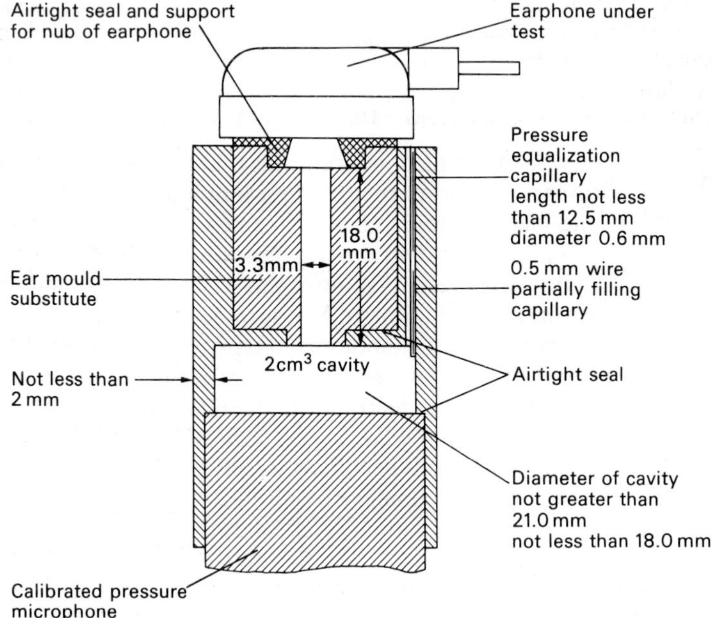

Fig. 10.11. A diagrammatic representation of the IEC 2cc acoustic coupler. For post-aural aids an adaptor is fitted to the top to allow a tube to be connected. For in the ear aids the earphone of the aid is led directly in the cavity. From BS 3171 (1968). (Courtesy British Standards Institution.)

The use of this coupler does not allow the actual performance of a hearing aid on a person to be obtained. However, the IEC recommends its use as a simple and ready means for the exchange of physical data on hearing aids.

If it is wished to indicate the sound pressure level that might be obtained in an average adult ear, corrections can be made from Fig. 10.12. An ear simulator for the measurement of simulated real conditions has now been agreed by IEC based on the work of Zwislocki (1970) which allows direct measurements to be made representing the effect of an average adult normal ear.

To any corrections would have to be added the diffraction effects of the head and torso and these will vary with the angle of incidence of the sound and its frequency. In addition to this the term average adult ear has been used which implies that the measurements are not necessarily representative of what happens on any individual ear. It might be argued that this makes hearing aid measurements rather useless, however this is not the case as it allows the objective performance to be measured in a systematic manner which can then be related to a subjective performance that may be measured at a different time.

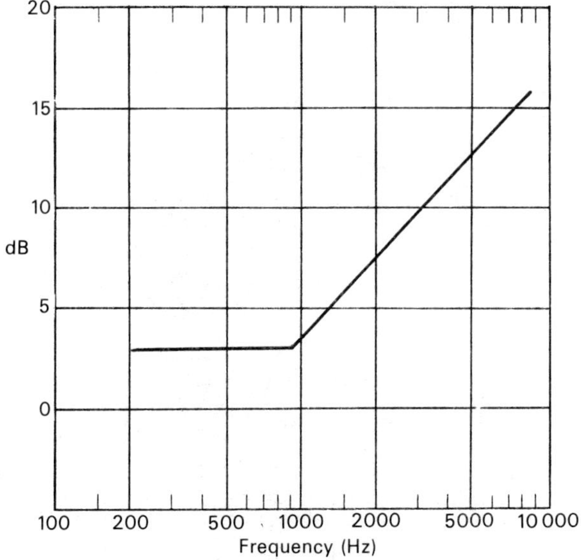

Fig. 10.12. Corrections to be added to measurements made in 2 cc acoustic coupler compared with adult real ears. (From Sachs and Burkhard (1972).)

PERFORMANCE CHARACTERISTICS

There are four main performance characteristics that are frequently reported, these are frequency response, amplification, maximum acoustic output, and, distortion. Each of these will be considered in turn.

Frequency response

When the frequency response is considered it is usually that at a linear position of the input–output characteristic of the hearing aid. Fig. 10.13 shows a family of frequency response curves that indicate what happens as the sound input is increased from a low to a high level. It may be seen that the frequency response can change completely with a change of input level, it is therefore important to know where a frequency response curve lies in relation to the maximum output. To ensure that the basic frequency response curve is in a linear portion of the input-output characteristic American Standard ANSI S3.22 (1976) instructs the tester to set the gain control so that the frequency response curve lies at an average value of 17 dB below the maximum acoustic output. IEC 118 (1959) requires that the gain control should be set such that with a 60 dB input at 1 kHz, 100 dB is measured in the acoustic coupler. A revision of IEC 118 now requires that the gain control be adjusted so that a 60 dB input at 1600 Hz provides an output sound pressure level of 15 dB less than that for a 90 dB input.

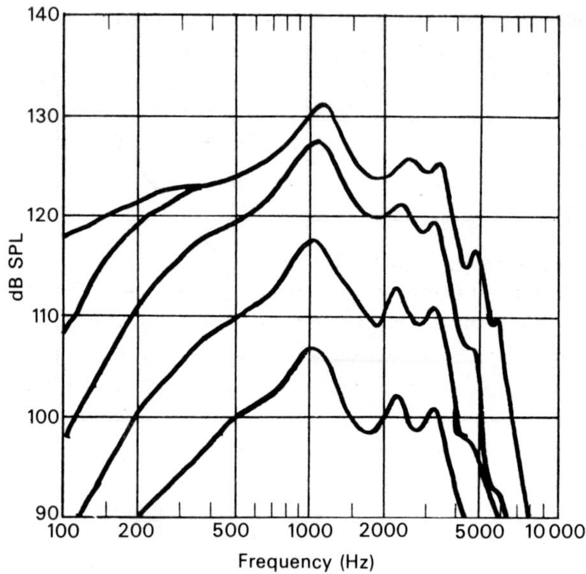

Fig. 10.13. Frequency response curves of post-aural hearing aid. Input levels 50 to 90 dB SPL from lower to upper curves.

Amplification

Amplification or gain is expressed in decibels (dB) and represents the ratio of input to output sound pressure. From Fig. 10.13 it may be seen that overall acoustic amplification may be deduced by subtracting the input sound pressure from the measured output sound pressure. Alternatively, it may be plotted as a frequency response curve for gain. For practical purposes it is very often better to have the basic information shown and to calculate the gain rather than plot gain itself. The sound pressure being presented to the listener is then directly indicated. Average values of gain are often quoted according to HAIC (1961) which is the average gain at 0.5, 1, and 2 kHz. More recently American Standard ANSI S3.22 (1976) specifies an average value of gain called the high-frequency average full on gain which is the average of 1, 1.6, and 2.5 kHz at the maximum setting of the gain control.

Maximum acoustic output

The maximum acoustic output from an aid is the highest output sound pressure measured when all possible input sounds are available. This may be seen in Fig. 10.13 or may be plotted on an input–output curve as in Fig. 10.5. A point to note is that in some aids the maximum output does not occur with the highest input sound level. This is due to the biasing-off effect of the signal on the amplifier circuit.

To achieve maximum acoustic output at low frequencies, i.e. below 250 Hz often requires very high input sound pressures which are not realistic for practical use. A lower level is therefore used and is now called SSPL 90. Standing for saturation sound pressure level with 90 dB input. IEC are proposing $OSPL_{90}$ as the new term standing for output sound pressure level for 90 dB input. This is the acoustic output measured for a constant input of 90 dB SPL and represents the type of levels that will be achieved in everyday life.

Distortion

Distortion is a term widely used and normally means non-linear distortion, i.e. that the input and output waveform are not the same. The most widely used measure is that of total harmonic distortion which measures the total level of harmonics left after the fundamental is removed and reported as a percentage. Fig. 10.14 shows the typical range of harmonic distortion found

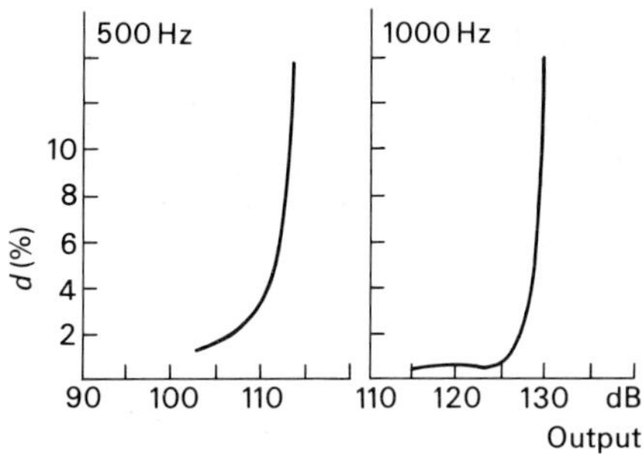

Fig. 10.14. Harmonic distortion at 500 and 1000 Hz for one position of the hearing aid controls. This method of presentation is widely used in commercial literature.

in many hearing aids at different frequencies for varying input levels. A point to note is that at frequencies above 2 kHz almost no harmonic distortion exists because of the sharp high-frequency cut off at the earphone, there can however be gross non-linear distortion. In general harmonic distortion does not occur in a well designed hearing aid at output levels 10 dB below the maximum acoustic output to any extent, i.e. distortion is less than 3 per cent.

A second form of distortion that is difficult to measure but may be of more importance than harmonic distortion is intermodulation distortion. With intermodulation distortion two tones are put into the aid and not only do the original tones appear at the output but all possible sum and difference frequencies may appear. Intermodulation distortion does not appear to any extent except near the maximum acoustic output where non-linearity occurs.

A further form of distortion is transient distortion. When a rapid change of input occurs then it is possible that the output change does not accurately follow the input, spurious signals are introduced usually in the form of overshoot or ringing.

CONTROL OF ACOUSTIC OUTPUT

Amplification

It is obviously essential to be able to control the acoustic output of a hearing aid and this is achieved by the gain control, usually called a volume control. The position of the gain control in the circuit is determined by two factors: (i) The need to ensure that the amplifying stages are not overloaded by the high input signals from a microphone, and (ii) To ensure that the signal-to-noise ratio is kept as high as possible. The first amplifying stage will generate electronic noise which will be amplified by the following stages, therefore if the gain control is situated after the first stage this ensures that the noise is reduced when the gain control is turned down. If the gain control is situated before the first stage the noise will be present at a constant level all the time.

The above considerations are basic to the siting of the gain control. The range of control on most hearing aids is about 40 dB which may be achieved in a near linear fashion, however at the upper and lower end of the control position the effect of rotation often becomes non-linear. The setting of the gain control alters the degree of amplification but from Fig. 10.15 it may be seen that it does not alter the maximum acoustic output of the aid.

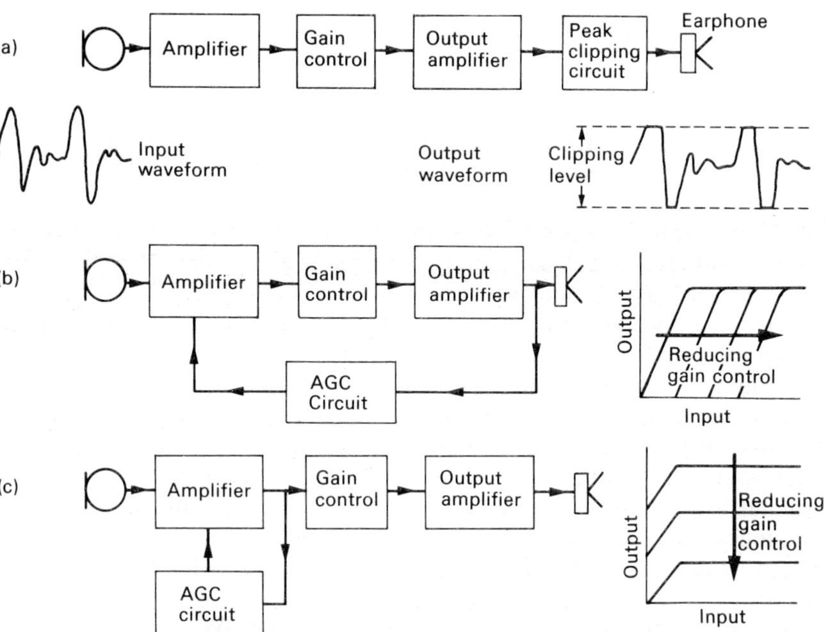

Fig. 10.15. (a). Normal position of peak-clipping circuit and its effect on a speech like waveform. (b). AGC circuit with the gain control inside the feedback loop. The input output characteristic of this circuit is shown and it can be seen that gain control variation does not affect maximum acoustic output. (c). AGC circuit with the gain control after the feedback loop. The input output characteristic shows that the maximum output is attained with the position of the gain control.

Maximum acoustic output

Maximum acoustic output is independent of amplification. It is possible to have high maximum output and low amplification and vice versa. Control of maximum output can be achieved by three methods: (i) output attenuator, (ii) peak clipping, and (iii) automatic gain control. The simplest form of output control is that of an output attenuator between the output stage of the amplifier and the earphone. The problem with this is that a separate control of gain is required and this is normally only found in large educational equipment. This does become possible however if automatic gain control systems are used, these will be described later.

Peak clipping as its name implies is a form of electronic circuit which clips the top and bottom off signals as in Fig. 10.16. The advantages of peak

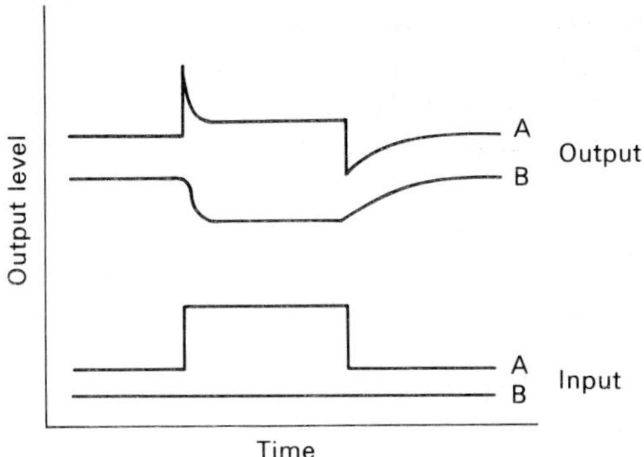

Fig. 10.16. The lower two lines represent two pure tones A and B. Tone A is increased in level while tone B remains constant. The output from an AGC system is shown in the upper part of the figure. The AGC action is clearly seen on tone A but as the gain is reduced on tone A it also effects the weaker tone B because it is passing through the same amplifier hence reducing the level of a signal that is already low. (From Barford (1978).)

clipping are that it is instantaneous in operation and simple in terms of circuitry. Its disadvantage is that it creates distortion due to the peak clipping action. It should be remembered that all hearing aids without AGC run into peak clipping at saturation, even AGC aids may run into peak clipping at very high input levels.

AGC is mainly used as a means of limiting the output of aids but without introducing distortion. Fig. 10.16 shows the action of an AGC system and a block diagram of the circuit operation. The position of the gain control considerably influences the input–output characteristic of the aid as can be seen from the figure.

In considering the action of an AGC aid it must be remembered that the highest amplitude signal is going to be the one that controls the AGC circuit hence the often loud low-frequency signals will cause a reduction in amplification which will also cause the lower level high-frequency sounds to be reduced and hence heard less well (as shown in Fig. 10.16).

RELATIONSHIP BETWEEN OBJECTIVE MEASUREMENTS AND THE HEARING AID USER

In the foregoing brief account of acoustic measurements, which might be termed objective as they involve no human appreciation of the sound, it might be considered by the uninitiated that these measurements could be directly related to what will happen on a hearing impaired person. Unfortunately this is not so for two fundamental reasons: (i) that the measurements do not accurately reflect what happens on any given individual and (ii) the hearing impairment of the individual will modify the perception of sound in a manner which is difficult to measure or predict. This does not mean that acoustic measurements are useless but that they have to be treated with both caution and a degree of background knowledge.

A major reason for making acoustic measurements on hearing aids is to ensure that they meet a specified performance and that this performance can be checked against its original performance at any time. Quite obviously there must be a relationship between the acoustic performance of a hearing aid and the effect on the hearing impaired person. However, in the author's opinion the only way to obtain this relationship is to measure it. These statements may appear to be a tautology but the vast majority of hearing aids are supplied and fitted without any measurement of the aided performance of the hearing impaired person.

It is not particularly difficult to measure the aided performance of a hearing impaired person (Fig. 10.17). The important features of such a test system are that the test arrangement is kept constant and that the test stimuli are appropriate and calibrated. Appropriate test stimuli for free or sound-field measurements are that they do not cause standing waves in the test room, therefore pure tones are not recommended. Warble tones, which

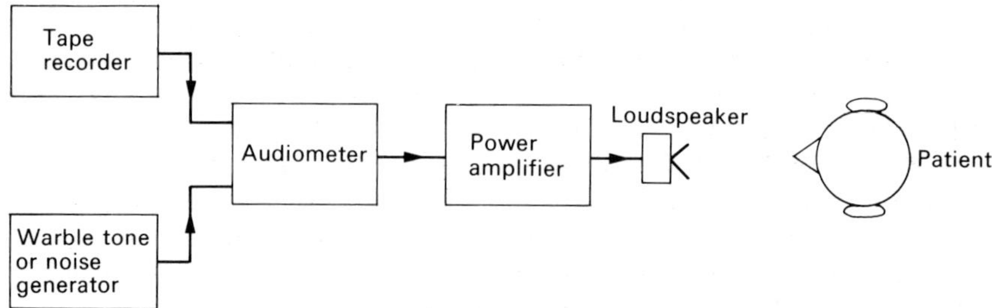

Fig. 10.17. An audiometer with facilities for electrical input and output can provide the basis of a free-field hearing aid evaluation system. Most modern audiometers have facilities for an external output but the signal can be taken from the earphone socket providing care is taken to provide correct impedance matching and to avoid earth loops. The sound field is calibrated by means of a sound level meter placed at the position to be occupied by the patient's head.

consists of frequency modulated pure tones, or bands of noise minimize the effects of standing waves and are widely used as stimuli for free-field measurements. Tests with speech or speech like material are of course undertaken and can be presented through the same equipment. The artificial stimuli, i.e. warble tones etc. and the speech signal, represent the two distinct and perhaps not well related test areas for hearing aid evaluation.

The first problem for the person fitting a hearing aid is to ensure that the hearing impaired patient can hear over an adequate frequency range to give him the opportunity to understand speech. Also to contain the output of the hearing aid so that it always lies within the dynamic range of the impaired ear. Following this it is necessary to ensure that the hearing impaired person is able to make maximum use of his ability to discriminate speech sounds. It is often the case that the first part of the problem can be easily resolved, but that the second part never can.

HEARING AID FITTING

The fitting of a hearing aid is considered by some as a minor matter that does not require much consideration. Experience has shown that the proper fitting of hearing aids require the services of someone who has a wide range of knowledge and the ability to understand the problems of a handicapped person. Many papers and books have been written on the subject and it is not the purpose of this chapter to review these. In essence the task of hearing aid fitting can be seen as overcoming a series of problems. The author has developed a flow diagram (Fig. 10.18) to illustrate the problems and to indicate how a logical approach might lead to at least an understanding of the patient's problems, if not a solution for them.

CROS HEARING AIDS

CROS stands for contralateral routing of signals and is a hearing aid system initially designed for people with profound unilateral hearing losses and normal or near normal hearing in the other ear. The principle is a simple one and consists of placing a microphone at the deaf ear and taking the signal to an amplifier and earphone on the good ear. Sound is conducted into the good ear by means of an open earmould, hence not blocking off that ear with normal hearing. The practical implementation of this system is either by means of a spectacle frame (Fig. 10.19) or by means of two post-aural hearing aids connected by a wire, one aid having the microphone the other the earphone, amplifier, and battery.

An extention of the CROS system is the BICROS where the good ear is not normal but has an aidable loss. In this case there is also a microphone on the better ear and the user has the input from both microphones fed into the hearing aid amplifier and earphone. A wide range of variations on the above system has been introduced.

CROS aids undoubtedly have a value but like all other hearing aid

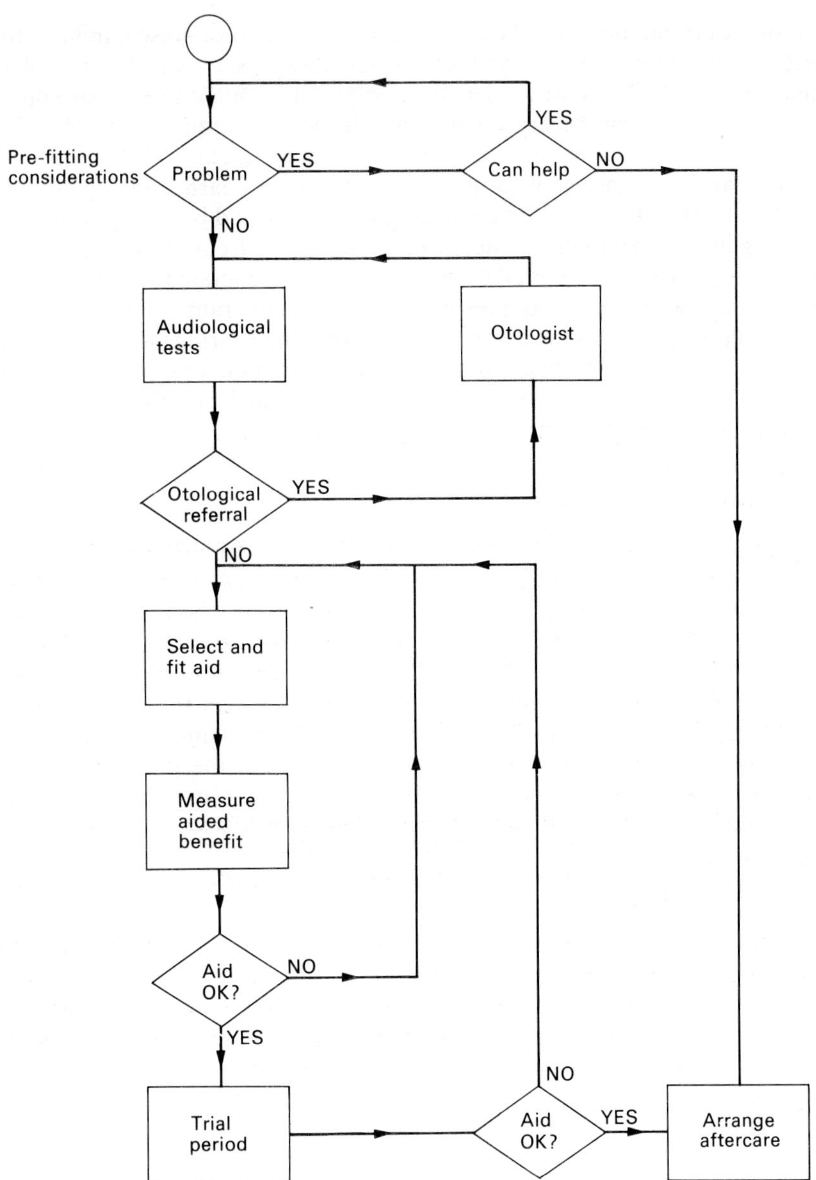

Fig. 10.18. A simplified flow diagram of the considerations required in hearing aid fitting. (Adapted from Martin (1978).)

systems have to be evaluated by the user in real-life situations before any certainty of their benefit can be determined. This presents a problem in the case of a spectacle fitting due to the practical difficulty of having the frames made before any user trials can be started.

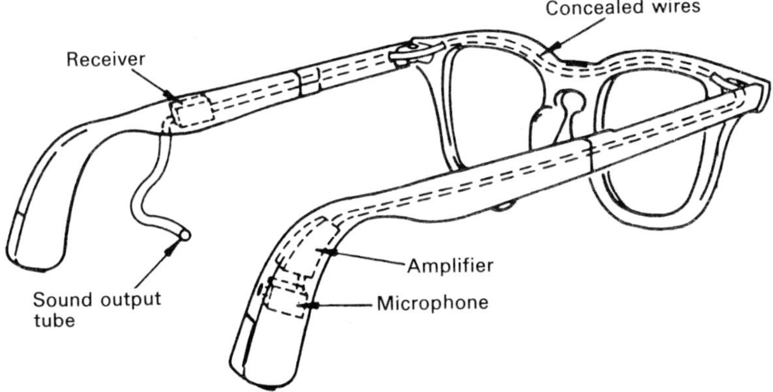

Fig. 10.19. CROS hearing aid fitted in spectacle frame. (Courtesy of Radioear Corp.)

FREQUENCY TRANSPOSITION AIDS

In a range of hearing losses it is quite likely that the high frequencies will be so reduced that they are beyond being helped by amplification. In frequency transposing hearing aids these high frequencies are moved down to a region where the ear has some useful hearing but still retaining normal low-frequency amplification. Fig. 10.20(a) shows the principle of frequency transposition, it should be noted, however, that what is important is the manner in which the sound is transposed. The system used by Johannson (1959) and available in the form of a body-worn hearing aid basically produces a noise burst when the high frequency sound is present. Fig. 10.20(b) is a block diagram of the hearing aid with its acoustical performance. An alternative approach (Velmans 1973) is to take the high-frequency signal and retain its spectral content when transposed down to lower frequencies.

The application of frequency transposition hearing aids has been limited and procedures have not been developed for fitting these aids in practice. An important feature is to ensure the correct ratio of direct to transposed channel signal. The effect of a frequency transposing aid is easy to demonstrate using a free-field warble tone (Fig. 10.21), this does not, however, indicate the ability to discriminate one high-frequency consonant from another.

EARMOULDS

Earmoulds can be obtained in a variety of shapes (Fig. 10.22) depending upon the type of aid being used and the particular needs of the user. Two methods of manufacturing an earmould may be termed the direct and indirect method. The indirect method is probably the most widely used and consists of taking an impression of the ear, usually with a self curing silicone material as a paste, and then sending the impression to a mould maker who

(a)

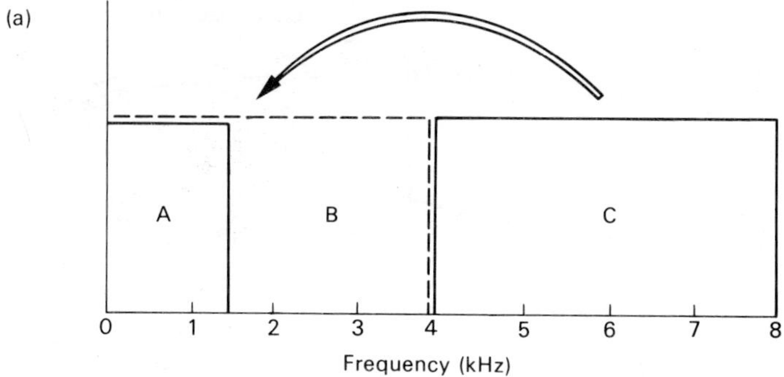

(b)

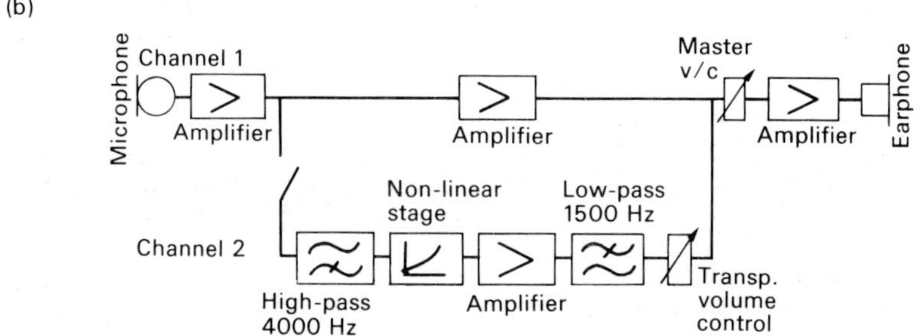

(c)

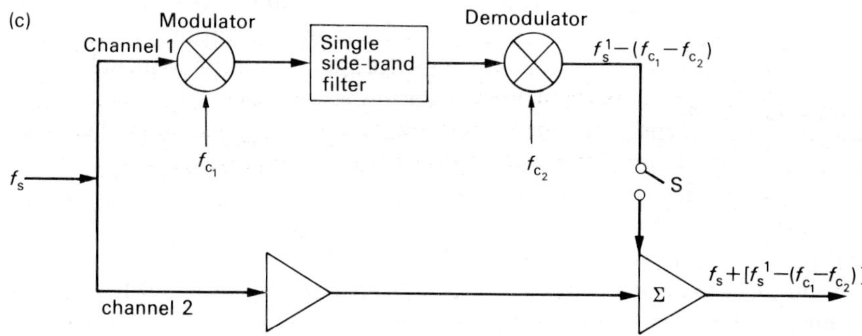

Fig. 10.20. (a). Example of frequency transposition. The high-frequency region, above 4 kHz is moved down to a low frequency. A represents the transposed range for the Oticon transposer while B is the range for the Velamns device. (b). Johansson type transposer. (Courtesy of Oticon Ltd.) (c). Block diagram of Velmans transposer where f_s is the input signal, $f_{s'}$ is a selected high-frequency band of the input signal, f_{c_1} is the modulating frequency, f_{c_2} is the demodulating frequency, $(f_{c_1} - f_{c_2})$ is the frequency 'shift' performed on each frequency component of $f_{s'}$, and $f_s + (f_{c_1} - f_{c_2})$ is the output signal.(From Valmens (1973).)

converts the impression into a finished mould in an acrylic or vynal material. The direct method used a self curing material that forms the mould itself. Hence the impression forms the mould.

As the ear mould is the means of acoustically coupling the aid to the ear it

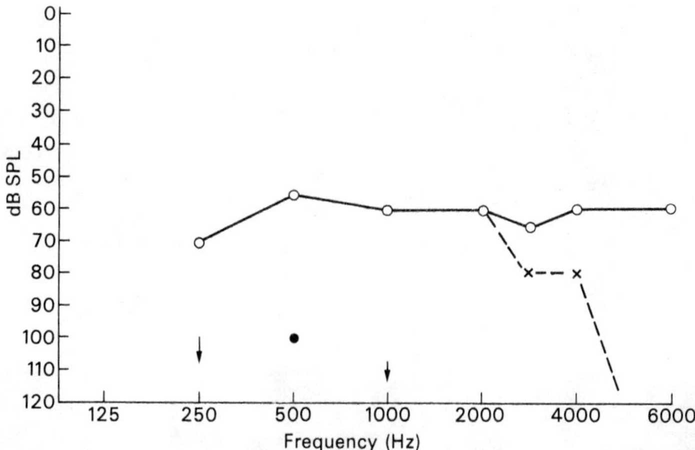

Fig. 10.21. Free-field threshold shift using warble tones for profoundly deaf person using a frequency transposing aid. Solid line shows threshold with transposition on, dashed line transposition off. Lower point and arrows indicate marked threshold. Using this technique it is possible to put transposition level to a required level.

is bound to influence the performance of the aid. Two parameters of the acoustic tube that can be altered are length and bore. In practice the length is largely determined by the size of the ear of the user, Fig. 10.9 shows the effect of length on frequency response and also variations in bore of the tube.

Acoustic leakage from the earmould gives rise to a loss of low frequencies and also to acoustic feedback if the amplification is too high. By introducing a hole in the earmould, called venting, some control of low frequency response can be achieved and may be found to be beneficial. Fig. 10.7(b) shows the effect of introducing different size vents into an earmould, it should be noted that the control of low frequencies is relatively coarse and can give an increase in amplification at some frequencies owing to resonance effects.

Acoustic filters may be inserted in the earmould itself or in the acoustic pathway from the earphone. A resistance element may be achieved by pulling wool or cotton threads through the tube to form a pad. Difficulties exists in predicting the effect of filters or resistance elements and their effect should always be checked objectively to ascertain that any subjective changes are due to the modification.

EDUCATIONAL HEARING AIDS

Educational hearing aids are identical in principle to conventional aids already discussed, they differ, however, in their construction and usually in the ease of changing the characteristics. Under this heading we shall briefly describe group hearing aids, auditory training units, inductive loop systems, radio systems, and infrared systems.

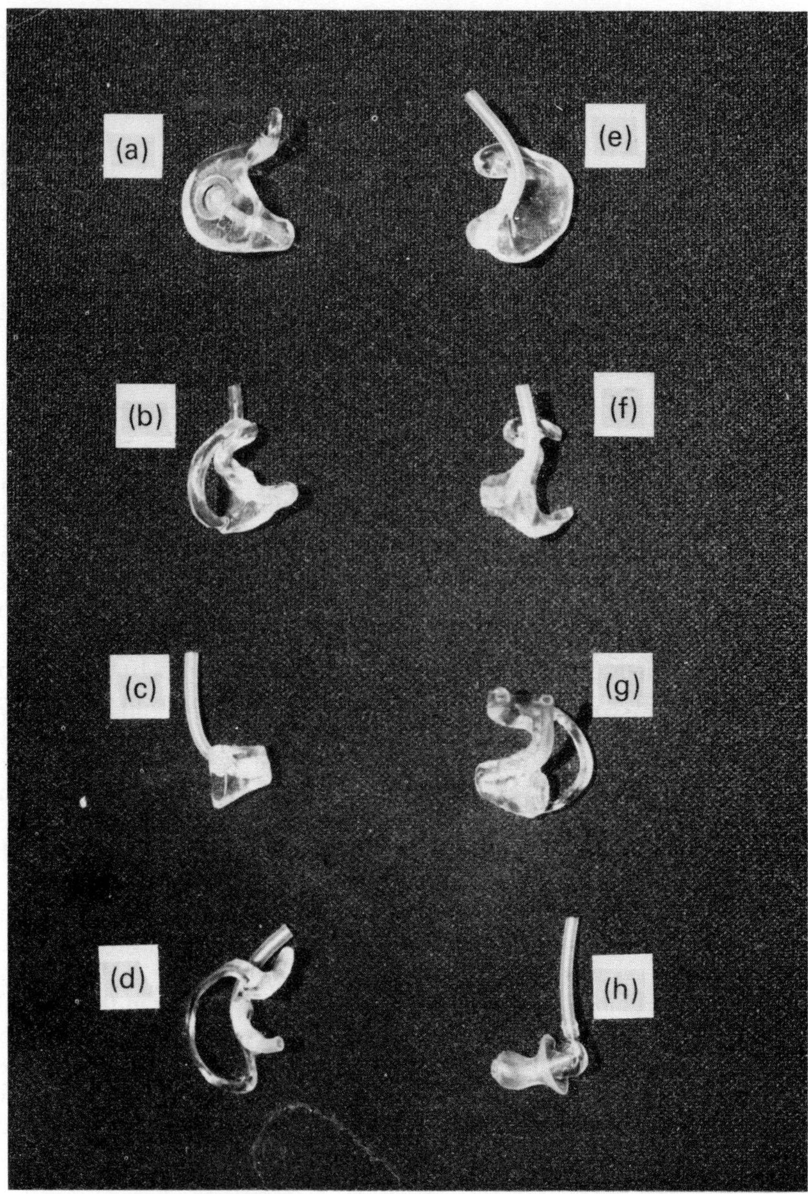

Fig. 10.22. Current types of earmould. (a). Mould button earphone. (b). Skeleton mould. (c). Meatal tip. (d). Open-ear fitting. (e). Shell mould. (f). Half skeleton. (g). Variable vent mould. (h). Temporary pip.

Group hearing aids/auditory training systems

The group hearing aid system was devised to enable deaf children to obtain good quality sound at a sufficient level for them to be able to make use of their residual hearing. In addition it was a requirement that all children should be able to hear the teacher's voice, their own voice, and the voices of other children in the group. Fig. 10.23 shows a block diagram of a typical modern group hearing aid.

The advantage of the group aid is that it picks up the speaker's voice near to the mouth and hence the speech is not mixed with any ambient noise or seriously affected by the acoustic environment. The teacher's console will allow signal levels to be controlled while output levels can be controlled by the children themselves. Large earphones are used in the United Kingdom because they represent the only means of obtaining high outputs at high frequencies. The use of button earphones, however, does enable a less cumbersome apparatus for the child provided the limitation in performance is accepted, if the child has no useful hearing beyond 3 kHz then this may be an acceptable criterion for using button earphones.

It is important to note in the group hearing aid that gain and output are controlled independently. The input from the microphone is adjusted to give a reference reading on the meter on the teacher's console and then the output to each child is adjusted by means of output attenuators. The monitoring meter therefore ensures effectively constant output signal and the output attenuators ensure both good signal-to-noise ratio and control of output. The output of the group aids does not necessarily have to be fed to earphones but may be fed as an electrical signal directly into the child's hearing aid or through individual inductive loops worn as halters for use with post-aural aids. With modern group aids each child has an individual channel in which frequency response and input–output characteristic can be adjusted to allow for the variation in need. The complexity of such systems does, however, require that teachers be instructed carefully in their use. The group hearing aid was designed for the formal teaching situation and modifications have been made to produce them in the form of mobile aids built into trolleys for less formal teaching.

The auditory training unit or speech trainer is a single channel of a group aid and some models can be connected together to form group aids. Performance requirements for group aids and auditory trainers have been agreed in the United Kingdom and published in the *Teacher of the Deaf*.

Induction loop system

Speech at the lips of a speaker can be as high as 90 dB SPL but at 1 metre has dropped to between 60 and 70 dB SPL. Given free-field conditions, the level will fall at 6 dB per distance doubled hence the signal may fall below the detection level of the hearing impaired listener who has a narrow dynamic range. As the level of signal falls so the signal-to-noise ratio becomes worse

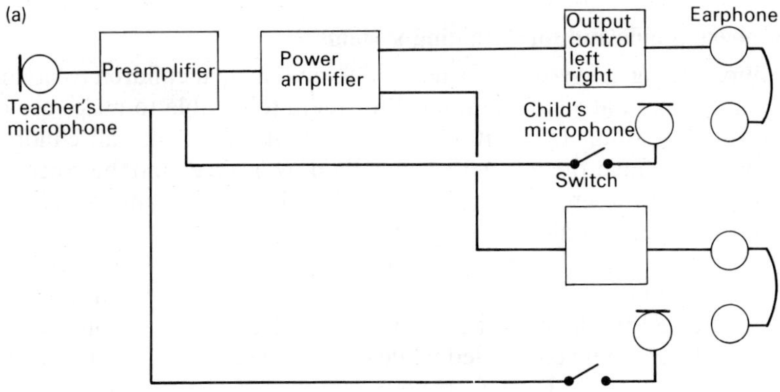

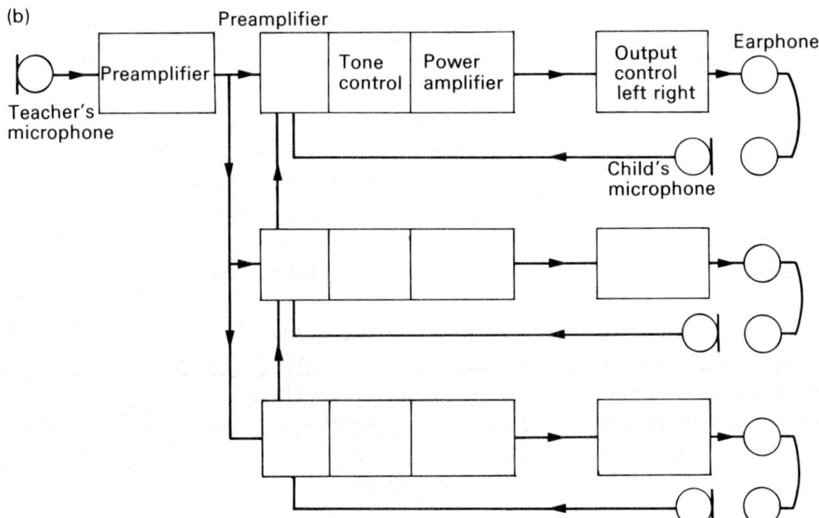

Fig. 10.23. (a). Basic group aid where teachers, and children's microphones are fed into a common preamplifier and mixer. One output amplifier drives all headphones which have independent control of output to each ear. A monitoring meter on the power amplifier ensures input levels are adequate to provide correct drive. A press to talk switch is provided on some children's microphones. Only two outputs are shown, up to ten are normally provided. (b). Modular group hearing aid with independent control of frequency response microphone level and output on each channel. Each channel in effect is an auditory training unit. (Adapted from Martin and Power (1967).)

and it is well know that hearing impaired people have considerable difficulties in understanding speech in noisy conditions.

The induction loop system was the first and simplest system devised to enable speech to be transmitted from a person speaking at a distance to a hearing aid user hence minimizing the adverse effects of distance and background noise. The induction loop system works on the principal of an electric current in a wire producing a magnetic field around the wire which is proportional to the current flowing. If a coil of wire is introduced into the magnetic field a current will be induced in that coil by any change in the magnetic field. Hence if the current in the wire is alternating an alternating signal will be induced in the coil. If the coil is put into a hearing aid in place of the microphone or in parallel with it the user will hear the signal that is creating the current in the wire.

To produce a magnetic field more easily the wire carrying the signal current is formed into a loop. The field strength at the centre of the loop can easily be calculated from the formula

$$H = \frac{I}{d} \text{ A/m}$$

where d is the diameter in metres and I the current in amps.

For a square loop for formula is

$$H = \frac{2\sqrt{2}}{\pi}\left(\frac{I}{a}\right) \text{ A/m}$$

Where 'a' is the length of one side.

The recommended magnetic field strength for hearing aid use is 100 mA/m corresponding to the long-term average of a 70 dB speech input signal to the microphone of the amplyfying system (IEC 1980).

Much adverse comment has been made against the loop system due to overspill problems and a lack of standardization for field strength. Overspill is the term used to denote the fact that the magnetic field is not contained closely within the loop but extends beyond it. Hence hearing aid users in adjacent rooms and particularly above and below the loop will pick up the signals if they are switched to the loop position and the correct field strength is not used. Field strength is proportional to current in the loop and hence the availability of power from the driving amplifier. In classroom conditions too much power is often used thereby aggravating the overspill situation.

A further difficulty has been the difference in frequency response between the aid on its loop position and that on the microphone position. Against standardization in the method of measurement IEC 118–1 (1975) has helped to ensure that the frequency responses are similar.

An essential feature for educational use of the inductive loop system is the combined position of the input selector switch, M denotes microphone input, T is the symbol for pick up coil input, and MT is the combined position when both microphone and pick up coil are operative. The combined position allows the teacher's voice to be heard clearly as well as the child hearing his own voice and other sounds. The relative sensitivity of the two inputs has been under consideration and the Department of Health and Social Security in the United Kingdom are recommending that when switching from the combined position (MT) to the microphone only position (M) the microphone sensitivity should be + 6 dB. When switching to the pick up coil only position (T) the pick up coil sensitivity should be + 3 dB.

While the inductive loop originated for school use it is now widely used by adults as a means of listening to television or radio and in some public places, notably churches and cinemas. Care has to be exercised in specifying loops and equipment for large areas such as churches and expert advice is recommended, however this is not a problem with smaller areas such as domestic rooms or classrooms providing the problems involved are understood.

Radio microphone systems

The induction loop system achieves the object of getting the speaker's voice to the hearing aid without the use of connecting wires. It does, however, have to be installed in a room and the microphone for the loop system has to be connected by means of a cable to the amplifier. The cable can cause difficulty in certain teaching situations and therefore for these situations a radio link is used to replace the wire.

The radio microphone has been in use in the entertainment world for some considerable while and this is what is basically used for deaf educational purposes. The radio microphone consists of a microphone connected into a small radio transmitter, often the two are housed in the same case. The radio transmitter is of low power and transmits to a radio receiver which then converts the signal back into an audio one which can be fed into the loop amplifier. In the United Kingdom all radio transmitting equipment must be approved by the Home Office and a licence obtained to operate on a given frequency. A frequency band in the 174 MHz region is set aside for deaf educational purposes but in other countries many different frequencies are used.

The use of radio systems with the inductive loop still retains the disadvantages of the loop and therefore radio receivers are now made small enough to be contained in an enlarged body-worn aid fed into aids by means of a direct contact pick up coil or electrical input. Fig. 10.24 shows a range of possible radio microphone and loop equipment combinations.

The ratio of signal from the radio input to the aid and the microphone is of the same importance as with the pick up coil input and in some radio hearing

Fig. 10.24. (a). Speaker (S) at a distance from a listener (L) using a hearing aid. The problems experienced by the listener will be due to the effects of distance and background noise. (b). The microphone from the hearing aid is extended to be close to the mouth of the speaker. (c). The microphone is fed into a loop amplifier which operates a loop system. The hearing aid picks up the signal from the loop thus giving mobility to the user. (d). In order to give mobility to the speaker the microphone has a radio transmitter attached to it (TX), a radio receiver (RX) picks up the signal, converts it to an audio signal and then operates a loop system. This gives both the speaker and the listener mobility. (e). To avoid installation of equipment the output from the radio receiver can be fed directly into the hearing aid either through and input socket or indirectly from a close contact pick up coil. (f). A radio microphone system in which the radio and audio amplifier are housed in one unit.

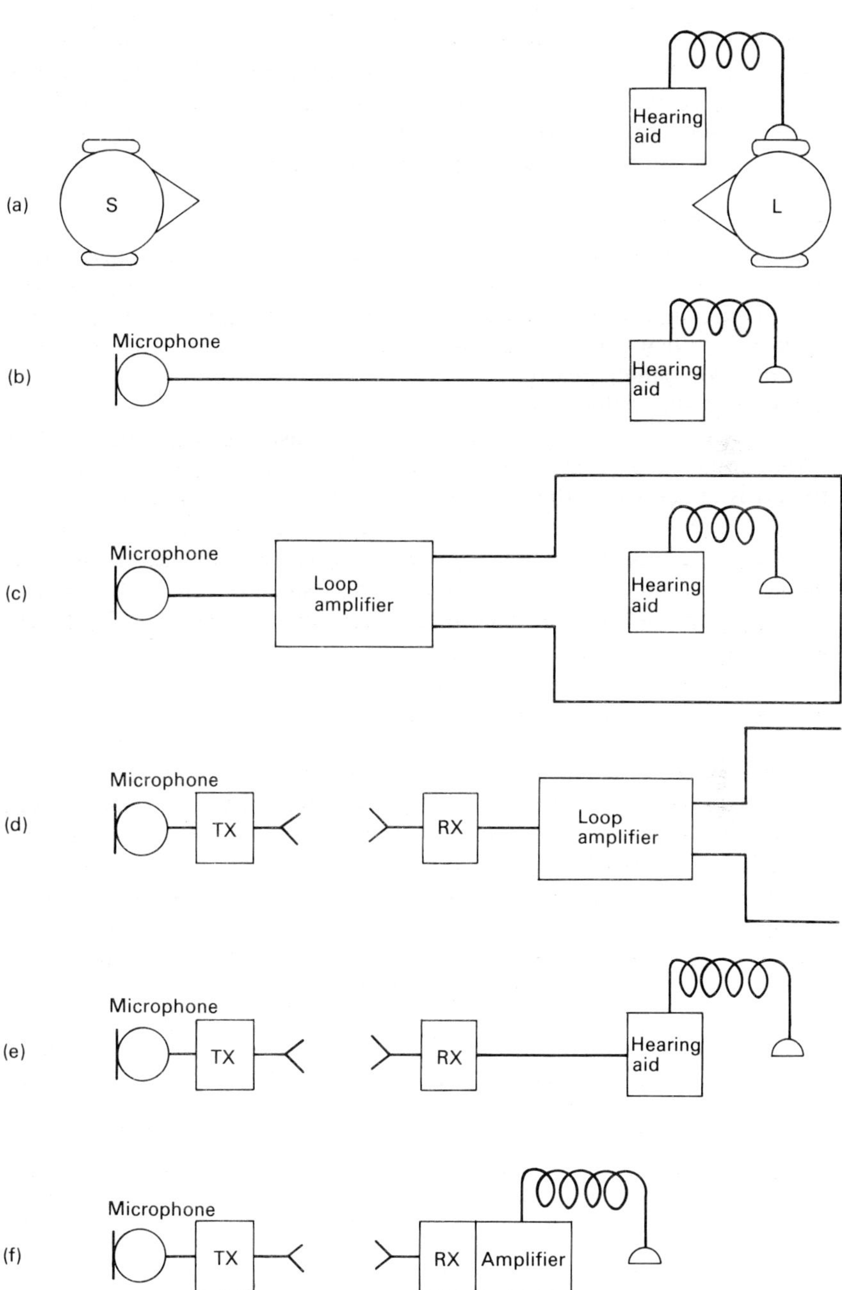
(a)
S
Hearing aid
L
(b)
Microphone
Hearing aid
(c)
Microphone
Loop amplifier
Hearing aid
(d)
Microphone
TX
RX
Loop amplifier
(e)
Microphone
TX
RX
Hearing aid
(f)
Microphone
TX
RX
Amplifier

aids an independent control is available on both channels. The radio hearing aid is becoming used in place of conventional group hearing aids because of their convenience and not needing installation. However, radio systems generally lack any means of allowing group discussion as the child's microphone will not pick up his neighbours voice adequately and certainly will not allow him to hear across a group. The exception to this is Siemens two-way system where each child's unit has a transmitter which transmits back to the teacher's unit, this in turn retransmits the signals to all the children.

The ideal situation for using a radio microphone hearing aid is for the hearing impaired child in a class of normal hearing children. Here the poor acoustics of the situation will make the use of the normal aid extremely difficult and the radio aid will minimize effects of distance and background noise. However, in a special school where a lot of money has been spent on obtaining quiet non-reverberant consitions and with small numbers of children it is difficult to understand the rationale for radio aids apart from mobility with small children.

It is often stated that children hear better with the radio aid than with their own aids. This is perfectly understandable at a distance, but there should be no advantage at a normal conversational distance. If the radio aid is better then it is obvious that there is some underlying difference in performance which could be found in a different non-radio aid. In other words there is nothing in the radio system that can give improvements that cannot be found in the performance of a conventional aid at small distances. The performance of radio aids may be measured in accordance with IEC 118–3 (1979).

ACOUSTIC AIDS

Although acoustic aids, i.e. ear trumpets and speaking tubes, may appear to be very old fashioned they do have a place in the rehabilitation of the deaf. Their main use is with the very elderly who cannot manage electronic aids. Due to the fact that there is little to go wrong and they are easy to use, they can be used by very elderly people and also carried around by professional people working with the hearing impaired elderly to provide ease of communication with those who do not have aids.

The speaking tube relies on picking up close sound close to the lips at high level and conducting it with little loss to the ear by means of a tube. Providing the tube is of some 1 cm diameter it can be made of almost any suitable material. The sound pressure delivered to the ear is therefore as high as with many moderately powered electronic aids. The ear trumpet is less efficient but does give some 20 dB gain over the range 500 to 4000 Hz. The acoustic aid could find an application in countries where the technology for maintaining electronic aids is not available if, even for educational purposes only, the willingness to experiment was there.

REFERENCES

ANSI S3.22 (1976). Specification of hearing aid characteristics. New York Acoustical Society of America.

Barford, J. (1978). Automatic regulation systems with relevance to hearing aids. *Scand. Audiol.* Suppl. **6,** 355–78.

Bogeskov-Jensen, O. (1978). World report on hearing aids. *Hearing Aid. J.* Nov. 6–7.

Burchard, M. D. and Sachs, R. M. (1975). Anthropometric manikin for acoustic research. *J. acoust Soc. Am.* **58,** 214–22.

Grover, B. C. (1976). Acoustic modifications to earmoulds. *Br. J. Audiol.* **10,** 8–12.

HAIC (1961). Method of expressing performance of hearing aids. Hearing Aid Industries Conference Inc., Washington DC.

IEC 118 (1959). Recommended methods for measurements of the electroacoustical characteristics of hearing aids. International Electrotechnical Commission, Geneva.

IEC 126 (1973). IEC reference coupler for the measurement of hearing aids using earphones coupled to the ear by means of ear inserts. International Electrotechnical Commission, Geneva.

IEC 118–1 (1975). Method of measurement of characteristics of hearing aids with induction pick-up coil input. International Electrotechnical Commission, Geneva.

IEC 118–3 (1979). Hearing aids not entirely worn on the person. International Electrotechnical Commission, Geneva.

IEC 118–4 (1980). Magnetic Field Strength in audio-frequency induction loops for hearing aid purposes. International Electrotechnical Commission, Geneva.

Johannson, B. (1959). A new coding amplifier system for the severely hard of hearing. *Proc. 3rd. Int. Con. Acoustics,* Stuttgart, Vol. 2, pp. 655–7.

Martin, M. C. (1970). Hearing aid batteries—a short or long life? *Hearing,* 52–4, February.

—— (1978). Individual hearing aids: selection and prescription. *J. Soc. Med.* **71,** 129–34.

—— and Power, R. (1967). A modular group hearing aid. *Sound* **1,** 33–6.

Sachs, R. M. and Burkhard, M. D. (1972). Earphone pressure responses in ears and couplers. Presented at 83rd Meeting of Acoustical Society of America.

Velmans, M. (1973). Speech imitation in simulated deafness, using visual cues and 'Recoded' auditory information. *Lang. Speech* **16,** 224–36.

Zwislocki, J. J. (1970). An acoustic coupler for earphone calibration. Report LSC-5-7. Laboratory of Sensory Communication, Syracuse University.

11 Acoustic impedance bridges

J. J. KNIGHT

INTRODUCTION

Although this chapter is entitled acoustic impedance bridges, its subject matter will include similar instruments variously called acoustic impedance meters, (acoustic) oto-admittance meters, middle-ear analysers, tympanometers, and impedance audiometers, used for measurements of the ear. The last name is an unfortunate one for these instruments are not concerned with measurements of hearing acuity but with malfunction of the component parts of the hearing system.

The concept of impedance was introduced into acoustics over 60 years ago after its use in the electrical field had been established. Then 20 years later came the acoustic impedance bridges of Schuster (1936) and Robinson (1937). The former was applied by Metz (1946) to measurements on normal and pathological ears, although West (1928) had already measured the acoustic impedance of normal ears at the level of the tympanic membrane using stationary waves in a tube connected to the ear. This latter work was conducted in connection with telephone development at the British Post Office Research Station.

In the application of acoustic impedance bridges to audiology, the distinction has been made between the Schuster and Metz bridges, which have been called electro-mechanical as they are balanced by mechanical adjustments, and the later compact electronic devices which have been called electro-acoustic. In reality both types could equally well be described as electro-acoustic but the distinction will be preserved in the following sections:

ELECTRO-MECHANICAL BRIDGES

The principle of the Schuster (and of the Metz) bridge is shown in Fig. 11.1.

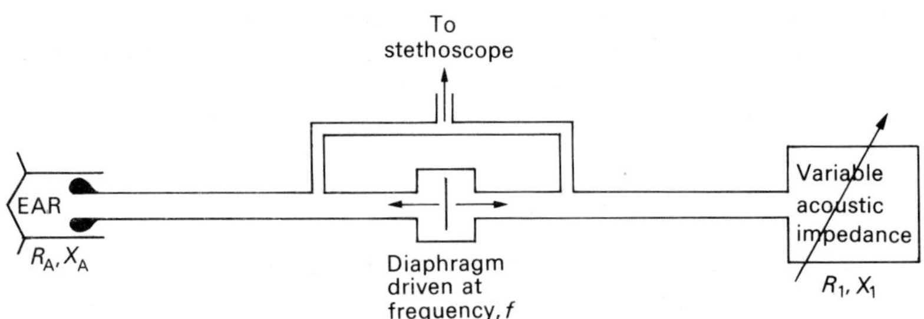

Fig. 11.1. Diagram of acoustic impedance bridge. (After Schuster (1936).)

The bridge consists of two equal lengths of tubing to feed sound waves of equal intensity, but of opposite phase, into the ear under examination at one end and into a variable impedance at the other. A centrally placed transducer connected to a pure-tone oscillator is the source of sound. Samples of the sound pressure at symmetrical points in the two tubes are combined at the connection shown for fitting a stethoscope. It can be understood that when the two controls of the variable impedance are tuned to match the impedance presented by the ear, a minimum of sound will be heard from the stethoscope. In this way the two components of the impedance at the end of the bridge fitted to the external auditory meatus can be determined in normal and pathological ears.

The impedance so determined includes the impedance of the air contained between the end of the bridge tube and the tympanic membrane, which is normally of little interest. A compensating volume was introduced into the measuring half of the bridge designed by Zwislocki (1963) as one of the improvements he made to the original design (see Fig. 11.2). Thus, with

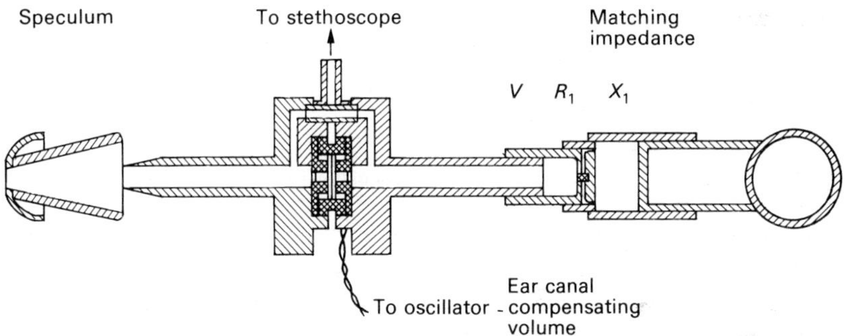

Fig. 11.2. Schematic diagram of Zwislocki's (1963) Acoustic Impedance Bridge.

a knowledge of the volume of the external meatus, the acoustic impedance at the plane of the tympanic membrane can be ascertained and compared with normal values as in Fig. 11.3.

Metz had noted the change in impedance caused by contraction of the middle-ear muscles as when a loud sound was applied to the ear contralateral to that fitted to the bridge, but measurement of the reflex threshold was difficult clinically before the advent of the electro-acoustic instruments.

The Zwislocki acoustic bridge was manufactured by Grason–Stadler in the United States and was introduced in Britain in 1965.

ELECTRO-ACOUSTIC INSTRUMENTS

While the Metz and Zwislocki bridges served to introduce acoustic impedance measurements into the field of audiological diagnosis, the clinical application of these devices as a routine procedure was limited. Measurement of the ear canal volume by filling with alcohol, though not difficult, was

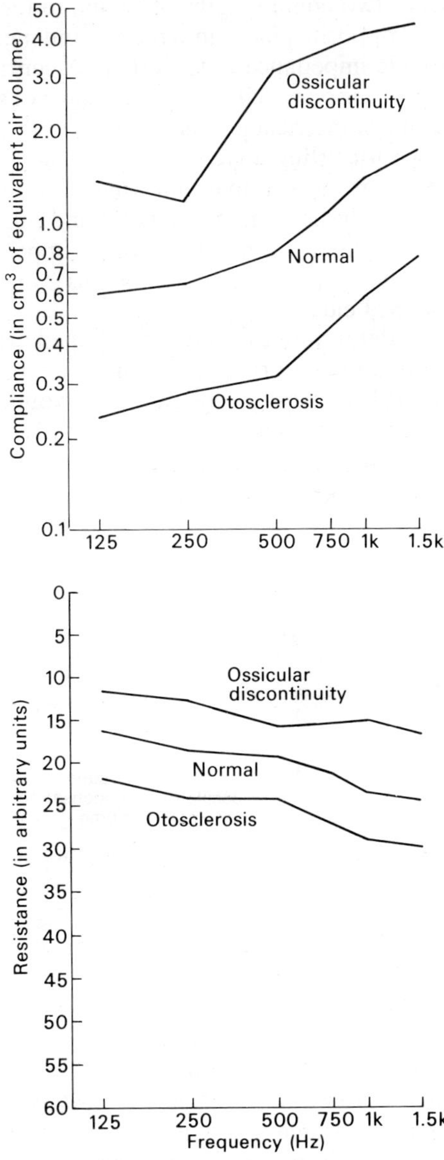

Fig. 11.3. Typical results using Zwislocki Acoustic Impedance Bridge in a case of otosclerosis and in another of ossicular discontinuity.

messy and tuning the two controls for minimum sound required low ambient noise levels and some degree of patience. The stimulus tone level needed to be kept well below that of the acoustic reflex threshold in order to avoid elicitation of the reflex. In all, this type of bridge was an eminently satisfactory research tool (and is still found to be a useful training aid) but its application was mainly in evaluation of cases of suspected ossicular disruption.

Terkildsen and Nielsen (1960) developed a more convenient form of (electro-acoustic) instrument with an acoustic probe, complete with a sound source and measuring microphone, mounted on a conventional headband. A low probe-tone frequency of 220 Hz was selected for clear definition of different disorders (see Fig. 11.3) by measurement of the components of the impedance. Two potentiometers enabled 'amplitude' and 'phase' to be adjusted in order to balance the bridge for a zero indication on a meter; the amplitude control covered a range from 200 to 2000 acoustic ohms and phase from 0 to 30°. A particular innovation was the introduction of a pump to enable measurements to be obtained with the tympanic membrane stressed by small positive and negative excess pressures; the procedure is called tympanometry. The Danish company, Madsen, undertook the manufacture of this instrument in 1957 and it was first used in Britain in 1960. A multiple-frequency oscillator was provided within the main instrument with suitable intensities for reflex threshold determination when applied to an earphone on the other (contralateral) end of the headband. A further novel feature of this instrument was the use of an inflatable cuff on the probe fitting to facilitate an airtight seal. A functional diagram of the Madsen Z061 is shown as Fig. 11.4.

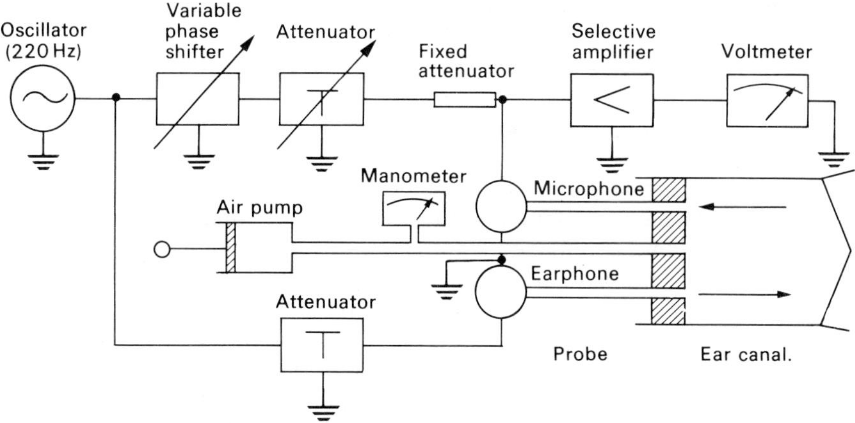

Fig. 11.4. Block diagram of Madsen Z061 Acoustic Impedance Bridge.

The next development in an instrument of this type took place in 1963 when the simplified Madsen Z070 (Fig. 11.5) became available using the same probe frequency of 220 Hz. The built-in reflex stimulating signal was dispensed with, as was the determination of the small resistive component of the ear impedance. The device was actually calibrated in terms of reactance, X_A where

$$X_A = -\frac{1}{2\pi f C_A}$$

and C_A is the compliance, and f is the frequency.

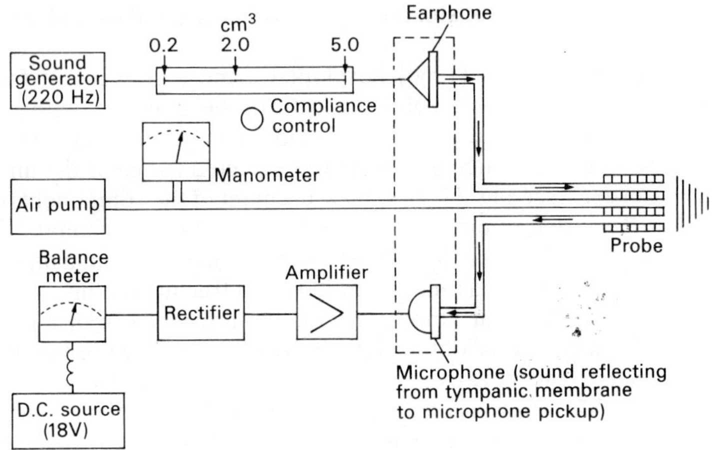

Fig. 11.5. Block diagram of Madsen Z070 Acoustic Impedance Meter.

A typical tympanogram of a normal ear obtained with this instrument is given in Fig. 11.6 where the compliance is plotted on the ordinate which is scaled in cubic centimetres of equivalent air volume. This relates to expressing the measured compliance of the ear in terms of the compliance of a volume of air contained in a simple hard-walled cavity

$$\text{as } C_A = \frac{V}{\varrho c^2}$$

where V is the volume and ϱc^2 is approximately 1.43×10^6 g/cm.s^2 at normal temperature and pressure.

Corrections are required for other ambient conditions and for change of humidity. An elegant solution to the problem of elimination of the external ear canal volume is obtained by stressing the tympanic membrane with a positive excess pressure of 200 mm of water when the membrane effectively becomes rigid and the compliance measurement *C_{200} under these conditions is the required volume (see Fig. 11.6). The middle-ear compliance, $C_{\text{middle ear}}$ is C_{peak}—C_{200}. The non-linear scale of the Z070 is calibrated in acoustic ohms for impedance as well as in equivalent cubic centimetres of air for compliance (0.2 cm^3 is approximately 5000 acoustic ohms, and 5 cm^3 is approximately 200 acoustic ohms). Although measurements in terms of acoustic impedance suggest greater scientific authenticity, complications ensue in the clinical situation in eliminating the external ear volume, Z_{200} with the formula

$$Z_{\textit{middle ear}} = \frac{Z_{\text{peak}} \times Z_{200}}{Z_{\text{peak}} - Z_{200}}$$

The advantage of using a compliance scale is apparent. At a fixed fre-

* This sometimes has been termed the *static* compliance although the compliance is essentially dynamic in this context.

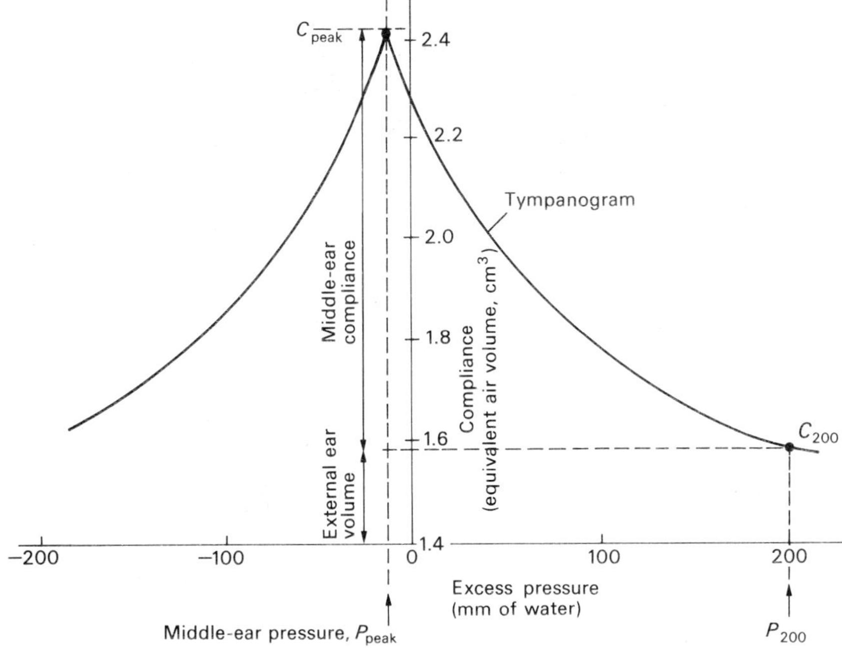

Fig. 11.6. Typical tympanogram of normal ear.

quency, compliance, C_A is inversely proportional to X_A or compliance is directly proportional to $1/X_A$. This is called acoustic susceptance, B_A which is the reactive component of admittance, Y_A(see chapter 6). Hence, some later instruments are called acoustic admittance meters as they really measure admittance rather than its reciprocal that is impedance.

The British firm of Peters later produced a similar instrument to the Z070 and gave it the Type Number A P61. A built-in tone generator was available for reflex threshold measurement and a 4000 Hz tone was provided at 25 dB HL for high-tone threshold measurement for application in school-screening tests using an impedance instrument rather than an audiometer (Brooks 1973). The Peters' range of instruments use a probe frequency of 275 Hz.

In 1971 Grason–Stadler in the United States introduced a precision grade oto-admittance meter Model 1720 (Fig. 11.7) which gave a write-out of a tympanogram on pre-printed charts with meaningful linear scales (Fig. 11.8). The two probe frequencies of 220 and 660 Hz were incorporated and both conductance G_A, and susceptance, B_A, could be measured at each frequency. Thus the 1720 was another research instrument for elucidation of special cases of middle-ear pathology where susceptance measurements at 220 Hz did not provide all the answers (Margolis, Osgathorpe, and Popelka 1978; Van Camp, Creten, Van Peperstraete, and Van Deheyning 1979; Knight and Chalmers 1979). Lutman (1976) and Lutman and Martin (1976,

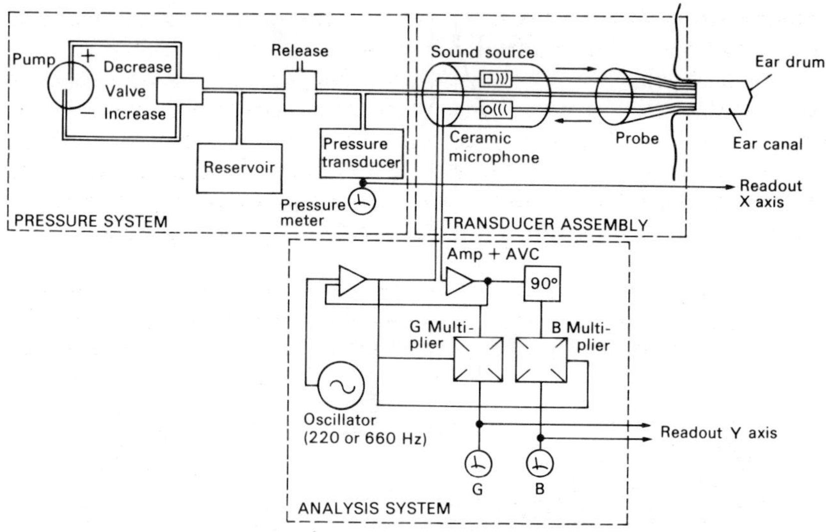

Fig. 11.7. Block diagram of Grason–Stadler Oto-admittance Meter Model 1720.

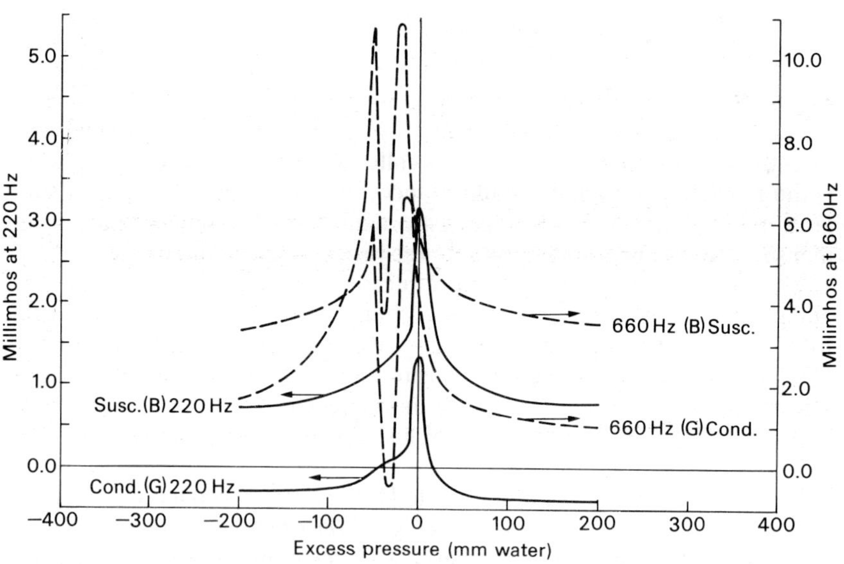

Fig. 11.8. Tympanograms from Grason–Stadler Oto-admittance Meter Model 1720.

1977a, b, 1978) have applied it to a number of important studies of the properties of the acoustic reflex. Chalmers and Knight (1976) reported on the use of the two-frequency, two-component measurements and normative data for clinical use was given by the same authors in 1979.

Liden, Peterson, and Bjorkman (1970, 1972) reported on the use of another instrument for tympanometry at the probe-tone frequency of 800 Hz but, as far as is known, it was never produced commercially.

Following Niemeyer and Sesterhenn's (1974) paper on the assessment of acoustic-reflex thresholds for noise and pure tones as a means of assessment of hearing acuity, Grason–Stadler for a time produced the Model 1721 Portable Oto-admittance Meter with 220 Hz probe tone, and a range of pure-tone and noise-band stimuli with cross-over frequency of 1600 Hz, according to the recommendations of Jerger, Burney, Maudlin, and Crump (1974).

1976 saw the appearance of a new generation of screening instruments with the production of the Grason–Stadler Model 1722 Middle-Ear Analyzer (Fig. 11.9). This device, which has a 220 Hz probe tone, tests the probe

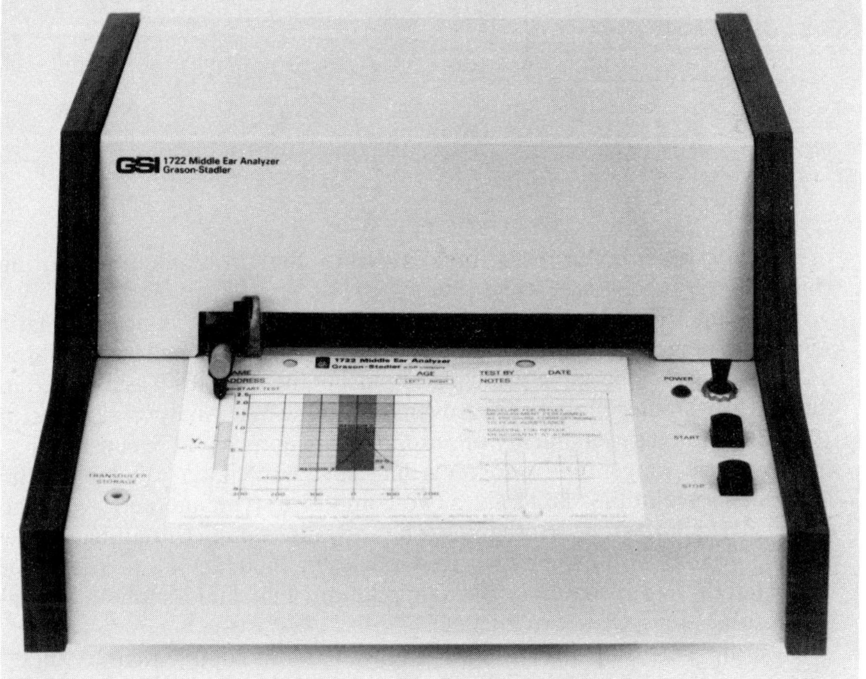

Fig. 11.9. Grason–Stadler Middle-ear Analyzer Model 1722.

seal in the ear, and automatically measures and subtracts the ear canal volume, traces a tympanogram and tests the reflex twice with ipsilateral stimulation for 1000 Hz at 95 dB HL in 35 seconds for each ear. A typical result is shown in Fig. 11.10 for a normal ear. Ipsilateral stimulation of the acoustic reflex was achieved for the first time in a commercial instrument by pulsing the stimulus tone for 45 ms with a 45 ms interval, during which interval time the probe tone is switched on to measure the susceptance. By this means the possibility is eliminated of artefactual responses from

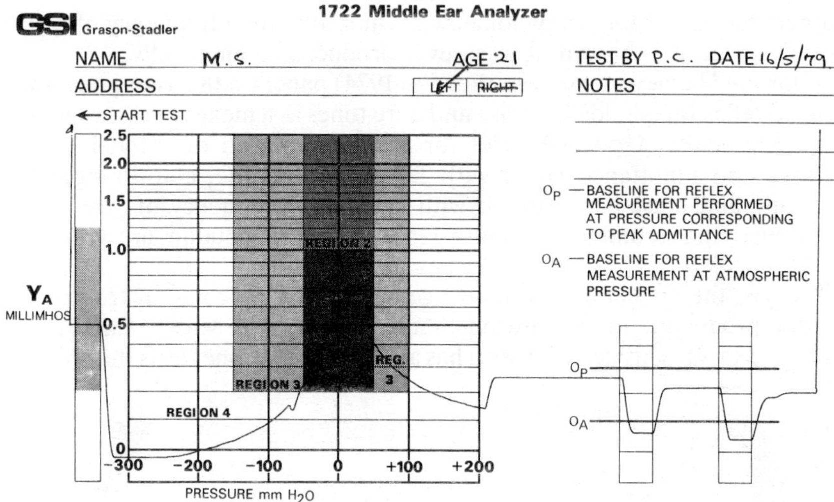

Fig. 11.10. Normal tympanogram and Acoustic Reflex at 1000 Hz (Model 1722).

the high-level stimulus tone breaking into the probe-tone measuring channel.

American Electromedic's Tympanometer Model 85R is an automatic screening device for producing tympanograms and reflex tests in three seconds per ear. The same principle of pulsing the stimulus was adopted in the Grason–Stadler Model 1723 Advanced Middle-Ear Analyzer released in 1978. It can be used manually or automatically and has three sensitivities, two pressure ranges and two recording speeds. A later version of the analyser shown in Fig. 11.11 gives two-component tympanometry with the extra 660 Hz probe tone. Both pure-tone and noise stimuli (broad-band, low and high bands with changeover frequencies of 1600 Hz) are provided for contralateral and ipsilateral reflex stimulation. Fig. 11.12 shows a typical test result.

Both the 1722 and 1723 models employ modern complementary metal oxide semiconductor (CMOS) circuits in 14–16 pin dual in line (DIL) packages and the 1723 contains at least 100 DIL packages. As the transistor density per package averages about 100, the total transistor count is in the order of 10 000. The use of CMOS in these instruments allows the power supply voltage tolerances to be wide (± 25 per cent) and the current requirements are much reduced. Digital circuits have been employed where possible to ensure freedom from temperature and voltage drift so that no preliminary set-up of the plotter is necessary. A closed-loop pressure system is incorporated so that when a pressure leak has been regained, the memory section of the control board automatically resets the pressure to the point at which the seal was lost. (Open-loop systems are likely to give a displaced

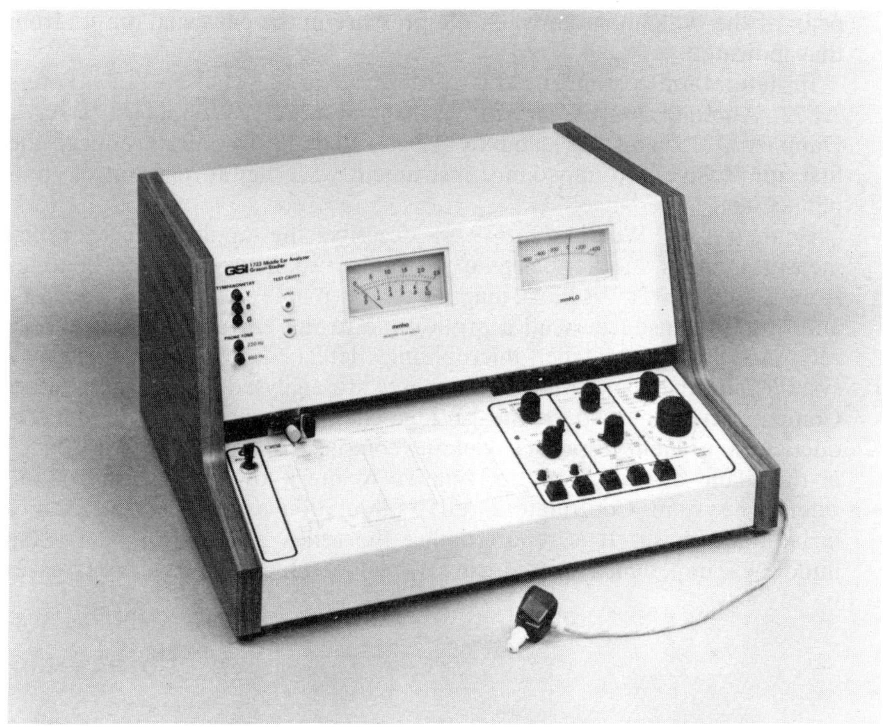

Fig. 11.11. Grason–Stadler Middle-ear Analyzer Model 1723.

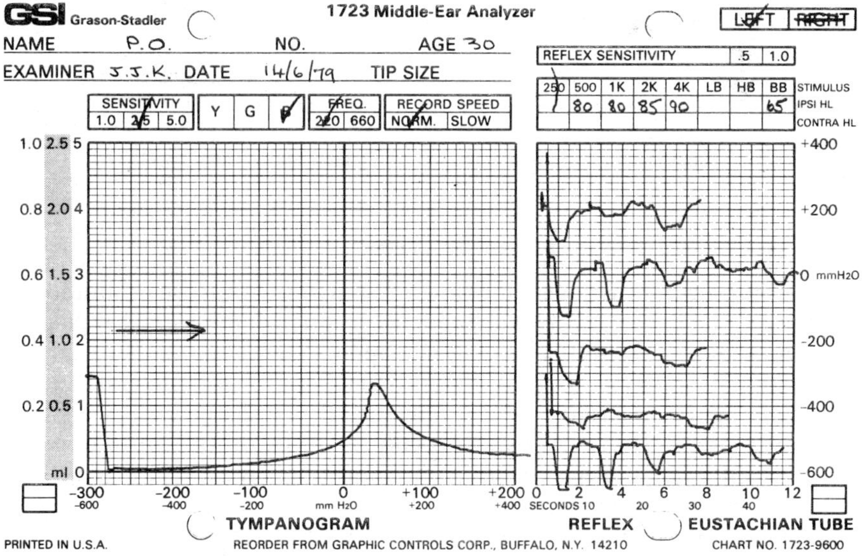

Fig. 11.12. Normal tympanogram and acoustic reflex responses for pure tones and broad-band noise (Model 1723).

peak of the tympanogram when the pressure in the ear canal differs from that indicated.)

Ipsilateral reflex stimulation is also offered in the Madsen Z073, Peters AP72, Amplaid 702, American Electromedics 85R, Interacoustics AZ3, Danplex D175, and the Kamplex AZ2. Teledyne Avionics produced the first admittance and impedance instrument with digital read-out of compliance and impedance.

Bennett and Weatherby (1979) describe the application to reflex measurement of another design of instrument to be used with probe tones from 220 to 2000 Hz. A block diagram is shown in Fig. 11.13. The oscillator and output transducer send a probe tone to the ear under test and to a reference system. Matched microphones detect the pressures in the two systems and their amplitudes and phases are analysed in the comparator. Comparison of the two identical bridge channels cancel any inherent frequency component responses, yielding complex components of impedance in the plane of the probe tip, relative to the known impedance of the reference system. Contralateral reflex stimulation is applied in the form of broad-band noise. It is reported that the reflex generally increases the middle-ear impedance for frequencies up to 700 Hz and thereafter decreases it.

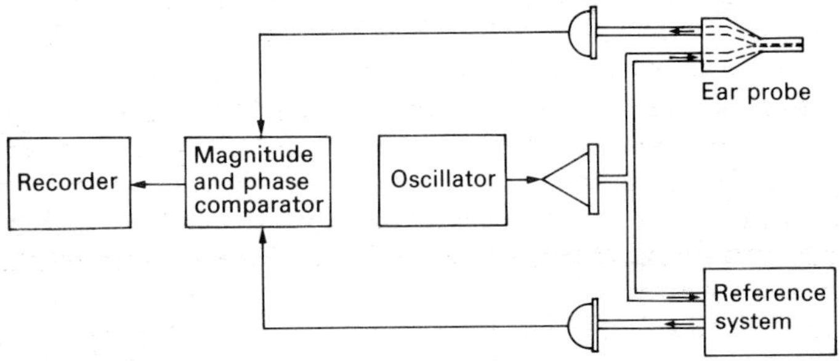

Fig. 11.13. Block diagram of apparatus used by Bennett and Weatherby (1979).

STANDARDIZATION AND CALIBRATION

No British or International Standards exist at present for the calibration of acoustic impedance bridges with the sole exception of the normal audiometric threshold standards (Chapter 8) that apply to reflex tones when supplied by external earphones for contralateral stimulation. For ipsilateral stimulation through the measuring probe, only the IEC126 2cc coupler (1961) is at all appropriate. However, the connection with the various forms of probe will be different and the resulting sound pressures will be subject to variation. Thus there is little hope of achieving by this means equality of stimulation levels for the contralateral and ipsilateral modes to normal audiometric degrees of accuracy.

It is understood that consideration is being given to the possibility of producing a standard within the IEC for the calibration of these instruments but there are obvious difficulties when rapid developments are taking place in the instrumentation and the different facilities offered. The American National Standards Institute (ANSI) is proceeding along the lines of a combined standard to specify several types of instrument together with recommended methods of calibration, preferred probe frequences, pressure range, etc. with suitable tolerances.

Even the units of measurements in use are diverse, e.g. millimetres of water pressure, cubic centimetres of equivalent air volume, c.g.s. and m.k.s. acoustic ohms, and acoustic mhos. It is likely that SI units will be adopted in the future with pascals for pressure, pascal seconds per metre to the third power for acoustic resistance, reactance and impedance, etc.

Lutman (1978) has reported on a Workshop on Ipsilateral Stimulus Calibration and Artefacts held recently in Britain where some of the problems were discussed and solutions proposed. The possibility of artefacts occurring in reflex threshold measurement has already been mentioned. Such artefacts were first reported by Danaher and Pickett (1974) with a Grason–Stadler Model 1720; they found a deflection in the *opposite* direction to that from a true reflex. However, Niswander and Ruth (1976) with an American Electromedics Model 81 found artefacts often in the *same* direction as true reflexes. Newall, Royall, and Lightfoot (1978) with measurements on cadavers using a Peters AP61C reported an artefact in the *same* direction as the reflex in all 49 cases. Kunov (1977) reported an 'eardrum' artefact in ipsilateral stimulation with a Madsen Z073. This is explained by the inherent non-linearity of the ear canal and tympanic membrane. It results in a deflection *opposite* to that of a true reflex. This eardrum artefact is distinct from the artefact which occurs in contralateral stimulation at high levels caused by inadequate filtering of the electrical signals in some acoustic impedance instruments.

Lutman and Leis (1980) have examined the reflex artefacts obtained in cadavers in six current instruments with ipsilateral stimulation. It appeared that the Grason-Stadler Model 1723 gave the least number of artefacts by use of its pulsed stimulus system, but even so an artefact was recorded only at 1000 Hz at 25 dB above the normal reflex threshold. It is important that due attention is given to the question of artefacts in both contralateral and ipsilateral stimulation for too often in the past a meter deflection synchronous with a stimulus presentation has been accepted as a genuine reflex.

The situation with calibration was equally bad a decade ago when Knight (1971) reported that in a sample of thirteen acoustic impedance meters in clinical use, eight showed gross calibration errors. Since that time, calibration cavities have often been supplied with the instruments to facilitate frequent local checks by those making the measurements, and the situation has improved. However, guidance is needed such as for the Regional Calibration Centres of the British National Health Service on the comprehensive calibration of these increasingly sophisticated instruments and it is already under consideration by the appropriate bodies. Instead of the instruction, which is now fairly general, to set up the probe tone to give 95 dB SPL (or a similar stated level) into an IEC 2cc coupler, it is likely that greater accuracy will result from adoption of the newly formulated draft IEC specification for the 'occluded ear simulator'. This improved device will probably supersede the 2cc coupler for appropriate calibrations. Advice will need to be given on the calibration of the pressure variation in tympanometers and the tolerances which can be allowed. In the meantime, emphasis is required on frequent and full personal checks on all impedance bridges in the same way that daily subjective checks are practiced by operators on their pure-tone and self-recording audiometers.

REFERENCES

BENNETT, M. J. and WEATHERBY, L. A. (1979). Multiple probe frequency acoustic reflex measurements. *Scand. Audiol.* **8**, 233.

BROOKS, D. N. (1973). Hearing screening. A comparative study of an impedance method and pure tone screening. *Scand. Audiol.* **2**, 67.

CHALMERS, P. and KNIGHT, J. J. (1976). Two component tympanometry in clinical investigation. British Society of Audiology Meeting, London 23rd April.

—— —— (1979). Diagnostic acoustic impedance measurements in the United Kingdom 1960–1980. *Proc. IV Int. Symp. Acoustic Imped. Measurements,* Lisbon.

DANAHER, E. M. and PICKETT, J. M. (1974). Notes on an artifact in measurement of the acoustic reflex. *J. Speech Hear. Res.* **17**, 305.

IEC PUBLICATION 126 (1961). IEC reference coupler. International Electrotech. Comm. Geneva.

JERGER, J., BURNEY, P. P., MAUDLIN, L., and CRUMP, B. (1975). Predicting hearing loss from the acoustic reflex. *J. Speech Hear. Dis.* **39**, 11.

KNIGHT, J. J. (1971). Acoustic impedance measurements in diagnosis of hearing disorders. *Proc. 7th Int. Cong. Acoustics,* Budapest, Paper 24 H7.

—— and CHALMERS, P. (1979). Two-component tympanometry. *Proc. Inst. Acoustics,* Winter Meeting, Windermere.

KUNOV, H. (1977). The 'eardrum artifact' in ipsilateral reflex measurements. *Scand. Audiol.* **6**, 133.

LIDEN, G., BJORKMAN, G., and PETERSON, J. L. (1972). Clinical equipment for measurement of middle ear reflexes and tympanometry. *J. Speech Hear. Dis.* **37**, 100.

—— PETERSON, J. L., and BJORKMAN, G. (1970). Tympanometry. *Archs Otol.* **92**, 248.

LUTMAN, M. E. (1976). The protective action of the acoustic reflex. Ph.D. thesis, University of Southampton.

—— (1978). Brief Proceedings of Workshop on Ipsilateral Impedance Meter Stimulus Calibration and Artefacts. Institute of Sound and Vibration Research Memorandum No. 583. University of Southampton.

—— and LEIS, B. R. (1980) Ipsilateral acoustic reflex artefacts measured in cadavers. *Scand. Audiol.* **9**, 33.

—— and MARTIN, A. M. (1976). The variability of acoustic reflex threshold measurements. J. Sound Vibr. **48**, 413.

—— —— (1977a). The acoustic reflex threshold for impulses. *J. Sound Vibr.* **51**, 97.

—— —— (1977b). The response of the acoustic reflex as a function of the intensity and temporal characteristics of pulsed stimuli. *J. Sound Vibr.* **54**, 345.

—— —— (1978). Adaptation of the acoustic reflex to combinations of sustained steady-state and repeated pulse stimuli. *J. Sound Vibr.* **56**, 137.

MARGOLIS, R. H., OSGATHORPE, J. D., and POPELKA, G. R. (1978). The effects of experimentally-produced middle ear lesions and tympanometry in cats. *Acta Oto-lar.* **86,** 428.

METZ, O. (1946). The acoustic impedance measured on normal and pathological ears. *Acta Oto-lar.* Suppl. 63.

NEWALL, ROYALL, R. A., and LIGHTFOOT, G. R. (1978). Some observations on the contralateral stapedial reflex artefact. *Br. J. Audiol.* **12**, 78.

NIEMEYER, E. and SESTERHENN, G. (1974). Calculating the hearing threshold from stapedius reflex threshold for different sound stimuli. *Int. Audiol.* **13**, 421.

NISWANDER, P. S. and RUTH, R. A. (1976). An artifact in acoustic reflex measurement: some further observations. *J. Am. Audiol. Soc.* **1**, 209.

ROBINSON, N. W. (1937). An acoustic impedance bridge. *Phil. Mag. J. Sci.* Suppl. 7, **23**, 665.

SCHUSTER, K. (1934). Eine Methode zum Vergluch akustische Impedanzen. *Physickal. Z.* **35**, 408.

TERKILDSEN, K. and NIELSEN, S. S. (1960). An electro-acoustic impedance measuring bridge for clinical use. *Archs Otol.* **72**, 339.

VAN CAMP, K. J., CRETEN, W. L., VAN PEPERSTRAETE, P. M., and VAN DEHEYNING, P. H. (1979). Tympanometry: how not to overlook middle ear pathologies. *The reflex.* Grason-Stadler, Littleton, Mass., USA.

WEST, W. (1928). Measurements of the acoustical impedance of human ears. *P.O. elect. Engrs' J.* **21**, 293.

ZWISLOCKI, J. J. (1963). An acoustic method for clinical examination of the ear. *J. Speech Hear. Res.* **6**, 303.

Section 3
Pathology of Deafness

12 Pathology of the ear

L. MICHAELS and MAHER WELLS

Despite many technological advances, the practice of medicine in the broad sense is still an art based on science. To understand and treat disease processes on a scientific basis, it is essential to appreciate the pathology of the disease so as to provide a three-dimensional view.

Aural pathology has been particularly difficult to study for many reasons, such as the problems involved in obtaining temporal bones at post mortem, the high degree of technical expertise involved in obtaining sections, and, of course, the lack of experience in interpretation of results.

The basis for an understanding of the pathology of the ear is the study of serial sections of temporal bones removed post mortem from patients whose ear condition has been studied clinically during life. The lesions so revealed can be correlated with clinical features so that a pathological basis can be derived for living patients with similar features. The study of temporal bone pathology is not as advanced as that of the pathology of other organs because the problems of access and processing of the specimen have resulted in far fewer specimens being available than with any other organ of the body. It would be a great help in the advancement of the subject if audiologists requested the removal of the temporal bone for pathological examination in any audiological patient whose death has come to their attention.

Most pathologists and post-mortem technicians are familiar with the technique of removal of temporal bones. As soon as the bone is removed it should be placed in 10 per cent formal saline until it is processed for histological examination. Processing should be carried out in histological laboratories that specialize in temporal bone work. Slow decalcification in weak acid is first necessary to soften the bone. Then, in order to protect the delicate structures of middle and inner ears, slow embedding in celloidin or some similar substance is carried out. The procedure is carried out at room temperature in contrast to the 60 °C heating required for the standard paraffin-wax embedding.

Sections of the temporal bone enable observation of the hair cells of the organ of Corti to be made; however, these cells are frequently not clearly delineated. A more accurate method of observation may be carried out by the surface specimen technique. By this method the cochlea is fixed in osmic acid solution, fragments of basilar membrane are removed, placed flat on the microscope slide, and examined by phase-contrast microscopy. This method has been used for human cochlear examination but is particularly valuable in experimental situations.

Aural pathology may be conveniently classified as: (i) congenital; (ii) traumatic; (iii) inflammatory; (iv) neoplastic; (v) disorders of growth, metabolism, and aging.

CONGENITAL LESIONS

Congenital lesions of the ear result in deafness present at birth. These lesions may be hereditary or acquired *in utero*. Congenital abnormalities of the external, middle, and inner ear may occur in isolation, or in various combinations, e.g. abnormality of the external auditory meatus may be associated with abnormalities of the middle ear.

The external ear

DEVELOPMENT OF THE EXTERNAL EAR

The auricle develops from six knob-like outgrowths from the first and second branchial arches. These evaginations fuse to form the various components (helix, antihelix, tragus, etc.) of the auricle. The external auditory meatus is derived from the first branchial groove, a depression of the ectoderm between the first (mandibular) arch and the second (hyoid) arch. The deep extremity of this groove meets the outer epithelium of the corresponding first pharyngeal pouch, separated only by a thin layer of connective tissue. The point of meeting produces the tympanic membrane, its ectodermal origin producing the outer squamous epithelial covering and its endodermal origin producing the cubical middle-ear lining of the tympanic membrane. The thin connective tissue layer separating the two epithelial layers produces the radial and circularly arranged (intermediate) sheets of the tympanic membrane.

Malformation of the external ear include: (i) partial or complete absence of the auricle; (ii) accessory auricles; (iii) pre-auricular sinus; (iv) atresia of the external auditory meatus, which may present as a blind protrusion or may be completely absent; and (v) abnormalities of the shape and size of the auricle. These may be ascribed to defects of fusion of the knob-like protrusions and hollowing out of the first branchial groove.

The middle ear

DEVELOPMENT OF THE MIDDLE EAR

The malleus and incus are developed from connective tissue of the first branchial arch of Meckel's cartilage. The stapes is formed from the connective tissue of the second branchial arch or Reichert's cartilage. The vestibular wall of the footplate of the stapes is derived from the otocyst. The ossicular chain is recognizable in cartilage by the twelfth week and the ossicles are of adult size at birth.

The cavity and lining of the middle ear (tympanic cavity) and of the Eustachian tube arise from the expanding terminal end of the first and possibly the second pharyngeal pouches which remains slit-like up to the 20th week and then proceeds to expand and cover the ossicles and tympanum proper by the 30th week. Subsequently the epitympanum and mastoid air cells become excavated and epithelialized.

MALFORMATION OF THE MIDDLE EAR

The malleus is more often malformed than the stapes and incus. It may be fused with the body of the incus, or fixed to the epitympanum by bone. The incus may also be fixed to the medial wall of the epitympanum or the long process can be short and in an abnormal position in the middle-ear cleft. The stapes may be congenitally fixed, or the crura distorted (Fig. 12.1). Occasionally there is complete absence of the stapes. Congenital dehiscence of the bony facial canal in the region of the oval window occurs not infrequently. Persistence of the stapedial artery and total absence of the round window are rare conditions. The whole middle-ear cavity may be incompletely developed leaving primitive mesenchymal tissue (Fig. 12.2). Anomalies of the internal and external ear are usually present in conjunction.

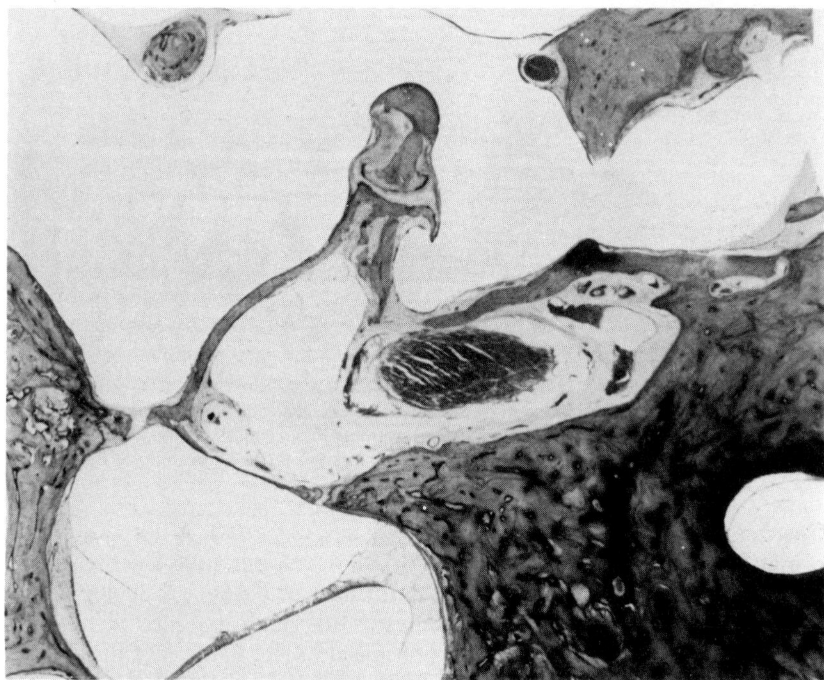

Fig. 12.1. Temporal bone section of foetus of 32 weeks. Cause of death was unrelated to the ear. The anterior crus of the stapes is markedly bowed and the posterior crus is shortened and abnormally closely related to the facial nerve. Abnormalities of the ossicular chain of this type have been seen frequently in our laboratory in perinatal deaths from causes unrelated to the ear. (H. & E. × 35.)

SYNDROMES INVOLVING THE MIDDLE EAR (see also Chapter 23)

A number of congenital syndromes are seen in which middle ear lesions are combined with abnormalities outside the ears.

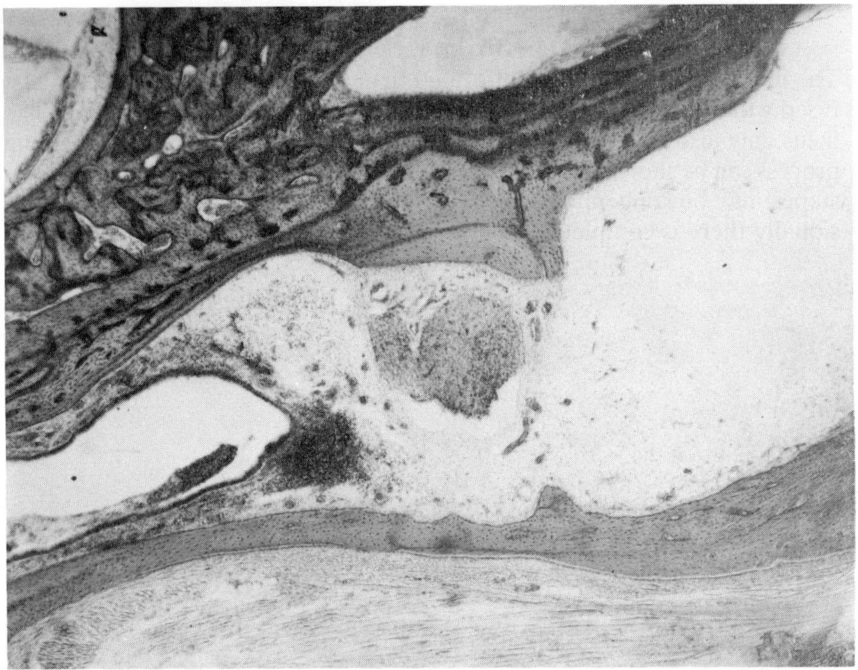

Fig. 12.2. Incomplete development of the whole middle ear. The Eustachian tube is seen on the left. The middle-ear cavity has not developed, but is composed of loose lying mesenchymal cells in the midst of which is the facial nerve. (H. & E. × 25.)

Treacher Collins' syndrome (*mandibulofacial dysostosis*). A hereditary malformation, predominantly due to abnormal development of the first branchial arch. The ossicles may be small, deformed, or absent producing mainly a conductive deafness. Other anomalies of this syndrome include notching of the lower eye-lids, diminished frontonasal angle, flatness of the cheeks, receding mandible, anomalies of the teeth, and deformity of the auricle. The defect is usually bilateral but may be unilateral.

Crouzon's syndrome (*craniofacial dysostosis*). This syndrome, first described by Crouzon in 1912, is characterized by hypertelorism, exophthalmus, optic atrophy, under-developed maxillae, and craniosynostosis. Convulsions and dementia can also occur.

Conductive deafness is due to fixation of the stapes footplate and deformed crura. The malleus and incus may also be fixed.

Hunter–Hurler syndrome (*gargoylism*). A hereditary disease characterized by skeletal deformity, blindness, deafness, low set ears, mental deficiency, and hepatosplenomegaly.

Deafness is conductive and sensorineural. The middle-ear cleft and bony cochlea may be filled with mesenchymal cell tissue containing 'gargoyle cells'.

Klippel–Feil syndrome. This consists of congenital fusion of the cervical vertebrae, causing shortening of the neck, low hair-line posteriorly, and deafness. The conductive element in the deafness is due to deformed and ankylosed ossicles. The sensorineural deafness is due to vestigial cochlea and labyrinth.

The inner ear

DEVELOPMENT OF THE INNER EAR

The inner ear develops in a different fashion from the external and middle ears, not being dependent on branchial arch structures, but on a specific entity—the otocyst. This is derived from ectoderm which grows in on each side, becomes separated from the surface, and by a system of branching and subdivision gives rise to the whole endolymphatic system. The bony labyrinth is formed from the surrounding mesoderm.

STRUCTURAL FORMS OF MALFORMATIONS OF THE INNER EAR

A large number of congenital pathological alterations of the inner ear have been described affecting large parts of the inner-ear structure in general or specific areas of the inner ear. Attempts have been made to classify these conditions into broad groups.

Thus Ormerod (1960) classified anomalies of the labyrinth associated with congenital deafness into four types based on historical descriptions:

1. Michel type—complete lack of development of internal ear.
2. Mondini–Alexander type—development only of a single curved tube representing the cochlea and similar immaturity of the vestibule and canals (Fig. 12.3).
3. Bing Siebenmann type—underdevelopment of the membranous labyrinth, particularly of the sense organ with a well-formed labyrinth.
4. Scheibe type—malformation restricted to membranous cochlea and saccule (Fig. 12.4).

Within this classification there are many defects which are not described fully. A large number of congenital lesions are listed in a recent review of the literature by Suehiro and Sando (1979) (Table 12.1). These indicate the range of possibilities in any case of congenital deafness resulting from inner-ear malformation. Suehiro and Sando proposed a new classification in which the letters A, B, and C indicate areas of the osseous labyrinth: both the cochlea and the vestibule, the cochlea only, and the vestibule only, respectively; the letters a, b, and c indicate areas of the membranous labyrinth: both the cochlea and the vestibule, the cochlea only, and the vestibule only, respectively. Underlining these letters indicates hypoplastic anomalies of the areas of the letters, e.g. $\underline{b}$ represents an anomaly of the membranous cochlea. Two subdivisions of these areas and their anomalies are indicated by a′ and a″: a″ indicates anomalies observed in the cochlea and saccule and a′ indicates anomalies in the cochlea and vestibule excluding anomalies categorized as a″. Thus hypoplastic anomalies of the inner ear can be classified into 16 groups as follows:

TABLE 12.1. *Anatomical classification of malformations of inner ear (1979)*

Inner ear as a whole
  Absence and underdevelopment of labyrinth
Cochlea
  (A) *Cochlea in general*
    Absent, underdeveloped, or anteriorly displaced
  (B) *Osseous cochlea*
    1. Osseous cochlea in general such as deformity
    2. Round window absent, displaced, or partitioned by a bony bar
    3. Scala tympani underdeveloped
    4. Scala vestibuli absent or underdeveloped
    5. Modiolus absent, underdeveloped, or focally thickened
    6. Cochlear aqueduct absent, underdeveloped, or widened
  (C) *Membranous cochlea*
    1. Cochlear duct in general absent or undeveloped
    2. Organ of Corti absent or undeveloped
    3. Tectorial membrane underdeveloped or rolled and covered by single epithelial layer
    4. Spiral limbus partially absent
    5. Stria vascularis absent, deformed, undeveloped or displaced
    6. Spiral ligament absent, deformed, or calcified
    7. Reissners membrane absent or displaced
    8. Basilar membrane elongated, absent, or displaced
    9. Ductus reuniens absent or enlarged

Vestibule
  (A) *Vestibule in general* undeveloped
  (B) *Osseous vestibule*
    1. Osseous vestibule in general underdeveloped or malformed
    2. Oval window absent, thin, malformed, calcified annular ligament
    3. Vestibular aqueduct underdeveloped or displaced
  (C) *Membranous vestibule*
    1. Utricle absent, underdeveloped, large, or malformed. Anomalies of macule
    2. Saccule absent, undeveloped, or malformed. Anomalies of macule.
    3. Endolymphatic duct and sac including undevelopment, shortening and widening, and anomalies of utriculoendolymphatic valve.

Semicircular canal
  (A) *Semicircular canal in general*
    Absent, underdeveloped, or enlarged
  (B) *Superior semicircular canal*
    1. In general. Absence of canal of parts of it
    2. Osseous superior circular canal. Undeveloped or widened
    3. Membranous superior circular canal. Absence of part or widening of part of it Absence or undevelopment of crista
  (C) *Posterior semicircular canal*
    1. Posterior semicircular canal in general absent, underdeveloped, displaced superiorly, or deformed
    2. Osseous posterior semicircular canal narrow or enlarged
    3. Membranous posterior semicircular canal absent, widened, narrowed, or crista malformed
  (D) *Lateral semicircular canal*
    1. Lateral semicircular canal in general absent, underdeveloped, or malformed
    2. Osseous lateral semicircular canal absent or underdeveloped and widened
    3. Membranous lateral semicircular canal absent, undeveloped, or flat. Crista undeveloped or flat and macula-like

TABLE 12.1 *continued*

Otic capsule

Bony anomalies owing to:
(a) Achondroplasia
(b) Craniofacial dysostosis
(c) Gargoylism
(d) Histiocytosis
(e) Hypophosphatasia
(f) Osteitis deformans
(g) Osteogenesis inperfecta
(h) Osteopetrosis
(i) Ostosclerosis
(j) Syphilis
(k) Endemic cretinism

Internal auditory meatus

Absent, undeveloped, displaced, or deformed

Nerve

(A) *Facial nerve*
Absent, underdeveloped, displaced
(B) *Eighth Nerve*
1. Eighth nerve in general absent or undeveloped
2. Cochlear nerve absent or displaced
3. Vestibular nerve absent or displaced

Vessels

Displaced, e.g. crossing perilymphatic space of cochlea

Subarcuate fossa

Absent, underdeveloped, displaced, or enlarged

Osseous and membranous labyrinth combined;
Aa, Ab, Ac, Ba, Bb, Bc, Ca, Cb, Cc.
Bony labyrinth only: A, B, C.
Membranous labyrinth only: a′, a′′, b, c.

Fig. 12.5 shows an example of an inner ear anomaly which under this system can be classified as Bb.

AETIOLOGICAL BASIS FOR MALFORMATIONS OF THE INNER EAR

Many of the malformations found in the internal ear represent part of a 'disease' or 'syndrome' in which other defects of the body are usually associated. These diseases may be classified on an aetiological basis. Table 12.2 summarized these aetiologies and gives some notes on important examples of some of the diseases. This table, like Table 12.1, is given as a guide only to the general range of congenital anomalies of the inner ear. Further details and references to papers on the pathology of these conditions will be found in Konigsmark (1969) and Suehiro and Sando (1979).

TABLE 12.2. *Aetiology of diseases with inner-ear anomalies*

Unknown aetiology

1. *Without associated anomalies*
   Congenital absence of round window
2. *With other associated anomalies*
   For example chromosomal anomalies, e.g. trisomy 13–15 syndrome and trisomy 18 syndrome—many abnormalities of cochlea vestibule and semicircular canals
   Congenital heart disease—abnormalities of cochlea, vestibule, and semicircular canals

Hereditary characteristics

Associated with heart disease

For example cardio-auditory syndrome (Jervell–Lange–Nielsen syndrome)—atrophy of organ of Corti, spiral ganglion, and cristae with P A S—positive hyaline deposits particularly in stria vascularis. Recessive inheritance

Associated with integumentary system disease

For example Waardenburg's disease in which there is widely spread medial canthi, flat nasal root, confluent eyebrows, and white forelock. The organ of Corti is absent.

Associated with eye disease

Recessive retinitis pigmentosa—Usher's syndrome. There are electron microscopical changes in the nasal cilia, sensorineural deafness is present, but the structural changes in the cochlea are not known

Associated with nervous system disease

For example dominant acoustic neuromas

Associated with skeletal disease

For example Paget's disease of bone—dominant with variable penetrance. Mosaic involvement of osseous labyrinth

Association with renal disease

For example dominant nephritis—Alport's disease. The cochlea shows atrophy of the organ of Corti and stria vascularis

Association with goitre

For example Pendred's syndrome—recessive. The cochlear defect is not known

Prenatal infections

Rubella showing a rolled up tectorial membrane and adhesions of saccular wall to otolithis membrane
Syphilis showing osteitis and/or osteomyelitis

Iatrogenic ototoxicity

For example chloroquine showing atrophy of organ of Corti or thalidomide showing absence of inner ear, thin membranous oval window, and absence of seventh and eighth cranial nerves.

TRAUMA

Direct injury by sharp objects to the pinna can cause laceration, haematoma, and, when infected, causes abscess formation and perichondritis, ultimately leading to a 'cauliflower ear' deformity. Haematoma and abscess spread easily in the loose perichondrial layer of the pinna.

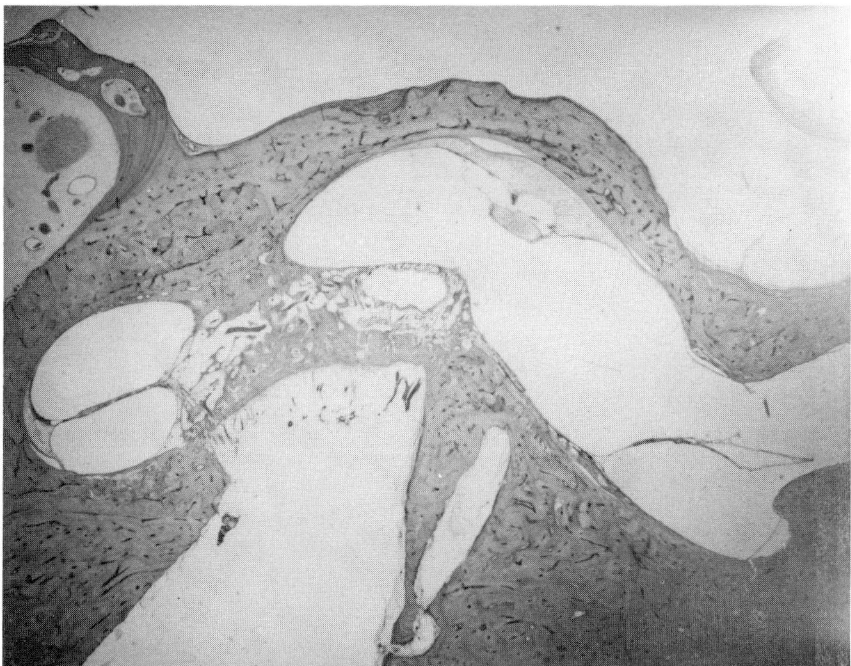

Fig. 12.3. The cochlea is represented only by a single tube which is continuous on the right with an abnormal vestibule. Note internal auditory meatus in the lower central part. The VIII nerve is (artefactually) not visible. This is an example of the anomaly usually referred to as Mondini–Alexander type (Suehiro and Sando—Aa). (H. & E. × 25.)

Foreign bodies may injure the ear and or the ossicular chain. Unskilled attempts at removal of foreign bodies with hairpins and needles cause further damage.

Fractures involving the cochlea

Trauma caused by automobile accidents is the commonest type of trauma in the Western world. It is the chief cause of death between the ages of one and 34 years and in the United States. 10 000 serious injuries were said to have taken place as a result of car accidents in 1974.

It is possible, and to be hoped, that enforced major changes in driving patterns will alter this epidemic of trauma, but in the meantime its effects are still with us. Three-quarters of automobile injuries are stated to involve the head, and fractures of the skull are extremely common. Fractures take place in the vault and/or the base of the skull. The vault fractures are usually of little significance unless, and this is rare, they are depressed onto the underlying brain. The base-of-skull fractures are very serious and an indication of the great severity of the trauma. In the majority of patients with fractures of the base of the skull, the rigid and more brittle wedge of bone

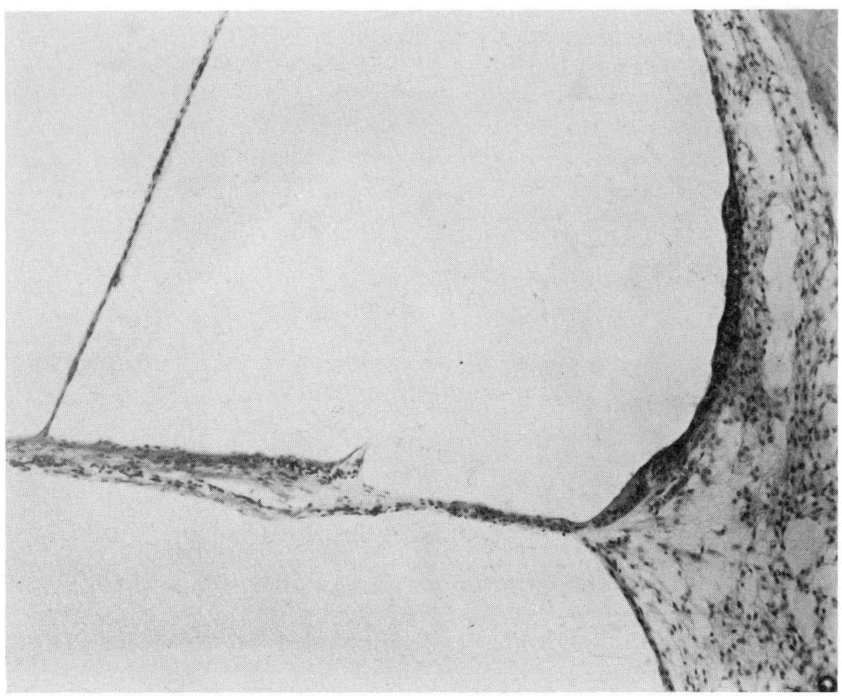

Fig. 12.4. Congenital anomaly of the cochlea in which the organ of Corti and tectorial membrane are absent. This particular anomaly has been referred to as the Scheibe type (Suehiro and Sando—b). (H. & E. × 100.)

occupying about one-third of the skull base—the temporal bone—is the seat of a fracture.

On the basis of radiological studies it has been found that fractures of the petrous temporal bone seem to fall within two anatomical groups: those in which the fracture line passes along the length of the petrous temporal bone—longitudinal fractures, and those in which the fracture line passes at right-angles to the length of the petrous temporal bone—transverse fractures (Figs. 12.7 and 12.8).

The effects on the cochlea of these two types of lesion are quite different. Longitudinal fractures arise as a result of direct blows to the temporal and parietal areas of the head. The fracture line starts in the squamous portion of the temporal bone and usually involves the external auditory canal, the tympanic membrane and one or more of the ossicles of the middle ear, and finishes up in the region of the foramen lacerum near the apex of the petrous temporal bone. The cochlea is not involved. The transverse fractures are caused by blows to the front or back of the skull producing a sideways tearing effect. The fracture line in these cases passes from the dural membrane on the posteromedial aspect of the petrous temporal, often through the internal auditory meatus to involve the seventh and eight cranial nerves and then into the cochlea in the region of the basal turn at its posterolateral

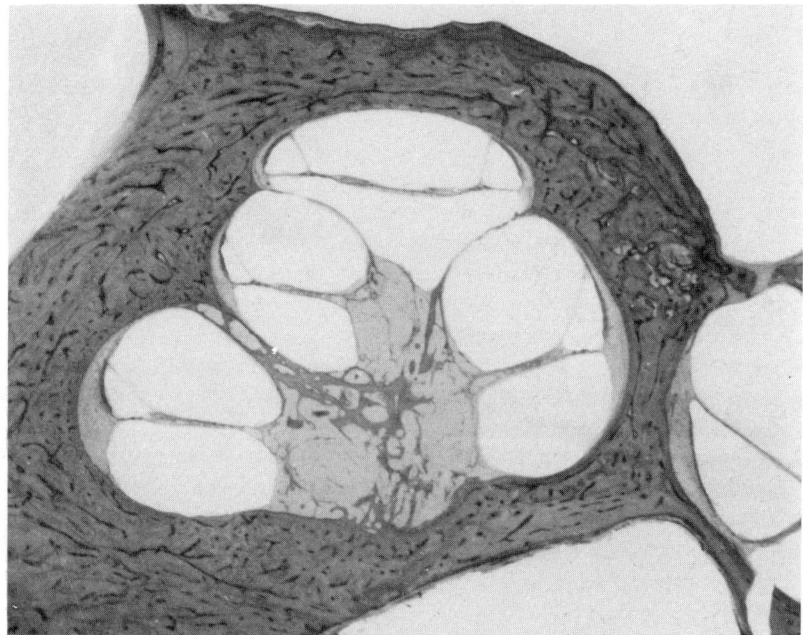

Fig. 12.5. Cochlea of 29-year-old male with deaf mutism and Friedreich's ataxia. A portion of a cochlear coil is absent as shown by the fact that the cochlea contains four compartments at this mid-modiolar level instead of five. Such an anomaly has been frequently observed in our laboratory in cases of perinatal death from causes unrelated to the ear (Suehiro and Sando—Bb). (H. & E. × 35.)

side. The adjacent vestibule and the round and oval windows are also frequently involved.

Thus, in the case of the longitudinal fractures, the hearing loss is usually a mild or moderate one of the conductive type which may be helped by surgery. The hearing loss caused by a transverse fracture, involving as it does both the sensory organ and the afferent nerve derived from it, produces a severe senorineural deafness from which little improvement is to be expected. A further serious side-effect of transverse fractures is the result of their establishing a communication between the meninges and the middle ear, so that there is a leak of cerebrospinal fluid which invariable leads to infection spreading to the meninges; this meningitis may cause death if it is not controlled by antibiotic therapy. Another form of fluid leakage in transverse fractures, that of perilymph, may be associated with the symptoms of Ménière's disease. The pathological changes in these cases come about from the lowering of perilymph pressure with secondary endolymphatic hydrops. Reissner's membrane is seen to be grossly distended throughout the cochlear duct and the saccule may be dilated.

The effect of a fracture in other parts of the body, e.g. in a long bone, is to give rise to local haemorrhage between the bone ends. This is soon invaded

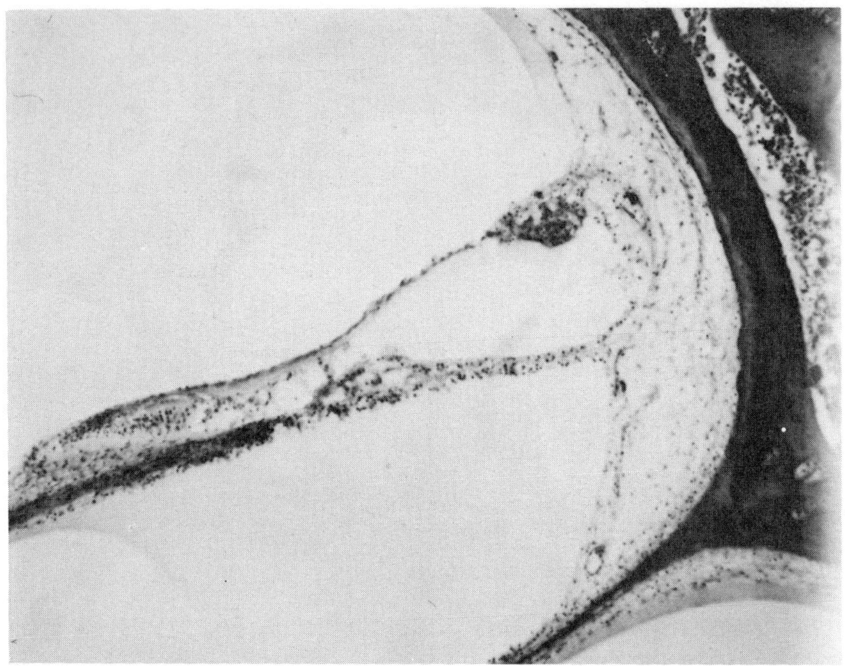

Fig. 12.6. Congenital rubella in foetal abortion specimen at 16 weeks. A granuloma-like group of cells is present at the junction of Reissner's membrane with the stria vascularis. (H. & E. × 100.)

by granulation tissue which then gives way to a primitive type of bone called callus, which acts as a splint to secure the two fractured ends. In the temporal bone, however, callus does not seem to form; moreover, the union of the two fractured portions is by fibrous tissue, not bone. This type of fracture healing seems to occur in skull fractures in general and may be related to the immobility of these fractures. Small fractures joined up by this type of fibrous union are often found in sections of temporal bone at post mortem in cases with no history of trauma and no symptoms related to the bone damage which usually is of insignificant degree. These healed fractures are found between the vestibule cochlea, or carotid canal and the middle ear. Their pathogenesis is unknown (Fig. 12.34).

Microscopic cochlear damage in head injury

After a head injury a sensorineural type of deafness may develop without any detectable microscopic damage to the cochlea. The hearing loss is in the higher frequency ranges from 3000 to 8000 Hz. The pathological changes giving rise to this functional loss have not been explored in human material. Experimental studies have revealed microscopic cochlear damage following direct head injury. Schuknecht, Neff, and Perlman (1951) trained ten cats to respond to auditory stimuli by walking forward in a rotating cage. The

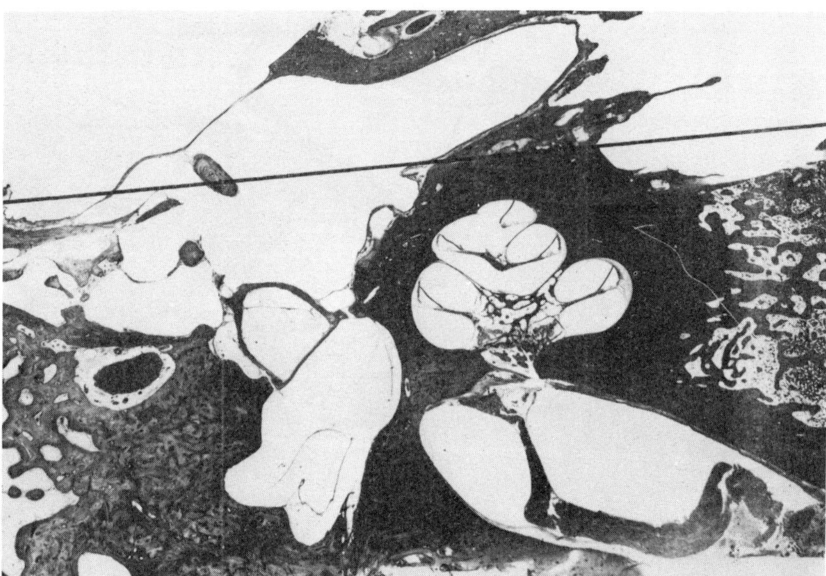

Fig. 12.7. Photomicrograph of horizontal section of temporal bone. A solid line has been drawn to illustrate the usual pathway of a temporal bone fracture of longitudinal type. This type of fracture passes though the tympanic membrane, ossicles (handle of the malleus is seen to be involved here) and goes anterior to the cochlea towards the foramen lacerum. (H. & E. × 6.5.) (Reproduced with the permission of Academic Press.)

anaesthetized animals were then given a blow to the exposed skull in the midline, via a 2 lb metal rod 1 inch in diameter by a 1 lb mallet. The animals were allowed to recover and then tested audiometrically until they were killed some weeks after trauma had been inflicted. All animals had hearing losses at least between 3000 and 8000 Hz, and some animals had even more widespread damage. The cochleae of all the animals were examined histologically by serial section. A constant change was found to be a loss of external hair cells in the upper basal coil region. In some animals damage was more marked and in a few there was a complete disappearance of internal and external hair cells in some areas. Nerve fibres and ganglion cells were correspondingly reduced in these cases. Microscopic haemorrhage was also frequently detected in cochlear sections. It did not provoke an inflammatory reaction and was thus not felt to be of any significance in producing the hearing loss.

Blast and gunshot injury

Peripheral damage to the ear, particularly rupture of the tympanic membrane, is the most striking result of explosive blast and gunshot injury and vestibular damage frequently takes place; however, permanent damage to the internal ear and its hearing mechanism is also a likely sequel. In the experimental study of injury from this source and other types of injury to the

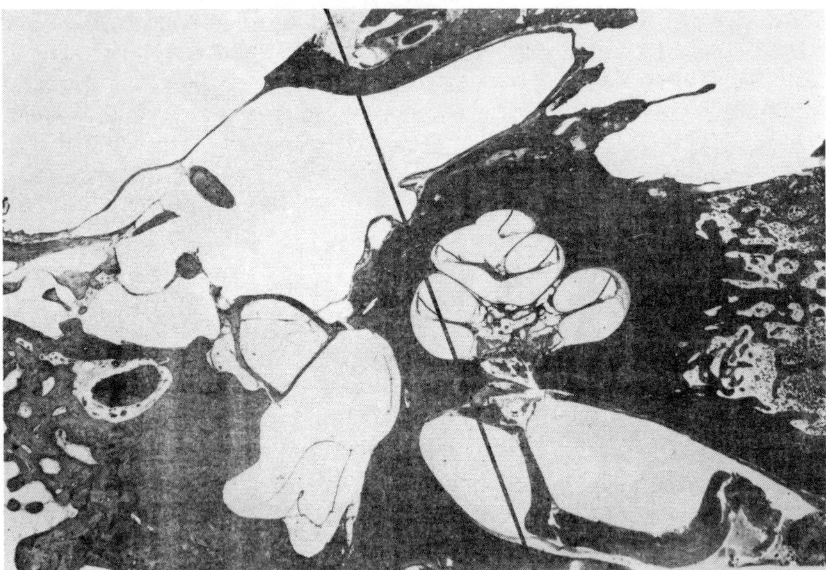

Fig. 12.8. Photomicrograph of horizontal section of a temporal bone. A solid line has been drawn to illustrate the usual pathway of a temporal bone fracture of transverse type. This type of fracture passes through the internal auditory meatus and VII and VIII cranial nerves, into the basal coil of the cochlea laterally and then into the middle ear. (H. & E. × 6.5.) (Reproduced with the permission of Academic Press.)

hair cells of the cochlea, a particularly valuable technique has been the examination of surface preparations of the spiral organ. By this method the exact distribution of hair cell damage can be mapped out easily and correlated with functional studies of sound reception. The effects of blast and gunshot injury are initially on the external hair cells of the basal coil. When this type of trauma is particularly severe, outer hair cells in long stretches of the cochlea may be damaged and the supporting cells in these areas may become disrupted.

Sound wave injury

Sound waves of high intensity can badly damage the cochlea. Again the pathological changes are those of microscopical destruction of hair cells. The earliest changes affect isolated external hair cells. As the intensity of the sound is increased, large groups of external hair cells die and their supporting cells are lost with them. The basal coil is once more the main centre for external hair cell loss. These findings have been obtained mainly in animal experiments but there is a little material from human pathology indicating that the same pattern of injury occurs.

Cytopathology of hair cells in conditions of 'stimulation' deafness

The changes in the inner ear following the trauma of direct blows to the head, of explosive blasts, and of high-intensity sound waves, together produce a condition which may be categorized as 'stimulation' deafness. All seem to be directed particulary to the external hair cells of the basal coil. Internal hair cells and higher cochlear coils may be affected to a greater degree by these insults to the inner ear. Light microscopical studies, whether by examination of stained sections or by surface preparations of osmic acid-fixed cochleae, show little more than loss of stereocilia and necrotic features of the cells, followed by disappearance of the hair cells.

INFLAMMATION

Otitis externa

The term otitis externa implies inflammation of the skin of the external ear. This may be acute or chronic. The acute form ('boil') usually subsides quickly on treatment. The chronic form has a number of possible aetiologies:

Infective
1. *Bacterial—Staphylococci, Staphylococcus aureus, Ps. pyocyaneus B. proteus.*
2. *Fungal—Aspergillus, Monilia.*
3. *Viral*—Herpes zoster and Herpes simplex.

Reactive
1. Eczema.
2. Seborrhoeic dermatitis.
3. Neurodermatitis.

Precipitating and aggravating factors include warm humid climates, sensitization to topical applications, bathing, and local trauma by scratching or unskilled syringing.

Pathological changes are those of chronic inflammation with marked hyperkeratosis of the epidermis of the ear. Blistering of the epidermis is common in the viral infections.

Malignant otitis externa

This is a disease which originates in the external auditory meatus at the junction of the bony and cartilaginous portions. The infective organism is said to be *Pseudomonas aeruginosa* (*Bacillus pyocyaneus*), but there is growing evidence that anaerobic organisms may be causative. The condition is most commonly seen in elderly diabetic patients.

The disease is not a malignant neoplasm in the pathological sense. It presents as granulations in the external auditory canal, which may extend to the tympanic membrane, middle ear, and mastoid air cells causing severe destruction. It may also spread to the parotid gland through the cartilaginous portion of the external auditory meatus. Further extension can involve the VII, VIIII, IX, X, and XII cranial nerves. Intracranial complications can also occur and mortality is high among these patients.

Otitis media

In the middle ear, bacterial infection with resultant inflammation presents its own characteristic pathological changes not only by virtue of the narrowness of the spaces that compose the middle-ear cleft, but also by the possibility of important structures such as the facial nerve, inner ear, lateral sinus, and brain becoming involved. The common form of the disease results from infection by one or more of a wide variety of organisms. In the acute phase Gram-positive organisms such as *Staphylococcus pyogenes*, and *B. haemolytic streptococcus* predominate. In the chronic phase Gram-negative organisms particularly *Proteus* and *Pseudomonas* are found although *Staphylococcus pyogenes* and *B. haemolytic streptococci* are sometimes isolated from the discharging pus of chronically inflamed ears.

The general pathological features of otitis media are those of the inflammatory reaction seen anywhere in the body. In the acute phase tissue is hyperaemic and destruction is rapid; the cellular reaction culminates in the production of numerous polymorphonuclear neutrophils which, discharged into the lumen of the middle ear together with necrotic material and bacteria, are seen as pus. In the chronic phase destruction is slower and fibrosis is frequently seen in reaction to it. Certain other changes particularly cholesteatoma are specific for the middle-ear inflammation, not being found in inflammatory conditions elsewhere in the body. In most cases, although one or more organisms can be isolated by bacterial culture of the aural discharge, the type of inflammatory reaction seen on histological examination of ear tissue is non-specific. On rare occasions the inflammatory reaction suggests a tuberculous origin. A special form of chronic otitis media is recognized known as seromucinous otitis media.

Thus, the following forms of otitis media may be considered: (i) acute suppurative otitis media; (ii) chronic otitis media; (iii) tuberculosis; (iv) seromucinous otitis media.

ACUTE SUPPURATIVE OTITIS MEDIA

The incidence of this condition as seen in hospital practice has declined in the past two decades, mainly because of readily available wide range of antibiotics and also improved socio-economic conditions of the general population in this country. Children are more often affected by this condition than adults.

The route of infection is via the Eustachian tube or as part of a generalized haematogenous spread. The common bacteria involved are Beta haemolytic streptococci, *Diplococcus pneumoniae*, and *Haemophilus influenzae*.

The mucosal lining of the Eustachian tube and middle-ear cleft is oedematous and congested or polypoidal; exudation of serous fluid, which soon becomes purulent, accumulates in the middle ear. The tympanic membrane is initially hyperaemic and then bulges as more pus collects in the middle ear.

As the disease progresses there may be avascular necrosis of the tympanic membrane which eventually perforates with discharge from the ear and relief of pain. The infection frequently also involves the mastoid air cells. The lining of the cells becomes congested and swollen, and pus accumulates. This is followed by osteitis and destruction of the bony partition of the cells. Gradually the pus may track to the surface and present as a sub-periosteal abscess. The infection may extend intra cranially causing meningitis, extradural abscess in middle or post-cranial fossae, or may burst through the mastoid tip and present in the neck (Bezold's abscess), or can cause lateral sinus thrombosis, facial palsy, and acute labyrinthitis.

CHRONIC OTITIS MEDIA

This disease represents one of the commonest infective conditions. The inflammatory process gives rise to serious complications and even mortality. The hearing loss that is a constant concomitant of the disease process also contributes to the immense socio-economic impact.

The histopathological changes of the disease take several forms and may affect any part of the middle-ear cleft. The hallmark of chronic otitis media as contrasted with the acute form is the presence of irreversible pathological changes in the tissue which have been produced by the destructive effects of the inflammation.

Perforation of the tympanic membrane. Some perforations of the tympanic membrane may be caused by trauma; the majority, however, are produced by outward pressure from within the middle ear by the products of inflammation, particularly pus. This leads to ischaemic necrosis of a focal area of the membrane followed by rupture at that point. At the rim of the perforation squamous epithelium usually grows in towards the middle ear and the junction between this epithelium and the columnar epithelium of the middle ear is situated at a variable distance on the middle ear side. Perforations frequently heal. In the process the normal structured arrangement of collagen in the middle layer of the tympanic membrane is lost and is often replaced by a thick unstructured layer of collagen between the middle ear and external auditory meatus epithelia (replacement membrane) (Figs. 12.9 and 12.10).

To the clinician an important sign of the presence of chronic otitis media is a perforation of the tympanic membrane. It comes therefore as a surprise that in a pathological study of 123 temporal bones with chronic otitis media only 19.5 per cent showed such a perforation (Meyerhoff, Kim, and Paparella 1978). Many of the 123 cases were not clinically active (the criteria for the diagnosis being histological ones in the post-mortem specimens). It seems likely that perforation of the ear drum is frequently a concomitant of particularly active otitis media although it should be remembered that mild forms frequently exist in which this structure is intact. Seromucinous otitis media (*vide infra*) would seem to be a form of such a condition with an intact tympanic membrane.

Inflammatory granulation tissue. The most specific feature of the pathology

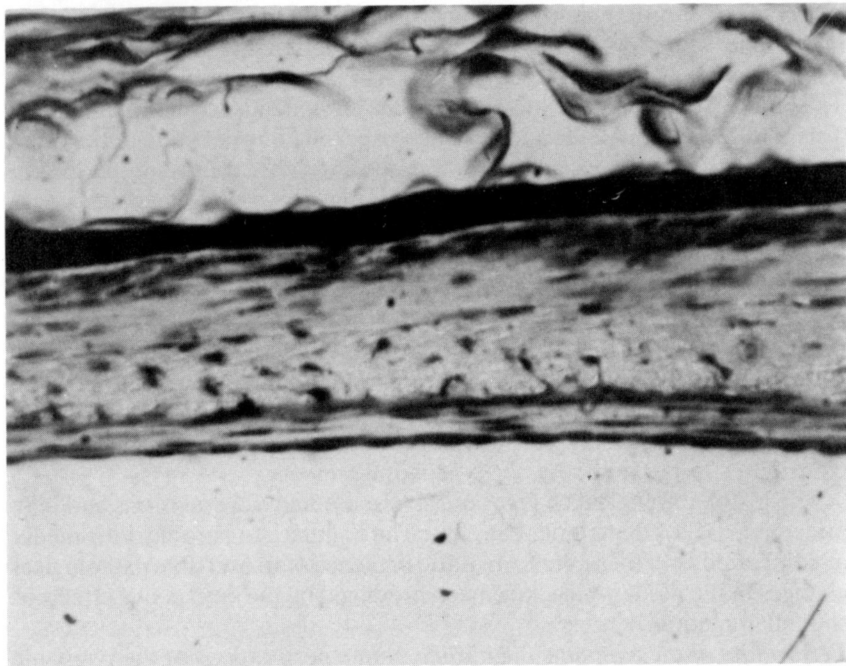

Fig. 12.9. Section of normal tympanic membrane. The ear canal stratified squamous epithelium is uppermost and is covered by a dark thick layer of keratin, external to which are loose lying keratin squames. The flattened epithelium of the middle-ear cavity is below. The layers of connective tissue can be seen between the epithelia. Their fibres run in different directions: the outer one parallel to the epithelium and the inner one at right angles to the epithelium. (H. & E. × 400.)

of chronic otitis media is the presence of inflammatory granulation tissue. This cellular reaction has two components. On the one hand there is the presence of leucocytes characteristic of chronic inflammation, i.e. lymphocytes, plasma cells, and histiocytes. The latter cells are characterized by their phagocytic propensity, continuing the work of polymorphonuclear neutrophils that has taken place early in the infection of taking up and destroying bacteria and also clearing up debris produced by the destructive effects of the inflammation. On the other hand there is granulation tissue, a specific combination of newly formed capillaries and fibroblasts. Granulation tissue represents an early stage of healing following inflammatory destruction of tissue. Either the chronic inflammatory leucocytes or the granulation tissue may be found in the middle ear in chronic otitis media independently of the other. The two forms of cellular reaction are seen together as the characteristic inflammatory granulation tissue of an aural polyp. This is usually a smooth protrusion of firm grey, vascular tissue that emanates from thickened mucosa on the medial wall of the middle ear in chronic otitis media. It pushes through a large perforation of the tympanic membrane and usually occludes the lumen of the external auditory meatus

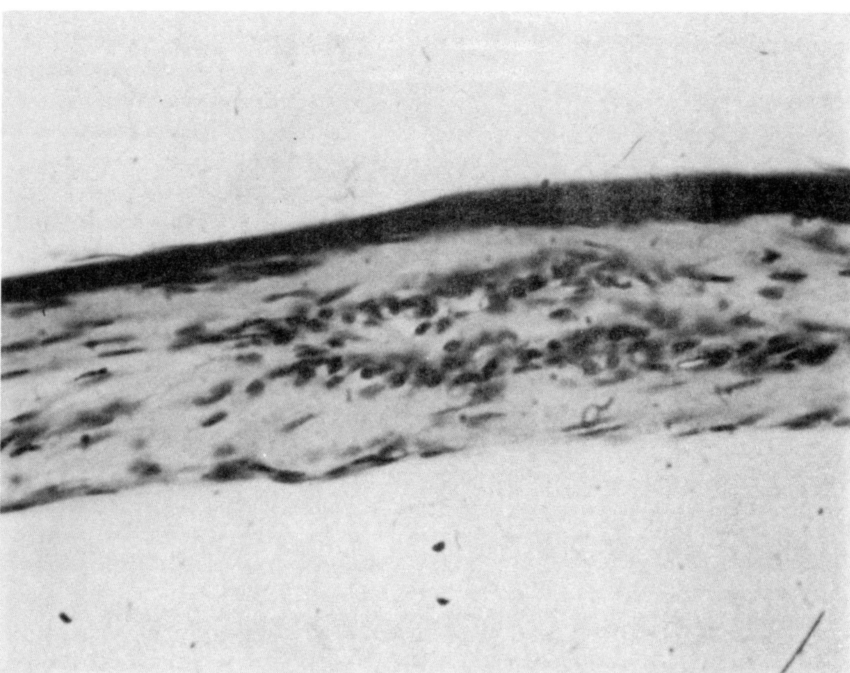

Fig. 12.10. Sections of tympanic membrane from a patient with chronic otitis media and a history of previous perforation. The epithelia are intact and are oriented in the photomicrograph similar to Fig. 12.9. There is no structured connective tissue between the epithelia but irregular vascular connective tissue is present. This is a manifestation of previous perforation of the tympanic membrane with healing (replacement membrane). (H. & E. × 400.)

where it is removed by the clinician by snaring. Histologically the aural polyp is covered by middle-ear epithelium, usually columnar, frequently ciliated. Sometimes squamous epithelium covers the surface, representing metaplasia incurred in the middle ear or by irritation of the surface of the polyp when it has reached the ear canal. The substance of the polyp is made up by chronic inflammatory granulation tissue. Chronic inflammatory granulation tissue is also found very frequently in chronic otitis media in the epitympanum, the round window niche, the oval window niche, and in the mastoid.

There is evidence that it is the chronic inflammatory granulation tissue which is largely responsible for the destructive effects of chronic otitis media. Collagenase is an enzyme which has been located in such tissue and is active in destroying collagen containing material particularly bone.

Bone changes. Histopathological study of temporal bones in cases of chronic otitis media shows bone changes of varying degree in all cases. These changes are produced mainly by the inflammatory reaction to infection. Some bone erosion may be caused by certain Gram-negative organisms; the endotoxins produced by such organisms are known to produce bone absorp-

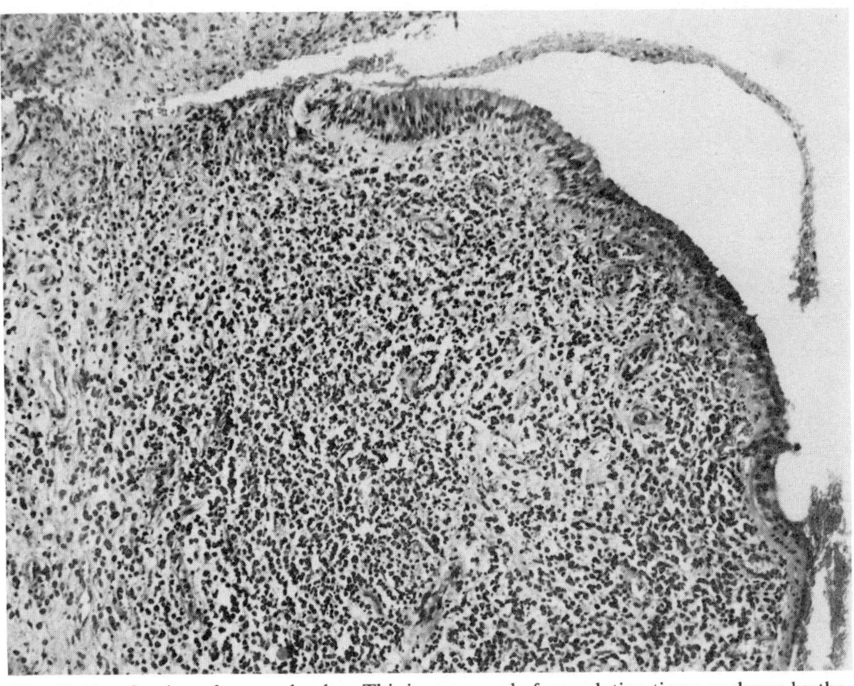

Fig. 12.11. Section of an aural polyp. This is composed of granulation tissue as shown by the capillaries and loose connective tissue. There is also an intense chronic inflammatory cellular exudate. Most of the cells are plasma cells. There are some lymphocytes. An epithelial covering of columner epithelium in which cilia are visible in the upper part of the field indicates a middle ear origin for this polyp. Squamous metaplasia is seen at the lower right corner. (H. & E. × 100.)

tion under certain conditions. The ossicles are most frequently involved. The incus particularly in the attic region is frequently severely eroded in inflammation as is the stapes and, less frequently the malleus. Thin bony partitions covering the mastoid air cells are usually inflamed and a characteristic reaction here is the development of new bone in the form of trabeculae of woven bone in reaction to the inflammatory irritant (Fig. 12.13). Inflammation with erosion of the periosteal layer of the lateral semicircular canal and of the bone covering the facial nerve are clinically important forms of osteitis which are also encountered.

When pathological studies are carried out on post-mortem temporal bones with chronic otitis media large surgically produced cavities are some-

Fig. 12.12. Section of an aural polyp. This polyp is rather more fibrous than the one seen in Fig. 12.11. and shows foci of foreign-body type giant cell in reaction to keratin squames. (H. & E. × 100.)

Fig. 12.13. Section of mastoid bone from a case of chronic otitis media. The mastoid air cells are filled with connective tissue which greatly narrows the air spaces which contain proteinaceous exudate. There has been considerable new bone formation in the walls of the air spaces as shown by the closely packed cement lines near their surfaces. (H. & E. × 25.)

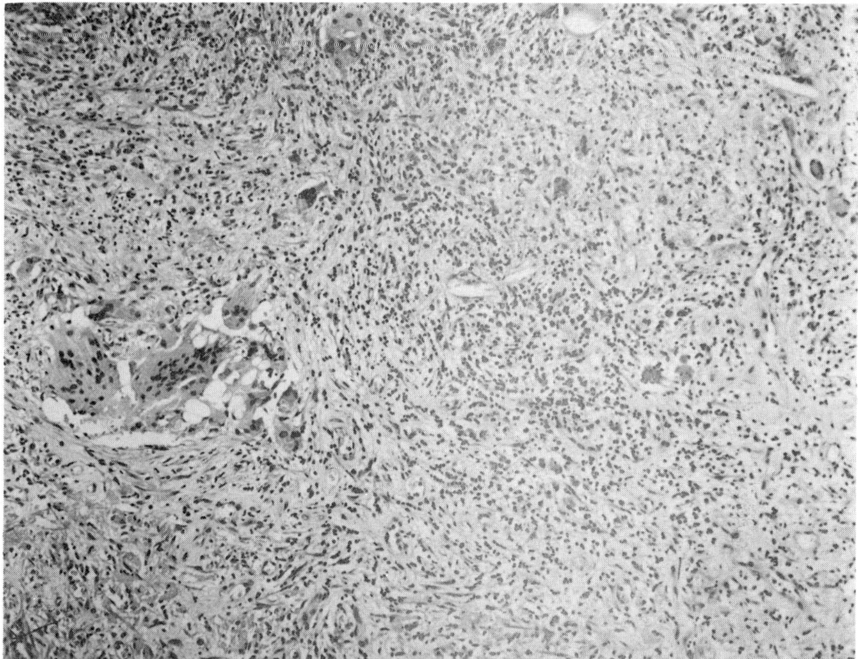

Fig. 12.12.

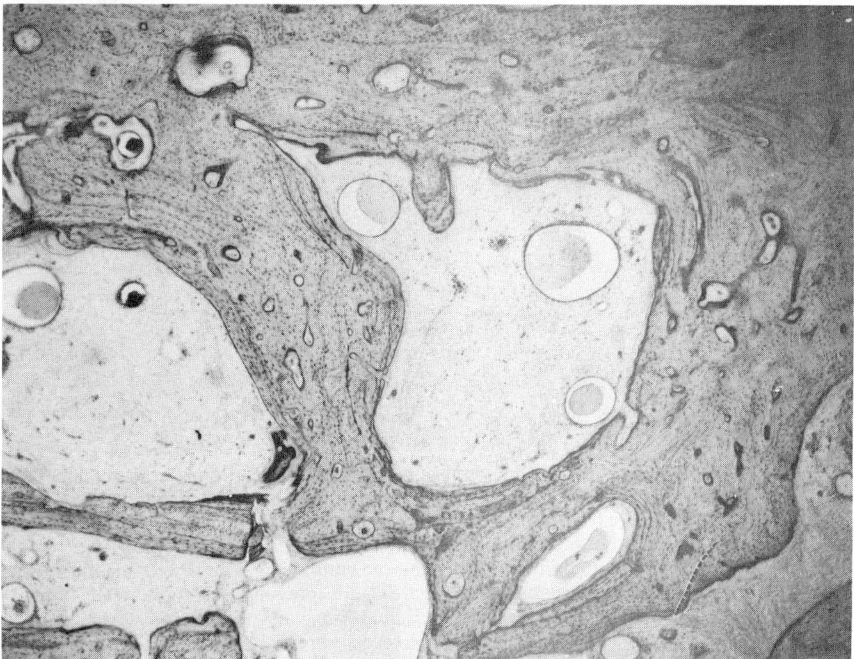

Fig. 12.13.

times found in the mastoid bones. These operations to drain the infected middle-ear cleft may or may not be accompanied by evidence of surgical procedures on the ossicles, depending on the severity of the 'clearance' of the middle ear used by the surgeon.

Glandular changes. The middle-ear cleft is normally lined by a single layer of cubical or columnar epithelium which may bear cilia. In chronic otitis media the epithelium frequently develops, as a result of the inflammatory irritation, glandular acini which are connected to the surface by small ducts. These small glands usually secrete mucus which may be found in their lumina. The secretion is an important component of the ear discharge in chronic otitis media. Glandular changes may be found in the mucosa lining the mastoid air cells as well as in the main middle-ear cavity (Figs. 12.14–12.16).

Haemorrhage and cholesterol granuloma. The granulation tissue so frequent

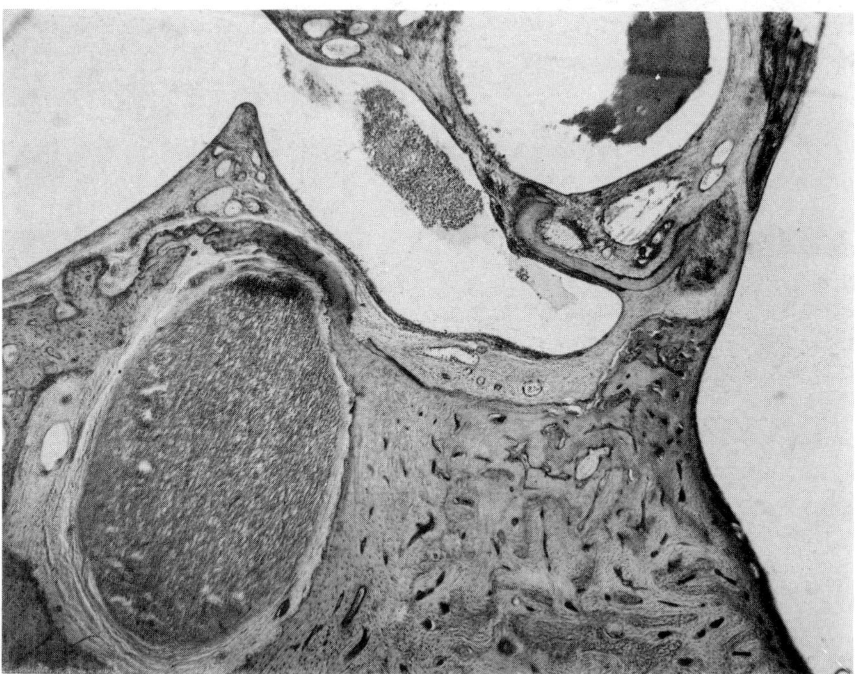

Fig. 12.14. Horizontal section of temporal bone from a case of chronic otitis media. The middle-ear mucosa over the facial nerve is lifted by the accumulation of glands and there are further glands in an adhesion traversing the middle ear adjacent to it. Pus cells are present in the middle-ear cavity. (H. & E. × 25.)

Fig. 12.15. Section of mastoid from a case of chronic otitis media. The air cells are filled with fibrous connective tissue and there are glands containing secretion. Newly formed bone is seen at the edges. (H. & E. × 100.)

Fig. 12.16. Section of middle ear mucosa from a case of chronic otitis media. Glands containing secretion are seen on the left. An area of cholesteatoma (hyperkeratotic squamous epithelium) is seen on the right. (H. & E. × 100.)

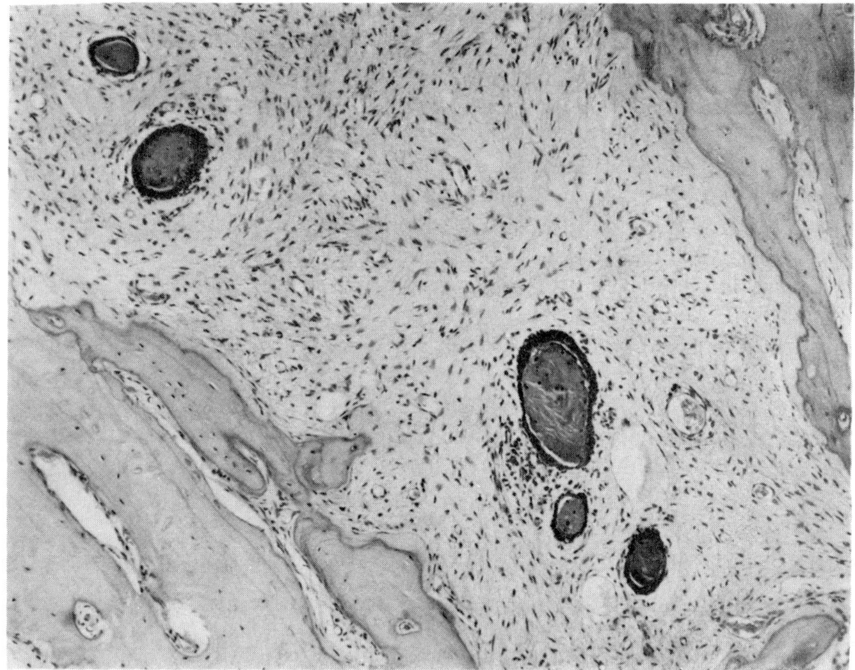

Fig. 12.15.

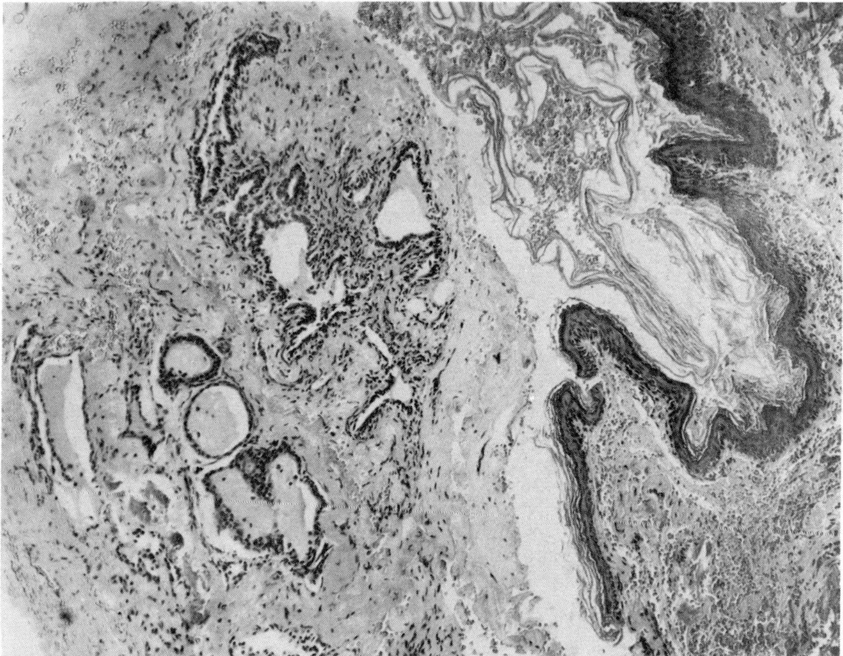

Fig. 12.16.

in chronic otitis media, being largely composed of thin-walled blood vessels, is a potent source of haemorrhage. Such haemorrhages are found in the mucosa of the middle ear in chronic otitis media.

Yellowish nodules of tissue are also found which are microscopically composed of cholesterol cyrstals (dissolved away to leave empty clefts in paraffin embedded histological sections) surrounded by foreign-body type giant cells and chronic inflammatory cells. Such cholesterol granulomas are almost always found in the midst of haemorrhage in the middle-ear mucosa and it seems likely that haemorrhage is causally related to the granuloma. It is possible that the cholesterol is derived from the lipid envelopes of red cells which, in the conditions of poor lymphatic drainage of the middle ear, are absorbed into the lymphatic stream with greater difficulty than the other more soluble contents of the red cells (Fig. 12.17).

Fibrosis. Areas of fibrosis are frequently seen in temporal bone sections of cases of chronic otitis media. This change represents the end result of healing following destruction of tissue wrought by the inflammatory pro-

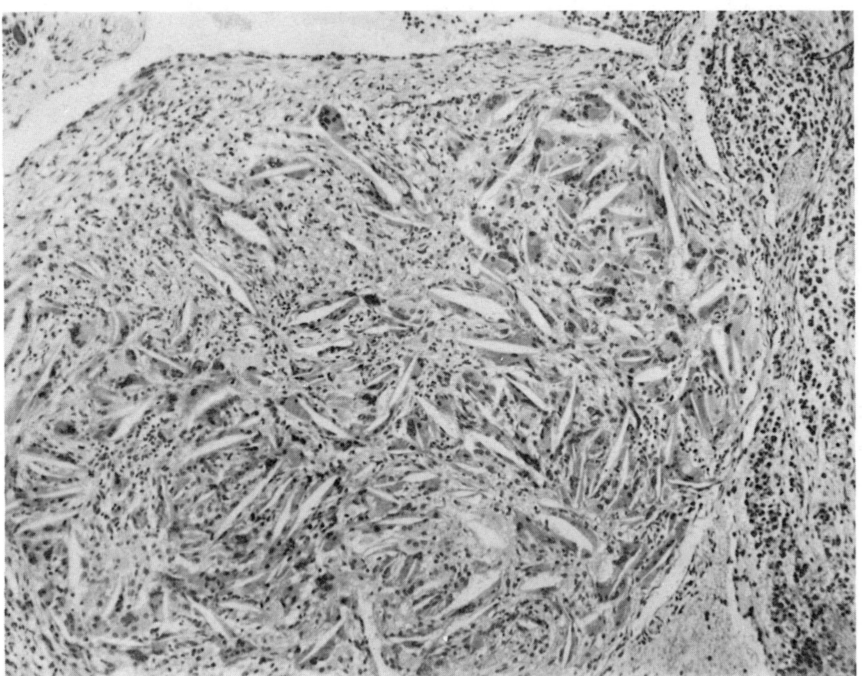

Fig. 12.17. Section of cholesterol granuloma from case of chronic otitis media. The needle-like spaces represent crystals of cholesterol esters which have been dissolved out in processing. These are surrounded by foreign-body type giant and inflammatory tissue. Red cells may be seen at the bottom right-hand corner and within the inflammatory tissue. The granuloma is situated in the mucosa of the middle ear and the cubical middle-ear epithelium extends across the top of the photograph. (H. & E. × 100.)

cess. Ankylosis of the malleus to the incus or the incus to the stapes may be present by fibrous connections.

Tympanosclerosis. A special form of fibrosis is often encountered in chronic otitis media known as tympanosclerosis. Deposits of this dense white tissue are seen in the middle-ear mucosa not only on the tympanic side of the ear drum but also on the ossicles, particularly the crura of the stapes, within the tympanic cavity and sometimes in the mastoid air cavity. Microscopically the material is composed of hyaline collagen with only an occasional fibroblast. Deposits of calcium salts impregnate this collagenous tissue (Figs. 12.18 and 12.19).

Cholesteatoma. Cholesteatoma is an important concomitant in from one-third to one-half of cases with chronic otitis media. It is composed of soft friable material witha pearly grey sheen or a yellowish coloration. Frequently a pale capsule is present, representing the immature squamous epithelium at the periphery. Cholesteatoma is frequently located in the upper part of the middle-ear cleft and discharges through a perforation of the pars flaccida portion of the tympanic membrane. The cholesteatoma may extend through the aditus into the mastoid antrum and mastoid air cells. It appears to conform in shape to normal structures, such as ossicles,

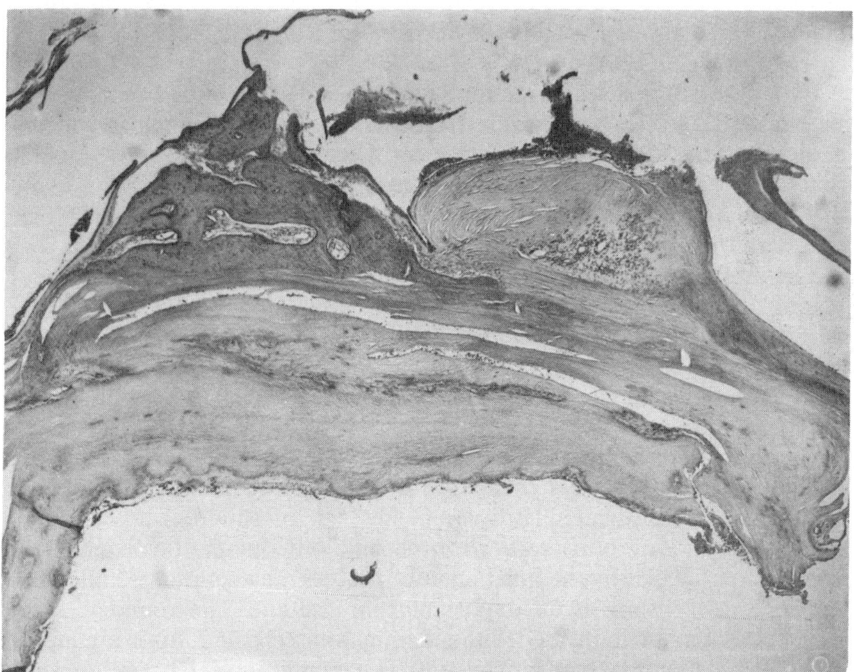

Fig. 12.18. Section of tympanosclerotic plaque from a case of chronic otitis media. The plaque is composed of hyaline collagen with area of darker staining representing deposits of calcium salts. There is also bone formation on the upper left. (H. & E. × 25.)

that it is in contact with. Frequently such ossicles are eroded, but other bony structures are rarely involved. Occasionally cholesteatoma is said to invade the bone of the facial nerve area or the area of the lateral semicircular canal, and very rarely it is said to erode the tegmen and burrow into the brain. It is impossible in these cases to dissociate these invasive properties from the above mentioned effects of chronic otitis media with which cholesteatoma is always associated.

In some cases of cholesteatoma the tympanic membrane is intact and the cholesteatoma forms an epidermoid cyst-like structure in the middle-ear cavity. Such cases are designated as 'congenital' cholesteatoma, but whether their origin is on a different basis from the more usual 'acquired' cholesteatoma is conjectural.

Under the microscope the pearly material consists of dead, fully differentiated keratin squames representing the corneal layer of the cholesteatoma. Sometimes biopsy material shows only such squames when the so-called capsule has not been removed. The capsule is composed of a fully differentiated stratified squamous epithelium similar to the epidermis of skin and resting on connective tissue. There is a basal layer of small cubical cells above which is a spinal or malpighian layer composed of five or six rows of cells in which intercellular 'prickles' or spines are present. A thin granular layer in which the cells display prominent cytoplasmic keratohyaline granules separates the malpighian layer from the corneal layer which is very extensive (Fig. 12.20).

Resorption of ossicles is frequently seen in cholesteatoma. In some cases the eroded ossicles are covered by the squamous epithelium of the cholesteatoma. Under the circumstances there is always a layer of granulation tissue between the squamous epithelium and the bone. It seems likely that it is the chronic inflammatory change, not the epithelium covering, that produces the erosion (Figs. 12.21 and 12.22).

The origin of cholesteatoma is doubtful. There is a widespread concept among otolaryngologists that the squamous epithelium of cholesteatoma is derived by migration from the external surface of the tympanic membrane. Such a migration is a unique one in non-neoplastic squamous epithelium. A more pathologically acceptable concept would be squamous metaplasia of the middle-ear mucosa.

Complications of chronic otitis media. The inflammatory process may extend from the middle ear to involve adjacent structures of the nervous system. As a result meningitis, brain abscess, or subdural abscess may result. In temporal bone sections of chronic otitis media involvement of inner ear structures by the inflammatory process may be found. Inflammation of the labyrinth is an important complication. The round window membrane may be infiltrated with inflammatory cells and this is an important route for labyrinthine inovlement. The membranous labyrinth in such cases may be distended with serous fluid or the fluid may be purulent (Fig. 12.23). In long standing cases of labyrinthitis the cochlea and vestibule may be partially replaced by new bone.

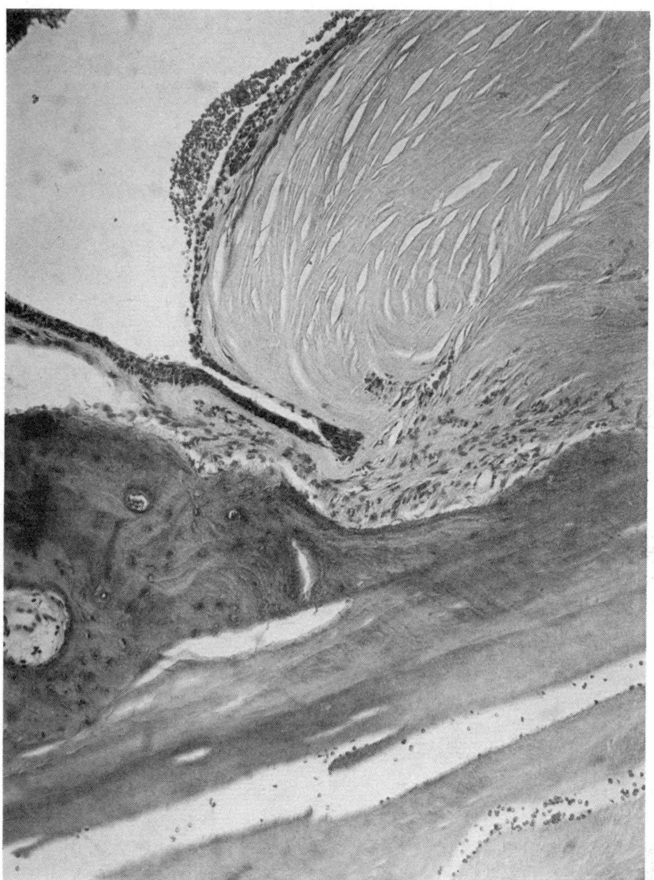

Fig. 12.19. Higher powered view of portion of Fig. 12.18. showing hyaline collagen, calcified areas and bone formation. (H. & E. × 100.)

Tuberculous otitis media. An unusual form of chronic otitis media, this condition is usually associated with pulmonary tuberculosis.

In the initial stages there are multiple perforations of the tympanic membrane. The granulations in the middle ear are pale and profuse and complications, especially facial palsy, are more frequent than in the commoner form of chronic otitis media.

Culture of middle-ear tissue may produce tubercle bacilli. Histological examination shows tuberculoid granulation tissue composed of epithelioid cells, Langhans giant cells, and caseation situated in the middle-ear mucosa. There is much destruction of bone (Fig. 12. 24).

SECRETORY OTITIS MEDIA OR 'GLUE EAR'

The condition is characterized by 'glue'-like fluid in the middle-ear cleft causing a conductive hearing loss of mild to moderate severity which is

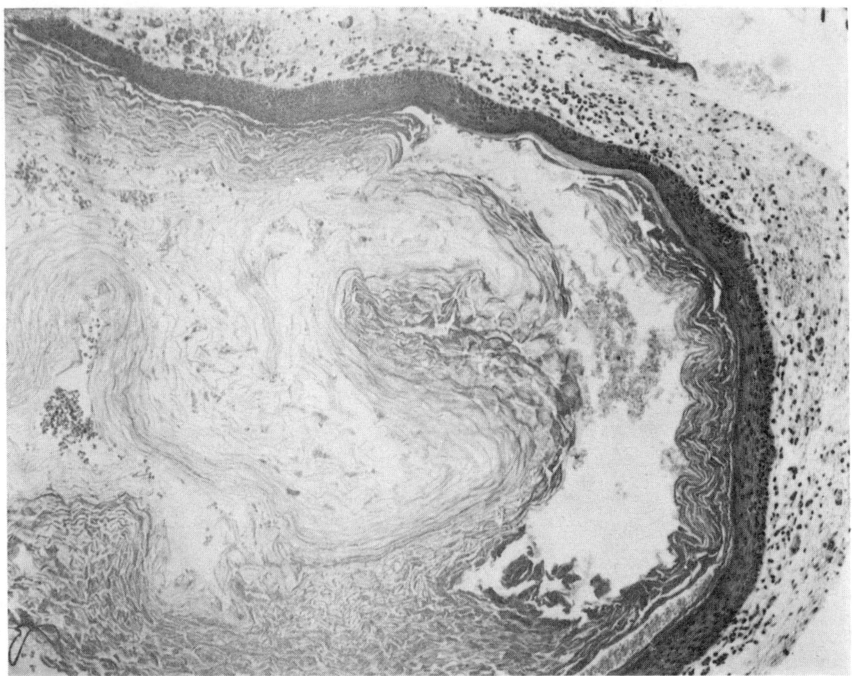

Fig. 12.20. Cholesteatoma sac. The wall of the sac is composed of stratified squamous epithelium with a well-marked stratum granulosum. The sac is filled with the products of the squamous epithelium, i.e. keratin squames. Deep to the basal layer of the epithelium there is a chronic inflammatory reaction. (H. & E. × 100.)

often fluctuant. It is the commonest cause of hearing loss in children between the age of three to eight years. It can also occur in adults. About 60 per cent of ear, nose, and throat hospital admissions in this age group in the United Kingdom are due to secretory otitis media.

There is thought to be a dysfunction of the Eustachian tube in this condition causing absorption of air in the middle-ear cleft and transudation of fluid from the blood vessels of the middle-ear mucosa. In the early stages this may be serous and later, due to glandular activity of the mucosal lining around the Eustachian tube, the fluid is seromucinous. It is sterile on bacterial and viral culture.

The aetiology of Eustachian tube dysfunction is debatable. Large adenoids and allergy-associated sinus infection are possible contributing factors.

If spontaneous resolution does not take place and no therapy is instituted, sequelae such as an atrophic tympanic membrane, retraction pockets, and adhesive otitis media can occur.

The pathological changes in serous otitis media have not been adequately investigated in temporal bone material. A few cases that have been studied

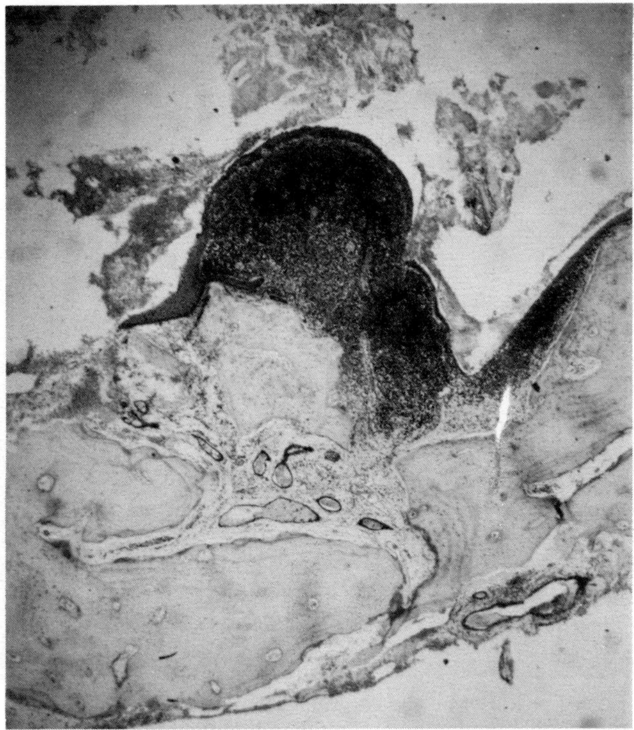

Fig. 12.21. Area of bone destruction of middle ear ossicle in chronic otitis media with cholesteatoma. The squamous epithelium of the cholesteatoma is separated from the eroded bone by a thick layer of chronic inflammatory tissue. Note the presence of glands and chronic inflammatory tissue within the eroded bone. (H. & E. × 25.)

have shown extensive cholesterol granuloma in the middle-ear mucosa. This is related to the intramucosal haemorrhage that is a feature of the disease. The middle-ear cleft contains an eosinophilic fluid with degenerated epithelial cells or foamy histiocytes and may be lined by cubical or columnar epithelial cells.

NEOPLASMS OF THE EAR

Primary neoplasms

A wide variety of neoplasms occurs primarily in the ear. Their type and effects are related particularly to their site of origin so that the different parts of the ear will each be considered in turn in describing the pathology of primary neoplastic diseases.

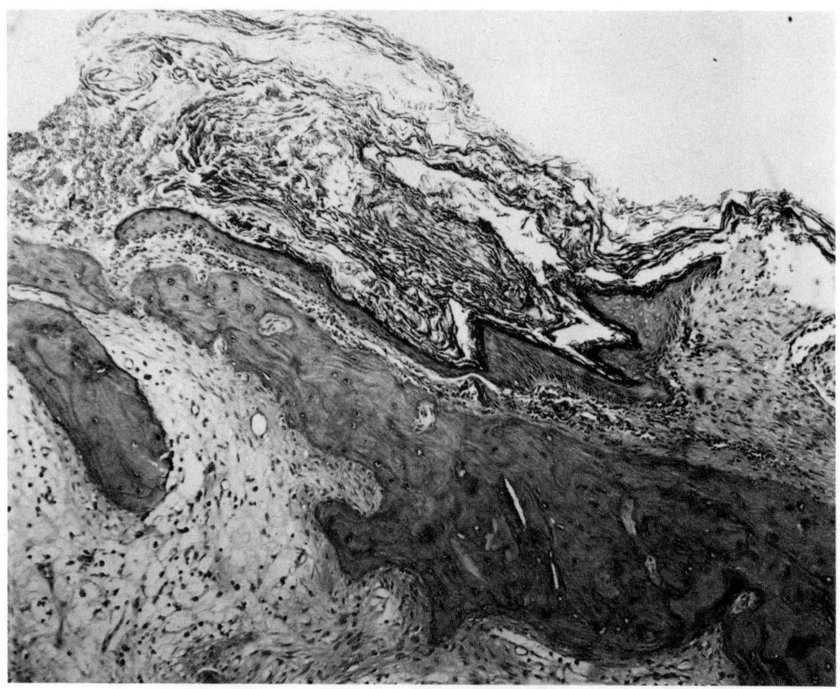

Fig. 12.22. Eroded ossicle of middle ear with cholesteatoma. The bone is infiltrated by chronic inflammatory tissue and although covered by a layer of cholesteatoma, i.e. hyperkeratotic stratified squamous epithelium, a thin layer of chronic inflammatory tissue can be seen between the cholesteatoma and the bone. (H. & E. × 100.)

EXTERNAL EAR—PINNA

The pinna is a specialized area of skin so that its neoplasms are those found in other parts of the skin. A wide variety of benign neoplasms presents in the pinna. In particular haemangioma (cavernous or capillary type) and verruca senilis are commonly seen. The malignant tumours are basal cell carcinoma, squamous carcinoma, and malignant melanoma. The features of all of these tumours are identical to those seen elsewhere.

EXTERNAL EAR—EXTERNAL AUDITORY MEATUS

Again this is a specialized area of skin. All of the above tumours may be found here too, except that the basal cell carcinoma, which is usually related to excessive sunlight, is very rare in the ear canal.

The external auditory meatus is distinguished from the rest of the external ear in its possession of wax-secreting ceruminous glands in the dermal layer. These specialized glands produce their own particular form of tumour—the *ceruminoma.* The normal ceruminal glands are apocrine glands. These glands consists of two layers, an inner layer which produces cerumen by a characteristic 'apocrine' method of pinching off part of the cytoplasm of the

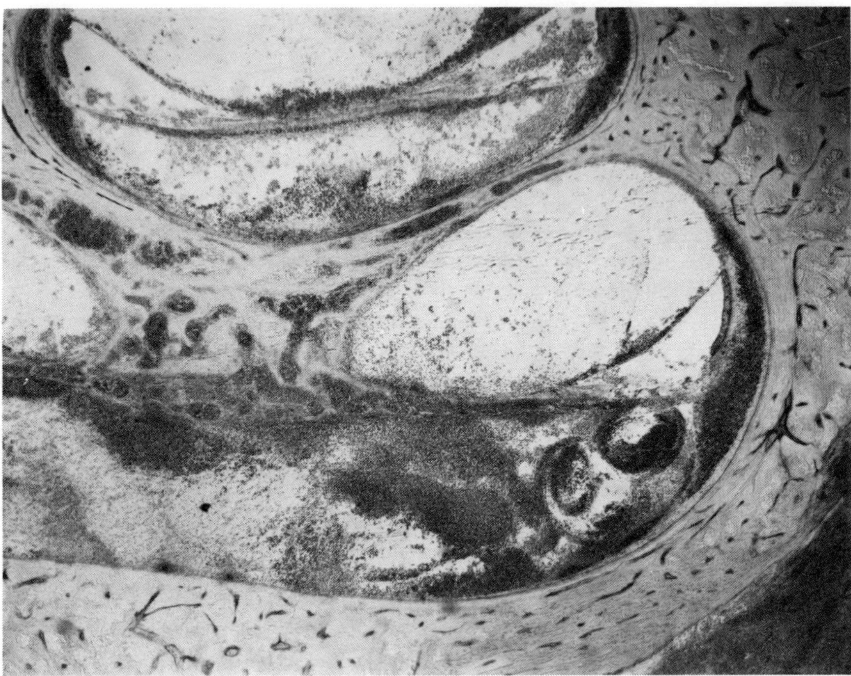

Fig. 12.23. Cochlea in horizontal section of temporal bone in case of acute suppurative labyrinthitis. There is an intense infiltration of polymorphonuclear leucocytes with destruction of cochlear tissue. (H. & E. × 25.)

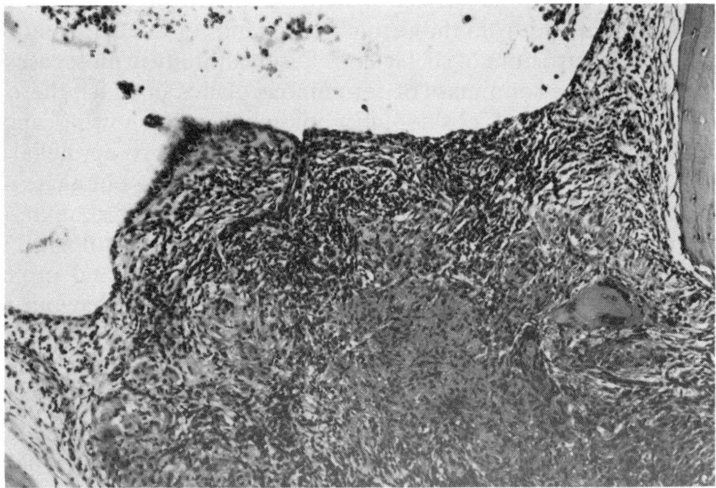

Fig. 12.24. Section of wall of mastoid air cell from a case of tuberculous otitis media. The air cell mucosa is thickened by tuberculous granulation tissue comprising epithelioid cells, occasional Langhans type giant cells and lymphocytes. Acid-fast bacilli were found in this inflammatory tissue on special staining. (H. & E. × 100.)

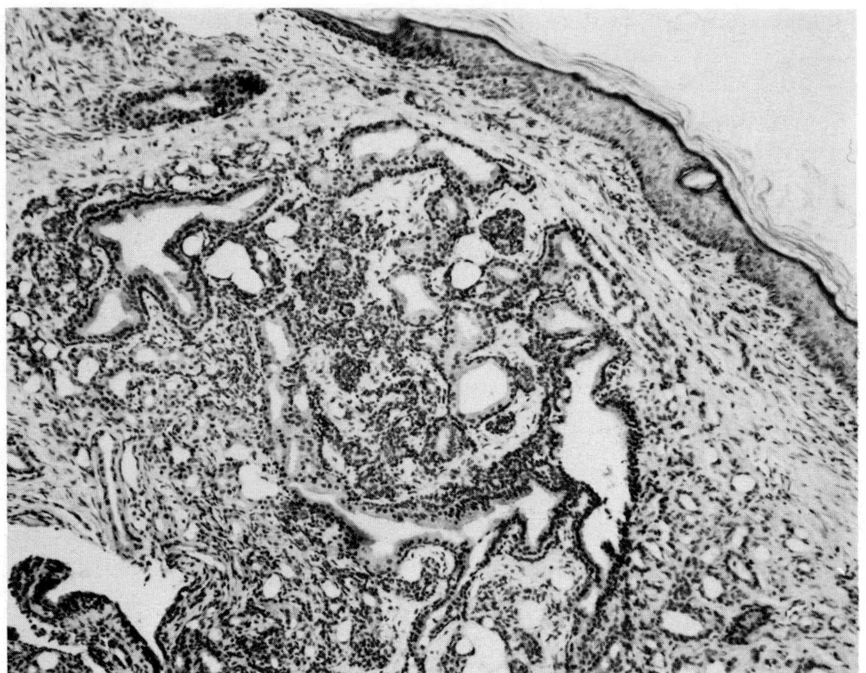

Fig. 12.25. Section of ceruminoma showing a collection of glands of apocrine type beneath the squamous epithelium of the external auditory meatus. (H. & E. × 100.)

cells bordering the glands, and an outer myo-epithelial layer. A duct conveys secretion through the surface squamous epithelium of the ear canal. The neoplasm derived from the ceruminous glands of the ear canal reproduces the normal structure of such glands fairly faithfully in most cases. The tumour consists of a solid mass of ceruminous glands in which there is an inner glandular layer of eosinophilic epithelial cells showing apocrine pinching-off of cytoplasmic fragments and an outer myo-epithelial layer (Figs. 12.25 and 12.26). Such tumours are slowly growing but have a tendency to recurrence if not adequately excised. Metastases are unknown.

Sometimes glandular tumours of the ear canal have a histological structure resembling the pleomorphic adenoma of salivary gland or 'mixed tumours'. Such neoplasms have a similar type of growth behaviour to the more usual ceruminomas (Fig. 12.27).

On rare occasions a glandular tumour of the external auditory meatus may have a histological appearance of *adenocystic carcinoma*, similar to this

Fig. 12.26. Glands from ceruminoma showing peg-like projections from inner surfaces of cells and flattened myoepithelial cells forming an outer layer around duct cells. (H. & E. × 250.)

Fig. 12.27. Neoplasm of ear canal with some resemblance to pleomorphic adenoma of salivary gland. The neoplasm is situated beneath the squamous epithelium of the external auditory meatus. It is composed of both glandualr structures and mesenchymal area. (H. & E. × 25.)

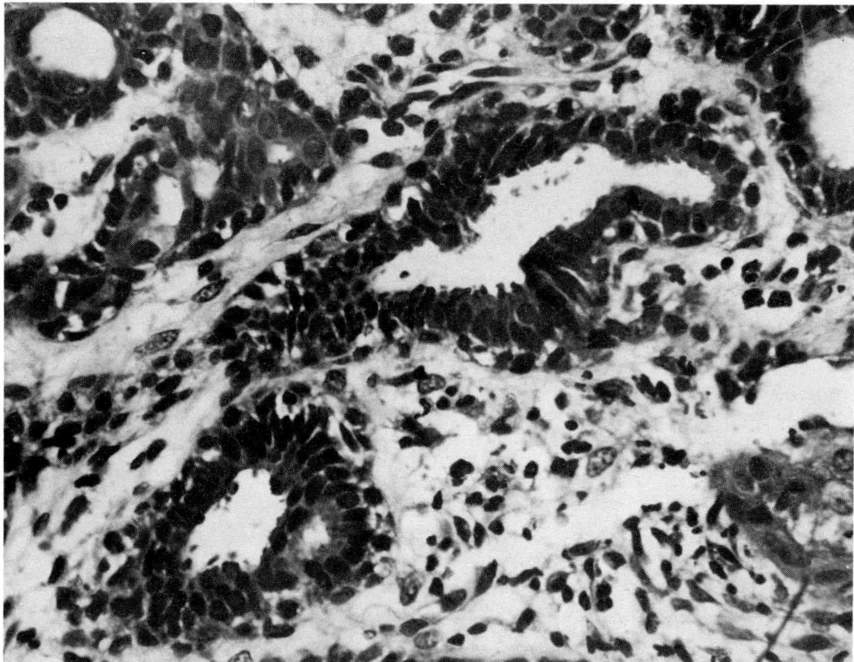

Fig. 12.26.

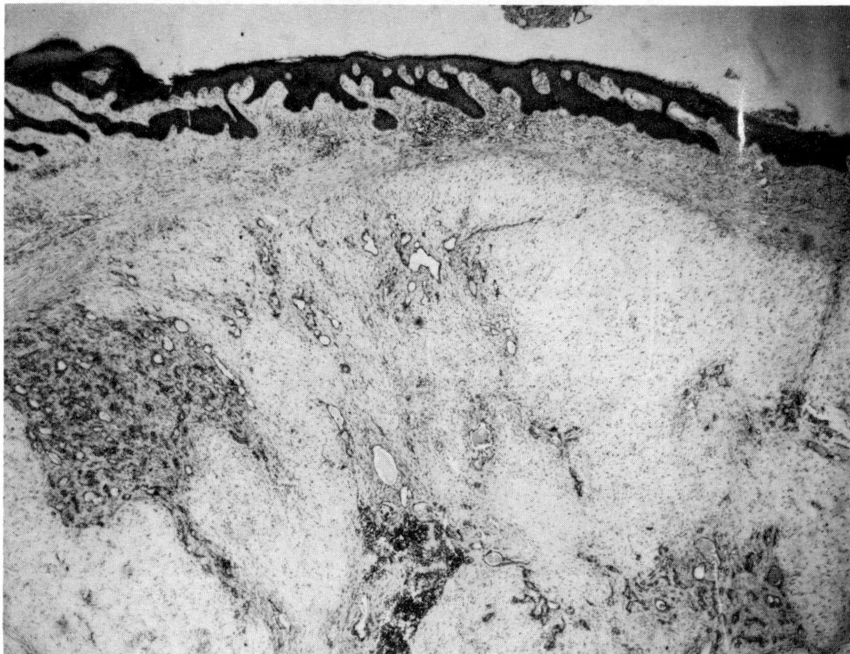

Fig. 12.27.

malignant neoplasm found in salivary glands and in the upper respiratory tract (Fig. 12.28). The behaviour of such a tumour is similar to that of adenocystic carcinomas found elsewhere, i.e. the tendency to produce metastases to the lung often after an interval of many years.

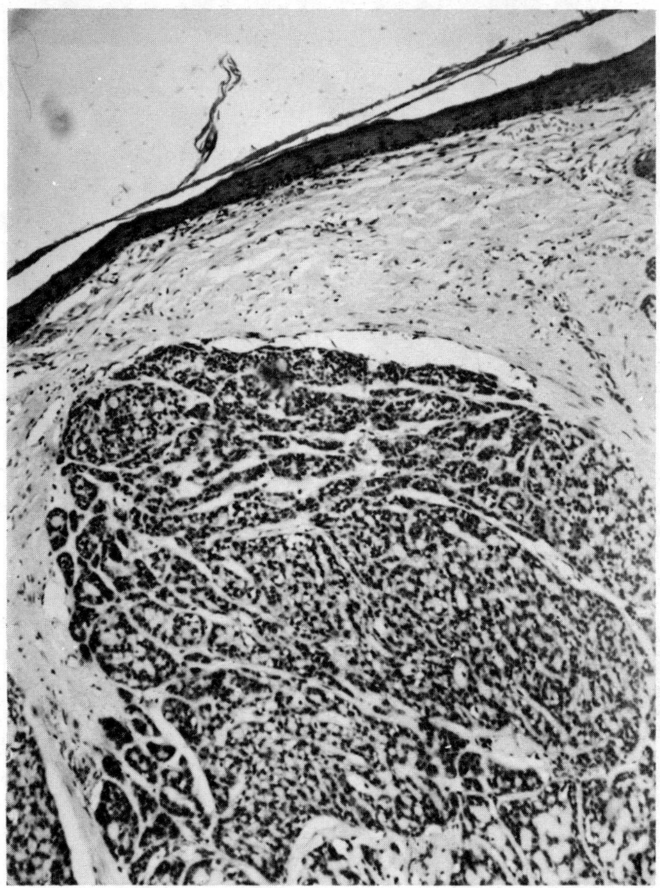

Fig. 12.28. Primary adenocystic carcinoma of the external auditory meatus. The tumour, situated beneath the squamous epithelium of the ear canal, shows a cribriform pattern of small darkly staining cells with intervening hyalinization in some areas. (H. & E. × 400.)

TEMPORAL BONE

Primary neoplasms arising in the temporal bone itself are found from time to time presenting usually in the ear canal or middle ear.

Osteoma of the ear canal is usually a spherical hard mass arising deeply from the bony portion of the external auditory meatus. It is composed of hard, compact bone covered by the normal squamous epithelium of the ear canal. Exposure to cold water is said to be a factor in its origin.

Fibrous dysplasia may be a solitary lesion, usually in the bone of the ear canal or may be a temporal bone manifestation of multi-osseous deposits. The deposit is composed of primitive osteoid and woven bone associated closely with cellular fibrous tissue. The lesion often does not progress and is likely to settle down after the neoplastic tissue has been curetted out surgically.

Histiocytosis X is a group term applied to the three conditions of eosinophilic granuloma, Hand–Schüller–Christian disease, and Letterer–Siwe's disease. The first two conditions are particularly liable to affect the temporal bone and present as a tumour mass in the external or middle ear. Letterer–Siwe's disease usually has a rapid and fulminating course particularly affecting lymph nodes so that it is the other two conditions which involve the ear. The histological appearance of eosinophilic granuloma and Hand–Schüller–Christian disease is similar. Eosinophil granuloma produces a single nodule and is found in older people. Hand–Schüller–Christian disease is characterized by multiple foci, particularly in the skull. It is a more serious condition that occurs in children and young people. Histologically the eroded area of bone shows histiocytic cells, often with a foamy cytoplasm occasional giant cells and numerous eosinophils. Neutrophils may be frequent (Fig. 12.29).

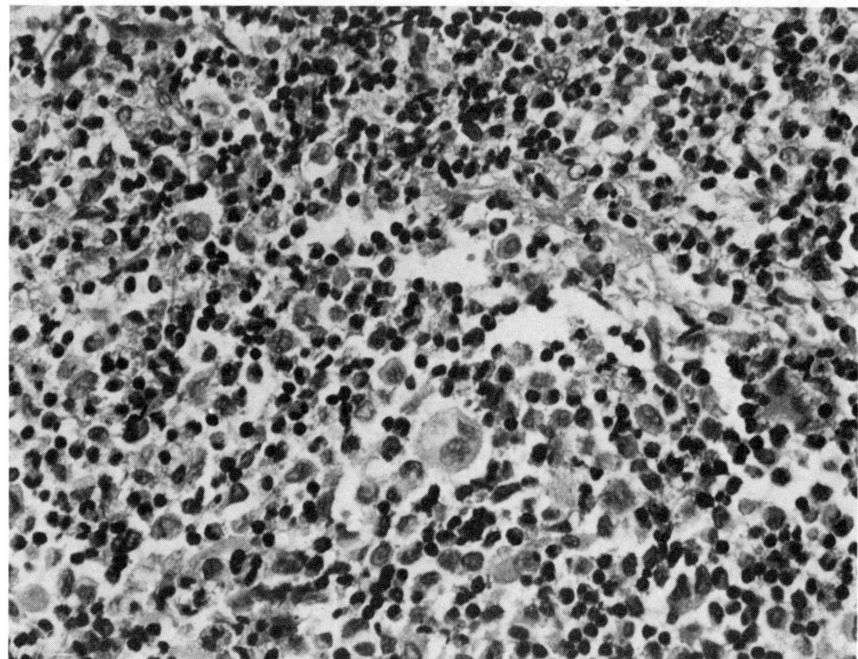

Fig. 12.29. Eosinophilic granuloma of the temporal bone. The cells of the infiltrating lesion are composed of foamy histiocytes with occasional giant cells. Numerous eosinophils are present among these cells, but are not easy to recognize in a black and white photograph. (H. & E. × 400.)

The malignant tumours of bone—*chondrosarcoma* and *osteosarcoma* rarely affect the temporal bone. Their pathological appearances and growth behaviour are similar to tumours of the same histological type found elsewhere.

MIDDLE EAR

A benign tumour of the middle ear has been described—the adenoma—which reproduces the glands formed in the middle-ear mucosa in chronic otitis media. Such a tumour is found only in the middle-ear mucosa and does not invade underlying structures such as bone and the facial nerve. Histologically it is composed of delicate gland structures forming a single layer on a thin reticular framework (Fig. 12.30).

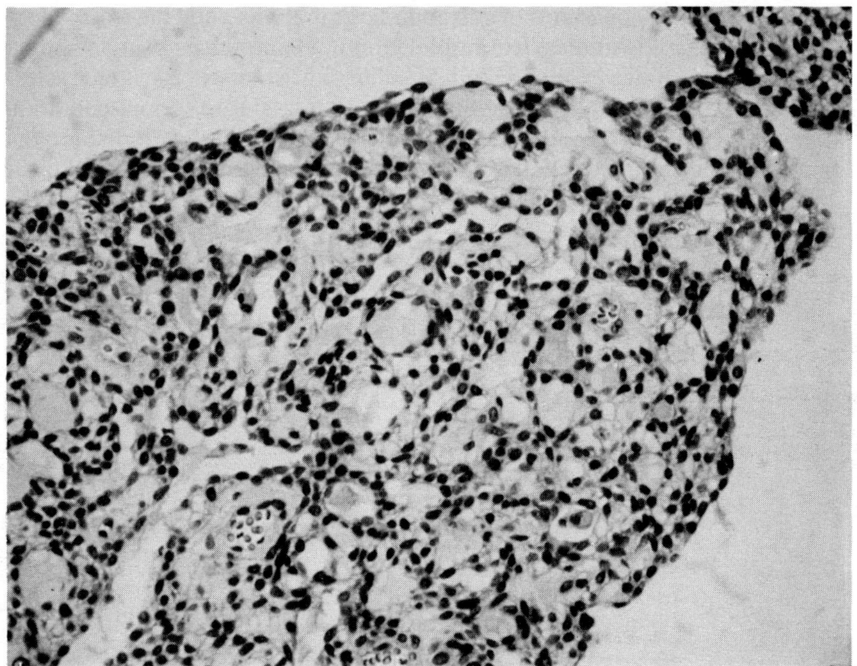

Fig. 12.30. Adenoma of the middle ear composed of glands lined by a single layer of uniform epithelial cells. (H. & E. × 250.)

Meningiomas are tumours that usually form intracerebral masses. They arise from fibrolastic cells in the arachnoid villi, which are protrusions of the arachnoid membrane into the venous sinuses. The function of these arachnoid villi is to enable the absorption of cerebrospinal fluid into the bloodstream. Arachnoid villi may be found in parts of the temporal bone including the middle ear and on occasion, meningiomas may arise from these structures as primary neoplasms of the temporal bone, particularly the middle ear. The histological appearances are those of a tumour with a whorled arrangement of cells: *meningiotheliomatous* if the tumour cells appear epithelioid, *psammomatous* if calcification of the whorled masses is prominent and *fibroblastic* if the tumour cells resemble fibroblasts. The meningioma is a slowly growing tumour of the temporal bone which is usually kept under control by careful local resection.

Paragangliomas or glomus body tumours are important neoplasms that represent a serious problem of treatment in otology. They arise from groups of cells known as paraganglionic or glomus bodies which are normally found in (i) in the jugular bulb region and (ii) in the mucosa of the middle ear over the promontory (Fig. 12.31). In these sites the glomus bodies are in relation to branches of the IX and X cranial nerves and on special staining are found to contain numerous ramifications of nerve fibres. The bodies consist of groups of epithelioid cells forming 'cell-balls' separated by blood vessels. The function of these glomus bodies is not known, but their structure is similar to that of the carotid body which serves as a chemoreceptor structure, i.e. changes in the blood relating to oxygen pressure or pH affect the cells and initiate impulses in the supplying nerves to affect reflexes in the brainstem producing alterations in respiration and cardiovascular state. The

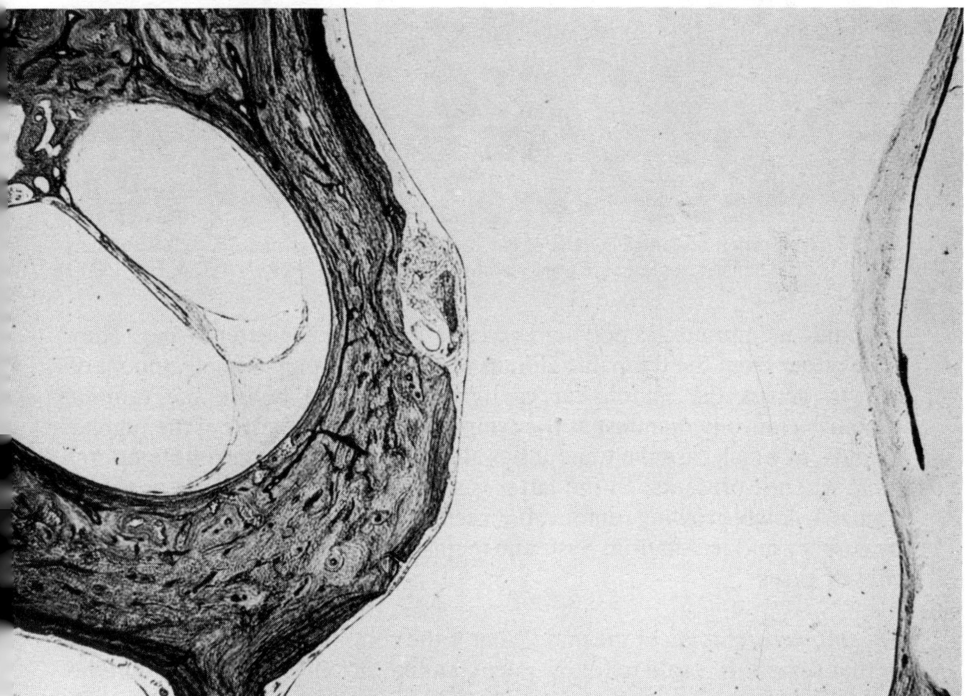

Fig. 12.31. Section of temporal bone showing basal coil of cochlea, promontory, middle ear, and tympanic membrane. A collection of cells and blood vessels in the middle-ear mucosa on the promonotory represents middle ear glomus body. (H. & E. × 25.)

glomus tumour histologically looks like a glomus body without the supplying nerves. There is a great vascularity and the epithelioid cells form tight clusters between the blood vessels (Figs. 12.32 and 12.33). These tumours present in the middle ear or even frequently, by breaking through the

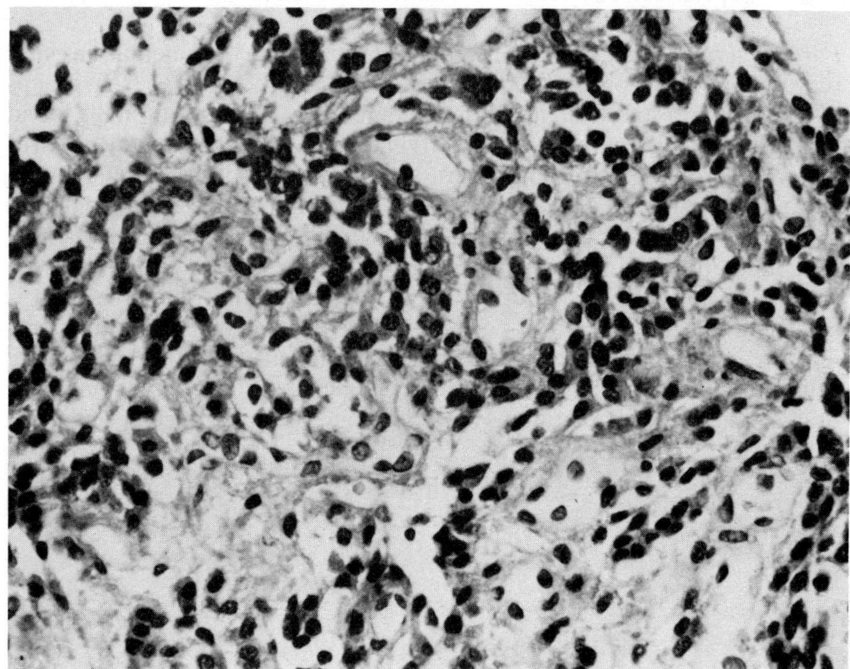

Fig. 12.32. Section of paraganglioma of ear. Collections of rather uniform cells with finely ganular cytoplasm are separated by numerous blood vessels. (H. & E. × 400.)

tympanic membrane, as polypoid vascular lesions in the external ear. They arise either from the tympanic glomus in which case only a small amount of growth across the middle-ear cavity has occurred before the tumour becomes clinically manifest at the tympanic membrane or from the jugular glomus, in which case the tumour has already invaded the petrous temporal bone when it presents. In the latter case surgical removal is not possible. This is a slowly growing tumour, but recurrence is frequent after treatment by surgery and irradiation. Systemic metastasis takes place in about 10 per cent of cases.

Squamous carcinoma of the middle ear is the commonest malignant tumour of that region. It is said to follow long-standing chronic otitis media, but the incidence of squamous carcinoma is very low in comparison with the great frequency of chronic otitis media. Histological studies have shown that the cancer may arise simultaneously from middle ear and ear canal, in which case growth takes place from a wide area of squamous change in the middle

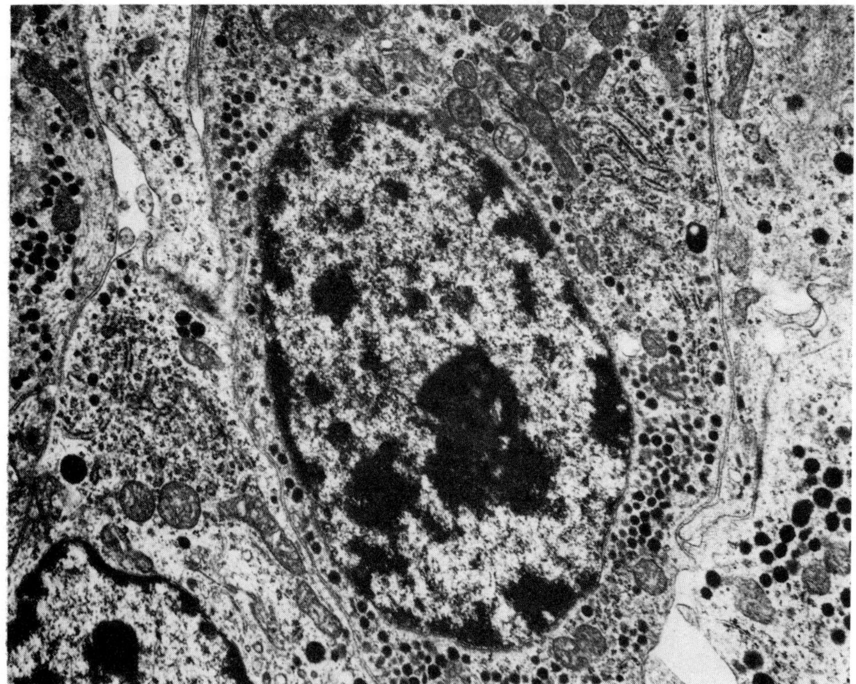

Fig. 12.33. Electron micrograph of paraganglioma of glomus jugulare showing tumour cells. The cytoplasm of each cell contains numerous membrane bound osmiophilic bodies probably related to catecholamine secretion. (H. & E. × 18 000.)

ear as well as from a malignant transformation of the external auditory meatus. The tumour soon erodes the thin bony plate on the medial wall of the middle ear separating it from the carotid canal and extends along the sympathetic nerves of the carotid canal. It also penetrates the thin bony walls of the posterior mastoid air cells and reaches the dura of the posterior surface of the temporal bone (Figs. 12.35–12.37). From there it travels medially and enters the internal auditory meatus and may invade the cochlea from the internal canal. These forms of growth take place silently without clinical symptoms, so that when the patient presents it is likely that the neoplasm has spread to this inoperable degree. There is no adequate means for the otologist to exclude such involvement. Thus surgical excision of large amounts of temporal bone with tumour is probably not indicated, leaving the clinician little choice of treatment but radiotherapy and perhaps cytotoxic drugs.

Rhabdomyosarcoma is a rare malignant neoplasm of children and young adults which forms polypoid fleshy masses in the middle ear presenting as a mass of tumour in the external ear with destruction of bone, the facial nerve and other structures. The histology is that of anaplastic usually somewhat

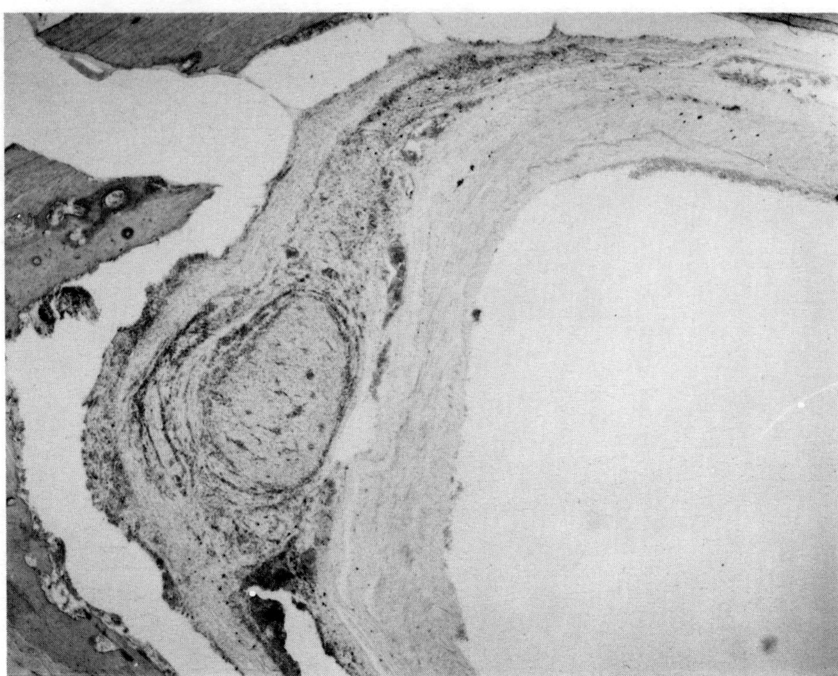

Fig. 12.34. Horizontal section of middle ear in a case of squamous carcinoma of the middle ear. The photomicrograph has been taken in the region of the carotid canal. Tumour tissue has entered the carotic canal and has infiltrated the nerve tissue surrounding the internal carotid artery. There is a microscopic fracture in the thin plate of bone separating the upper Eustachian tube from the carotid canal in the upper left hand corner of the photograph. (H. & E. × 25.)

fusiform cells. The presence of an occasional large cell with granular eosinophilic cystoplasm characteristically enables the correct diagnosis to be made. The presence of transverse striations may be detected in a rare cell on light microscopy, but electron microscopy will enable this diagnostic observation to be made more easily.

INNER EAR

Schwannomas of the vestibular branch of the VIII nerve are the only important primary neoplasms arising in the inner ear. Occasionally a similar tumour may arise from the cochlear branch of the VIII nerve or from the facial nerve. The common form of acoustic neuroma arises on the peripheral

Fig. 12.35. Posterior wall of the middle ear in a case of squamous carcinoma. A tumour has infiltrated the air cells and bone and has reached the dura which stretches along the upper left corner. The facial nerve seen at the lower right corner. (H. & E. × 25.)

Fig. 12.36. Section of stapes in squamous carcinoma of the middle ear. The vestibule is in the upper left corner of the picture. The stapes has been disrupted by squamous carcinoma arising from the middle-ear mucosa, but the adjacent osseous vestibule has not been invaded by tumour. (H. & E. × 25.)

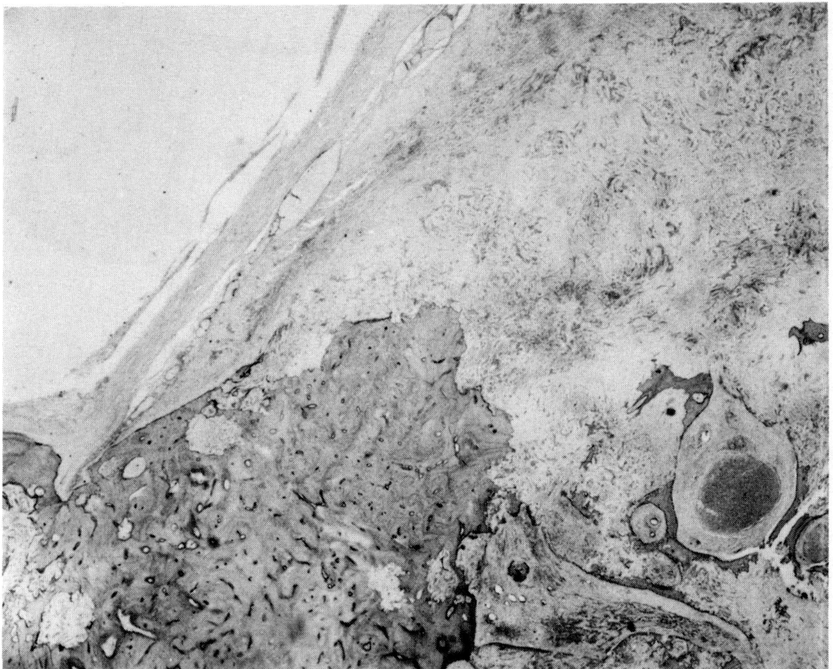

Fig. 12.35.

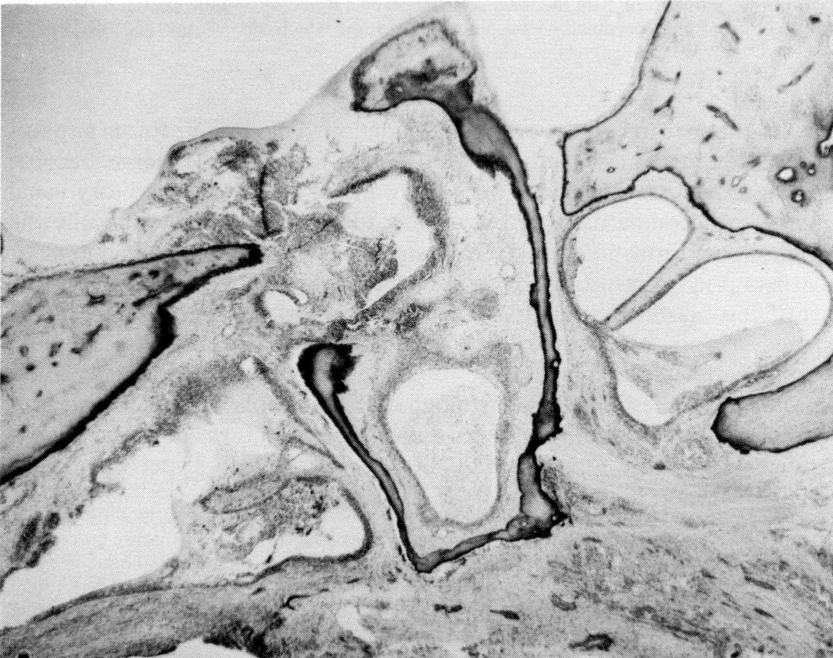

Fig. 12.36.

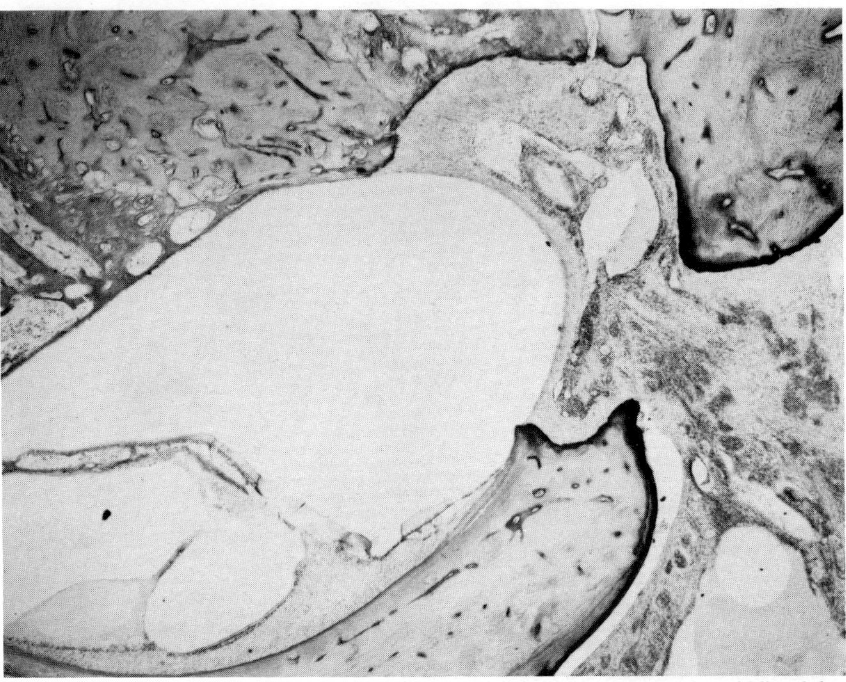

Fig. 12.37. Section of round window membrane which forms an arc near the middle of the photograph with the scala tympani on its left and the middle ear on its right. The latter is occupied by squamous carcinoma which has not invaded the bony or membranous cochlea. (H. & E. × 25.)

side of and near the glialneurilemmal junction. The tumour forms a spherical well-defined mass and as it grows the fibres of the nerve become stretched over the surface. The bony walls of the interal auditory canal enlarge to accommodate the expanding tumour mass. Histologically the neoplasm conforms to the pattern designated by the term Schwannoma or neurilemmona (Fig. 12.39). It shows a well-defined almost organoid structure of fibroblastic-like cells patterned in such a way that their nuclei become aligned in rows, a process known as palisading. These cells also exhibit a swirling pattern resembling tactile corpuscles and known as Verocay bodies. Antoni in 1920 described the histology of these neoplasms and the areas of fibroblastic-like palisading and Verocay bodies are known as Antoni Type A arrangement of the tumours (Fig. 12.40). The Antoni Type B areas are

Fig. 12.38. Invasion of the bony cochlea (note globuli ossei) by poorly differentiated squamous carcinoma (below). This is a late occurrence in the disease process and takes place after infiltration of the posterior dura of the temporal bone from the middle ear. (H. & E. × 100.)

Fig. 12.39. Section of acoustic neuroma of the VIII nerve in the internal auditory meatus. The latter is enlarged to accommodate the neoplasm. The vestibule (right) contains proteinaceous fluid and there is a thin layer of the same material lining cochlear scala. (H. & E. × 10.)

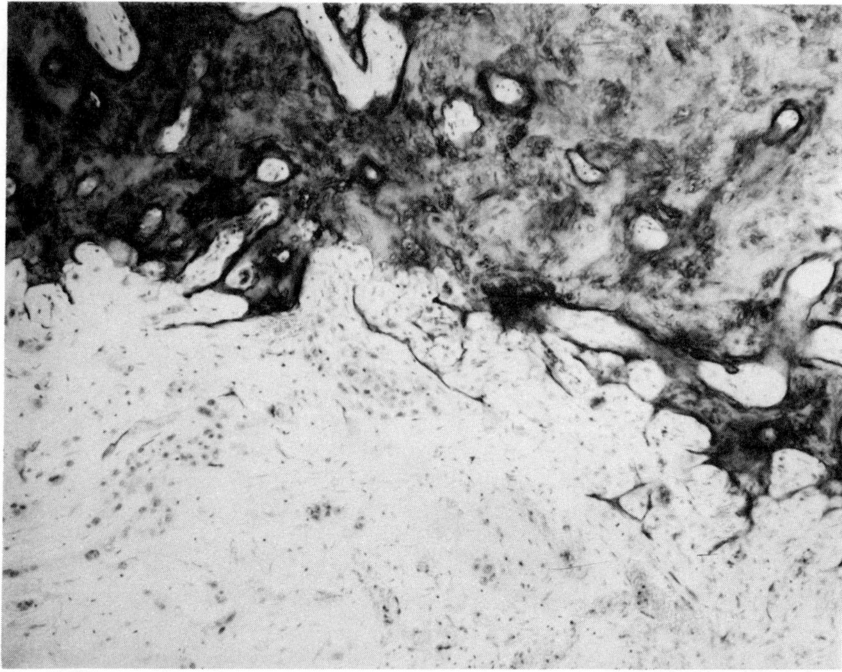

Fig. 12.38.

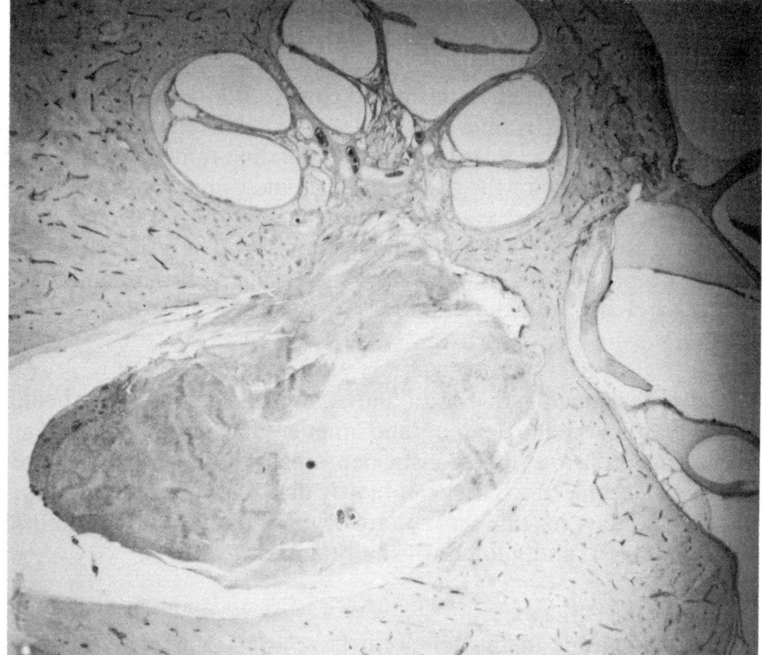

Fig. 12.39.

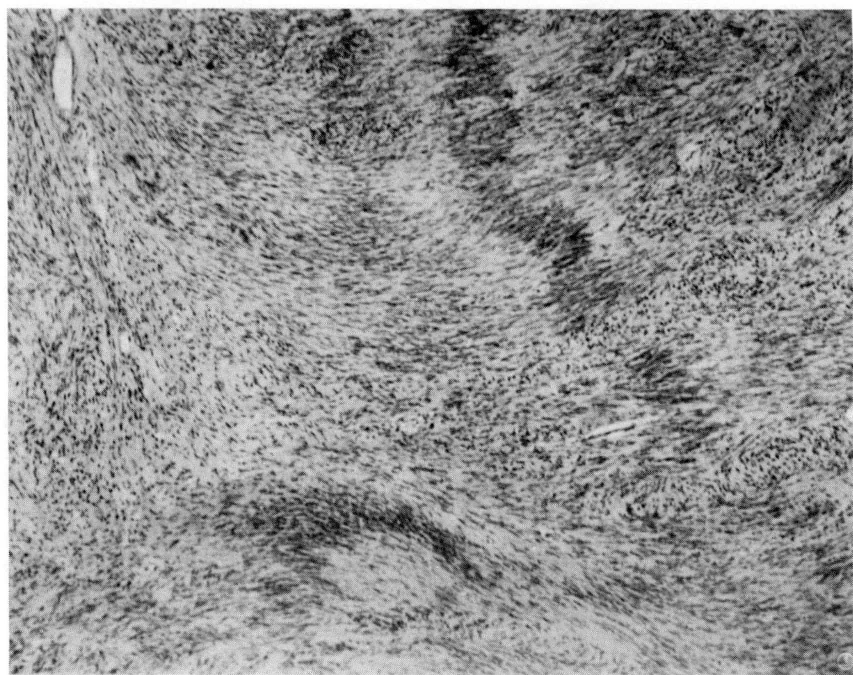

Fig. 12.40. Acoustic neuroma of VIII nerve showing Antoni A arrangement. There is palisading of nuclei of the fibroblast-like cells comprising of the tumour. (H. & E. × 250).

usually found in the same neoplasm and consist of looser areas containing foamy histiocytes and hyaline foci (Fig. 12.41). Histological changes are found in the inner ear in relation to this expanding tumour of the internal canal. There is atrophy of the organ of Corti and often of the maculae and cristae. These changes are caused by the damage of both branches of the VIII nerve produced by the expanding tumour. There is also seen the exudation of proteinaceous fluid into the scala vestibuli and tympani perilymph, and also into the vestibule.

TUMOURS OF THE CEREBELLOPONTINE ANGLE

It should be mentioned at this point that other tumours of the cerebellopontine angle may give rise to deafness and other cranial nerve symptoms and so cause clinical confusion with acoustic neuromas. Neurosurgical procedures will usually be required to carry out biopsy diagnosis of such tumours. The commoner lesions in this group are meningiomas, epidermoid cysts ('cholesteatomas'), and gliomas of the brainstem.

METASTATIC NEOPLASMS

Malignant neoplasms in the temporal bone are frequently the result of haematogenous dissemination from a primary site in one of the following

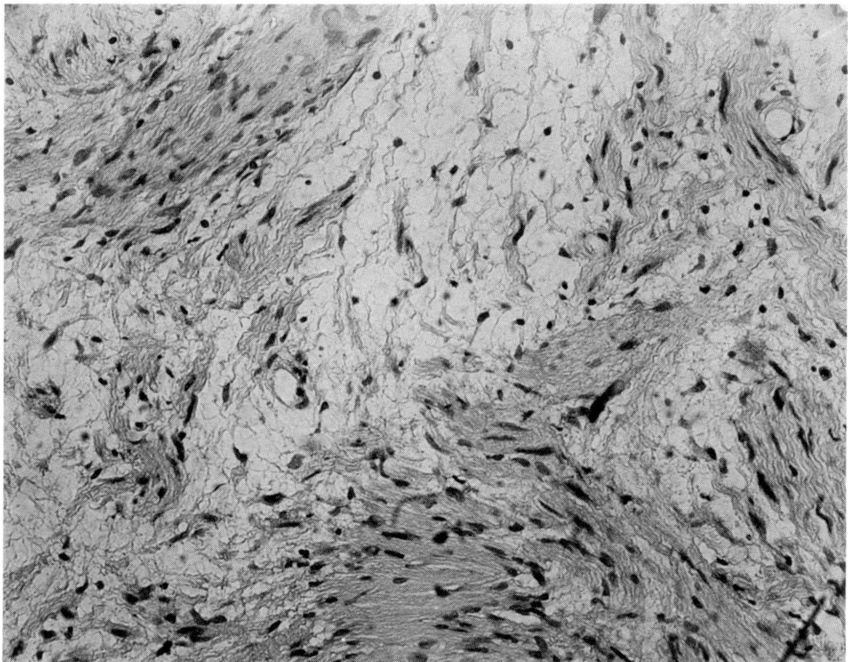

Fig. 12.41. Acoustic neuroma of VIII nerve showing Antoni B arrangement. There is a loose arrangement of corrective tissue with some foamy histiocytes. (H. & E. × 250.)

organs: breast, kidney, lung, stomach, larynx, prostate, and thyroid. The internal auditory canal is a common location for metastatic growth and the neoplasm may invade the inner ear by this route. The bony labyrinth is resistant to neoplastic involvement so that the sensory structures of the inner ear are uncommonly affected. The temporal bone elsewhere may be widely invaded and occasionally secondary neoplasm may invade and thicken the tympanic membrane.

LEUKAEMIA AND LYMPHOMA

Apart from the temporal bone marrow in cases of leukaemia, leukaemic deposits are frequently found in the inner ear, both in the cochlea and vestibule. A common cause of deafness in these conditions is haemorrhage into the internal ear. In Waldenstrom's macroglobulinaemia the increased viscosity of the blood is associated with hearing loss which is relieved after therapy. The exact mechanism of the inner-ear change is not known. Permanent hearing loss may also result from haemorrhage in this condition (Figs. 12.42–12.44).

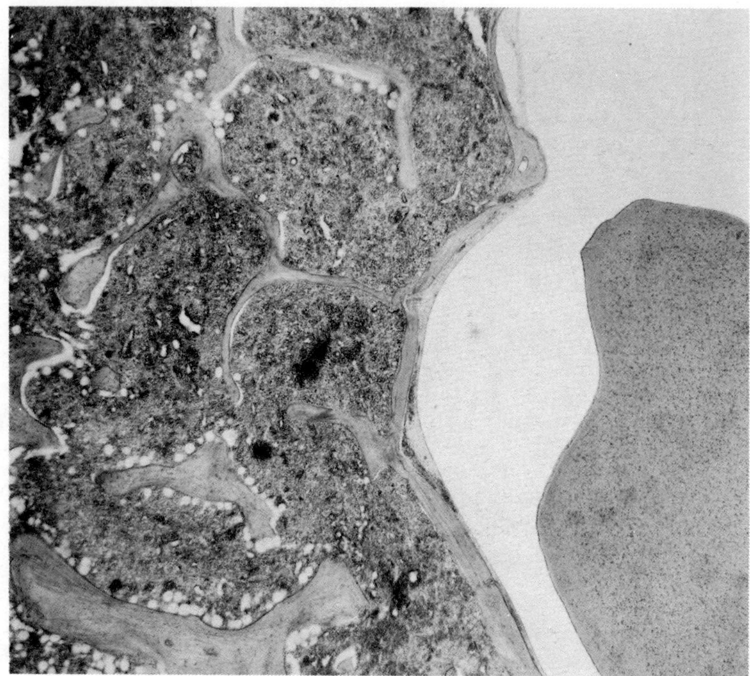

Fig. 12.42. Section of temporal bone in a case of Waldenstrom's macroglobulinaemia. The condition is essentially a lymphomatous one. The bone contains greatly dilated marrow spaces filled and lymphomatous tumour. The middle ear space on the right contains a proteinaceous fluid. (H. & E. × 25.) (By courtesy of the editor, *Clinical Otolaryngology*.)

DISORDERS OF GROWTH, METABOLISM, AND AGING

Ostosclerosis

This is a disorder of the otic capsule, causing fixation of the stapes and deafness. The bony otic capsule consists of an outer periosteal layer of dense lamellar bone which continues to thicken during adult life; a middle endochondral layer which consists of cartilaginous rests within bone (globuli ossei) and a thin inner endosteal layer of lamellar bone. Otosclerotic foci commonly commence in the residual cartilage of the fissula ante fenestram anterior to the foot plate of the stapes. Further development of the disease causes fixation of the stapes. Other foci may occur posterior to the stapes, on the promontory or around the round window (Fig. 12.45). Clinical mani-

Fig. 12.43. Cells of lymphamatous tumour from marrow space of temporal bone in case of Waldenstrom's macroglobulinaemia. The neoplastic cells are intermediate between lymphocytes and plasma cells in appearance. (H. & E. × 400.) (By courtesy of the editor *Clinical Otolaryngology*.)

Fig. 12.44. Cochlea in case of Waldenstom's macroglobulinaemia showing disruption by haemorrhage which was a terminal event in the patient's condition. (H. & E. × 25.) (By courtesy of the editor, *Clinical Otolaryngology*.)

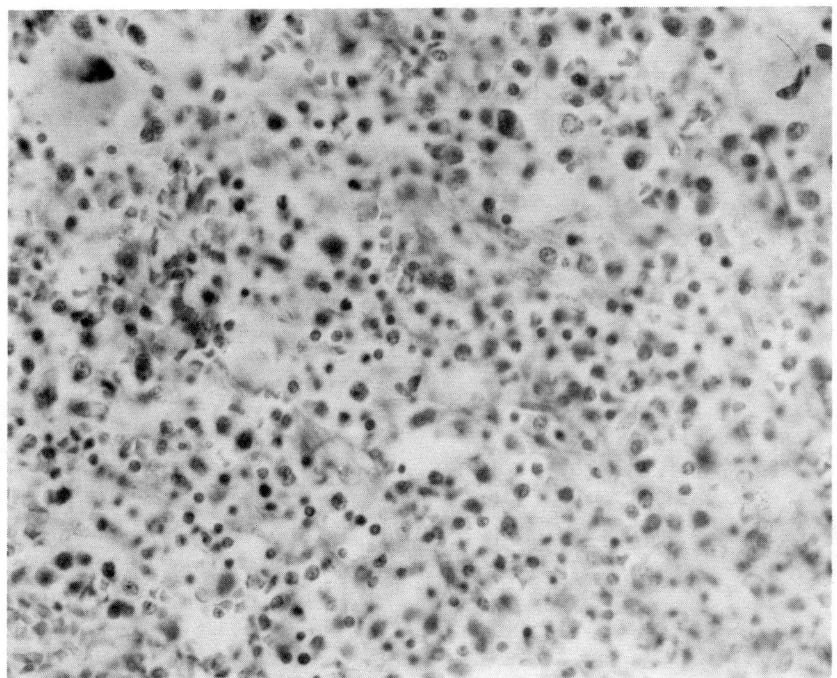

Fig. 12.43.

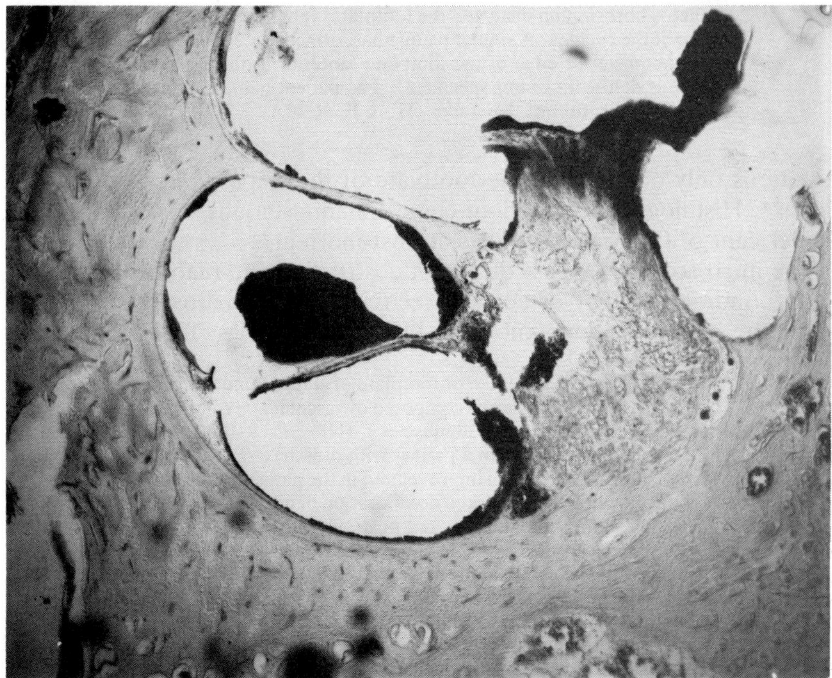

Fig. 12.44.

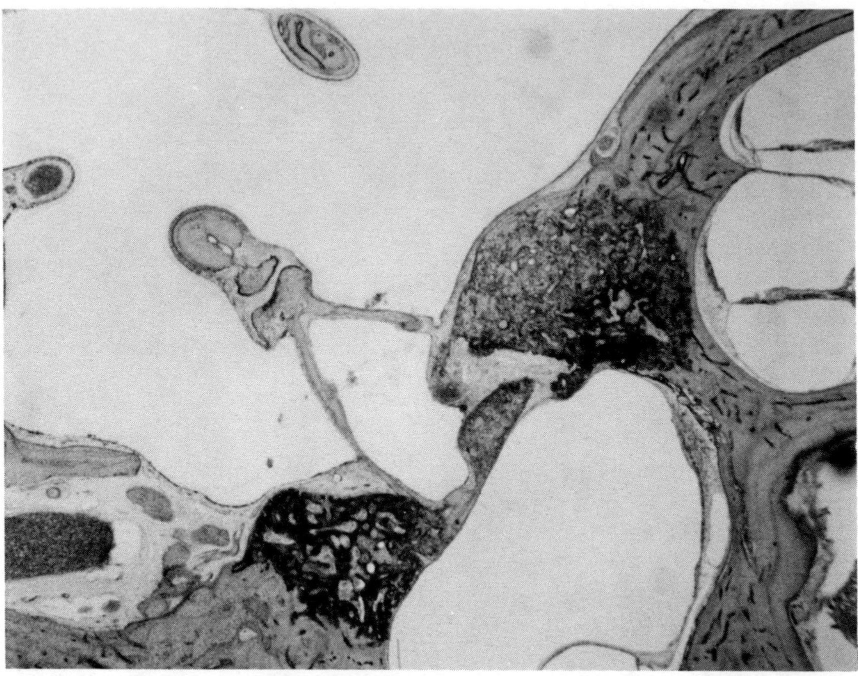

Fig. 12.45. Section of temporal bone in a case of otosclerosis is present anterior to the anterior crus and footplate of the otosclerotic bone stapes. It has replaced the annulus fibrosus and distorted the footplate. It has grown as far as the endosteal bone of the cochlea. A similar plaque has formed in relation to the posterior crus and the posterior edge of the footplate (anterior to the facial canal, and nerve which is dehiscent in this specimen). The patient had a conductive hearing loss due to the fixation of the stapes (H. & E. × 20.)

festations only occur when the footplate of the stapes is involved by the disease. Histological foci without clinical manifestations are seen in about 10 per cent of Caucasian subjects at post-mortem.

The microscopic changes consists of destruction and reabsorption of the endochondral bone, by osteoclastic activity and formation of tongues of immature basophilic bone known as blue-mantles (Figs. 12.46 and 12.47).

Fig. 12.46. Section of surgical specimen of footplate of stapes removed at stapedectomy for otosclerosis. The footplate is composed of vascular and cellular bone which stains in a basophilic fashion ('blue mantles'). (H. & E. × 100.)

Fig. 12.47. In this temporal bone from a patient with otosclerosis a stapedectomy had been carried out which led to an improvement in the patient's hearing loss. However, a sudden and permanent marked deterioration of hearing took place. The otosclerotic plaques are seen anterior and posterior to the footplate. A prosthesis has been removed from the specimen. Its position can be seen from the V-shaped connective tissue layer that had covered it. However, there is a fistula immediately beneath the prosthesis, extending from the middle-ear cavity above to the vestibule below. This is a complication of stapedectomy which ruins the beneficial effect of the operation. (H. & E. × 40.) (By courtesy of Update Publications Ltd.)

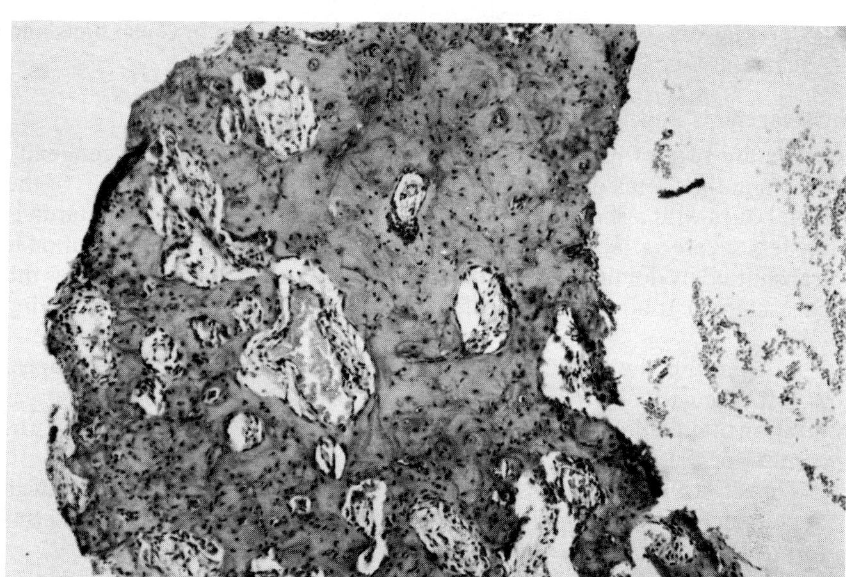

Fig. 12.46.

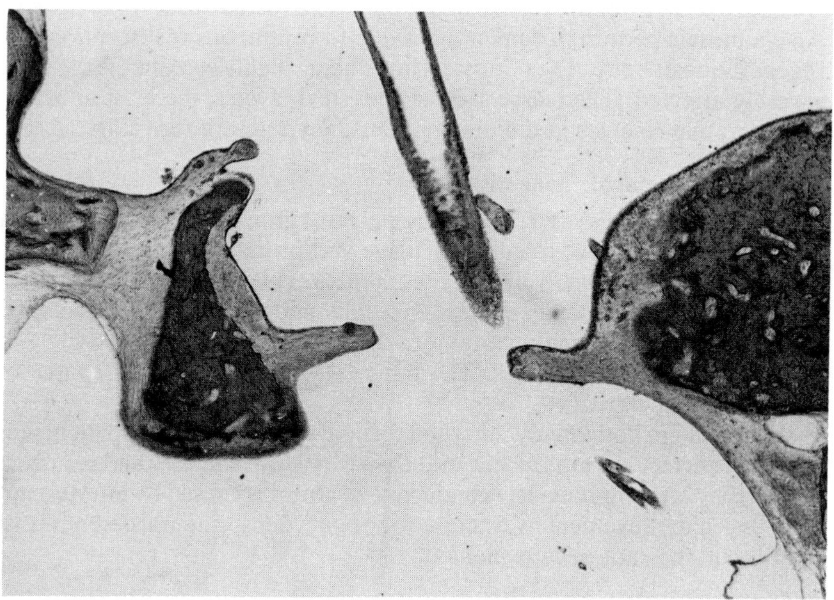

Fig. 12.47.

Otosclerosis is more common in females, and is seen in Caucasians and Asians only; negroes are not affected by this condition.

Osteogenesis imperfecta

There are two forms of this disease: (i) osteogenesis imperfecta congenita occurs in the foetus or newborn, characterized by multiple fractures of the long bones with a short survival time; (ii) Osteogenesis imperfecta tarda is the less severe variety. The affected individuals survive and the condition is transmitted by dominant inheritance. The Van der Hoeve syndrome has the characteristic triad of the blue sclera, fragile bones, and conductive hearing loss.

At operation the middle ear shows hyperaemic mucosa and a fixed stapes. A soft vascular bone fills the oval window niche. Basically there is disorganization of the collagen fibres at the reticular stage. Calcium and phosphorus content of the bone is normal.

The site of lesions in this condition and to some extent the histological appearances are similar to that of otosclerosis, but results of surgery in this form of stapedectomy are not as good.

Osteitis deformans (Paget's disease)

This common disease affects the skull, pelvis, spine, and femur. Frequent involvement of the temporal bone causes impaired hearing which may be conductive or sensorineural. Tinnitus and vertigo are not uncommon symptoms. The serum calcium and alkaline phosphatase are raised with low phosphorus levels.

Histopathology of the temporal bone shows affected parts of the bone to have a mosaic pattern of cement lines due to continuous reabsorption and regeneration of bone. The periosteal layer being highly vascular, is the most severely affected. The least vascular endosteal layer is the least affected. Degenerative changes in the membranous labyrinth are rare (Fig. 12.48).

Osteopetrosis (marble bone disease)

This is a rare bone disorder. The abnormal bone growth is characterized by a failure of resorption of calcified cartilage and primitive bone.

In its malignant recessively inherited form the children die at an early age. Optic atrophy, splenomegaly, hepatomegaly, poor growth, frontal bossing, fractures, loss of hearing, mental retardation, and facial palsy are some of the common clinical features. The bony labyrinth and ossicles consist of dense calcified cartilage.

In the benign dominantly inherited form of the disease many patients for the most part are asymptomatic and survive longer. Fractures and recurrent facial palsy are common. The conductive deafness is caused by interference with ossicular movement by osteopetrotic bone. Sensorineural deafness that also occurs has not been explained.

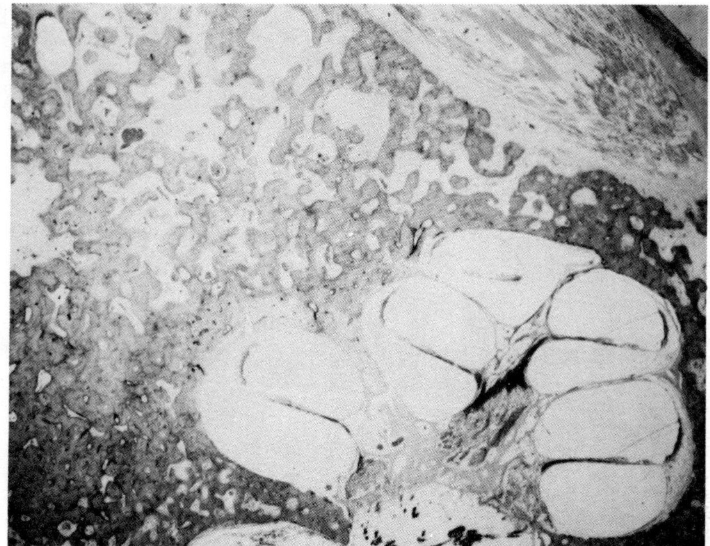

Fig. 12.48. Advanced Paget's disease of bone affecting the temporal bone. There is a loss of the normal structure of the bony cochlear capsule and replacement by a loose arrangement of bony trabeculae with a mosaic pattern of cement line. (H. & E. × 10.)

Diabetes mellitus

Clinically it is known that some patients with diabetes mellitus have progressive bilateral sensorineural hearing loss. This is by no means consistent in all patients affected with diabetes mellitus.

The impairment of hearing is attributed to changes in the capillaries of the stria vascularis ranging from internal thickening of capillaries, which stain positively by the PAS method and atrophy of the stria. Varying degrees of neuronal degeneration and atrophy of the spiral ligaments also occur.

Presbyacusis

Aging is an inevitable biological phenomenon. Presbyacusis implies a hearing loss caused by the degenerative changes of aging.

It usually commences in middle age and is progressive. The hearing loss is essentially sensorineural. The type of audiological pattern can be correlated with the histopathological findings in the temporal bone.

TYPES OF PRESBYCUSIS

(i) *Sensory*. Deafness commences in middle age and is very slowly progressive. The audiogram shows an abrupt high-tone hearing loss. The cochlea shows atrophy of the organ of Corti in the basal turn. The supporting and basal cells are atrophied. These changes may be associated with secondary degeneration.

(ii) *Neural*. This form of presbycusis can commence at any age. Speech

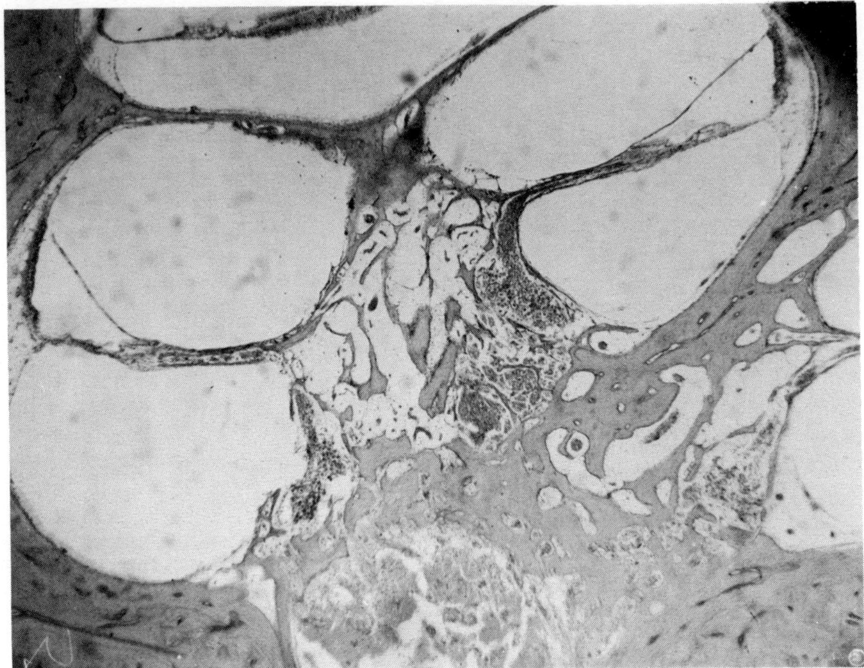

Fig. 12.49. Basal coil of cochlea in sensory presbycusis. There is a marked diminution of nerve cells in the spiral ganglion. These usually fill the spaces between the bony trabeculae of the modiolus. Some are still present adjacent to the scala tympani of the basal coil, but elsewhere they have vanished. (H. & E. × 25.)

discrimination is poor as compared to thresholds on pure-tone audiogram. There is degeneration of cochlear neurones in the entire cochlea, worse in the basal turn.

(iii) *Vascular*. Hearing loss is insidious in onset between the third and sixth decades of life and is progressive. Audiometric pattern is flat with good speech discrimination. The stria vascularis may show partial or diffuse atrophy. Cystic structures may sometimes be seen in the stria vascularis.

Ménière's disease (endolymphatic hydrops)

This is characterized by paroxymal episodes of vertigo and unilateral or bilateral sensorineural hearing loss associated with tinnitus. The essential histopathological features include generalized hydrops or swelling of the endolymphatic system. There is ballooning and sometime rupture of Reissner's membrane so that it distends the scala vestibuli and eventually lies against the bony wall. The hydrops of the saccule may be so great that it touches the footplate of the stapes (Fig. 12.51). There may be atrophy of the maculae (Fig. 12.52). Rupture and collapse of the membranous labyrinth can occur. Escape of potassium from the endolymphatic system to scala vestibuli and then via the helicotrema to the scala tympani may cause metabolic damage to the hair cells in the organ of Corti at the apical turn,

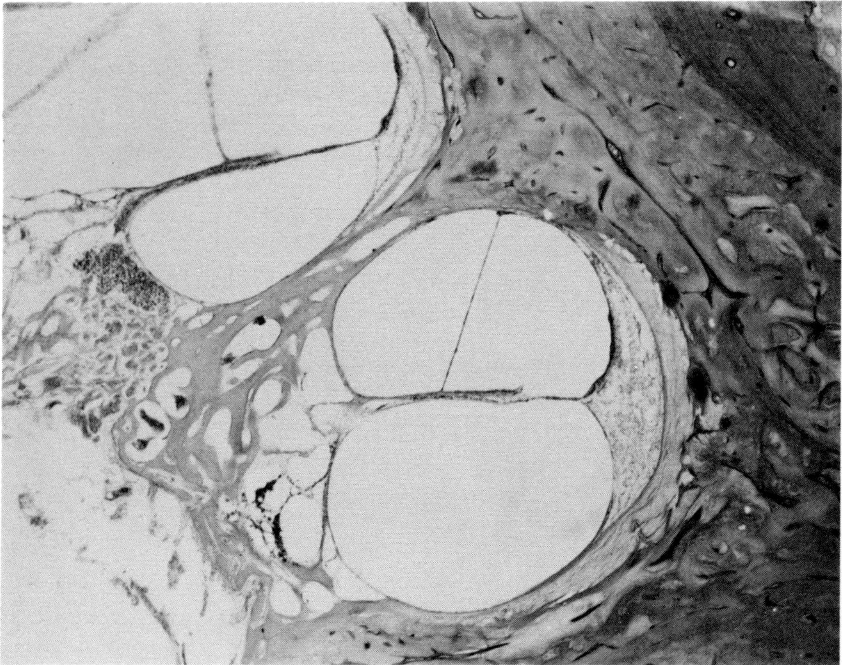

Fig. 12.50. Hydrops of the cochlear duct in Ménière's disease. There is ballooning of Reissner's membrane so that it distends the scala vestibuli and lies abnormally against the bony wall. (H. & E. × 25.)

thus causing hearing loss in the lower frequencies. The hair cell population and cochlear neurons are usually normal in Ménière's disease and the impaired hearing may be attributed to metabolic, biochemical, and mechanical dysfunction. Other changes that are found in temporal bones with Ménière's disease are: (i) a fibrous proliferation between the distended saccular wall and the footplate of the stapes; (ii) the presence in some cases of papillary structures in the dilated vestibular end of the cochlear duct, and (iii) the fibrous thickening of the endolymphatic duct and sac found in some cases. This has been held to represent the basic lesion accounting for the increase in endolymphatic fluid pressure (Fig. 12.53).

Ototoxic injury to the cochlea

Ototoxic injury is produced by the effects of molecular or chemical change. Although many therapeutic substances have been incriminated as causes of ototoxic injury, the most important ones fall into two main groups: certain antibiotic substances and certain diuretic substances. The usual target effect of the ototoxic antibiotics in therapeutics is on 70 S-ribosomes of bacteria leading to a paralysis of the reproductive capacity of the organism. The two diuretics frusemide and ethacrynic acid are used in medicine for their inhibition of certain enzyme activities of the renal tubules, thereby

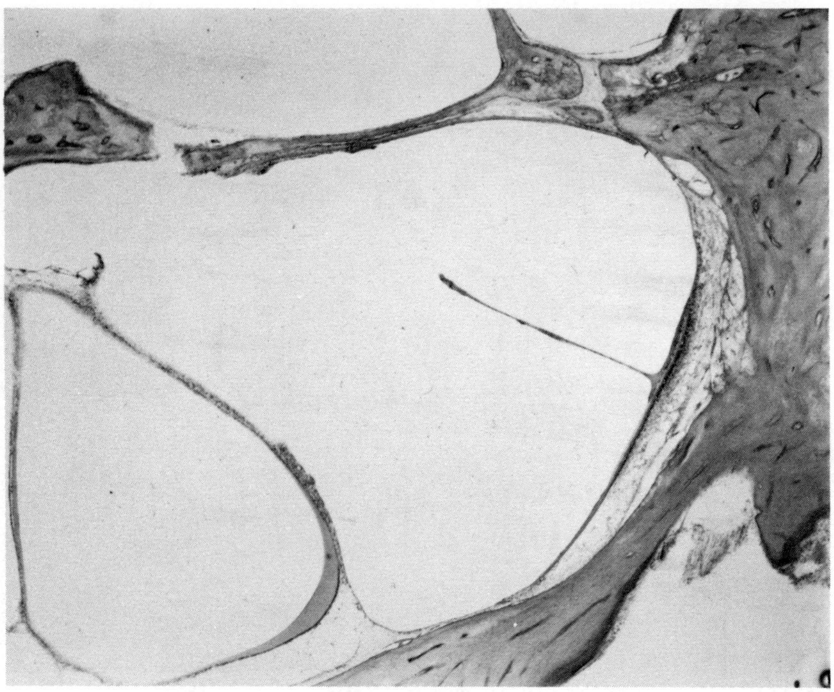

Fig. 12.51. Hydrops of the saccule in Ménière's disease. The distended saccular lining has been pushed up against the vestibular surface of the footplate of the stapes (which shows a fracture probably originating at post mortem). A projection into the saccular lumen is present. This is characteristically seen in Ménière's disease. (H. & E. × 25.)

diminishing water absorption. It is unfortunate that these two groups of drugs are among the most important in the modern pharmacopoeia; infection and heart failure with oedema, the condtions treated by the two types of drugs respectively, are among the most prevalent serious illnesses (see also Chapter 23).

Possible means of transport of any of these ototoxic substances to the cochlea are shown here. The commonest route is through the bloodstream after administration by mouth or by injection. The damage is done to the hair cells, but the exact means by which these structures are reached by the ototoxic substances is not known. It is possible that they enter the endolymph by diffusing from blood vessels in the stria vascularis or even the spiral lamina. There seems to be microcirculation among the outer hair cells so that ototoxic substances—indeed all substances, nuitritive as well as toxic—most diffuse from surrounding fluids.

During the early years of the treatment of tuberculous meningitis with streptomycin until about the middle 1950s, it was felt that daily injections of antibiotics into the subarachnoid space were necessary in order to achieve adequate contact between antibiotic and tubercle bacillus. Such treatments

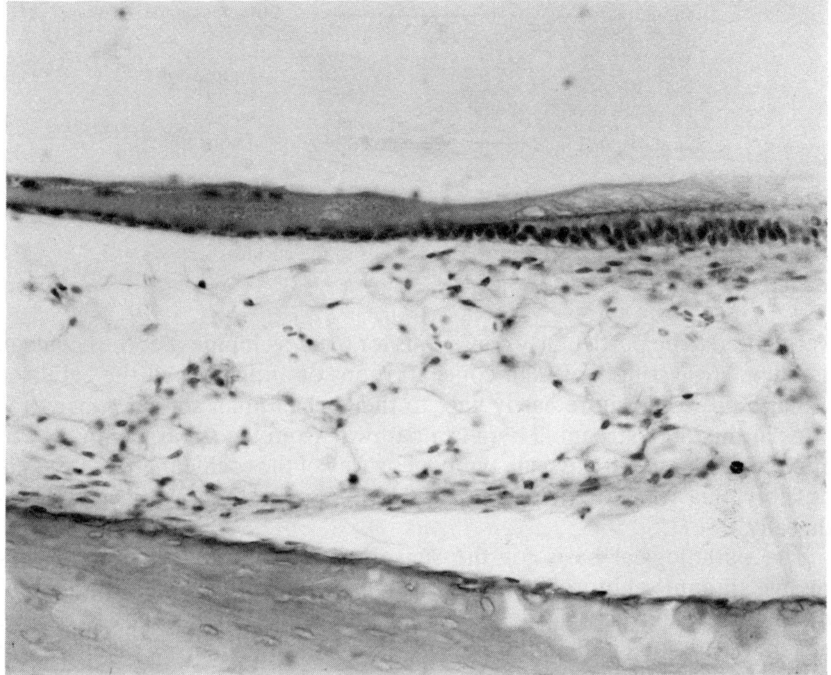

Fig. 12.52. Atrophy of the sensory cells of the saccular macula and underlying nerve fibres in Ménière's disease. (H. & E. × 250.)

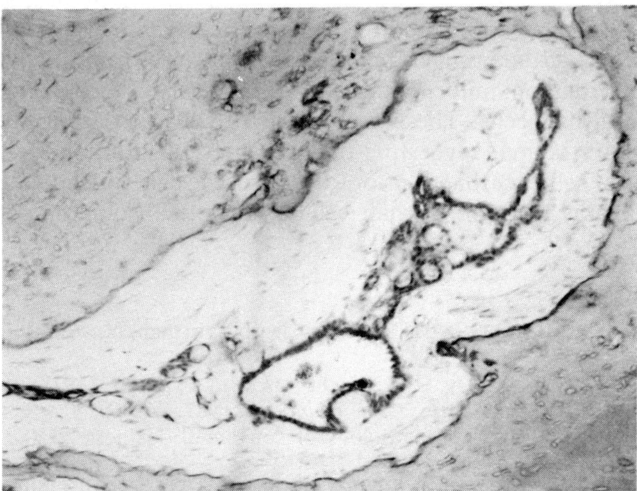

Fig. 12.53. Endolymphatic duct from a case of Ménière's disease. There is an abnormal proliferation of fibrous tissue beneath the duct lining.

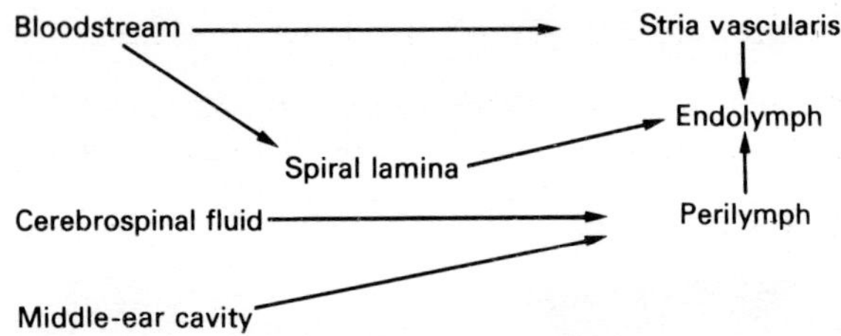

Fig. 12.54. Routes of access of ototoxic substances to the cochlea.

were noted to be particularly dangerous for the development of the cochlear damage, suggesting that high concentrations of antibiotics in the cerebrospinal fluid would more easily pass to the cochlea than similar concentrations in the bloodstream. There is a pathway from the subarachnoid space into the perilymph at the scala tympani by way of the cochlear aqueduct. It is possibly this route that is taken by ototoxic substances injected intrathecally.

The pathological basis for the sensorineural deafness induced by excessive amounts of ototoxic drugs is curiously similar to that of 'stimulation' trauma (see above). The lesion produced in the early stages is one of degeneration and death of the external hair cells principally of the basal coil of the cochlea. In the later stages internal hair cells, supporting cells and nerve elements may be involved. The examination of surface preparations of the spiral organ is on the cochlea. In ototoxicity by some antibiotics, sensory cells in other parts of the membranous labyrinth may be involved, notably the maculae of the utricle and the saccule. The surface preparation method may be adapted to the study of cellular damage in these situations.

Electron microscopical studies of the spiral organ in experimental animals, which had been given an excess of ototoxic drugs, showed apical lysosome formation, mitochondrial degeneration, and vacuole formation in the external hair cells. These are similar to changes described following 'stimulation' trauma, suggesting that these lesions are non-specific manifestations of cell disturbance prior to death of the cell. Indeed, both types of insult probably work on the hair cells through final common path.

REFERENCES

Konigsmark, B. W. (1969). Hereditary deafness in man. *New Engl. J. Med.* **281**, 713–20; 774–8; 827–32.

Meyerhoff, W. L., Kim, C. S., and Paparella, M. M. (1978). Pathology of chronic otitis media. *Ann. Otol. Rhinol. Lar.* **87**, 749–60.

Ormerod, F. (1960). The pathology of congenital deafness. *J. Lar. Otol.* **74**, 919–50.

Schuknecht, H. F. (1974). *Pathology of the ear*. Harvard University Press, Cambridge, Mass.

—— Neff, W. O. and Perlman, H. B. (1951). An experimental study of auditory damage following blows to the head. *Ann. Otol. Rhinol. Lar.* **60**, 273–89.

SUEHIRO, S. and SANDO, I. (1979). Congenital anomalies of the inner ear. Introducing a new classification of labyrinthine anomalies. *Ann. Otol. Rhinol. Lar.* Suppl. 59.

13 Genetically determined hearing defects

G. R. FRASER

INTRODUCTION

The emphasis of this chapter is directed towards forms of hearing loss which are present at birth or are of childhood onset mainly because far more is known about the hereditary aspects of such forms. This emphasis in no way implies that the far more common occurrence of hearing loss with onset in adult life is unimportant from the hereditary point of view and, in the final section, this problem is discussed both in the case of otosclerosis and of sensorineural hearing loss. It should be noted that hearing loss of childhood onset represents a much greater handicap to the individual in that it may, when of sufficient severity, interfere with normal education and with the acquisition of speech, thereby leading to lifelong problems in communication which are far graver than in the case of adult hearing losses. In addition, substantial amelioration or mitigation of hearing loss of adult onset is often possible, whether by surgery or through the use of hearing aids.

THE AETIOLOGY OF HEARING LOSS IN CHILDHOOD

Approximately half of all cases of hearing loss in childhood, which are of sufficient severity to interfere with education, are due to Mendelian genetical causes. This is not to say that hereditary factors play no role in the causation of hearing loss among the remainder but their influence is more complex.

In the first, Mendelian, group, a single gene locus is involved and the hearing loss may be dominant where one abnormal allele is sufficient to cause the damage, the paired allele being normal (i.e. the affected person is a heterozygote), or autosomal recessive where both of a pair of alleles at a particular chromosomal locus are abnormal, and the affected individual is therefore a homozygote. A special case is that of X-linked recessive hearing loss which forms a small proportion of all cases. Essentially only males are affected and they carry on abnormal allele on the X-chromosome. Since the X-chromosome is unpaired in the male, there is no normal allele to counteract its effects. Such affected male individuals are known as hemizygotes; females who are heterozygous for such alleles on the X-chromosome enjoy normal hearing.

It should be noted that possession of the genes under discussion, whether in heterozygous or homozygous form, may lead to a very wide variation of hearing loss; sometimes hearing may even be completely spared. This phenomenon is known as variability of expressivity of the gene in question and, when hearing is spared altogether, as failure of penetrance. Such variation in the effects of abnormal genes responsible for profound hearing loss in childhood is especially marked in connection with dominant forms of deafness (i.e. in heterozygotes with one normal and one abnormal allele, who may be totally and bilaterally deaf, may have mild or unilateral hearing loss, or may even hear normally).

Thus, as stated at the outset of this discussion, this first group comprises cases whose hearing loss is due primarily to Mendelian genetical causes, the term primarily indicating that the presence of the abnormal gene is necessary but not sufficient, the degree and even the existence of the hearing loss being dependent to a minor degree on modifying factors which may, to some extent at least, also be hereditary, forming part of the residual genotype, but may be exogenous in nature.

In the second, non-Mendelian group, which is approximately equal in size, exogenous factors, whether they act prenatally, such as maternal rubella, perinatally, such as profound jaundice or administration of ototoxic drugs to weakly premature neonates, or in infancy and childhood, such as meningitis, are the primary causes of the deafness, whereas modifying factors which may again be hereditary, at least in part, and complex in nature, determine the extent of the hearing loss due to the exogenous insult, or indeed whether any hearing loss occurs at all.

Autosomal recessive forms of hearing loss in childhood

Thus, the presence and, secondarily, the degree of profound hearing loss in childhood can never be attributed exclusively to hereditary or to exogenous factors but are always the resultant of an interaction between the two. Within these semantic limitations, however, it is possible to discuss and to define the forms which are primarily genetically determined in that they follow Mendelian laws of transmission. In the majority of cases, these are autosomal recessive conditions, and it is striking that all the evidence indicates that there are several dozen quite distinct such forms determined by genes at different chromosomal loci. This evidence is of three types. Firstly, those who are profoundly deaf from childhood tend to marry similarly affected persons and many families have been described where unions between individuals both of whom are affected by autosomal recessive hearing loss give rise only to normally hearing offspring. This is to be expected on the hypothesis that the autosomal recessive hearing loss in the two marriage partners is determined at different gene loci, since the offspring would then be double heterozygotes. If there is only one form of autosomal recessive deafness, then all the offspring would be expected to be of the same genotype as the parents and would also suffer from hearing loss. Such marriages have been reported but are far less common than those of the first type where the offspring have normal hearing.

The second type of evidence in favour of the existence of multiple gene loci determining autosomal recessive hearing loss is derived from a theoretical relationship between the incidence of an autosomal recessive condition in the population and the proportion of consanguineous marriages among the parents of affected individuals. The rarer such a condition, the higher should be the rate of consanguinity, and the anomalously high rate found among the parents of those with autosomal recessive hearing loss is readily explicable by the fact that multiple such forms exist, each sub-group so defined obviously being much rarer than the entity taken as a whole.

The most important and interesting evidence regarding multiplicity of gene loci concerns clinical associations of profound hearing loss in childhood in a variety of autosomal recessive syndromes, and this evidence will now be considered in some detail. A complete enumeration and description of such syndromes may be found in the books of Fraser (1976) and of Konigsmark and Gorlin (1976) and only a few will be discussed within the brief compass of this chapter.

One of the more common types of autosomal recessive hearing loss is that which is associated with a block in the synthesis of thyroid hormones and is known as Pendred's syndrome. The enzymatic defect is at the stage of conversion of inorganic iodide, trapped by the thyroid gland, to organic form (Fig. 13.1). This defect is fortunately usually only partial rather than complete, so that most individuals with Pendred's syndrome can compensate for its effects by feedback stimulation of the thyroid gland through the pituitary. Thus, they are euthyroid, though they often suffer from goitre which is potentially troublesome but can readily be controlled by long-term administration of exogenous thyroid hormone which eliminates the pituitary stimulation.

Another relatively common type of autosomal recessive hearing loss (though somewhat less common in most populations than Pendred's syndrome) is that which is associated with retinitis pigmentosa. This usually goes under the name of Usher's syndrome though it was clearly described more than half a century before Usher's publication in a paper by the noted German ophthalmologist Albrecht von Graefe in 1858.

A third autosomal recessive syndrome to be found among children with profound hearing loss, which is less common that the other two but of which many examples have been described in the literature, is that where the deafness is accompanied by disturbances of cardiac conduction which result in a unique anomaly of the electrocardiogram characterized by bizarre biphasic T waves and marked prolongation of the QT interval (Fig. 13.2). This condition is known as the cardio-auditory or surdocardiac syndrome of Jervell and Lange-Nielsen (1957) and is associated with attacks of cardiac syncope during which ventricular fibrillation occurs; in a substantial proportion of cases one of these attacks eventually proves fatal. Now that the characteristic features of this syndrome of 'deafness with fainting attacks' are better known, long-term drug therapy can be instituted and a fatal outcome is less common, but Friedmann, Fraser, and Froggatt (1966, 1968) were able to report the pathological findings in the organ of Corti of three affected children who had died while under observation. The organ of Corti was entirely disorganized with retraction of the tectorial membrane, and

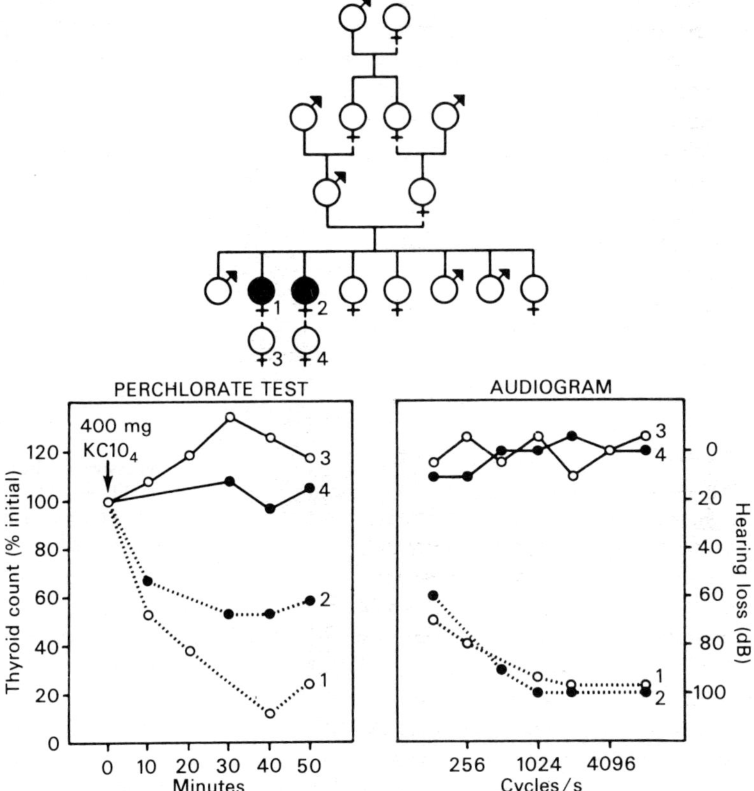

Fig. 13.1. Recessive inheritance of the syndrome of deafness with goitre in two sisters born of a marriage of first cousins. The response of the thyroid counting rate of the two sisters to $KClO_4$ given one hour after radioactive iodide is abnormal. The rate falls dramatically as iodide still in unbound inorganic form is discharged from the thryroid gland. The heterozygous daughters of the affected sisters show normal responses to $KClO_4$ and normal audiograms. The audiograms of their mothers show the typical greater loss of hearing in the high tones. ● indicates subject with Pendred's syndrome. (Reproduced by courtesy of the Editor, *Journal of Medical Genetics*.)

both the cochlear and vestibular portions of the membranous labyrinth were involved. The most striking anomaly was the presence of widespread PAS-positive deposits throughout the membranous labyrinth, particularly in the vascular stria, where many appeared to lie within the greatly distended vessels. The deposits also lay on the spiral prominence and sometimes extended quite deeply into the region of the organ of Corti. The region of the crista of the horizontal canal was practically unrecognizable and contained huge masses of PAS-positive material. These pathological findings more closely resemble those of Siebenmann and Bing (1907), Nager (1927), and Buch and Jørgensen (1963) in cases of the syndrome of deafness

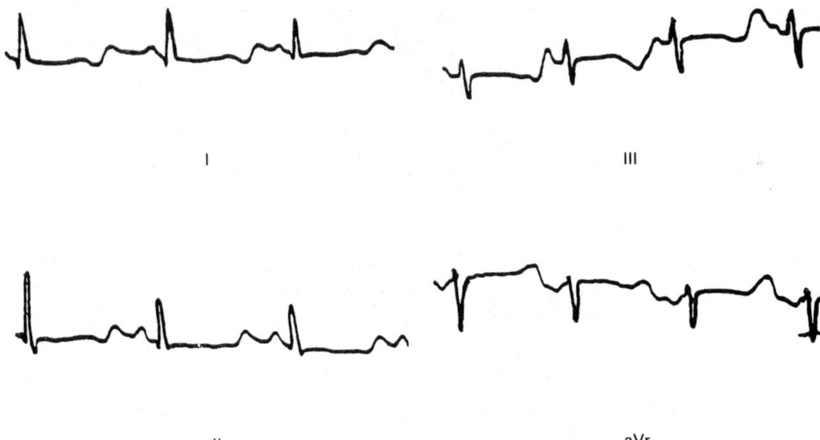

Fig. 13.2. Electrocardiogram (cardiac cycle = 0.80 s) of a case of the recessive syndrome of deafness with fainting attacks, electrocardiographic abnormalities, and sudden death. The tracing shows the distinctive features characteristic of this condition—the extreme prolongation of the Q–T interval and the bizarre, often biphasic, T waves. (Reproduced by courtesy of the Editor, *Journal of Medical Genetics*.)

with retinitis pigmentosa than the cochleosaccular type of degeneration (Scheibe 1892) often found in cases of clinically undifferentiated genetically determined deafness.

In general, histological post-morten material coming from well-defined types of genetically determined deafness is sparse, and only one autopsy of a documented case of Pendred's syndrome has been described (Hvidberg-Hansen and Jørgensen 1968). In this case a malformation of the bony labyrinth consistent with the description of Mondini (1791) was reported. Thus, it does not seem that the histological lesions of the organ of Corti of the type described by Scheibe (1892) are characteristic of any of these three syndromes even though it is generally stated that such lesions are typical of autosomal recessive hearing loss in childhood. It should be emphasized, however, that there is insufficient material available in general to establish a firm correlation between the clinical and pathological features of genetically determined forms of hearing loss.

It has already been stated that it is not proposed to provide an exhaustive enumeration of all the autosomal recessive syndromes which may include hearing loss. They are all less common than the three discussed above, and it is not surprising that a very large number of such syndromes exist, since the embryological development of the auditory apparatus and the biochemical mechanism of normal hearing are both very complex processes and, therefore, vulnerable to many different types of abnormal gene action, resulting in recessive as well as dominant modes of Mendelian transmission. In these syndromes, as well as in most forms of clinically undifferentiated autosomal recessive profound deafness, the hearing loss is characteristically symmetrical in the two ears and of a predominantly high-tone type with the retention of an island of hearing of variable extent in the low tones which can be of great practical importance with respect to the potential for amplification with electronic hearing aids.

Profound hearing loss, as defined above in the sense that it is of sufficient severity to interfere with normal education, occurs in economically developed countries in about 1 per 1000 of the childhood population and, of this total, as stated above, about one-half is due to Mendelian inheritance. The contribution of autosomal recessive forms to this genetically determined moiety is about two-thirds so that the population frequency of autosomal recessive profound hearing loss in childhood is about 33 per 100 000. In populations of British origin in Great Britain, the Republic of Ireland, and South Australia studied by Fraser (1976) the frequency of Pendred's syndrome (with goitre) is 6–8/100 000, that of Usher's syndrome (with retinitis pigmentosa) is 2–4/100 000, and that of the syndrome of Jervell and Lange-Nielsen (with anomalies of cardiac conduction) is less than 1/100 000. The remainder of the figure of 33/100 000 mentioned above is accounted for by rarer syndromes and also, in the majority, by clinically undifferentiated forms of hearing loss (that is to say unaccompanied by recognizable clinical features involving other organ systems).

In the vast majority of cases of these autosomal recessive syndromes, the hearing loss is sensorineural in nature but it need by no means always be profound. Thus, milder losses may exceptionally be seen in the syndromes of Pendred, of Usher, and of Jervell and Lange-Nielsen; in many other autosomal recessive forms, whether it occurs as part of a syndrome or not, the hearing loss is habitually mild, so that such conditions are only infrequently found among profoundly deaf children and are not included in the population incidence of 1 per 1000 mentioned above. In the case of both the mild and severe hearing impairments associated with autosomal recessive forms, there is little evidence about the possibly progressive nature of the loss. This question is of considerable potential importance from the point of view of future mitigation and prevention and is discussed further below.

In a few cases, autosomal recessive hearing losses may be conductive in nature, usually due to malformations of the ossicles of the middle ear. As an illustration of such a condition, the cryptophthalmos syndrome may be cited. This entity owes its name to the fact that the cleft between the eyelids does not form, and behind the unopened lids only disorganized remnants of the ocular globe are to be found. This is an autosomal recessive multiple malformation syndrome and, among these malformations, ossicular deformities may be present, giving rise to hearing impairment which may be profound, though this is by no means invariably the case. Because of the gravity of visceral maldevelopment usually associated with such multiple malformation syndromes, they are often fatal. In the case of the cryptophthalmos syndrome, renal hypoplasia of variable degree may be found and is frequently so pronounced as to constitute virtual aplasia; such infants are stillborn or survive only a few hours. Where survival does occur, a basic difference between such conditions and sensorineural forms of deafness is that the former are frequently amenable to middle-ear surgery which can restore a substantial degree of hearing.

It should be noted in passing that many malformation syndromes exist which include hearing impairment as one of their facultative features. These may be autosomal recessive, as in the case of the cryptophthalmos syndrome, or autosomal dominant, as discussed below. In addition, most major chromosomal anomalies are associated with some derangement of the structure of the auditory apparatus leading to hearing impairment. In the majority of cases, however, malformations associated with hearing impairment are not due to simple Mendelian or chromosomal causes but, as is the case with congenital malformations in general, have a complex aetiology.

THE POTENTIAL IMPORTANCE OF SYNDROMES FROM THE POINT OF VIEW OF PREVENTION AND TREATMENT OF HEARING LOSS

In general, the existence of so many genetically determined syndromes which combine hearing loss with multiple clinical associations, varying so widely from syndrome to syndrome is of considerable potential biological significance. It has frequently been shown to be the case that an autosomal recessive pathological trait, whether in Man or in other mammals, can be attributed to interference with a metabolic pathway through the failure to produce an enzyme or through the production of an abnormal molecule, whether an enzyme or, as in the case of sickle-cell anaemia, another type of protein, which is inactive or which acts in an inappropriate manner.

Unfortunately virtually complete ignorance prevails concerning the biochemical and metabolic basis of normal hearing. Thus, we are unable even to hazard a guess concerning the possible site of action of the various abnormal alleles which in homozygous form can cause loss of hearing. There is little doubt, however, that if we are able in one or more cases eventually to unravel the mode of action of the genes involved in the causation of autosomal recessive hearing loss, this will clarify many aspects of the basis of normal hearing. Perhaps our best hope of unravelling the modes of action of the abnormal genes lies in the study of individuals affected with the syndromes which have been discussed, for the specific nature of the features associated with hearing impairment in these conditions may afford important clues to these modes of action. For example, a specific inborn error of metabolism must lead concomitantly to hearing loss and to a well-defined defect of thyroid hormone synthesis, another such error to the association of hearing loss with retinitis pigmentosa, and yet a third to that with a seemingly unique disturbance in cardiac conduction. Our present inability to take advantage of these clues stems from the sheer vast extent of our ignorance of human metabolism, but this need not always be so. In the future, one or other of these associations may suggest to an astute investigator specific areas in which to seek an aberrant metabolic pathway and in this way to make a breakthrough of substantial importance. To take a possible analogy, deficiency of the action of the enzyme galactose 1-phosphate-uridyl transferase, determined in an autosomal recessive manner, leads to the disease galactosaemia of which the cardinal features are early cataracts and hepatic dysfunction. While this was not in fact the mode of discovery of this inborn error of metabolism, retrospectively it is possible to envisage a situation in which an astute clinical investigator might have been encouraged by the observation of a group of infants with this particular constellation of clinical abnormalities to study the metabolism of galactose, since this substance is known to be of considerable importance to the biochemical functioning both of the liver and of the lens.

As has been pointed out above, another question of considerable potential importance in this context is the timing of the damage to the organ of Corti or other vital parts of the auditory apparatus in these hereditary forms of hearing loss. Extensive histological studies in laboratory mammals have shown wide variations in this respect which depend on the particular gene locus, the animal, and the strain involved. On the analogy of the dietary treatment of phenylketonuria, once the biochemical basis of a particular type of hereditary hearing loss is elucidated, steps could possibly be contemplated to counteract completely or at least to mitigate the deleterious effects on hearing of the inborn error of metabolism. The potential effectiveness of such therapy would depend very much on the usual timing of the damage. Thus, the success of the dietary treatment of phenylketonuria is dependent on the fact that the foetus seems to be protected from the effects of the genetical defect by maternal metabolism, and brain development is therefore virtually normal at birth, the associated mental subnormality being essentially postnatal in origin. We are completely ignorant of the timing of the damage to the auditory apparatus in the various hereditary forms of hearing loss in Man and whether, if postnatal, they are progressive and to what extent. The acquisition of such knowledge, however, is vital since, if the damage is in fact already far advanced at birth, the hopes for eventual cure, or at least mitigation, are much reduced.

HETEROZYGOTES FOR GENES CAUSING AUTOSOMAL RECESSIVE HEARING LOSS

It has been stressed that the most common forms of genetically determined hearing loss are inherited in an autosomal recessive manner, that is to say in homozygotes for abnormal alleles. There are many gene loci at which such abnormal alleles may occur giving rise to multiple forms of autosomal recessive deafness whose existence has been discussed above. It should be appreciated that while these forms of autosomal recessive deafness are rare, the alleles which cause them are by no means so. Thus, to take as an illustration population frequencies of 7/100 000, 3/100 000, and 1/100 000 as applicable to the three syndromes of Pendred, of Usher, and of Jervell and Lange-Nielsen, these incidences would imply frequencies for the abnormal alleles of approximately 0.008, 0.006, and 0.003 respectively. This in turn means that 1.6, 1.2, and 0.6 per cent respectively of the population are carriers for these alleles. Since these calculations involve only three of the many types of autosomal recessive deafness which are known to exist, it is clear that a substantial proportion of the population must be carriers for one or another of the many abnormal alleles capable of causing autosomal recessive hearing loss in homozygous form.

Suggestions have been made that possession of one of these alleles in heterozygous carriers may lead to minor deviations from the normal in hearing function which, while clinically insignificant, can perhaps be elicited by sophisticated otological testing (Anderson and Wedenberg 1968). It would clearly be of importance to establish if this is so, and to what extent, since it might be possible to base genetical counselling on such evidence in the all-too-common situation where a single hearing-impaired child is born in a family without a history of deafness in the relatives, and the parents wish to know the recurrence risks. These are 25 per cent if the impairment is autosomal recessive, but may also be zero if it is due to an acquired but unrecognized cause as is often the case.

In addition, the question must be left open (and is discussed further below) to what extent heterozygosity for such alleles contributes to the variable hearing loss which seems an inescapable accompaniment of aging, and even to susceptibility to exposure to exogenous insults such as noise in an industrial environment.

X-linked hearing impairment in childhood

A small proportion of cases of hereditary hearing loss are determined by genes on the X-chromosome. In such families, the pattern of inheritance is similar to that seen in conditions such as haemophilia and colour-blindness. The hearing impairment is seen in males and is transmitted through heterozygous females who themselves enjoy normal hearing. Several distinct types of X-linked hearing impairment exist. Some are sensorineural in nature, whereas at least one is primarily conductive (with an additional sensorineural component.

This condition, first described by Nance, Setliff, McLeod, Sweeney, Cooper, and McConnell (1971), although very rare, shows characteristic features which are of some importance from the point of view of attempts to remedy the defect by surgery. A malformation in the middle ear consists of fixation of the footplate of the stapes and operations are invariably complicated by a profuse flow of perilymphatic fluid, thought to be under increased pressure due to an abnormal patency of the cochlear aqueduct.

Exceptional families have been described in which X-linked deafness has been associated with clinical features involving other organ systems. Thus, it may occur with pigmentary anomalies, an association discussed at some length in the following section on autosomal dominant hearing impairment.

Autosomal dominant forms of hearing impairment in childhood

About one-third of all cases of profound hereditary hearing impairment in childhood is due to autosomal dominant inheritance. In a typical case, such hearing impairment can be traced through several generations and approximately one-half of the offspring of a parent with hearing impairment will also be affected. However, while in the case of recessive hearing impairment, whether autosomal or X-linked, the familial pattern conforms well to Mendelian laws, there are several complications in the case of autosomal dominant inheritance which may give rise to deviations from this pattern.

Firstly, as pointed out in the Introduction, the phenomena of variable expressivity and failure of penetrance of the abnormal alleles involved may lead to mild or unilateral deafness in persons who carry such alleles and may even result in their having normal hearing despite the fact that the pathological allele is inherited from a deaf parent. Such persons, however, may in turn transmit the allele in question to offspring who are bilaterally and profoundly deaf, thus giving rise to irregularities in the dominant pattern of inheritance of the hearing loss.

Secondly, a certain proportion of individuals with autosomal dominant hearing loss owe their handicap to fresh mutation. This implies that neither parent was carrying the abnormal allele in question but that it arose through a process of mutation in gametogenesis and was transmitted in a single cell, either a spermatozoon or an ovum. In such individuals, therefore, the hearing impairment may represent a *de novo* phenomenon from the family point of view, and they may have no affected relatives. They are, however, at risk for passing on the abnormal allele, and hence hearing impairment, to their offspring.

It should be noted that, in general, even when autosomal dominant hearing loss is bilateral, profound, and of childhood onset, it tends to be less severe than in autosomal recessive forms. In addition, although correspondence is not absolute, the audiogram tends to show a relatively flat or gently sloping form, the high-tones being only slightly more affected than the low, in contrast to the predominantly high-tone loss mentioned above as being characteristic of autosomal recessive inheritance.

Emphasis has been placed in the discussion of recessive hearing impairment on biological heterogeneity and the multiple genetically distinct forms which may exist. The same applies to autosomal dominant forms also. Thus, they may be clinically undifferentiated in that the hearing impairment is apparently an isolated effect of the action of the abnormal gene or it may occur as part of a syndrome. The most common associations of this type to be found with autosomal dominant deafness are pigmentary anomalies, and sufficient heterogeneity exists within this sub-group to indicate that more than one genetic entity is involved. Thus, several distinct abnormal alleles, which may be at the same or at different gene loci may give rise in heterozygous form to dominantly inherited associations of hearing impairment with pigmentary anomalies. In one variety, which may be denoted as the classical form of Waardenburg's syndrome, an additional component is a morphological abnormality of facial and skull development whose main feature is a lateral displacement of the medial canthi of the eyelids. This form tends to be associated with the most striking pigmentary anomalies including heterochromia of the irides and partial depigmentation of the hair (white forelock). It should be noted in this context of the genetical heterogeneity of these syndromes that, as well as the several abnormal alleles determining autosomal dominant associations of hearing impairment with pigmentary anomalies in Man and in many other mammals, at least one such gene in Man is situated on the X-chromosome as mentioned in the preceding section.

The association of genetically determined autosomal dominant hearing impairment with pigmentary anomalies has been the subject of extensive histological studies in the cat (Bosher and Hallpike 1965, 1966). This work suggests the possibility that the degeneration of the organ of Corti in these animals takes place shortly after birth rather than being truly congenital and, although these results cannot be extrapolated directly to Man, they are of the utmost potential significance in view of the discussion above of the possibilities of postnatal prevention or mitigation of the effects of abnormal genes causing hearing impairment, once their biochemical mode of action is elucidated. The sparse post-mortem evidence which is available in Man in the case of Waardenburg's syndrome does suggest that the damage to the organ of Corti is at the microscopic cellular level, and that the structure of the osseous labyrinth is normal. The situation is, however, somewhat complicated by the fact that at least some of the effects of the abnormal gene, such as the pigmentary anomalies and the morphological facial deformities, must be determined during embryogenesis, even though this by no means excludes the possibility that the damage to the hearing apparatus which is the only significant handicap in Waardenburg's syndrome may indeed be postnatal in its genesis, as it may also be in the case of many autosomal recessive syndromes involving hearing impairment.

These autosomal dominant syndromes involving pigmentary anomalies give rise to sensorineural hearing impairment by causing damage to the auditory mechanism at the cellular level. As in the case of recessive forms of hearing impairment, both autosomal and X-linked, autosomal dominant syndromes exist which cause hearing impairment, which is at least in part conductive in nature, through malformations. A prototype of such a syndrome is the mandibulofacial dysostosis (Treacher–Collins syndrome). In this condition, many different types of malformations may occur during embryogenesis in various organ systems but the most consistent feature is a maldevelopment of the branchial arches and of the facial skeleton which may lead to hearing impairment by causing deformities of the outer or middle ear, or even sometimes of the osseous labyrinth. All the phenotypic expressions of this gene including those which affect hearing are very variable in their expression. Fortunately, the auditory anomalies, at least those affecting the outer and middle ears, are amenable to surgical repair which often leads to dramatic improvement in hearing.

It should be noted that the mandibulofacial dysostosis is only one of a whole gamut of malformation syndromes affecting branchial arch development and hence involving hearing loss as a facultative feature. Some of these are inherited in an autosomal dominant manner, while others are not transmitted in any simple Mendelian pattern, this being the case in the majority of congenital malformations.

GENERAL CONSIDERATIONS CONCERNING GENETICALLY DETERMINED HEARING LOSS IN CHILDHOOD AND IN ADULT LIFE

In this very brief review of genetically determined forms of profound hearing loss in childhood, only a small number of syndromes have been mentioned to illustrate specific points and principles, and it has been noted that exhaustive lists of such syndromes which run into many score are to be found in extensive compendia. It has also been pointed out that the existence of this multitude of different types of genetically determined hearing loss is not surprising when it is considered how very complex the embryogenesis of the auditory apparatus and the mechanisms of conduction of the auditory impulses are. In fact, this complexity leads to a vulnerability to the effects of a very great number of abnormal genes, and hearing loss may be only a minor component of the pathological burden which some of them cause. A good example of such a phenomenon is the mild to moderate hearing loss of adolescent onset to be found in the relatively common autosomal dominant Alport's syndrome. The main handicap in this condition is the renal defect which may be fatal in males, in whom the hearing loss is also more pronounced. The reasons for this more severe expression in males of the gene responsible are not known.

In fact, hearing loss of some degree is a virtually inescapable accompaniment of the aging process and, while, in most cases, this development of hearing loss with time is under the control of complex factors, many relatively common types are simply determined genetically. This applies to several forms of sensorineural hearing loss of adolescent or adult onset, unaccompanied by other clinical features, which are progressive in character, and possibly also to otosclerosis although the formal pattern of inheritance of this relatively common condition is not easy to define (see, for example, Morrison (1967)).

Reasonably reliable figures exist concerning the prevalence of profound hearing impairment in the childhood population. In economically developed countries, this figure may be estimated as mentioned above as about 1 per 1000. Far less reliable figures are available about significant hearing impairment in adult life, though, depending on the definition of significance adopted, it may be as much as 5–10 per cent. In fact, predominantly high-tone loss of variable extent involves most individuals in adult life but fortunately causes significant difficulty only in a minority. Perhaps the term significance in this context should be equated with inconvenience, hardship, or handicap, and it is at this level that the figure of 5–10 per cent is applicable.

Of these, a substantial proportion suffer from otosclerosis and it is thought that this condition in general is inherited in an autosomal dominant manner, but there are several unsolved problems in this respect. Clinically manifest otosclerosis occurs in about 2 per cent of the white population while histological features may be seen in as many as 10 per cent. It is much rarer among blacks. Women are affected twice as frequently as men, and the expression of the gene concerned must presumably be subject to hormonal influences to account for this excess. Corroborative evidence for this point of view is provided by the fact that pregnancy and childbirth are known to lead to clinical deterioration in many cases.

There have been virtually no studies to determine in what proportion of cases significant sensorineural hearing losses in adults are due to simple hereditary factors. The proportion is likely to be high and the mode of inheritance is usually autosomal dominant. In other cases such losses are due to exposure to exogenous insults which may be long-term such as noise in factory workers and possibly in dance-band musicians, or of brief duration, as when sudden hearing losses occur after viral illnesses. In such cases, whether the aetiology is occupational, infectious, or other, the question of genetically determined susceptibility must be raised and this point has been discussed above, especially in connection with the high proportion of the population who are heterozygous carriers for one or other of the alleles which can cause autosomal recessive profound hearing loss in childhood in homozygous form. In addition, the problem may be analogous to that discussed above with respect to the susceptibility to profound hearing loss in childhood determined by such agents as foetal infection with rubella or administration of ototoxic drugs in infancy.

In conclusion, in the field of genetically determined forms of hearing loss we are at present largely at the stage of descriptive epidemiology and this is because our knowledge of the mechanism of normal hearing and of its deviations is so fragmentary. We know very little about the embryogenesis of the auditory apparatus, the biochemistry of normal hearing or the nature of the maintenance of normal bone structure in later life. Thus, we can only describe the malformations which take place during embryogenesis, the otological and radiological features of profound childhood hearing losses and the clinical accompaniments which characterize many hereditary forms, and the osseous changes which occur during adult life and lead to otosclerosis, without being able to further to define the chain of causation.

Many more studies are needed both in the area of childhood hearing impairment and of those types which have their principal impact in adult life. Such studies should be conducted along methodological lines which combine the epidemiological population approach with the biological one so that fruitful interactions may develop between the geneticist, the audiologist, the epidemiologist, the clinician, the biochemist, the physiologist, the pathologist, and scientists from other disciplines who are interested in this multifaceted problem of hearing loss.

In a singularly perspicacious vein, William Harvey wrote in 1657:

> Nature is nowhere accustomed more openly to display her secret mysteries than in cases where she shows traces of her workings apart from the beaten path; nor is there any better way to advance the proper practice of medicine than to give our minds to

the discovery of the usual law of Nature by careful investigation of cases of rarer forms of disease. For it has been found, in almost all things, that what they contain of useful or applicable nature is hardly perceived unless we are deprived of them, or they become deranged in some way.

Thus, Harvey clearly indicated more than three centuries ago how much it behoves us to make use of these experiments of Nature which lead to genetically determined abnormal deviations to throw light on the mechanisms of the normal of which in the context of hearing we are so woefully ignorant today.

REFERENCES

ANDERSON, H. and WEDENBERG, E. (1968). Audiometric identification of normal hearing carriers of genes for deafness. *Acta oto-lar.* **65**, 535.

BOSHER, S. K. and HALLPIKE, C. S. (1965). Observations on the histological features, development and pathogenesis of the inner ear degeneration of the deaf white cat. *Proc. R. Soc.* **B162**, 147

—— —— (1966). Observations of the histogenesis of the inner ear degeneration of the deaf white cat and its possible relationship to the aetiology of certain unexplained varieties of human congenital deafness. *J. Lar. Otol.* **80**, 222.

BUCH, N. H. and JØRGENSEN, M. B. (1963). Pathological studies of deaf-mutes. *Archs Otolar.* **77**, 246.

COLLINS, E. T. (1900). Congenital abnormalities. 8. Case with symmetrical congenital notches in the outer part of each lower lid and defective development of the malar bones. *Trans. opthal. Soc. U.K.* **20**, 190.

FRASER, G. R. (1976). *The causes of profound deafness in childhood. A study of 3,535 individuals with severe hearing loss present at birth or of childhood onset.* John Hopkins University Press, Baltimore.

FRIEDMANN, I., FRASER, G. R., and FROGGATT, P. (1966). Pathology of the ear in the cardio-auditory syndrome of Jervell and Lange-Nielsen (recessive deafness with electrocardiographic abnormalities). *J. Lar. Otol.* **80**, 451.

—— —— —— (1968). Pathology of the ear in the cardio-auditory syndrome of Jervell and Lange-Nielsen: report of a third case with an appendix on possible linkage with the Rh blood group locus. *J. Lar. Otol.* **82**, 883.

HVIDBERG-HANSEN, J. and JØRGENSEN, M. B. (1968). The inner ear in Pendred's syndrome. *Acta oto-lar.* **66**, 129.

JERVELL, A. and LANGE-NIELSEN, F. (1957). Congenital deaf-mutism, functional heart disease with prolongation of Q-T interval, and sudden death. *Am. Heart J.* **54**, 59.

KONIGSMARK, B. N. and GORLIN, R. J. (1976). *Genetic and metabolic deafness.* Saunders, Philadelphia.

MONDINI (Mundinus), C. (1791). Anatomia surdi nati sectio. In *De Bononiensi Scientiarum et Artium Instituto atque Academia Commentarii,* Vol. 7, 28, (comment), p. 419. (opusc.). Bologna.

MORRISON, A. W. (1967). Genetic factors in otosclerosis. *Ann. R. Soc. Coll. Surg. Engl.* **41**, 202.

NAGER, F. R. (1927). Zür Histologie der Taubstummheit bei retinitis pigmentosa. *Beitr. path. Anat.* **77**, 288.

NANCE, W. E., SETLIFF, R. C. MCLEOD, A., SWEENEY, A., COOPER, C., and MCCONNELL, F. E. (1971). X-linked mixed deafness with congenital fixation of the stapedial footplate and perilymphatic gusher. *Birth Defects: Orig. Art. Ser.* **7**(4), 64.

PENDRED, V. (1896). Deaf-mutism and goitre. *Lancet* **ii**, 532.

SCHEIBE, A. (1892). A case of deaf-mutism, with auditory atrophy and anomalies of development in the membranous labyrinth of both ears. *Archs Otol., N.Y.* **21**, 12.
Also in German: Ein Fall von Taubstummheit mit Acusticustrophie und Bildungsanomalien in häutigen Labyrinth beiderseits. *Z. Ohrenheilk.* **22**, 11.

SIEBENMANN, F. and BING, R. (1907). Über den Labyrinth- und Hirnbefund bei einem an Retinitis pigmentosa erblindeten Angeboren-Taubstummen. *Z. Ohrenheilk.* **54**, 265.

USHER, C. H. (1914). On the inheritance of retinitis pigmentosa with notes of cases. *R. Lond. ophthal. Hosp. Rep.* **19**, 130.

VON GRAEFE, A. (1858). Vereinzelte Beobachtungen und Bemerkungen. 6. Exzeptionelles Verhalten des Gesichtfeldes bei Pigmentenartung der Netzhaut. *Albrecht v. Graefes Arch. Ophthal.* **4** (ii), 250.

Section 4

Adult audiology

14 Clinical tests of auditory function in the adult and the schoolchild

R. HINCHCLIFFE

INTRODUCTION

The clinical examination of auditory function in the adult and in the schoolchild is based upon tests developed in the nineteenth century. This has permitted time for the accumulation of a considerable data base and, with the introduction of the modern type of audiometer in the 1930s, the possibility of validating the tests against more precise electro-acoustic measures. Nearly a hundred years ago, however, reports were appearing of comparisons of the results obtained with tuning forks and the watch and the whisper tests (Eitelberg 1886).

The clinical examination of auditory function uses six sound sources, some thirty auditory phenomena and two reflexes. The six sound sources are finger movement, speech, tuning forks, the monochord, the whistle, and the lever pocket watch. It is convenient to classify the tests according to their use of these sound sources.

FINGER FRICTION TESTS

Successive rubbing or snapping of a finger and thumb is an acoustic stimulus which is more commonly used by neurologists (DeJong 1967) than by other specialists. It is a convenient sound source not only for screening for defects in the *threshold of hearing* but also for screening for defects in *sound localization* (localization encompasses both directionalization and distance perception).

The mechanism of sound localization appears to have been broached first by Müller (1838) in his *Handbook of physiology*. Experimental studies reported by von Kries and Auerbach and by Thompson in 1877 and 1878 respectively provided evidence for the importance of intensity differences and phase differences respectively. Von Hornbostel and Wertheimer (1920) subsequently showed the importance of time differences which were reflected in phase differences at the two ears. The relative importance of intensity and phase were demonstrated by the subsequent experimental studies of Stevens and Newman (1934, 1936). Dysstereoacusis (impaired sound localization) as a clinical symptom was reported by Politzer in 1876.

Klingon and Bontecou (1966) reported the use of the finger friction/snapping test to examine localization in the *horizontal* plane. They examined 156 patients, of whom 154 had a neurological disorder,* together

* Two suffered from aural disorders (see later).

with a comparison group of 50 'neurologically normal nurses'. In each case, the thumb and forefinger 'were successfully rubbed or snapped until the patient touched them or obviously could not locate them'. Care was taken to have the fingers closer to the patient than any other part of the examiner's arm. The sound was produced in a minimum of three locations. These locations were all in the horizontal plane; two of the locations were in the acoustic axis of the ear being tested, one adjacent to the auricle and the other within the patient's own arm length. The third location was at an intermediate distance but anterior to the acoustic axis and at an angle of just less than one radian subtended at the meatal orifice. Each stimulus was given at least three times. Thirty-three of the forty-two patients with supratentorial neurological disease had defects in localization on the side opposite to the involved hemisphere; in three cases the localization defect was bilateral. None of the patients with neurological disease which was not supratentorial showed localization defects. Klingon and Bontecou also reported two other patients with localization defects. One had had the 'external ear virtually amputated because of a basal cell carcinoma'; the other had had 'an external and middle ear removal for malignant parotid tumour'. In the first case, 'gross acuity was bilaterally equal, but the patient could not localize the stimulus on the opposite side'. The second case was 'totally deaf on the operated side' but sounds loud enough to be heard on the normal side could not be localized. Among the fifty nurses, only one showed a defect in localization; this was associated with a chronic suppurative otitis media.

Sound directionalization or localization in the *vertical* plane should also be tested since this function may be impaired when that in the horizontal plane is normal, and vice versa. Different mechanisms are involved for the two planes.

In 1881, Laborde had already suggested that stereoacusis was dependent on normal vestibular function. Both Young (1931) and Wallach (1940) subsequently showed that satisfactory vertical plane directionalization requires the ability to move the head.

Vertical plane directionalization also requires the possession of normal high-frequency auditory acuity. For example, normal horizontal plane directionalization, but impaired vertical-plane directionalization, has been observed in a patient with a bilateral abrupt high-tone loss (90 dB HL at 6 kHz; 75 dB at 8 kHz) above 4 kHz; the converse ability was observed in a patient with a total unilateral hearing loss (Butler 1970).

Vertical-plane directionalization thus depends on the ability to correlate head movement with high-frequency acoustical clues. Neurological cases may similarly show different behaviour in the two planes. For example, a man with a parietal glioblastoma showed normal (or near normal) vertical plane directionalization, but impaired horizontal plane localization. The converse behaviour is sometimes associated with brainstem lesions (Walsh 1957).

In the author's experience screening hearing with finger friction or finger snapping noise is an extremely sensitive test, especially with regard to localization in the sagittal plane.

One form of audiometry, directional audiometry (Nordlund 1964; Nilsson, Lidén, Rosén, and Zöller 1973; Tonning 1975), has already been used for measuring some aspect of sound localization for clinical purposes. More sophisticated approaches (Damper 1976a) to the psychoacoustical bases of binaural hearing, i.e. binaural fusion and separation, permit the use of Békésy type tracking procedures for complex binaural images (Damper 1976b).

Dysstereoacusis must be distinguished from what Heilman, Pandya, Karol, and Geschwind (1971) term *auditory inattention*. The latter applies to conditions in which the subject reacts as though acoustic stimuli (whether unilateral or bilateral) were coming from one side only. The condition occurs in certain hemisphere lesions. In parietal lesions, there is no response to contralateral stimuli, in frontal lesions, no response to ipsilateral stimuli.

SPEECH TESTS

Clinical tests have been used:
(i) to measure hearing impairment;
(ii) to detect feigning; and
(iii) to determine the nature of an organic hearing impairment

Measuring hearing impairment

Since their introduction by Wolf (1871, 1879) and recommendations regarding their quantification by Lucae (1907), clinical speech hearing tests have been subject to criticism (Hartmann 1877; Fowler 1947; Trowbridge 1947). Hartmann said that they were too complicated to ensure accuracy.

Despite early attempts, such as those by Reuter (1904) and by Bezold (1897), to standardize the tests, King (1953) ranked the failure to standardize as still the principal source of variability. Reuter advocated limiting the use of speech material to monosyllables. Bezold suggested that only the residual air, i.e. the volume of air left in the lungs after an ordinary, but not enforced, expiration, should be used for whispering; this characterizes the *forced whisper* test. Difficulty in controlling the intensity and frequency content of a whisper, lack of control of ambient noise, and differing acoustical properties of test rooms are the other three factors which King (1953) points to as contributing to the variability of responses to the forced whisper test. The last item may, however, not be responsible for as much variability as was hitherto believed (see Fig. 14.1).

Fowler (1947) also pointed to the reflex raising of the voice by examiners when they increased their distance from the patient; such an effect can be responsible for paradoxical results. However, one expects to find that the greater the hearing loss, the nearer must the examiner be to the patient in order to be heard.

In a truly free field where sound can spread spherically in all directions

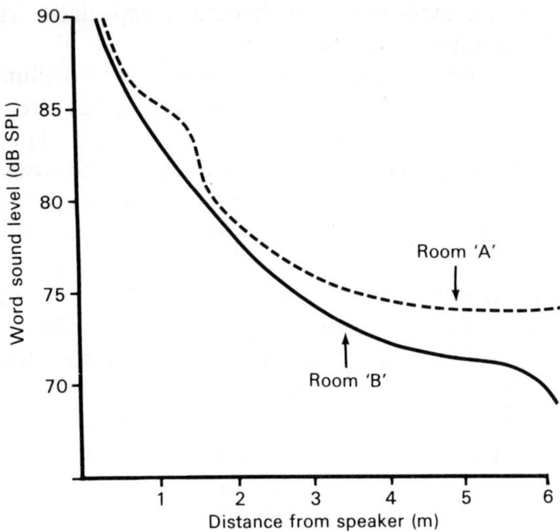

Fig. 14.1. The decay in sound pressure of prerecorded words replayed at a constant level through a loudspeaker 1.7 m above the ground in two separate rooms, 'A' and 'B'. Both rooms were 6.7 m long and 2.9 m wide. Room 'A' had smooth, glossy painted walls and a light carpet; the average ambient noise level was 60 dB SPL. Room 'B' had walls and ceiling lined with acoustic tiles and was furnished with a thick carpet; the average ambient noise level was 45 dB SPL. (After King 1953.)

without encountering any reflecting surfaces the sound pressure decreases as the distance from the source increases. The form of the relationship between sound pressure and distance is given by the equation:

$$p_i = p_1\ (r_1/r_i) \tag{14.1}$$

where p_i = sound pressure at point of measurement, p_1 = sound pressure at some particular distance r_1 from the acoustic centre of the source, and r_i = distance from acoustic centre at which sound pressure p_i is measured; therefore

$$p_i = k_1/r_i. \tag{14.2}$$

This equation is the mathematical expression of the inverse distance law. It is a special case of spherical divergence. Since the intensity of a sound, I_i, is proportional to the square of its pressure, then

$$\sqrt{I_i} = k_2/r_i, \tag{14.3}$$

i.e.

$$I_i = k_2^2/r_i^2; \tag{14.4}$$

therefore

$$I_i = k_3/r_1^2. \tag{14.5}$$

In other words, the intensity of a sound decreases in proportion to the square of the distance from the sound source (Poisson 1808). The inverse distance law is therefore sometimes referred to as the inverse square law. Rayleigh invoked the law to calculate the amplitude of minimal audible sound.

As Young (1957) pointed out, because of reflections from the walls, the sound pressure from a source in most rooms does not decrease as rapidly as would be predicted from the inverse distance relationship. If the law were obeyed the sound level would drop by 6 dB with doubling of the distance. This under-attenuation with distance is illustrated in Fig. 14.1. With increase in distance from 1 to 5 m, the sound level of the words in each room falls by 11.5 dB instead of the predicted 14 dB.

King reported that he had attempted to standardize the test

> by placing the examinee at 20 ft from the examiner. The eyes are shielded by an assistant to prevent lip-reading, the ear under test is towards the examiner, while the other ear is blocked by light intermittent pressure of the assistant's index finger on the tragus. This does produce efficient masking, which is as important in testing monaural hearing in this as in other tests of auditory acuity. The distance at which the examinee can repeat all words correctly is then found.

Despite the imprecision of the forced whisper and the conversational voice tests many clinicians find them useful as clinical screening tests. For example, Søhoel (1956) found that whispered and conversational voice tests detected 75 per cent of audiometrically demonstrable hearing losses in children after otitis media.

A modification of the test which can be performed without an assistant is as follows. The examiner uses one hand to shield the patient's eyes to prevent lip-reading and the index finger of the other hand masks the non-tested ear by intermittent pressure on the tragus. With this method, the maximum distance at which clinical speech tests can be given is about 50 cm. Nevertheless, it would appear that a forced whisper at this distance will screen out subjects with any significant degree of hearing impairment. If the subject fails to respond to a forced whisper at this distance, the hearing impairment may be quantified by an examiner bringing his lips progressively nearer to the subject. The conversational voice test is employed if the subject fails the forced whisper test at 50 cm.

Detecting feigning

There are five clinical speech tests which are helpful in exposing a feigned (simulated) unilateral hearing loss, i.e. Erhard's (1872) loud voice test, Lombard's (1911) test, Hummel's (1898) double conversation tests, Teuber's two-tube test, and Callahan's (1918a) test.

Erhard's loud voice test is suitable for suspected feigned total unilateral hearing loss. The test is based upon the watch test of the same name. The test depends on the fact that occlusion of the meatus of a normally-hearing ear does not cut out sound completely. Experimental studies indicate that occlusion by firm finger-tip pressure on the tragus would attenuate speech by less than 30 dB (Hinchcliffe 1955) (see Fig. 14.2).

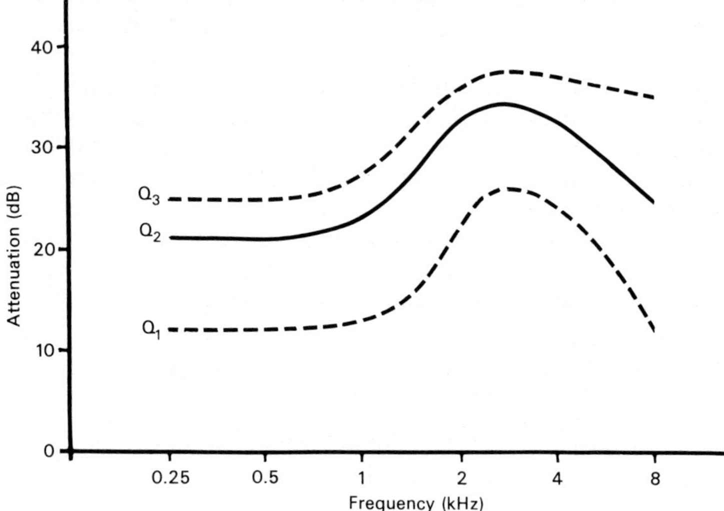

Fig. 14.2. Attenuation achieved by finger-tip pressure on the tragus. Measurement by binaural free-field audiometry. Twenty normal subjects. The lines are the curves of best fit to the upper quartile (Q_3), median (Q_2), and lower quartile (Q_1) values at the indicated frequencies (Hinchcliffe 1955).

The suspected malingerer is asked to close his eyes and to repeat the words which he hears. He is told that the normal ear will be blocked up. The examiner then presses the tip of his index finger on the subject's tragus. The words are delivered in a loud voice to the suspected ear. Failure to respond indicates malingering since even with the head shadow effect, there would be insufficient attenuation to prevent the normal ear from hearing.

Lombard's (1911) voice reflext test is also appropriate to a feigned total unilateral hearing loss. The test was first described by Bárány in 1910. It depends on the normal monitoring of the sound level of speech by the auditory system; the level is governed by the perceived signal-to-noise ratio. Thus an increase in the ambient noise level results in a speaker raising the intensity of his voice, e.g. as in a factory. The patient who is suspected of malingering is asked to read a piece of prose. A Bárány noise box is applied to the good ear. After the patient has started to read, the noise box is switched on. If there is an organic hearing loss in the suspected ear the patient's voice level is appreciably raised. If there were a feigned hearing loss, the normal monitoring would be unimpaired.

Hummel's double conversation test depends upon the confusing effect of different voices giving different messages to the two ears. If one ear is totally deaf, the subject will hear only one speaker. The test is performed with two speakers, each using a speaking tube to one ear. Each speaker asks different questions of the subject.

Teuber (quoted by Müller 1869) used two tubes, one end of each being coupled to an ear of the patient. The tubes were led to the examiner who stands behind the patient and asks the patient to repeat the words that he hears. The examiner speaks into the free ends of the tubes. During the period that he is speaking he compresses alternate tubes. The patient, being unable to realize what is happening, often repeats a word that could have been coming only through the tube coupled to the ear with the alleged hearing loss.

The stethoscope test applies to Coggin's (1879) description of a similar procedure using this instrument.

Callahan (1918a) based his test upon the phenomenon of binaural fusion which is used in the Stenger test (see p. 332). The test compared responses of the subject to speech delivered monaurally and binaurally via lengths of tubing. Callahan used 0.6–0.9-m lengths of rubber tubing of 5-mm internal diameter and 2-mm wall thickness. These lengths could be coupled to one another with short metal tubes. One end of each length of tubing was coupled to an aluminium funnel which was held adjacent to, but not touching, one ear of the subject. The distal end of each length of tubing was 'attached to what was once an ether cone which has been covered at one end with tin. Two tubular extensions are fitted to this end and the rubber tubing is connected to these. The other end of the ether cone is placed over the mouth and nose of the examiner so that it fits closely to the face.' Callahan cites a subject who was simulating a total left hearing loss. The subject responded to a whisper delivered to the good ear through a 4.5-m tube. With a 4-m length of tubing connecting the good ear with the facepiece, together with a 0.6-m length connecting the bad ear to the facepiece, the subject denied hearing anything (see Fig. 14.3).

Determining the nature of an organic loss

Information regarding the nature of an organic loss of hearing may be derived from (i) comparing the relative hearing impairment for low tone words with that of high-tone words, (ii) comparing results for the forced whisper with the conversational voice test, and (iii) comparing the ability to hear speech with the ability to hear tuning forks.

In disorders characterized by *low-frequency hearing losses*, the patient may give a relatively poor response to words such as *moon*, *room*, *rude*; with *high-frequency losses*, there will be a relatively poorer response to words such as *seize*, *six*, *tease*.

Gradenigo (1912) proposed the *index vocalis* as a method for determining the presence or absence of loudness recruitment. The index is the ratio of the distance that a subject hears a forced whisper to the distance that he hears a conversational voice. Ears showing a recruiting hearing loss are considered to have a smaller index than those not recruiting. The frequency pattern of the hearing loss will, however, influence this index. The distance at which a forced whisper can be heard correlates best with the pure-tone threshold at 4 kHz and the conversational voice with that at 1 kHz

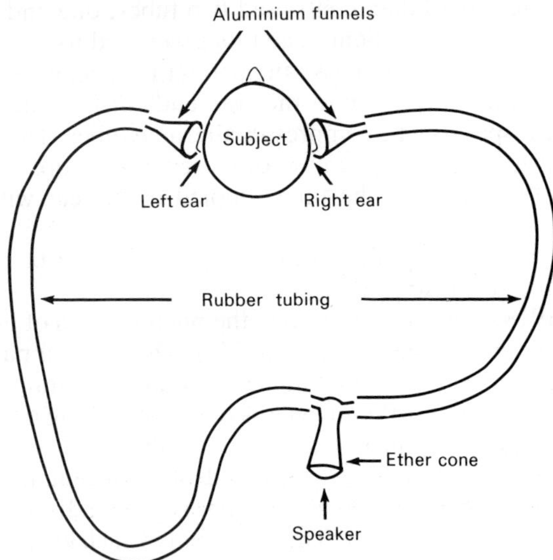

Fig. 14.3. Callahan's (1918) voice test to detect malingering. The examiner is positioned behind the subject. His voice is delivered to the subject's ears via two separate different lengths of rubber tubing. In a normally hearing subject, the examiner's voice appears to come from the ear coupled to the shorter tube. In the above diagram, this would therefore be from the right side. If this subject were feigning deafness on that right side he would deny hearing anything. However, if he were really deaf on that right side he would say that he heard the voice on the left side.

(Hinchcliffe 1967). Because of this dependence upon the frequency pattern of the hearing loss (Fig. 14.4), the results for clinical speech tests may show poor correlations with those for other clinical tests, e.g. watch tests, of auditory function. According to Feldmann (1960), this observation had already been made by Frank in 1849.

A patient who shows a very poor performance on speech tests but whose response to tuning-fork tests is not so poor should be suspected of having a *neuronal lesion*, particularly a vestibulocochlear schwannoma. An apparently normal response to tuning-fork tests but no response at all to speech tests indicates an aphasia.

TUNING-FORK TESTS

The tuning fork

The basic transverse vibration pattern of a straight rod or bar is such that, with both ends free, it vibrates about two nodes (points at rest in a vibrating structure). If the bar is bent on itself, the nodes approach each other at the point of flexion.

In all cases of rectangular bars vibrating transversely, the frequency of vibration (f) is given by

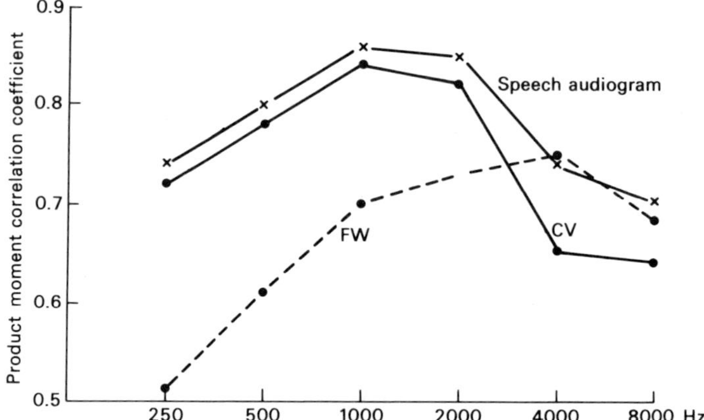

Fig. 14.4. Correlation with pure-tone audiometric thresholds of distances at which a forced whisper (FW) and a conversational voice (CV) could be heard. The graph also shows the correlation with the pure-tone audiometric threshold of the hearing loss for speech measured by monosyllabic speech audiometry (Speech audiogram). Data from a group of 70 consecutive patients complaining of vertigo (Hinchcliffe 1967).

$$f = (kt^2/l^2) \sqrt{} (E/\rho) \qquad (14.6)$$

where f = frequency in hertz; k = a constant; t = thickness of bar in metres; l = length of bar in metres; E = Young's modulus of elasticity; ρ = density of bar material.

Thus, for a given material, the fundamental frequency of a vibrating rectangular bar is proportional to the square of the thickness and inversely proportional to the square of the length of the bar.

Overtones generated by vibrating bars are not harmonics as in the case of vibrating strings. For a bar clamped at one end only ('clamped-free' condition), the frequencies of the first three overtones, expressed as the ratios of the fundamental frequency, are 6.3, 17.6, and 34.4. Rayleigh regarded the tuning fork to be equivalent to two 'clamped-free' bars mounted on a heavy stiff block of metal (Wood 1942).

A tuning fork is produced by attaching a U-shaped metal bar to a straight piece, termed the *stem* (see Fig. 14.5). In respect of medical tuning forks, such as the Gardiner–Brown, it is advantageous to have (i) a disc-like portion of the stem for the examiner to grip between the fingers, and (ii) an expansion (*footpiece*) at the otherwise free end; the footpiece provides a suitable surface of the tuning fork for the transmission of sound to the skull and, at the same time, it enables the fork to be applied firmly to the skull without discomfort. The limbs (tines) of the U are termed the *prongs*, the portion of the fork joining these, the *base*, and the point at which the prong joins the base is known as a *shoulder*. The sides of the prongs which face one another are termed the *inner normal faces*; the other pair of sides which are

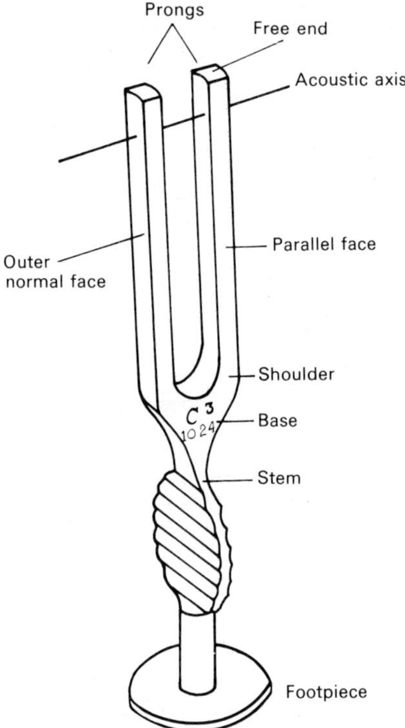

Fig. 14.5. A Gardiner–Brown tuning fork.

parallel to these are termed the *outer* normal faces; the sides of the prongs which are at right angles to these are known as the *parallel faces* of the fork. When a force is applied to an outer normal face and at right angles to it, the prongs are set in transverse vibration, and they alternatively approach and separate from each other. The two nodal points which are situated in the shoulders remain stationary and the *internodal segment* vibrates in the plane of the long axis of the prongs; this vibration is transmitted as a longitudinal vibration, to the attached stem. If struck correctly, the tuning fork produces a comparatively pure tone whose frequency is remarkably constant. Although it is now half a century since, in Britain, the Section of Otology of the Royal Society of Medicine set up a Committee for the Consideration of Hearing Tests, their findings in respect of the use of tuning forks remain valid to this day. The Committee deliberated for four years before publishing their Report in 1933. The Committee recommended, *inter alia*, that the prong should be struck at a point about one third of its length from the free end. By this means, a pure tone is produced and overtones are kept to a minimum. Overtones are more prominent when a prong is struck nearer the shoulder; the first overtone is usually about six times greater than the fundamental frequency of the fork, which is a constant frequency for a given fork. Miller (1979) has referred to this first overtone as the strike frequency. The Committee also recommended that a prong should be struck sharply against some resistant, but elastic, object, e.g. a mass of hard rubber; failing the availability of this, the tester may strike the tuning fork on his thenar eminence, or over one of his femoral condyles.

When testing hearing by air conduction, the fork should be held as close to the auricle as possible, without touching protruding hairs, and such that the *acoustic axis* of the fork is coincident with the anatomical axis of the external acoustic meatus. The acoustic axis corresponds to a line which is perpendicular to the normal faces of a fork and which passes through the point that is equidistant from both the free end and the parallel faces of the corresponding prong (Fig. 14.5).

As with any other instrument, tuning forks can, and should, be calibrated. When this has been done, the capital letters, *A*, *B*, and *C*, will be engraved one under the other on the base of the fork. Against each letter there will be a number. The numbers opposite *A* and *B* specify the decay rates of the generated tone when the fork is used in the air conduction mode or the bone conduction mode respectively. The number against *A* or *B*, refers, in each case, to the time in seconds which is required for the sound intensity to fall 3 dB when sound is being transmitted by air or bone conduction respectively.* The letter *C* stands for what Lowndes Yates (1933) referred to as the *characteristic* of the fork, and which Hallpike (1933) said would be better termed the *stem-transmission factor*. This was defined as the number of *half-intensity periods* for which the fork could be heard by air conduction after hearing by bone conduction had ceased. A *half-intensity period* is the time required for the sound intensity to fall to a half, i.e. undergo a 3-dB change. Thus, if a tuning fork is heard for 42 s by air conduction after it has ceased to be heard by bone conduction, and the value of *A* is 7 s, then the characteristic, *C*, of the fork is 6. This is equivalent to $6 \times 3 = 18$ dB.

There are cogent arguments for calibrating tuning forks but the values for *A* and *B* should now be expressed in decibels per second (dB/s) and the value for *C* in decibels. Further studies are required to determine the optimum values for *A*, *B*, and *C* at specified frequencies. These values should then be standardized.

Measurement of hearing loss

Tuning forks can be used not only qualitatively to determine the type of hearing impairment, but also quantitatively to measure the degree of hearing loss. Rudolph Koenig (1832–1901) had a set of 150 tuning forks ranging in frequency from 16 Hz to nearly 22 kHz (Boring 1942). Both Fletcher (1925) and Hallpike (1927) proposed a graphic method for representing the results of tuning-fork tests.

In measuring the amount of hearing loss, tuning forks can be accurate to within 10 dB, which is a level of accuracy obtainable with audiometry

* The intensity of sound generated by a tuning fork decays exponentially so that the change in decibels is linear with time.

(Lumio and Arni 1949). When used to measure the degree of hearing loss by either air conduction or bone conduction, the 1933 Report recommended that the sound be applied intermittently, in the appropriate mode, for durations of one second, with three second intervals; this would enable the clinician to reduce the effect of any auditory adaptation on the measurement of threshold. Hopefully, the examiner has essentially normal hearing, and can compare the patient's hearing with his own hearing to obtain a measure of the hearing loss. By means of the *A* and *B* values on the fork, the time difference between the patient's end-point of hearing and the examiner's, for both air conduction and bone conduction, can be converted to a hearing loss in dB HL (decibels re the normal threshold of hearing at the frequency tested).

Diagnostic tests

There are more than 20 tuning fork tests available to the clinician to distinguish feigned hearing loss from organic hearing loss, conductive hearing loss from sensorineural hearing loss and cochlear hearing loss from neuronal hearing loss.

Non-organic hearing loss

Apart from detecting inconsistencies in responses, a bilateral non-organic hearing loss is difficult to diagnose with tuning-fork tests, especially if a total bilateral hearing loss is simulated.

UNMASKED BONE CONDUCTION

Should a patient deny hearing by both air and bone conduction on one side, the vibrating tuning fork is then applied to the opposite mastoid process. Should the patient then acknowledge hearing the fork, it is then applied to the mastoid process on the suspected side. Failure of the subject to acknowledge the sound on this side indicates a non-organic hearing loss. The explanation for this is that there is little or no attenuation across the skull for bone conducted vibrations (Reger and Lierle 1946). As a corollary of this, a vibrating tuning fork applied to any point on the skull is providing an essentially similar acoustic stimulus to both cochleae. Consequently, a masking sound must be applied to the ear not being tested whenever valid bone conduction hearing measurements are required. Feldmann (1970) reminds us that Wheatstone* (Fig. 14.6) already knew about the occurrence, under certain conditions, of cross-hearing from the mastoid process of one side to the opposite ear.

TEAL TEST

Should the patient acknowledge hearing bone-conducted, but not air-

* Sir Charles Wheatstone (1802–75) was a British physicist who might rightly be regarded as the founder of audiology. He made notable contributions to many aspects of knowledge, including that of speech and vision. He was generally known as the inventor of the bridge for measuring electrical resistance. However, this instrument was invented by Christie in 1833, and Wheatstone acknowledged this (Bowers 1975).

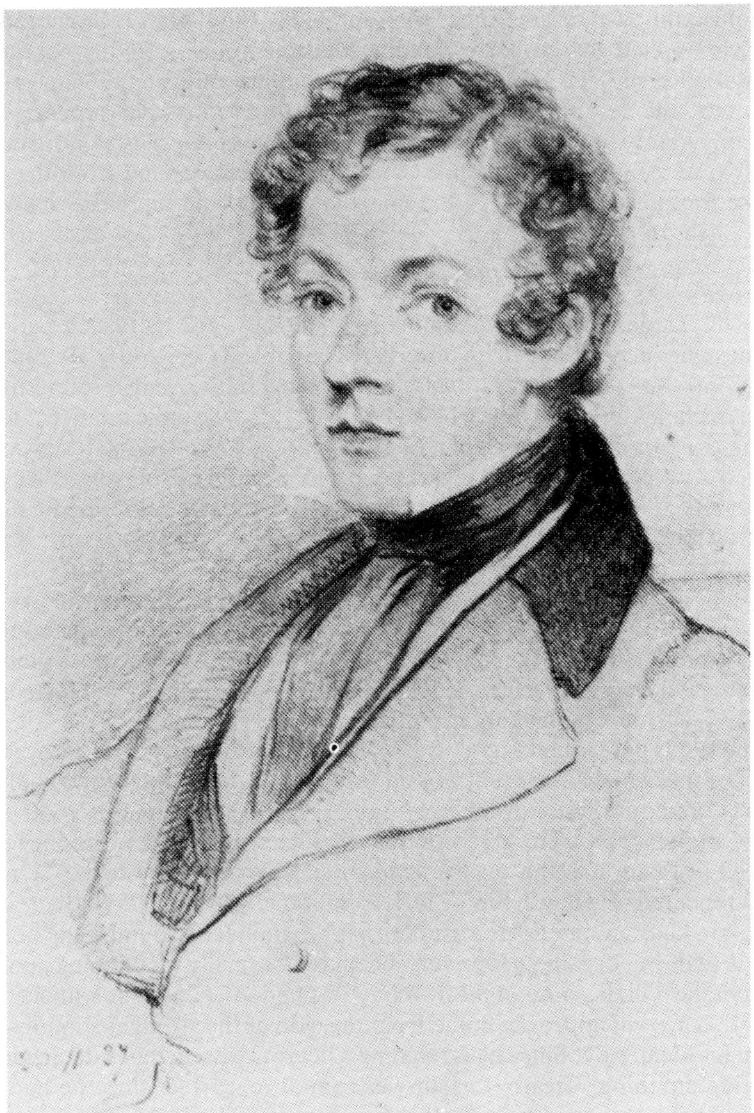

Fig. 14.6. Wheatstone at the age of 35 years, i.e. a year after his election as a Fellow of the Royal Society. (From a drawing by William Brockedon in the National Portrait Gallery, London.)

conducted, sound on one side, use should be made of the Teal (1918) illusion. The patient is asked to close his eyes, the examiner adding 'so that you can concentrate on hearing the sound better'. Two tuning forks of the same frequency are now used, but one only is set into vibration. The prongs of the latter fork are brought up to to the ear to deliver an air-conducted stimulus and, at the same time, the footpiece of the other (non-vibrating) fork, is applied to the corresponding mastoid process. If his hearing is normal, the subject perceives a sound stimulus and, at the same time, perceives the footpiece of a fork applied to the mastoid process. Not realizing that two tuning forks are being used, he usually does not dissociate the two perceptions. He assumes that the sound is coming from the fork whose footpiece is applied to the mastoid process and therefore acknowledges hearing a sound.

STENGER TEST

In 1878, Tarchanow reported an experiment in which he placed two earphones one on each side of an observer. He noticed that, with pure tones of equal intensity, the bilateral stimulation 'fused' into a single sound in the median plane. Urbantschitsch (1881) showed that, when the relative intensities in the two earphones changed, the apparent source of the fused sound moved towards the louder side. Bloch (1893) pointed out that this phenomenon could be used as a test for simulated unilateral hearing loss. The application of the phenomenon to the detection of malingering is now known as the Stenger (1900) test.

A pair of tuning forks (256 or 512 Hz) is required for the clinical application of the test. During the course of the test these forks are separately or concurrently disposed one on either side of the head. Differences in intensity are achieved by placing the forks at different distances from the corresponding ear, i.e. by making use of the inverse distance law.

The test is performed as follows. The subject is asked to close his eyes and told 'so that you can concentrate on listening to the sounds'. His ability to hear a tuning fork at a distance of, say, 14 cm distant from his good ear is confirmed; his refusal to acknowledge anything when the same tuning fork is placed just lateral to the auricle on the 'bad' side is also verified. The test is then repeated using both tuning forks simultaneously, and the subject asked if he can hear anything. He signifies that he can hear a sound if the hearing loss is real, i.e. organic. However, if he has a normally functioning auditory system, he will, because of the Tarchanow phenomenon, hear a single fused sound. This will appear to come from the side of the stronger stimulus, i.e. from his 'deaf' side. Since he is feigning a hearing loss on that side, he denies hearing anything. Clearly this answer cannot be correct since he had previously acknowledged hearing that one tuning fork alone and at the same distance from his good ear.

In practice, when the two vibrating tuning forks are used simultaneously, the examiner would bring the fork on the side of the good ear a little nearer (say 10 cm) to the head. If the subject previously could hear the vibrating fork at a distance of 14 cm, then there should be no doubt about his being able to hear now at a distance of 10 cm (Fig. 14.7).

The Stenger test can be done with an audiometer provided that this instrument can deliver tones of identical frequency and preferably cophasic to the two ears but with separate attenuators for each ear. Frenzel (1932) in

Germany and subsequently, MacKenzie (1940) in the USA reported the use of an audiometric Stenger test; Cheesman and Stephens (1965) showed how Békésy audiometry can also be adapted for this purpose. Auditory thresholds determined using the principle of the Stenger test are referred to as *minimum contralateral interference levels* (Martin 1972).

Bergman (1964) has used what might be termed a reversed Tarchanow–Urbantschitsch phenomenon for monaural threshold determinations.

CALLAHAN'S TUNING-FORK TEST

This test employed the same principle used in the Stenger tuning-fork test. Again using 2-mm thick, 5-mm internal diameter rubber tubing, Callahan (1918b) coupled each end of a 2.1-m length of tubing to a funnel; each funnel was fixed about 2.5 cm distant from one auricle of the subject (to eliminate bone-conduction hearing). Using a principle of sound transmission which was reported by Bonnier (1890), Callahan tested hearing by applying the footpiece of a vibrating 256-Hz tuning fork to the tubing. A normally hearing ear was found able to hear sound delivered in this way at a distance of 2.3 m. Each ear was initially tested separately by disconnecting the tubing from the funnel corresponding to the ear not under test. The tube was then connected to both funnels and the hearing re-tested in the binaural situation with the footpiece of the fork applied to the tube at varying distances along it. With normal hearing, the tuning fork is heard in the right ear when applied to the right half of the tubing, and in the left ear when applied to the left half of the tubing. However, in the centre of the tube in normally hearing subjects, Callahan found a 10–15 cm 'neutral space' where sound almost disappeared.

A subject with a suspected simulated total right hearing loss was tested with the tube coupled first to each ear funnel separately. The subject responded to the tuning fork at a distance of 2 m when the tube was coupled to the left ear, but denied hearing on the right side, even when the fork was at a distance of 10 cm. The two funnels were then connected one to each end of the tubing. The footpiece of a vibrating tuning fork was then placed on the tubing near the left ear. The subject admitted hearing sound in the left ear until a point 1 m from that ear was reached. From that point on the subject denied hearing any sound. Had the subject suffered from an organic hearing loss on that right side, he would have acknowledged hearing a sound the full length of the tube.

CHIMANI–MOOS

This test depends on a phenomenon discovered by Wheatstone (1827). In a normally hearing subject, a bone-conducted sound is lateralized to an ear when its external meatus is occluded. It also depends on the presumption that this phenomenon would appear paradoxical to the layman. The test was first reported by Moos in 1869.

Let us consider the case of a man who acknowledges hearing in, say, the right ear but is simulating a total hearing loss on the left side. A 256-Hz tuning fork is applied to the skull and he is asked 'where do you hear that, left, right, or centre?' If he wishes to demonstrate that he can hear only with the right ear, he may say 'right'. The examiner then says 'I shall now block up that right ear', as he applies firm pressure with his finger to the right tragus. 'Where do you hear the sound now?' Although hearing the sound in the right ear, the subject may think this unlikely, and deny hearing any sound at all. A truthful person would of course acknowledge the sound in the right ear. In practice, the Chimani–Moos test has not been found to be as helpful as other tests for malingering.

Conductive hearing loss

WOLLASTON'S TEST

Wollaston was a British chemist and physicist, as well as a medical practitioner. In 1820 he reported that some hearing-impaired patients have a loss which is predominantly low frequency; others have a predominantly high-frequency loss. Moreover, he showed that these frequency impairments were correlated with conductive and sensorineural hearing losses respectively. Although this is a good generalization, exceptions spring to mind. Thus endolymphatic hydrops is a low-frequency sensorineural hearing loss and a ossicular chain disruption may give rise to a high-frequency conductive hearing loss.

SCHWABACH (OR CAPIVACCI–SCHMALZ–SCHWABACH) TEST

The principal evidence for a conductive hearing loss is the patient's ability to hear sound by bone conduction. This ability has been referred to as *Ingrassia's Phenomenon*, after Giovanni Philippo Ingrassia, a fifteenth-century Italian professor of anatomy who discovered the phenomenon. However, as Feldmann (1960) point out, Ingrassia himself never published these findings. They were published by his grandson around 1602. Thus recognition for the discovery of the phenomenon is often accorded to Cardano

Fig. 14.7. The Stenger test. The subject is tested with the eyes closed. In this illustrative case, the subject, who otherwise hears normally, is pretending to be deaf in the right ear. He therefore acknowledges hearing the vibrating tuning fork when it is at a distance of 14 cm from the left ear (a), but denies hearing anything when the fork is at a distance of 2 cm from the right ear (b). When two identical forks are applied simultaneously (c), a normally hearing subject would, because of the Tarchanow phenomenon, perceive only a single sound source. Assuming that the forks had been struck with the same force, the direction of this fused sound source would be from the louder, i.e. nearer, fork. Thus in (c), a normally hearing subject would hear a sound coming from his right side. In fact, from the perception of sound point of view, he would experience the same acoustic sensation as in (b). Consequently, if this normally hearing subject were pretending to be deaf in that right ear he would deny hearing anything. Clearly he would be lying since he had previously acknowledged hearing the tuning fork on the left side when it had been presented on its own (b). To make the test more convincing, the tuning fork on the left side is moved a little nearer to the ear when both forks are presented simultaneously (c). A subject who is suffering from a real deafness in the right ear would acknowledge hearing a sound in (c) since the only sound that he would hear would be that from the tuning fork on the left side.

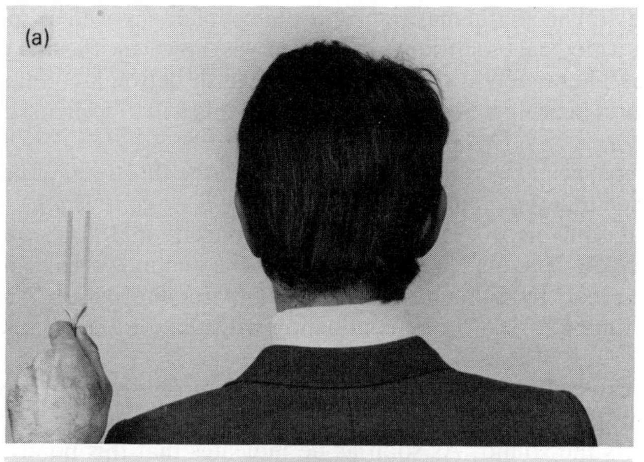

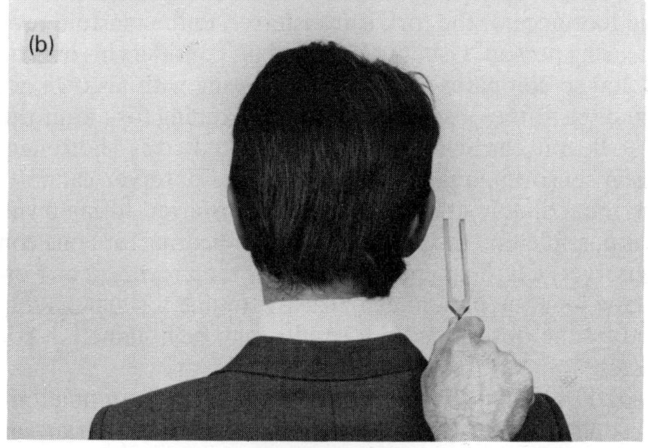

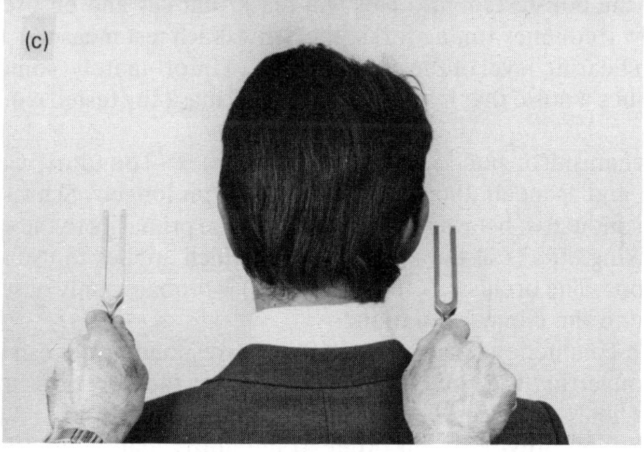

(1550), an Italian mathematician and philosopher, as well as physician. Capivacci, a medical practitioner of Padua, was, however, the first person to employ the phenomenon clinically to distinguish between conductive and sensorineural hearing loss. Further developments had to wait another three centuries.

The Schwabach (1885) test is the measure of the threshold of hearing by bone conduction of an *unoccluded* ear (*relative bone conduction*). It is thus the clinical equivalent of what is done in conventional bone conduction audiometry. As Huizing (1975b) points out, the method was also described as early as 1846 by Schmalz. The test compares the patient's ability to hearing a tuning fork by bone conduction with that of a normally hearing person.

The test is usually performed by placing the footpiece of a vibrating tuning fork on the patient's mastoid process and asking him to say when he no longer hears the sound. As soon as he indicates that this point has been reached the footpiece of the fork is transferred to the mastoid process of a normally hearing person. Usually the examiner considers his own hearing to be normal and so compares the patient's hearing with his own hearing by bone conduction. If the observer can hear the tuning fork after the patient has ceased to hear it, the Schwabach test is designated as 'shortened'. This is the finding in sensorineural hearing loss. If the observer cannot hear the tuning fork immediately after it has been transferred to his own mastoid process, it is possible that the patient has better hearing for bone conduction than the observer. The sequence of testing is then reversed and one determines for how long the patient can hear the tuning fork after it has ceased being heard by the observer. Such results may be obtained in conductive hearing losses.

Because of the absence of any appreciable interaural attenuation for bone conducted sound, the test should be repeated with a Bárány noise box applied to the non-tested ear. This will mask that ear and ensure that, at least for low frequency tuning forks, the Schwabach test measures the bone conduction hearing level of the ear under test. Unfortunately, some Bárány boxes produce a noise that is so loud that it may mask the tested ear (Dieroff 1958).

The mechanism of bone conduction is complex (Tonndorf, Campbell, Bernstein, and Reneau 1966). However, the 'prolonged' Schwabach response on conductive hearing loss is probably due primarily to the exclusion of the masking effects of the ambient noise which applies to usual clinical test situations. The occlusion effect (see later) is probably only of secondary importance in the clinical situation.

The bone-conduction hearing level of the corresponding ear can be calculated by converting the time difference between the two thresholds to a value in decibels using the *B* calibration on the tuning fork.

As mentioned previously, in order to minimize adaptation effects, the Royal Society of Medicine 1933 Report recommended that the fork be applied intermittently.

POMEROY'S TEST

Pomeroy's (1883) test is a measure of the threshold of hearing by bone conduction of the *occluded* ear (*absolute bone conduction*). The value of the test has been stressed by Hallpike (1927) and others. The test is performed in the same manner as the Schwabach test except that the examiner applies firm pressure to the tragus of the ear being tested. The effect is thus to standardize by 'giving everyone a conductive hearing loss' and excluding the masking effects of the usual clinic ambient noise; the latter is the principal factor accounting for the variability of bone-conduction hearing levels determined by tuning forks in the clinic. Because of this attenuation of room masking noise and the operation of the occlusion effect, the Pomeroy test will normally give lower i.e. better, thresholds than the Schwabach test. Patients with conductive hearing losses will show either a reduced difference between the thresholds determined by the two tests, or identical thresholds. Like the Schwabach test, a 'shortened' Pomeroy test is indicative of a sensorineural component in the hearing loss.

The Pomeroy test may also be performed as an audiometric procedure. In this case it is usual to occlude the meatus with the earphone used for air conduction testing. Forty years ago, Aubry and Giraud (1939) stressed the importance of measuring both absolute and relative bone-conduction levels. Judging from the results of studies made with bone conduction audiometry, it would appear that variability in the results of the Pomeroy test will arise, *inter alia*, from differences in the pressures used to occlude a meatus as well as in applying the fork footpiece to the mastoid process.

Intra-individual comparison of air- and bone-conducted sound

A number of tuning-fork tests have been described which compare the perception of air– and bone-conducted sound in the same subject. These are the Bing, the Rinne, the Lewis, and the Federici tests.

BING TEST

Comparison of occluded and unoccluded bone-conduction thresholds in the same subject constitutes what has become known as the Bing or occlusion test. Bing (1891) was the first to report the use of the test for the diagnosis of disorders of hearing although the phenomenon on which the test is based was known to Rinne (Huizing 1975b).

The phenomenon whereby a bone-conducted sound is perceived to be louder when the ipsilateral meatus is occluded was first described by Wheatstone in 1827. The phenomenon is primarily due to the elimination of the normal high-pass filter effect produced by the unoccluded external acoustic meatus (Tonndorf *et al.* 1966).

The test may be performed by either a *loudness comparison method* or by a *threshold method*. In either case, the footpiece of a vibrating tuning fork is applied to the mastoid process. After ensuring that the patient hears it, the corresponding external acoustic meatus is occluded by pressing a finger tip

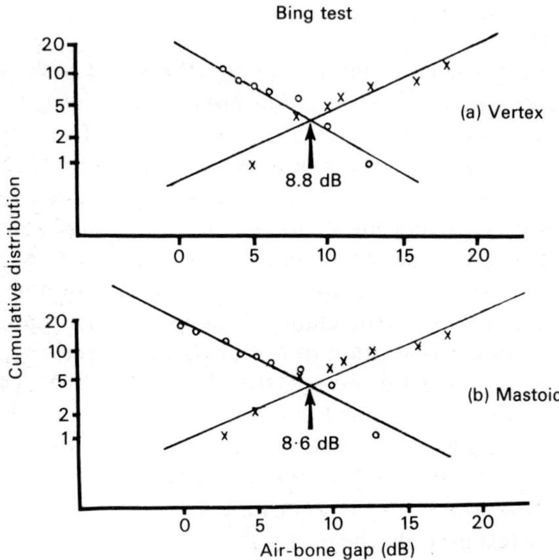

Fig. 14.8. The cumulative distributions of the air–bone gaps at 500 Hz for either positive or negative Bing responses when either the vertex (a) or the mastoid process (b) is used to perform the test. A 512–Hz tuning fork was used for the test (Golabek and Stephens 1979).

on the tragus. The patient is then asked: 'Does that make the sound quieter, louder, or no change?' If the subject says that the sound becomes louder, the Bing test is said to be *positive*; other responses are termed *negative Bing responses*. An increase in loudness after occlusion of the meatus occurs with normal sound conducting mechanisms; defective sound conducting mechanisms, i.e. those producing conductive hearing losses, are associated with negative Bing response.

With the threshold method, the tuning fork is intermittently applied to the mastoid until it is no longer heard. The ipsilateral meatus is then occluded by pressure on the tragus. The patient is then asked whether or not he hears anything. In an assessment of the Bing test using the loudness comparison method, Golabek and Stephens (1979) found that this test could detect conductive hearing losses of 9 dB or more at 512 Hz (see Fig. 14.8). Sheehy, Gardner, and Hambley (1971) say that they find the Bing test more valuable than the Rinne test (see p. 339) in differentiating between a conductive and a sensorineural hearing loss.

A quantitative expression of the occlusion phenomenon can be obtained by audiometry. It is, of course, the difference between Aubry and Giraud's (1939) COA (conduction osseuse absolue) curve and their COR (conduction osseuse relative) curve. Previous audiometric studies by Kelley and Reger (1937) had showed that this shift was of the order of 20 dB for frequencies below 1000 Hz. Csovanyos (1961) has also used audiometry to study the occlusion phenomenon on more than 300 ears seen in audiological practice. The bone conduction hearing levels were determined with masking. Meatal occlusion was obtained with wet cotton wool. The phenomenon was quantified using the occlusion index of Sullivan, Gotlieb, and Hodges (1947). This index is the sum of the differences between the absolute and relative bone-conduction thresholds at 250, 500, 1000, and 2000 Hz. The value of this index ranged from 0 to 60 dB, normal ears giving an average value of 34 dB. As well as the test being negative in conductive hearing losses, the test was negative in the majority of 28 ears with Ménière's disease. The response to the test was associated with the activity of the disorder. During periods of remission, the test became positive. A possible explanation is that a dilated saccule (or other part of the membranous labyrinth) splints the stapes base.

The test can also be done using acoustically evoked potentials (see Chapter 31). An increase in the amplitude and a reduction in the latency of the slow cortical response can be demonstrated in subjects with normal sound transmitting mechanisms; no effect is demonstrated in subjects with conductive losses (Bochenek and Bochenek 1972).

RINNE (OR POLANSKY–RINNE) TEST

This is perhaps the best known of the tuning-fork tests used to distinguish conductive from sensorineural hearing losses. Rinne, a general practitioner in Göttingen who later became a psychiatrist, described all the details of the tests in 1855. However, Huizing (1975a) points out that the principles of the test were first described by Polansky (1842), a Viennese otologist.

In the Rinne test, the patient's ability to hear by bone conduction is compared with that by air conduction. The clinician can simply ask 'Which is louder, number one sound (as he holds the vibrating fork with the prongs near the ear) or number two sound' (as he transfers the same vibrating tuning fork to press the footpiece gently but firmly on the corresponding mastoid process)? A normally hearing subject will say 'Number one sound'; so will a subject with a sensorineural hearing loss in the affected ear, unless the loss is marked; a subject with an incipient conductive loss, or with a conductive component (up to 20 dB) in a mixed loss, will also give the same response. The response in which a sound is heard better by air conduction than by bone conduction is referred to as a *Rinne positive* response.

If the tuning fork is heard better by bone conduction than by air conduction then the test is termed a Rinne negative response. Such cases may be due either to (i) the bone conduction sounds being heard in the opposite ear (in cases of severe or total hearing loss in the tested ear), or to (ii) an appreciable impairment of sound transmission in the affected ear, i.e. a conductive hearing loss in that ear in excess of about 15–20 dB HL. The two conditions can be differentiated by applying a Bárány noise box to the opposite ear. This masking noise raises the threshold of hearing in the non-tested ear to such a level that the tuning fork cannot be heard in that ear by cross-hearing. Thus if the Rinne test is repeated with noise applied to the opposite ear and it abolishes hearing by bone conduction on the tested side, the Rinne response is said to be a *false negative Rinne* response. If the Rinne negative response (bone conduction better than air conduction) is still obtained with a noise box applied to the opposite ear, then the result is said to be a *true Rinne negative* response.

Repetition of the test with contralateral masking is still required in bilateral Rinne negative responses since such a result may be found in a patient with a pure conductive loss on one side and a total sensorineural hearing loss on the other side. Responses of a subject indicating a bilateral false negative Rinne response indicate a non-organic hearing loss.

In a patient with a unilateral hearing loss showing a negative Rinne response, the direction of lateralization of the Weber test (see p. 342) would indicate to the examiner the nature of this hearing loss without recourse to contralateral masking; in practice, owing to the vagaries of the Weber test, a Rinne test giving a negative response should always be repeated with contralateral masking.

The paradoxical terminology by which the normal response to the test is termed 'positive' and an abnormal response 'negative' is attributed to Bezold. As early as 1885, a plea (by Politzer) was made to end the confusion but the terminology has stuck (Tschiassny 1946).

The *validity* of the Rinne test has been investigated by comparison with both otoscopic appearances (Hinchcliffe and Littler 1961) and autopsy findings (Polvogt and Bordley 1936). Studies on a random sample of a rural population in the UK indicated a negative Rinne response was invariably associated with abnormal otoscopic appearances. Exceptions would correspond to otosclerosis. The clinicopathological study showed that a negative Rinne response was associated with one or more lesions involving the ossicular chain in every ear of a sample of subjects who had had impaired hearing during life.

Erroneous true Rinne negative responses may be obtained with tuning forks of frequencies 128 Hz and below. These erroneous responses are due to responses to vibrotactile stimulation (DeWeese and Saunders 1973; Gelfand 1977).

The *reliability* (*reproducibility*) of the test has also been investigated in a sample of the rural population. A total of 75 individuals were re-tested one month after the initial test. Twelve of the ears had given a negative response on the first occasion, the remainder a positive response. On the second occasion, one of these 12 showed a positive response, another a neutral response (tuning fork heard as long by air conduction as it is on the mastoid process). All the ears (144) that had given a positive response to the first test gave a positive response on the second test (Hinchcliffe and Littler 1961).

The *sensitivity* of the test has been investigated by comparing test response with audiometric measurements. Bunch (1941) compared the Rinne response for a 512-Hz tuning fork with the difference between the air- and bone-conduction thresholds at the same frequency. The air–bone gap was taken as a measure of conductive hearing loss. The differences between the two thresholds showed two distinct distributions depending upon whether the Rinne response was positive or negative. The two distributions intersected at a point equivalent to about 20 dB of conductive hearing loss, with little or no overlap. Other reports on the sensitivity of the Rinne test using the standard (loudness comparison) technique have given values, at 512 Hz, of 17 dB (Hinchcliffe and Littler 1961), 25 dB (Crowley and Kaufman 1966), 15 dB (Sheehy *et al.* 1971), and 19 dB (Golabek and Stephens 1979). The differences are not surprising when one considers that different patterns of tuning forks made of different materials were used in rooms of varying acoustic treatment (untreated clinic rooms to 'sound insulated and absorbent rooms'). The construction of the fork will clearly influence the characteristic of the fork.

Sheehy and his colleagues (1971) point to a number of other factors which may account for varying results, i.e. placement (the footpiece should be over the suprameatal triangle), whether or not the fork touches the auricle, force of application, force with which fork is excited (if too strong, overtones may be produced), and whether or not spectacle frames are interfering with the conduct of the tests. A systematic study of some of these factors has been made by Feldmann and Sann (1967).

The sensitivity of the Rinne test can be improved, and quantification provided, by following Bezold's suggestion (Feldmann 1960) of measuring the time which elapses between cessation of bone-conduction excitation and cessation of air-conduction excitation. For example, if the A value of the particular fork used is 4, and the C value, 6, then a normally hearing person would be expected to hear the fork by air conduction for

$$A \times C = 4 \times 6 = 24\,\text{s} \tag{14.7}$$

after it had become inaudible by bone conduction. This period of time would correspond to a fall in sound intensity of

$$3C = 18\,\text{dB}. \tag{14.8}$$

A hearing-impaired person who is able to hear the fork for t seconds by air conduction after ceasing to hear it by bone conduction will have a conduction loss given by

$$H_c = 3(C - t/A)\,\text{dB} \tag{14.9}$$

where H_c = conductive loss in dB, A = decay rate of fork in air conduction mode expressed as the time required for a fall in intensity of 3 dB, and C = characteristic of fork.

For a patient with a Rinne negative response, the results can correspondingly be quantified by measuring the time for which the fork can be heard by bone conduction after ceasing to be heard by air conduction. In this case, the degree of conductive loss is given by

$$H_c = 3(C + t/B)\,\text{dB} \tag{14.10}$$

where H_c = conductive loss in dB, B = decay rate of fork in bone-conduction mode expressed as the time required for a fall in intensity of 3 dB, and *C* = characteristic of fork.

As Golabek and Stephens (1979) have shown, the quantification of the Rinne negative response by this method is a more valid procedure in conductive losses than is quantification of the Rinne positive response.

As indicated by Golabek and Stephens' report, timing of Rinne test responses on a group of conductive hearing losses of varying severity can be used to determine the *A*, *B*, and *C* values for a particular tuning fork. The duration by which hearing by sound transmission in one mode exceeds that in the other mode is plotted against the corresponding audiometric measure of hearing loss. The slopes of the two curves (one for Rinne positive responses, the other for Rinne negative responses) will be measures of the *A* and the *B* values respectively. The point of intersection will correspond to the value of *C* in decibels.

Gelfand's (1977) paper indicates that the probability of obtaining a Rinne negative response in a group of conductive hearing losses decreases from 0.78 for a 128-Hz tuning fork to 0.06 for a 2048-Hz fork. Unfortunately, it is not clear whether or not this group is representative of conductive losses seen in clinical practice. Although there was audiometric control, it is not clear to what extent this decreasing probability of a negative response is related to the decreasing sensitivity of the test and to what extent it is related to the, in general, decrease in conductive loss with increase in frequency. The paper is also marred by misinterpretations of previous reports on the sensitivity of the Rinne test.

LEWIS TEST

In the Lewis (1925) test, a vibrating tuning fork is applied to the posterior root of the zygomatic process of the temporal bone. As soon as it ceases to be heard in that location, the footpiece is applied to the ipsilateral tragus. Lewis claimed that the sound of the fork was again heard in all cases of sensorineural hearing loss and of conductive hearing losses except those due to stapedial ankylosis. In the author's experience this abnormal response is also observed in cases of conductive loss other thant those due to stapedial ankylosis.

The Lewis test would appear to be less sensitive than the Rinne test.

FREDERICI TEST

In this modification of the Lewis test the tuning fork is applied to the mastoid process, instead of the zygomatic process, of the temporal bone. Hlaváček (1968) has reported the use of this test in the assessment of otosclerotics and of the operative results.

WEBER (OR SCHMALZ–WEBER) TEST

The literature consistently refers to Weber (1795–1878) as the originator of the tuning fork test which bears his name. However, according to Huizing (1973), Weber's (1834) book shows that he described only (i) the occlusion phenomenon and (ii) lateralization to the occluded ear. Huizing says that there was no mention of any test nor any suggestion that the lateralization phenomenon could be used to differentiate conductive from sensorineural hearing loss. This is understandable since Ernst Heinrich Weber (1795–1878) was Professor of Anatomy and Physiology in Leipzig.* His principal contribution to knowledge is the law which was developed in his book. Weber's Law states that, in order for a stimulus to appear just noticeably different from a preceding stimulus, the necessary increment in the stimulus dimension must be a constant fraction of the original stimulus.

The discovery of both the occlusion effect and the lateralization phenomenon (for both the tuning fork and the voice) must be attributed to Wheatstone (1827).

Huizing points out that Schmalz appears to have been the first to apply Wheatstone's lateralization phenomenon to clinical medicine. Schmalz (1846), who may well have been the first audiological physician, gives a complete description of the test and its application to the differential diagnosis of hearing disorders. Nevertheless, according to Feldmann (1960), Schmalz gave credit to Weber for having encouraged him in this work.

The Weber test is valuable in cases of unilateral hearing losses, and usually only in such cases. In this test, the examiner applies the vibrating fork to the head in the midline (forhead or vertex) and asks the subject 'Where do you hear that sound, left, right, or centre?' If the patient has a left hearing loss and he lateralizes to that side, then this indicates that the loss is conductive (sound transmission loss) in type; if the patient lateralizes the sound to the normally hearing ear, then the hearing loss on the affected side is sensorineural. Responses obtained with the Weber test should be used only in the context of the results of the battery of hearing tests as a whole; anomalous results are obtained not infrequently, e.g. lateralizing to a 'dead' ear.

The mechanism of the test is complex. When a tuning fork is lateralized to a conductively-impaired ear, two situations must be distinguished (Tonndorf 1976). First, with otitis media, for example, there is a combination of ossicular loading, due to the oedema of the tissues covering the ossicles and increased damping owing to the presence of free fluid in the middle ear, giving the audiometric curve the peculiar shape that was first described by Lierle and Reger (1946). Secondly, with stapes ankylosis, there are considerable phase advances at low frequencies, and some phase lags at higher ones. The cause of this lies in the elimination of the middle-ear bone conduction component and the consequent prevention of sound leakage through the fenestra ovalis. The phase advance leads, of course, to a lateralization towards the involved ear and is capable of overcoming the loss that, being due to a so-called Carhart notch, is still small at low frequencies.

The *validity* of the Weber test has been assessed by comparing lateraliza-

* Two other brothers were also famous scientists. Eduard Friedrich Weber (1806–71) also worked on sound localization; Wilhelm Eduard Weber (1804–91) was the physicist after whom the SI unit of magnetic flux is named.

tion with the Rinne response for 722 ears of a random sample of rural population (Hinchcliffe and Littler 1961). For the purposes of this analysis, lateralization was accepted only if there was lateralization to one and the same side when the fork footpiece was applied to the forehead and the vertex. A χ^2 value of 108.6 with Yates' correction was significant at the 0.1 per cent probability level. Thus there was confirmation of the clinical experience that ears which are unequivocably lateralized on this test also tend to give a true unilateral negative Rinne response.

The *reliability* of the test was assessed by the same authors on 78 unselected individuals from the same sample. These individuals were tested after an interval of one month. For forehead applications of the fork, the initial results were duplicated in 72 per cent of cases; for vertex applications, the results were duplicated in 86 per cent of cases. For cases (about 75 per cent of the sample) where the first test response was the same for both forehead and vertex applications, replication occurred in about 75 per cent of cases. It should be emphasized that these results apply to the general population; higher reliability obtains for a predominantly hearing-impaired clinic population.

The Schmalz–Weber Test can, of course, be performed using an audiometer (Bunch 1943). The bone conduction transducer is applied to the forehead in the midline. Rubinstein and Klein (1957) used this method to assess the sensitivity of the test. They claimed that patients with an 'air–bone gap' of as little as 5 dB could lateralize easily and correctly. These authors also presented a formula based upon the air conduction and the bone conduction thresholds by means of which it is possible to predict the side that will be lateralized. The high predictability has, however, not been borne out by the studies conducted by Golabek and Stephens (1979). These authors, however, determined lateralization with the tuning fork; Rubinstein and Klein did so with the audiometer. Moreover, for a variety of reasons, Rubinstein and Klein rejected 150 of their initial sample of 250 subjects before analysing the results. Since lateralization involves interaural phase (Christian and Roser 1957) as well as intensity differences (Spoor, Schmidt, and van Dishoeck 1957), it would appear unlikely that a simple consideration of air and bone conduction thresholds alone could provide a valid prediction of lateralization.

Groen (1962) considered that the results of the lateralization test were not valid for frequencies in the range of 1000 Hz to 3000 Hz; paradoxical results often occur in this region.

Analysis of results for the lateralization test in four positions (upper incisor teeth, nasal bridge, forehead, vertex) showed that the greatest consistency occurred with a tuning fork on the upper incisors and the least when on the forehead (Golabek and Stephens 1979).

ESCAT'S TEST

This little-used tuning-fork test consists of asking the patient to perform an auto-inflation (Valsalva) manoeuvre whilst listening to a vibrating tuning fork by air conduction. A decrease in loudness of the fork accompanying the manoeuvre is held to indicate combined normal auditory tubal and normal tympano-ossicular function. Absence of any change in loudness will of course occur if the patient is unable to perform the manoeuvre (whether or not the auditory tube is functioning normally) and/or there is stapedial ankylosis (Escat 1914).

GELLÉ TEST

This test is based upon a phenomenon which was first discovered by Wheatstone (1827). The significance of the absence of the phenomenon was first described by Gellé (1881), a Parisian otologist, who also first reported its application to clinical diagnosis (Gellé 1885). The phenomenon consists of the decrease in the loudness of a bone-conducted sound when the pressure in the ipsilateral external acoustic meatus is increased. This effect is found in individuals with a normal sound conducting mechanism. The phenomenon is absent in patients with stapedial ankylosis.

Tonndorf (1976) says that the change in air pressure mechanically biases the tympanic membrane by displacing it inwards (increased pressure) or outwards (decreased pressure). It is the only test in which lateralization occurs away from the tested ear.

By conducting the test with an audiometer, it may be shown that the absolute bone-conduction threshold is impaired by about 7 dB for frequencies lower than 2 kHz. Arnold and Schindler (1963a) adapted Békésy audiometry to do the test. Nevertheless, doubts are still expressed regarding the validity, reliability, and sensitivity of the test. Dankbaar (1970) found considerable variation. He re-emphasized that special attention needs to be paid to the influence of the occlusion effect and the necessity for masking in the bone conduction measurement. De Wit and van Dishoeck (1959) emphasized the converse effects on bone conduction of meatal occlusion (Bing test) and meatal pressure (Gellé test). The effects of meatal pressure change are much greater on air conduction than on bone conduction and negative pressure was more effective than positive pressure. Maximum effects were at 250 Hz; a 6 kPa negative pressure at that frequency impaired the air conduction threshold by 15 to 25 dB.

There is also the confounding effect of auditory tubal malfunction. With slight degrees of malfunction, negative pressure becomes less effective than positive pressure in shifting both the air conduction and the bone-conduction threshold; with severe degrees, negative pressure may actually improve these thresholds, the effect on air conduction being more marked than on bone conduction (Arnold and Schindler 1963b).

Judged by changes in the bone conduction threshold at 1 kHz, the Gellé is an insensitive test. At this frequency, Jones and Edmonds (1949) found that the test was unable to detect conductive hearing losses unless there was at least a 30 dB air–bone gap. Half a century ago, Clarke (1929) also queried the sensitivity of the test when conducted with tuning forks. Moreover, Clark also reported a third type of response to the Gellé test. This response, which he termed the reversed response, was characterized by an increase in loudness occurring with increase in metal pressure.

RUNGE TEST

Runge's test (1923) is also based upon a phenomenon first described by Wheatstone (1827). In individuals with a normal sound transmission mechanism, bone conduction for low frequencies is enhanced by filling the external meatus with water. Tonndorf (1976) says that the effect is due to increased ossicular loading.

Sensorineural hearing loss

If it has been demonstrated that a hearing loss is not feigned and, if organic, not conductive, then it must be sensorineural. A number of tests are available to distinguish a cochlear hearing loss from a neuronal hearing loss.

Cochlear hearing loss

In cochlear disorders there are abnormalities of both frequency coding and intensity coding which may be detectable with tuning-fork tests.

FREQUENCY CODING ABNORMALITIES

Frequency coding abnormalities in auditory disorders became recognized in the nineteenth century. Tuning-fork tests to recognize these abnormalities were also employed then although their precise pathophysiological bases were not (and still are not) completely understood. Because of the nature of these abnormalities they may also constitute symptoms for which a person, especially one who is musical, may seek medical attention.

A classification of these frequency coding paracuses is shown in Fig. 14.9. Unlike other auditory tests, and the phenomena underlying them, those relating to frequency coding have no particular eponyms attached to them.

PARACUSIS SCLEROTICA

Itard (1821) was perhaps the first to recognize the phenomenon of sound distortion which characterizes certain auditory disorders. He wrote: '. . . .

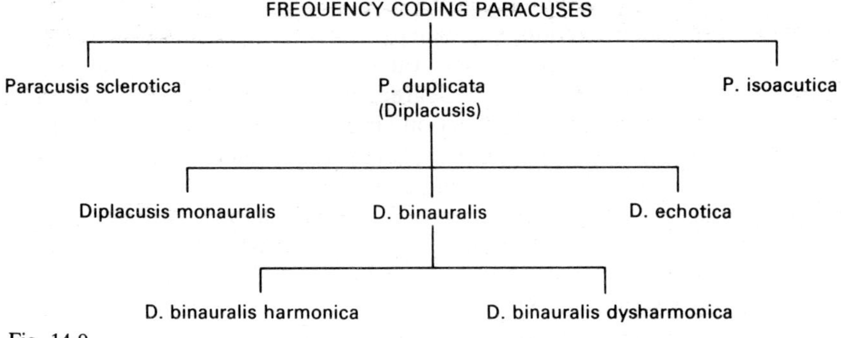

Fig. 14.9.

j'ai pu observer chez un acteur qui vint me consulter . . . Toutes les fois qu'il voulait chanter dans le haut, les sons de sa voix produisaient sur son oreille une sensation confuse qui le faisait continuellement détonner. Les mêmes sons tirés d'un instrument à vent ou à corde produisaient sur lui le même effet.'

This phenomenon of sound distortion is detected by presenting a vibrating tuning fork first to one ear and then to the other ear of the patient. He is asked if the musical note sounds the same on the right side as on the left side. If this form of paracusis is present the patient will say that the sound is distorted, harder (hence the term, paracusis sclerotica), harsher, rougher or out of tune on one or other side. Daae's (1894) first case, a 32-year-old man who had sustained a direct injury of the left internal ear, perceived tones as a scratching of metallic substances against one another. In this case, as in many other cases, the phenomenon was associated with diplacusis.

Clinically, the phenomenon is characteristic of cochlear disorders. Even the cochlear hair cells of *Pseudemys scripta elegans* (a turtle) are sharply tuned (Crawford and Fettiplace 1979) so that P. sclerotica, along with other frequency coding abnormalities, probably arises from hair cell dysfunctions.

PARACUSIS DUPLICATA

This was the term used by Sauvages to describe a phenomenon which is now generally known as diplacusis (Itard 1821). The first of Sauvages' cases 'est celui d'un donneur de cor . . . Lorsqu'il donnait de son instrument, il entendait le son qu'il voulait en tirer; plus un autre son du même rhythme, quoique tout différent, ce qui lui rendait l'ouie double. Ce n'était pas un echo, puisque les deux sons se faisaient entendre simultanément; ce n'était pas non plus deux consonnants, car ils eussent été agréables.' Thus Sauvages clearly characterizes this case as one of *diplacusis dysharmonica*, distinguishing it from both *diplacusis echotica* and *diplacusis harmonica* which came to be recognized by Gruber (1888) and by Gradenigo (1892) respectively. However, from the description, it is not clear whether either of Sauvages' cases had binaural or monaural diplacusis. This distinction was not clarified until Gradenigo's paper in 1892. Nevertheless, from the description of Itard's fourth case it would appear that that was one of *binaural diplacusis*. Itard wrote '. . . car, en bouchant alternativement l'une et l'autre oreille, elle entend séparément, ou le son naturel, ou le son aigu.'

MONAURAL DIPLACUSIS

In *harmonic monaural diplacusis* the affected ear perceives not only the fundamental tone but, particularly when the fundamental is not intense, one of the harmonics also, so that in one ear there is a double and synchronous perception of sound (Gradenigo 1892). In reporting the phenomenon in his first case, i.e. that of a 29-year-old violinist and composer 'with catarrhal otitis media' but 'no symptoms pointing to disease of the internal ear', Gradenigo emphasized its dependence upon intensity. He said that when a fork of middle or higher register is held before the ear, the tone is heard single so long as its intensity is great; but as the intensity diminishes a second tone is clearly heard which is usually harmonic and represents a higher or lower major or minor third or quarter. The interval varied with different fundamentals but was constant for the same tone.

Gradenigo's second case was a 28-year-old woman with bilateral 'catarrhal otitis media' and involvement of the internal ear. The forks 'c^3, c^4 and c^5' were heard double in the last 10 seconds before coming inaudible. The interval between the true tone and the pseudo-tone was harmonic.

Steinbrügge's (1882) case must also have been one of monaural diplacusis since the hearing was said to be completely lost on one side. Moreover, it was of the harmonic type since the patient observed that 'along with each tone he heard also the major third'.

Shambaugh (1940) reported a 25-year-old male with cochlear otosclerosis and stapedial ankylosis who exhibited what he termed *diplacusis monauralis dysharmonica*. The pitch from a 1024-Hz tuning fork appeared to be double on one side.

Gradenigo pointed out that the phenomenon can be elicited by bone-conduction testing. He considered that the site of this distortion was in the cochlea. The precise mechanism is, however, uncertain. Nevertheless, even in normal subjects, as Wegel and Lane (1924) first pointed out, a single pure tone generates harmonics because of the non-linear characteristics of the cochlea. Cochlear mechanical non-linearities exist for both moderately high (Tonndorf 1958; Rhode and Roubles 1974) and very low (Kemp 1979; Anderson and Kemp 1979) sound stimulus levels. Despite his inability to find other evidence for internal ear dysfunction in his first case, it may well be that Gradenigo's phenomenon has its basis in normal low level non-linearities.

Indeed Flottorp (1953) has speculated that monaural diplacusis is related to the idiophonic effect (pure-tone tinnitus evoked by acoustic stimulation). This in turn shows remarkable similarities to Kemp's stimulated acoustic emissions from the cochlea. More recent biochemical studies by Macartney, Comis, and Pickles (1980) have demonstrated the presence of myosin in the stereocilia of cochlear hair cells. It has therefore been suggested that these cochlear acoustic emissions may be the result of actin–myosin interactions as in muscle cells. As with binaural diplacusis, the validity of differentiating between harmonic and dysharmonic monaural diplacusis may be questioned. Interpretations based upon the idiophonic effect would indicate that the presence or absence of consonance would depend, *inter alia*, on the frequencies of the stimulus (test) tone and of the idiotone (Flottorp 1953), and how many of the latter existed in a particular individual.

BINAURAL DIPLACUSIS

Although, as pointed out previously, Gradenigo (1892) and others have differentiated between harmonic and dysharmonic diplacusis, the value of this distinction is questionable. Daae (1894) pointed out that, in a given patient, discordant double hearing may be present in one part of the musical scale, and harmonic may be present in another part. Moreover, during the course of the disorder, the interval between the tone and the pseudo-tone may be changed. Indeed, a gradual decrease in the interval may herald recovery. As such a test of binaural diplacusis may be of prognostic as well as diagnostic value. Williams (1952) says that it is the first sign to disappear in Ménière's disorder in response to successful treatment.

The diagnostic value of the binaural diplacusis test in Ménière's disorder has been emphasized by Shambaugh. In 1935, he reported three cases of Ménière's disorder in which the patient reported that a tuning fork of a given frequency was perceived as being of a different pitch in the two ears when heard by air conduction. In two of the cases, low frequency tuning forks were heard at a higher pitch on the affected side. Subsequently, Shambaugh (1940) reported 43 more cases where binaural diplacusis was demonstrated with tuning forks. The pitch was invariably perceived to be higher on the affected side.

Studies by Jones and Pracy (1971) showed that there is not normally a difference of more than 4 per cent for a pair of tones that are matched to give the same pitch perception to the two ears. In Ménière's disorder, the difference may amount to 37 per cent (maximum at 250 Hz) and, in high-frequency hearing losses, 17 per cent (maximum at 4000 Hz). These authors also confirmed the upward shift in perceived pitch on the affected side.

Binaural diplacusis occurs in a number of cochlear disorders other than endolymphatic hydrops. Moos (1866) reported a patient who inhaled chloroform for an asthmatic attack. This produced tinnitus, impaired hearing, and 'all the notes of the scale from A appeared doubled'. Diplacusis was observed in another asthmatic who took 35 mmol potassium iodide daily for six weeks (Moos 1882). Spalding (1881) himself sustained binaural diplacusis following exposure to factory noise. In the affected ear the sounds from a flute were observed to be a 'minor third higher'. Subsequently, experimental studies by Elliott, Sheposh and Frazier (1964) on noise-induced temporary threshold shift demonstrated an upward shift in pitch for the frequencies 2800 Hz and 5000 Hz after fatiguing at 2000 Hz and 4000 Hz respectively.

Rossberg (1954) reported observing binaural diplacusis in two fenestrated otosclerotics. The tones in the operated ear were of a higher pitch. Bracewell (1966) observed diplacusis as a temporary phenomenon following stapedectomy. At a level of 20 dB SL, all subjects with diplacusis matched a 500-Hz tone in the operated ear to a tone of 540 ± 10 Hz in the unoperated ear. The phenomenon was most noticeable 10–14 days following operation, negligible after one month, and had disappeared by 6 weeks. It is of note that the most severely affected case was a patient who developed acute vertigo on the fourth post-operative day. This post-stapedectomy diplacusis probably indicates a temporary endolymphatic hydrops which itself reflects a serous labyrinthitis.

The experiments of Brandt (1967) have a bearing on the clinical demonstration of binaural diplacusis even when there appears to be little or no hearing loss. In studies on noise-induced temporary threshold shift, Brandt demonstrated impaired binaural pitch matching even at frequencies which did not show a threshold shift.

The clinician must test for the presence of diplacusis since, as Knapp (1869) pointed out over a hundred years ago, few patients recognize its presence.

Albers (1965) has reported that binaural diplacusis can be measured conveniently by an adaptation of Békésy audiometry, i.e. by diplacusimetry.

ECHOIC DIPLACUSIS

On reading the description of his first case of diplacusis, it would appear that Sauvages was mindful of the possible occurrence of *diplacusis echotica.* However, we shall never know whether or not he had observed such a phenomenon. Nevertheless, the occurrence of *diplacusis echotica* is clearly referred to by Gruber (1888). The condition was also recognized by Treitel (1891).

In echoic diplacusis, the true tone and the false tone (pseudo-tone) are separated by an interval of time. The phenomenon is not infrequently associated with binaural diplacusis (Gradenigo 1892).

Shambaugh (1940) reported a 42-year-old male with acute suppurative otitis media and serous labyrinthitis who perceived the sound from a tuning fork as a distinct echo in one ear.

Flottorp (1953) has suggested that some cases of diplacusis echotica, like diplacusis monauralis, may be manifestations of the idiophonic effect. There are indeed broad similarities to Kemp's stimulated acoustic emissions from the cochlea.

ISOACUSIS [Gk. 'equal hearing']

This is a condition in which all frequencies in a particular frequency band are perceived as being of the same pitch. The condition is sought clinically by using a set of tuning forks of different frequencies. Daae (1894) reported the case of an adult male who was afflicted with progressive hearing loss and tinnitus. Examination showed that tones ranging from 60 to 128 Hz were perceived correctly and with equal intensity in both ears. On the left side, however, tones between 128 and 2048 Hz were perceived as one and the same tone, i.e. *f*.̈ Above 2048 Hz, the tones were heard alike and correctly on the two sides.

Bunch (1942) reported a patient in which all frequencies above 512 Hz 'sounded exactly alike'. Bunch considered the condition to be a special case of binaural diplacusis. The condition could of course occur not only bilaterally but also to a similar degree on the two sides so that no binaural diplacusis might be demonstrable.

The condition is associated with cochlear dysfunction. The pathophysiological basis could be the loss of 'tips' of the tuning curves of cochlear neural elements (Evans 1975) with degradation to a very broad tuning.

ALTERED PITCH–INTENSITY FUNCTION

Pitch is primarily a function of the frequency of a tone (Galilei 1638). However, it is secondarily a function of the intensity of the tone. This phenomenon was recognized by Urbantschitsch (1881) long before Zurmühl (1930), followed by Stevens (1935) and by Morgan and Garner (1947), put it on an experimental basis. Urbantschitsch observed that, even in normally hearing subjects,a given tone seemed lower in pitch as it became more intense and higher as it grew weaker.

Gradenigo (1892) reported that his first patient with monaural diplacusis showed an accentuation of this pitch–intensity relationship. The monaural diplacusis affected both ears, the left more than the right, where the hearing was almost normal. However, the altered pitch–intensity relationship affected the right ear. 'The tone of g^2 which was heard normally for 45 seconds by the right ear seemed more than a half-tone higher as its intensity diminished.'

INTENSITY CODING ABNORMALITIES

Intensity coding abnormalities in cochlear disorders are classically held to show themselves in the phenomenon that was first described by Pohlman and Kranz (1924). The phenomenon is generally termed loudness recruitment (Fowler 1937). However de Bruïne-Altes (1946) referred to it as *regression,* since the term describes what happens to the hearing loss; this regresses, i.e. decreases, with increase in loudness. Moreover, to the neurophysiologist, the word 'recruitment' has a specific neurological connotation. The phenomenon may be defined as a change in the growth of loudness of a tone as a function of sensation level in which the growth is more rapid than normal. Thus notwithstanding that a patient may have a unilateral hearing loss for say 30 dB at a given frequency, at 80 dB HL the tone may appear equally loud in the two ears.

CHANDLER'S TEST

Chandler (1958) describes his test for loudness recruitment as follows. The tuning fork is struck to produce threshold, or near threshold, sound in the ear under test. The two ears are then compared by presenting the fork to the other (better ear). Sound is heard much louder in the better ear. The fork is then maximally activated and immediately presented to each ear in turn. The patient is asked 'in which ear is the sound louder now?'. If the patient answers that the loudness is the same, or similar, in the two ears, then loudness recruitment has been demonstrated.

Paradoxically, audiometric methods for examining loudness recruitment were reported at an earlier stage than the tuning-fork method. A manual audiometric procedure for demonstrating the phenomenon was presented by Fowler in 1936; this was termed the *alternate binaural loudness balance test.* Self-recording (Békésy type) audiometric methods for measuring loudness recruitment were reported by Miskolczy-Fodor (1964). The phenomenon can also be demonstrated using acoustically evoked potentials (Knight and Beagley 1969; Portmann, Aran, and Lagourge 1973).

Dix, Hallpike, and Hood (1948) demonstrated that the phenomenon of loudness recruitment was characteristic of cochlear, as opposed to neuronal, auditory dysfunction. In this connection one must distinguish between the 'site of the auditory defect' and the 'site of the causative lesion'. Failure to do this has brought some hearing tests into disrepute in audiological diagnosis, e.g. if failure to recognize that a cochlear auditory defect may be associated with a tumour of, or pressing on, the vestibulocochlear nerve.

A current interpretation of loudness recruitment is that it is due to loss of the 'tips' of the tuning curves of the neural elements (Evans 1975). However, such a mechanism could not account for the recruitment of the conductive element which is sometimes seen in early otosclerosis. A simpler, and more likely, explanation to account for many recruitment results is the one based upon the 'summation' principle (Simmons and Dixon 1966). As the intensity of a low-frequency tone increases, longer and longer segments of the basilar membranes are excited, with extention towards the basal turn. Thus loudness recruitment is characteristically associated with low-frequency hearing losses, e.g. endolymphatic hydrops, or early otosclerosis with a 'stiffness tilt' of the audiogram. It may not be irrelevant that early (reversible) hydrops also has an essentially mechanical basis.

At specific locations on the basilar membrane, and for lower levels of stimulation, abnormal loudness growth may be due to increased firing rate of neurones which are tuned closely around the stimulus frequency (Coles and Johnstone 1974).

As well as being able to demonstrate loudness recruitment, Chandler's test might also be used to demonstrate *loudness decruitment* (Fowler 1965; Davis and Goodman 1966). This is the converse of loudness recruitment, i.e. it is the condition of an abnormally slow growth in loudness. The phenomenon has also been referred to as *loudness reversal* (Dix 1965) and *loudness decrement* (Simmons and Dixon 1966). In contrast to loudness recruitment, loudness decruitment is characteristic of vestibulocochlear nerve lesions, particularly those due to tumours, or demyelinating disorders.

UNCOMFORTABLE LOUDNESS LEVELS

Chandler (1958) mentioned the common observation that a maximally activated tuning-fork produces obvious discomfort when it is presented to an ear with a cochlear disorder.

In normal ears when a 1000-Hz tone reaches a level of about 100 dB SPL* it becomes uncomfortably loud. An audiometric threshold of uncomfortable loudness was first used systematically by Watson (1944). Subsequently, Bangs and Mullins (1953) recommended the audiometric mea-

*Such levels are within the range of tuning forks since, when struck forcibly against the heel of the shoe without regard to generating distortion products, 110 dB SPL may be reached (Chandler 1958).

sure as an index of the recruitment phenomenon. As such, Hood and Poole (1966) emphasized the value of the measurement in distinguishing Ménière's disorder from vestibulocochlear nerve disorders. Patients with cochlear disorders show similar uncomfortable thresholds (measured in SPL) to normal subjects. Conductive and neuronal disorders show elevated thresholds. The measurement has been variously referred to as the uncomfortable loudness level (ULL) or the loudness discomfort level (LDL). Clearly, however, there are a number of such levels. Moreover, LDL is the abbreviation used by physicians for low-density lipoproteins. It would, therefore, be more appropriate to refer to this measurement as the threshold of uncomfortable loudness (TUL).

Audiometric studies have shown that there is considerable variation in the TUL (Stephens, Blevgad, and Krogh 1977). It depends on the noise experience of the individual (Niemeyer 1971) and, unlike the most comfortable loudness level, it is influenced by psychological measures (Fuller and Stephens 1979; Stephens and Anderson 1971).

WEBER RECRUITMENT TEST

Responses to the Weber test may also be used as an index of the recruitment phenomenon. The prerequisite for this test is that a just audible tuning fork positioned on the head in the midline should be lateralized to the normal ear in a case of unilateral hearing loss. These cases are clearly those of sensorineural hearing loss. If the fork footpiece is then removed from the head and struck forcibly before being replaced on the head, the patient may then be unable to lateralize the sound generated by the fork. In such a case, loudness recruitment is being exhibited by the impaired ear.

Under the term 'audiometric Weber test', Markle, Fowler, and Moulonguet (1952) reported the procedure as a method for determining loudness recruitment. However, they commented 'Unfortunately the relatively low maximum output of the audiometer for bone conduction restricts the use of this recruitment test to slight or moderate losses.'

Neuronal

CORRADI'S TEST

Stephens (1974) recounts how Lord Rayleigh (J. W. Strutt) demonstrated the phenomenon of auditory adaptation at threshold to Helmholtz in 1881. Auditory adaptation may readily be demonstrated at high frequencies even in normally hearing individuals. Corradi (1890) was the first to describe the phenomenon with bone-conducted sound from a tuning fork. Historical accounts of auditory adaptation frequenctly cite Gradenigo's (1893) work. However it would appear that Gradenigo's test was much more akin to examining for abnormal fatiguability than to examining for abnormal auditory adaptation.

Later manual audiometric studies by Schubert (1944) in Germany and by Carhart (1957) in the USA and Békésy type studies by Reger and Kos (1952) and by Jerger (1960) in the USA and by McLay (1959) in the UK showed that marked auditory adaptation at threshold is characteristic of neuronal lesions.

Abnormal auditory adaptation may be demonstrated by a tuning fork as follows. The audibility of an ear to air-conducted sound is tested in the usual way with the tuning fork. The patient is asked to raise his hand as long as he hears a musical note. As soon as it stops he is told to lower his hand immediately. Should he hear a note again he must raise his hand immediately, and so on. As soon as the patient indicates that he no longer hears the sound, the tuning fork is brought briskly away from the ear to a distance of about half a metre and then quickly back again to its original position with the prongs of the fork near to the meatus. The sequence is repeated until such time as the patient indicates that he can no longer hear the fork. At the same time that the patient first indicated that he could no longer hear the fork a stop-watch was started. As soon as the patients indicate that he can no longer hear the fork when the tuning fork has been restored to its testing position, the watch is stopped. A quantitative measure of auditory adaptation is thus available.

MONOCHORD TESTS

With recent emphasis on the importance of high frequency hearing threshold levels in audiological diagnosis (Dieroff 1976; Osterhammel 1979), it is possible that clinicians may now retrieve from museums the monochord and the whistle. These are the two clinical instruments which were formerly used to measure the upper frequency limit of hearing.

Struycken's monochord (Schulze 1908) consists of a steel string under tension. In contrast to the tuning fork and musical string instruments which are activated to generate transverse vibrations, the monochord is activated to generate longitudinal vibrations. The frequency of the sound generated is controlled by varying the tension and/or the length of the wire.

Equipment is now available for determining high-frequency hearing threshold levels in the range 8 kHz to 20 kHz and data have been reported on normal thresholds in respect of sex and age (Northern, Downs, Rudmose, Glorig, and Fletcher 1971; Osterhammel and Osterhammel 1979). The means are therefore now at hand for assessing the validity and sensitivity of the monochord and other measures of high-frequency hearing sensitivity.

WHISTLE TESTS

The Galton whistle is essentially a closed organ-pipe filled with an obturator which enables the length of the contained air column to be varied. This manoeuvre changes the resonant frequency. A sound (whistle) is generated by propelling air through the tube by means of an attached rubber bulb. As Feldmann (1960) points out, the Galton whistle was introduced into medicine by Burckhardt-Merin (1885). However, Sonnenschein (1933) considered the monochord the instrument of choice in determining the upper frequency limits of hearing.

LEVER POCKET-WATCH TESTS

Prior to the introduction of the quartz watch a lever pocket watch was used by patients and doctors alike to test the hearing. For some years after the Second World War, ex-servicemen in the USA were compensated on the basis of watch and whisper tests of hearing (Suter and von Gierke 1976). In his text-book on *The neurological examination,* DeJong (1967) says, 'but for more critical evaluation a watch is used'.

Of equal importance to Tarchanow's fusion property of binaural hearing is the property of sound separation. This property was reported by Weber in 1848. Weber observed that, when two watches were placed one either side of the head of an observer, each could be heard separately and could be referred to its correct side of the head. A single watch, like finger friction, can be used to test sound localization.

The ability to hear a lever watch is particularly sensitive to high-frequency hearing losses. The author was recently consulted by a 38-year-old woman who complained that she was unable to hear a watch ticking in one ear. Pure-tone thresholds of hearing in that ear were normal up to 4 kHz. Had the auditory examination covered only that range of hearing an erroneous diagnosis of cophophobia (fear of losing hearing) might have been made. Sweep frequency Békésy-type audiometry showed that threshold sensitivity of that ear fell off above 4 kHz.

Miyazaki (1975) used a watch in an industrial screening test. 8 per cent of 4393 adult male workers in a metal industry in Japan were found to have a hearing loss. The loss was confirmed by audiometry in 96 per cent of cases.

Not only can the watch be used to obtain a quantitative measure of hearing loss (Knapp 1898; Keen 1929), but it can also be used to distinguish between a conductive and a sensorineural hearing loss. Stephens (1979) points out that Astley Cooper's (1801) test may prove invaluable if one is caught off balance by an unexpected domiciliary visit. In referring to the auditory status of a young male patient, Astley Cooper wrote: 'The auditory nerves, however, were perfect; for he could distinctly hear the beating of a watch if placed between the teeth or against the side of the head; and he never had perceived any buzzing in the ears'.

In 1827, Tortual described the occlusion phenomenon using a pocket watch. He performed the test with the watch in his mouth.

A watch test for feigned unilateral hearing loss was described by Erhard (1872) and is similar to the loud voice test that bears his name. Erhard observed that a chiming pocket watch could be heard at a distance of 3 m even when the meatus was occluded.

REFLEXES

In suspected feigned bilateral deafness, the clinician must have recourse to physiological tests. The *cochleopalpebral reflex* (blinking in response to a sudden loud sound) was known to Müller (1838) and used by Gault (1916) in the First World War to identify feigned bilateral deafness. The *cochleopupillary reflex* (transitory pupillary contraction followed by more sustained dilatation in response to loud sounds) was described by Holmgren (1876) and has been used by Ungar (1939) and others.

The *cochleostapedial (acoustic stapedius)* reflex, which cannot be detected clinically, can be detected by acoustic impedance technique (see Chapter 29). This technique was introduced as a test for feigned hearing loss by Jepsen in 1953.

CONCLUSIONS

There are clearly a plethora of clinical tests of hearing which can prove invaluable not only in the quantification of hearing loss but also in the differential diagnosis. Only those tests which can with advantage be used in current clinical practice have been selected for discussion. Other tests have been described, e.g. those of Eitelberg (1887), of Gruber (1885), of Jankau (1897) and of Müller (1869), which, for a variety of reasons, have no application in present day clinical audiology. Nevertheless, it is hoped to have shown that the specialist in disorders of hearing need not feel naked or helpless without his audiometer nor be unable to make a diagnosis without knowing the response pattern of some particular acoustically evoked potential.

REFERENCES

Albers, G. D. (1966). Diplacusimetry. *Proc. VIII Int. Congr. Otolaryngology*, Tokyo, 1965, p. 401. Excerpta Medica, Amsterdam.

Anderson, S. D. and Kemp, D. T. (1979). The evoked cochlear mechanical response in laboratory primates. *Arch. Otorhinolar.* **224**, 47–54.

Arnold, G. E. and Schindler, P. (1963a). Gellé test with Békésy audiometry, I method and procedure. *Acta oto-lar.* **56**, 33–50.

—— —— (1963b). Gellé test and Békésy audiometry. III Findings with salpingitis. *Acta oto-lar.* **56**, 55–64.

Aubry, M. and Giraud, J. C. (1939). Etude de la conduction osseuse. *Presse méd.* **47**, 653–5.

Bangs, J. L. and Mullins, C. J. (1953). Recruitment testing and its implications. *Archs Otolar.* **58**, 582–92.

Bárány, R. (1908). Lärmapparat zum Nachweis der einseitegen Taubheit. *Verhandlung Deutsche Otologische Geselleschaft* 84–5.

—— (1910). Neue Methode zum Nachweis der Simulation ein-und doppelseitiger Taubheit. *Verh. Dt. Otol. Ges.* 109–10.

Bergman, M. (1964). The Fit test. *Archs Otolar.* **80**, 440–9.

Berthold, E. (1902). Ueber diplacusis monauralis. *Arch. Ohrenheilk.* **55**, 17–25.

Bezold, F. (1897). *Ueber die functionelle Prüfung des menschlichen Gehörorgans.* Bergmann, Wiesbaden.

Bing, A. (1891). Ein neuer Stimmgabelversuch. *Wiener med. Bl.* **14**, 637–8.

Bloch, E. (1893). Das binaurale Hören. *Z. Ohrenheilk.* **24**, 25–85.

Bochenek, W. and Bochenek, Z. (1972). Evoked response audiometry in patients with peripheral hearing loss. *Audiology* **11**, 294–300.

Bonnier, P. (1890). *Le sens auriculaire de l'espace.* Lille.

Boring, E. G. (1942). *Sensation and perception in the history of experimental psychology.* Appleton-Century, New York.

Bowers, B. (1975). *Sir Charles Wheatstone.* Science Museum, London.

Bracewell, A. (1966). Diplacusis binauralis—a complication of stapedectomy. *J. Lar. Otol.* **80**, 55–60.

Brandt, J. F. (1967). Frequency discrimination following exposure to noise. *J. acoust. Soc. Am.* **41**, 448–57.

Bressler, H. (1840). *Die Krankheiten des Kopfes und der Sinnesorgane,* Vol. 2 *Die Krankheiten des Seh-und Gehörorgans,* p. 375. Voss, Berlin.

de Bruine-Altes, J. C. (1946). The symptom of regression in different kinds of deafness. Thesis, University of Groningen.

Bunch, C. C. (1941). The Rinne test and the audiometer. *Ann. Otol. Rhinol. Lar.* **50**, 47–54.

—— (1942). Hearing aids. *Trans. Am. Acad. Ophthal. Otolar.* 170.

—— (1943). *Clinical audiometry.* Mosby, St Louis.

Burckhardt-Merian, A. (1885). Vergleichende Ergebnisse verschiedenartiger Hörprüfungen. *Archs. Ohrenheilk.* **22**, 177–94.

Burnett, S. M. (1877). Ein Fall von Diplacusis binauricularis mit Erläuterungen. *Arch. Augen heilk.* **6**, 241–5.

Butler, R. A. (1970). The effect of hearing impairment on locating sound in the vertical plane. *Int. Audiol.* **9**, 117–26.

Callahan, J. F. (1918*a*). Hearing test with voice to detect malingering. *Boston. med. surg. J.* **179**, 423–5.

—— (1918*b*). Hearing test to detect malingering. *Boston. med. surg. J.* **179**, 236–9.

Cardano, H. (1550). De subtilitate. Norimbergae. [Quoted by H. Feldmann (1960).]

Carhart, R. (1957). Clinical determination of abnormal auditory adaptation. *Archs Otolar.* **65**, 32–9.

Chandler, J. R. (1958). A simple and reliable tuning fork test for recruitment. *Archs Otolar.* **67**, 67–8.

Cheesman, A. D. and Stephens, S. D. G. (1965). A new method for the detection of functional hearing loss. *Charing Cross Hosp. Gaz.* vii–xii.

Christian, W. and Roser, D. (1957). Ein betrag zum Richtungshoren. *Z. Lar. Rhinol. Otol.* **36**, 432–45.

Clarke, T. A. (1929). Hearing tests. *J. Lar. Otol.* **44**, 83–104.

Coggin, D. (1879). Eine neue Prüfungsmethode auf simulierte einseitige Taubheit. *Z. Ohrenheilk.* **8**, 294–5.

Coles, R. R. A. and Johnstone, B. M. (1974). [Quoted by Priede and Coles (1974).]

Committee for the Consideration of Hearing Tests (1933). Report of Committee for the Consideration of Hearing Tests. *J. Lar. Otol.* **48**, 22–48.

Cooper. P. A. (1801). Further observations on the effects which take place from the destruction of the membrana tympani of the ear; with an account of an operation for the removal of a particular species of deafness. *Phil. Trans. R. Soc.* 440.

Corradi, C. (1890). Zur Prüfung der Schallperception durch die Knochen. *Arch. Ohrenheilk.* **30**, 175–82.

Crawford, A. C. and Fettiplace, R. (1979). An electrical tuning mechanism in cochlear hair cell. Proc. Nonlinear and Active Mechanical Processes in the Cochlea. Institute of Laryngology and Otology, University of London.

Crowley, A. C. and Kaufman, R. S. (1966). The Rinne tuning fork test. *Archs Otolar.* **84**, 406–8.

Csovanyos, L. (1961). The Bing test in the diagnosis of deafness. *Laryngoscope, St. Louis* **71**, 1548–60.

Daae, H. (1894). Ueber Doppelhören. *Z. Ohrenheilk.* **25**, 251–68.

Damper, R. I. (1976a). Lateralisation of binaural images in a computer-controlled experiment. *Br. J. Audiol.,* **10**, 21–30.

—— (1976b). Tracking of complex binaural images. *Audiology* **15**, 488–500.

Dankbaar, W. A. (1970). The diagnostic value of Gellé's test. *Acta oto-lar.* **69**, 266–72.

Davis, H. and Goodman, A. C. (1966). Subtractive hearing loss, loudness recruitment, and decruitment. *Ann. Otol. Rhinol. Lar.* **75**, 87–94.

DeJong, R. N. (1967). *The neurologic examination*, 3rd edn, p. 270. Hoeber, New York.

DeWeese, D. and Saunders, W. (1973). *Textbook of otolaryngology*. Mosby, St. Louis.

Dieroff, H. G. (1958). Ueber Schalldruckmessungen auf der Bárány-Lärmtrommel. *Arch. Ohrenheilk.* **172**, 281–5.

Dieroff, H. G. (1976). Erfahrungen mit der Hochfrequenzaudiometrie und ihre Einsatzmöglichkeit. *Laryngol. Rhinol.* **9**, 739–42.

Dix, M. R. (1965). Observations upon the nerve fibre deafness of multiple sclerosis, with particular reference to the phenomenon of loudness recruitment. *J. Lar. Otol.* **79**, 695–706.

—— Hallpike, C. S., and Hood, J. D. (1948). Observations upon the loudness recruitment phenomenon, with a special reference to the differential diagnosis of disorders of the internal ear and eighth nerve. *Proc. R. Soc. Med.* **41**, 516–26.

Eitelberg, A. (1886). Comparative tests of the hearing of one hundred persons by means of tuning forks, watch and whispering. *Archs Otol.* **15**, 299–329.

—— (1887). Zur Differential diagnose der Affectionen des schalleitenden und des schallempfindenden Apparates. *Wien. med. Press* **28**, 341–3.

Elliott, D. N. Sheposh, J., and Frazier, L. (1964). Effect of monaural fatigue upon pitch matching and discrimination. *J. acoust. Soc. Am.* **36**, 752–6.

Erhard (1872). Das Gehörorgan als Object der Kriegsheilkunde. *Dt. Militärärztl. Z.* 157–9.

Escat, E. (1914). Applications à la physiologie et à la pathologie de l'audition. *Annls. Mal. Oreille Larynx* **4**, 329–48.

Evans, E. F. (1975). The sharpening of cochlear frequency selectivity in the normal and abnormal cochlea. *Audiology* **14**, 419–42.

Feldmann, H. (1960). *Die Geschichtliche Entwicklung der Hörprufungsmethoden.* Thieme, Stuttgart.

—— (1970). *A history of audiology*. [English translation of the 1960 monograph by the Beltone Institute for Hearing Research, Chicago.]

—— and Sann, P. (1967). Physikalische and physiologische Grundlagen des Rinneschen Versuches. *Archiv klin. exp. Ohren.-, Nasen.- u. Kehlkopfheilk.* **188**, 624–37.

Fletcher, H. (1925). New methods and apparatus for testing the acuity of hearing. *Laryngoscope, St. Louis* **35**, 501–24.

FLOTTORP, G. (1953). Pure-tone tinnitus evoked by acoustic stimulation: the idiophonic effect. *Acta oto-lar.* **43**, 396–415.

FOWLER, E. P. (1936). A method for the early detection of otosclerosis; a study of sounds well above threshold. *Archs Otolar.* **24**, 731–41.

—— (1937). The diagnosis of diseases of the neural mechanism of hearing by the aid of sounds well above threshold. *Archs Otolar.* **26**, 627.

FOWLER, E. P., Jr (1947). Discovery and evaluation of otic cripples. *Archs Otolar.* **45**, 550–61.

—— (1965). Some attributes of loudness recruitment. *Trans. Am. Otol. Soc.* **53**, 78–84.

FRANK, M. (1849). *Ueber den gegenwärtigen Standpunke der objektiven otiatrischen Diagnostik.* München.

FRENZEL, H. (1932). [Quoted by Feldmann (1960).]

FULLER, H. and STEPHENS, S. D. G. (1981). Experimental studies on the comfortable and uncomfortable loudness levels. To be published.

GALILEI, G. (1638). *Discorsi e dèmonstrazioni mathematiche intorno a due nuove scienze.* [Quoted by Boring (1942).]

GAULT (1916). Note sur l'utilisation de réflexe cochléo-orbiculaire pour la surdité. *Presse méd.* **24**, 424.

GELFAND, S. A. (1977). Clinical precision of the Rinne test. *Acta. oto-lar.* **83**, 480–7.

GELLÉ, M. (1881). L'épreuve de pression. *Trans. Int. Congr. Med.* **3**, 370.

—— (1885). Valeur de l'épreuve des pressions centripètes. *Annls Mal. Oreille Larynx* **11**, 63–70.

GOLABEK, W. and STEPHENS, S. D. G. (1980). Some tuning fork tests revisited. *Clin. Otolar.* **4**, 421–30.

GRADENIGO, G. (1892). Ueber Diplacusis monauralis. *Z. Ohrenkeilk.* **23**, 251–3.

—— (1893). In *Handbuch der Ohrenheilkunde* (ed. H. Schwartze) Vol. 2, p. 403. Vogel, Leipzig.

—— (1912). Index vocalis: Sprach-index. *Arch. Ohrenheilk.* **87**, 252–79.

GROEN, J. J. (1962). The value of the Weber test. In *International symposium on otosclerosis* (ed. H. F. Schuknecht) Chap. 14. Little Brown, Boston.

GRUBER, J. (1885). Zur Hörprüfung. *Mschr. Ohrenheilk. Lar.-Rhinol.* **19**, 33–5.

—— (1888). *Lehrbuch der Ohrenheilkunde.* Carl Gerold's Sohn, Vienna.

HALLPIKE, C. S. (1927). Suggested graphic method of representing the tuning fork tests. *J. Lar. Otol.* **42**, 322–7.

—— (1933). Critical review: The Hearing Tests Committee Report. *J. Lar. Otol.* **48**, 114–20.

HARTMANN, A. (1877). Ueber Hörprüfung und über Politzer's einheitlichen Hörmesser. *Arch. Augenheilk.* **6**, 467–75.

HEILMAN, K. M., PANDYA, D. N., KAROL. E. A., and GESCHWIND, N. (1971). Auditory inattention. *Archs Neurol., Chicago* **24**, 323–5.

HINCHCLIFFE, R. (1955). Sound hazards and their control. Unpublished Dissertation, University of Manchester.

—— (1967). Intercorrelation of some auditory measurements on a vertiginous population. *Int. Audiol.* **6**, 63–7.

—— and LITTLER, T. S. (1961). The detection and measurement of conductive deafness. *J. Lar. Otol.* **75**, 201–15.

HLAVÁČEK, V. (1968). Naše výsledky s federiciovou a lewisovou zkouškou u otosklerózy. *ČS. Otolar.* **17**, 152–5.

HOLMGREN (1876). Undersökning af iris' rörelser. Kort meddelande Uppsala läkareförenings förhandlingar.

HOOD, J. D. and POOLE, J. P. (1966). Tolerable limits of loudness: its clinical and physiological significance. *J. acoust. Soc. Am.* **40**, 47–53.

HORNBOSTEL, E. M. VON and WERTHEIMER, M. (1920). Ueber die Wahrnehmung der Schallrichtung. *Sber. Akad. Wiss. Wien.* **15**, 388–96.

HUIZING, E. H. (1973). The early descriptions of the so-called tuning fork tests of Weber and Rinne. I The "Weber Test" and its first description by Schmalz. *ORL* **35**, 278–82.

—— (1975a). The early descriptions of the so-called tuning fork tests of Weber, Rinne, Schwabach, and Bing. II The "Rinne Test" and its first description by Polansky. *ORL* **37**, 88–91.

—— (1975b). The early descriptions of the so-called tuning fork tests of Weber, Rinne, Schwabach, and Bing. III The development of the Schwabach and Bing Tests. *ORL* **37**, 92–6.

HUMMEL, E. (1898). Ueber die Funktions prüfung des Ohres durch den ärztlichen Praktiker. *Dt. militärärztl. Z.* **27**, 515–32.

ITARD, J.-M.-G. (1821). *Traité des maladies de l'oreille et de l'audition,* p. 42. Méquignon-Marvis, Paris.

JANKAU, L. (1897). Zur Perceptions fähigkeit des normalen menschlichen Ohres. *Mtschr. Ohrenhlk.* **31**, 56–7.

JEPSEN, O. (1953). *Studies on the acoustic stapedius reflex in man.* Aarhus University.

JERGER, J. (1960). Békésy audiometry in analysis of auditory disorders. *J. Speech Hearing Res.* **3**, 275–87.

JONES, M. F. and EDMONDS, F. C. (1949). Acoustic and vestibular barometry: air pressure effects on hearing and equilibrium of unoperated and fenestrated ears. *Ann. Otol. Rhinol. Lar.* **58**, 323–44.

JONES, R. O. and PRACY, R. (1971). An investigation of pitch discrimination in the normal and abnormal hearing adult. *J. Lar. Otol.* **85**, 795–802.

KEEN, J. A. (1929). Intensity perception in monaural and in binaural hearing. *J. Lar. Otol.* **44**, 315–23.

KELLEY, N. H. and REGER, S. N. (1937). The effect of binaural occlusion of the external auditory meati on the sensitivity of the normal ear for bone conducted sound. *J. exp. Psychol.* **21**, 211–17.

KEMP, D. T. (1979). Evidence of mechanical nonlinearity and frequency selective wave amplification in the cochlea. *Archs Otorhinolar.* **224**, 37–45.

KING, P. F. (1953). Some imperfections of the free-field voice tests. *J. Lar. Otol.* **67**, 358–64.

KLINGON, G. H. and BONTECOU, D. C. (1966). Localisation in auditory space. *Neurology, Minneap.* **16**, 879–86.

KNAPP, H. (1869). Ein durch die Nasendouche verursachter und von Doppelthören begleiteter Fall von Otitis media purulenta. *Arch. Augenheilk.* **1**, 93–100.

—— (1898). On the functional examination of the ear. With an exhibition of Bezold's continuous-tone series. *Archs Otol.* **27**, 325–34.

KNIGHT, J. J. and BEAGLEY, H. A. (1969). Auditory evoked response and loudness function. *Int. Audiol.* **8**, 382–6.

KRIES, J. VON and AUERBACH, F. (1877). Die Zeitdauer einfachster psychicher Vorgänge. *Arch. Anat. Physiol.* **1**, 297–378.

LABORDE, J.-V. (1881). Essai d'une détermination expérimentale et morphologique du rôle fonctionnel des canaux semi-circulaires. *Bull. Soc. Anthrop. Paris* **4**, 797–840.

LEWIS, E. R. (1925). Observations in bone-conduction and a differential test for stapes fixation. *Laryngoscope, St. Louis* **35**, 109–10.

Liebermann, P. von and Révész, G. (1914). Die binaurale Tonmischung. *Z. Psychol.* **69**, 234–55.

Lierle, D. M. and Reger, S. N. (1946). Correlations between bone and air conduction acuity measurements over wide frequency ranges in different types of hearing impairments. *Laryngoscope, St. Louis* **56**, 187–224.

Lombard, E. (1911). Le signe de l'élévation de la voix. *Annls Mal. Oreille Larynx* **37**, 101–19.

Lucae, A. (1907). Die chronische progressive Schwerhörigkeit. Ihre Erkenntnis und Behandlung. Springer, Berlin.

Lumio, J. S. and Arni, P. (1949). Comparison of the hearing examination with the audiometer and with a set of Struycken's tuning forks. *Acta oto-lar.* **37**, 71–9.

Macartney, J. C., Comis, S. D., and Pickles, J. O. (1980). Is myosin in the cochlea a basis for active motility? *Nature, Lond.* **288**, 491–2.

MacKenzie, G. W. (1940). An infallible test for the detection of simulated unilateral deafness. *Eye Ear Nose Throat Mon.* **18**, 361.

McLay, K. (1959). The place of the Békésy audiometer in clinical audiometry. *J. Lar. Otol.* **73**, 460–5.

Markle, D. M., Fowler, E. P. Jr, and Moulonguet, H. (1952). The audiometer Weber test as a means of determining the need for, and the type of masking. *Ann. Otol. Rhinol. Lar.* **61**, 888–94.

Martin, F. N. (1972). Nonorganic hearing loss. An overview and pure-tone tests. In *Handbook of clinical audiology* (ed. J. Katz) Chap. 19. Williams and Wilkins, Baltimore.

Miller, G. W. (1979). Tuning Fork Decay. *Laryngoscope, St. Louis* **89**, 459–72.

Miskólczy-Fodor, F. (1964). Automatically recorded loudness balance testing. *Arch Otolar.* **79**, 355–65.

Miyazaki, S. (1975). Experience on hearing test with a stop-watch in reference to improvement of practice and evaluation of accuracy. *Sumitomo Bull. Industr. Hlth* No. 11, pp. 30–4.

Moos, S. (1866). *Klinik der Ohrenkrankheiten: ein Handbuch fur Studirende und Aerzte.* Wilhelm Braumüller, Vienna.

—— (1869). Ein einfaches Verfahren zur Diagnose einseitig simulierter Taubheit. *Arch. Augenheilk.* **1**, 240–4.

—— (1882). Doppelthoren in Folge einer Jodkaliumcur. *Z. Ohrenheilk.* **11**, 52–3.

Morgan, C. T. and Garner, W. R. (1947). Further measurements of the relation of pitch to intensity. *Am. Psychol.* **2**, 433.

Müller, J. (1838). *Handbuch der Physiologie des Menschen.* Koblenz.

Müller, L. (1869). Zur Feststellung einseitiger Taubheit. *Berl. klin. Wschr.* 155–6.

Niemeyer, W. (1971). Relations between the discomfort level and the reflex threshold of the middle ear muscles. *Audiology* **10**, 172–6.

Nilsson, R., Lidén, G., Rosén, M., and Zöller, M. (1973). Directional hearing, three different test-methods. *Scand. Audiol.* **2**, 125–31.

Nordlund, B. (1964). Directional audiometry. *Acta oto-lar.* **57**, 1–18.

Northern, J. L., Downs, M. P., Rudmose, W., Glorig, A., and Fletcher, J. L. (1971). Recommended high-frequency audiometric threshold levels (8000–18 000 Hz). *J. acoust. Soc. Am.* **52**, 585.

Osterhammel, D. (1979). High-frequency audiometry and noise-induced hearing loss. *Scand. Audiol.* **8**, 85–90.

—— and Osterhammel, P. (1979). High-frequency audiometry. Age and sex variations. *Scand. Audiol.* **8**, 73–5.

POHLMAN, A. G. and KRANZ, F. W. (1924). Binaural minimum audition in a subject with ranges of deficient acuity. *Proc. Soc. exp. Biol. N.Y.* **21**, 335–7.

POISSON, S. D. (1808). Mémoire sur la théorie du son. *J. Ec. polytech.* **7**, 319–29.

POLANSKY, P. (1842). *Grundriss zu einer Lehre von den Ohrenkrankheiten.* Vienna.

POLITZER, A. (1876). Studien über die Paracusis loci. *Arch. Ohrenheilk.* **11**, 231–6.

—— (1887). Lehrbuch der Ohrenheilkunde. Enke, Stuttgart.

POLVOGT, L. M. and BORDLEY, J. F. (1936). Pathologic changes in the middle ear of patients with normal hearing and of patients with a conduction type of deafness. *Ann. Otol.* **45**, 760–8.

POMEROY, O. D. (1883). *Diagnosis and treatment of diseases of the ear,* p. 337. Appleton, New York.

—— (1885). Otological contribution. *N.Y. Med. J.* **41**, 435–8.

PORTMANN, M., ARAN, J. M., and LAGOURGE, P. (1973). Testing for "recruitment" by electrocochleography. *Ann. Otol.* **82**, 36–43.

PRIEDE, V. M. and COLES, R. R. A. (1974). Interpretation of loudness recruitment tests—some new concepts and criteria. *J. Lar. Otol.* **88**, 641–62.

REGER, S. N. and KOS, C. M. (1952). Clinical measurements and implications of recruitment. *Ann. Otol. Rhinol. Lar.* **61**, 810–20.

REUTER, C. (1904). Beitrag zur Prüfung der Gehörschärfe mit der Flüsterstimme. *Z. Ohrenheilk.* **47**, 91–9.

RHODE, W. S. and ROUBLES, A. L. (1974). Evidence from Mossbauer experiments for nonlinear vibration in the cochlea. *J. acoust. Soc. Am.* **55**, 588–96.

RINNE, A. (1855). Beiträge zur Physiologie des menschlichen Ohres. *Vjschr. prakt. Heilkunde. Med. Fak. Prag.* **12**, 71–123.

ROSSBERG, G. (1954). Beobachtungen von Diplacusis binauralis nach Fensterungsoperation bei Otosklerose. *Z. Lar. Rhinol. Otol.* **33**, 236–42.

RUBENSTEIN, M. and KLEIN, L. (1957). The Weber test. Its significance in assessing the true value of bone conduction.. *Acta oto-lar.* **48**, 266–75.

RUNGE, H. G. (1923). Ueber die Lehre der Knochenleitung und über einen neuen Versuch zu ihrem weiteren Ausbau. *Z. Hals- Nasen- u. Ohrenheilk.* **5**, 306–8.

SAUVAGES. [Quoted by Itard (1821).]

SCHMALZ, E. (1846). *Erfahrungen über die Krankheiten des Gehörs und ihre Heilung.* Teubner, Leipzig.

SCHUBERT, K. (1944). Hörermüdung und Hördauer. *Z. Hals- Nasen- u. Ohrenheilk.* **51**, 19–74.

SCHULZE, F. A. (1908). Monochord zur Bestimmung der oberem Hörgrenze und der Perzeptionsfähigkeit des Ohres für sehr hohe Töne. *Z. Ohrenheilk.* **56**, 167–73.

SCHWABACH, P. (1885). Ueber den Werth des Rinne'schen Versuches für die Diagnostik des Gehörkrankheiten. *Z. Ohrenheilk.* **14**, 61–148.

SHAMBAUGH, G. E. Jr. (1935). Syndrome of diplacusis and nerve deafness for low tones. *Archs Otolar.* **21**, 694–702.

—— (1940). Diplacusis: a localising symptom of disease of the organ of Corti. *Archs Otol.* **31**, 160–4.

SHEEHY, J. L., GARDNER, G., and HAMBLEY, W. M. (1971). Tuning fork tests in modern otology. *Archs Otolar.* **94**, 132–8.

SIMMONS, F. B. and DIXON, R. F. (1966). Clinical implications of loudness balancing. *Archs Otolar.* **83**, 449–54.

SNOW, W. B. (1936). Change of pitch with loudness at low frequencies. *J. acoust. Soc. Am.* **8**, 14–19.

SØHOEL, T. (1956). Acute suppurative otitis media in children 0–10 years of age. *Acta oto-lar.* **46**, 422–38.
SONNENSCHEIN, R. (1933). Fundamental principles of functional hearing tests. *Archs Otolar.* **18**, 599–613.
SPALDING, F. A. (1881). Diplacusis binauralis. Eine Selbstbeobachtung. *Z. Ohrenheilk.* **10**, 143–6.
SPOOR, A., SCHMIDT, P. H., and VAN DISHOECK, H. A. E. (1957). The location on the skull of a bone conduction receiver and the lateralization of the sound impression. *Acta oto-lar.* **48**, 594–7.
STEINBRÜGGE, H. (1882). Ein Fall von Diplacusis. *Z. Ohrenheilk.* **11**, 53–5.
STENGER (1900). Ein Versuch zur objectiven Festellung einseitiger Taubheit bzw. Schwerhörigkeit mittelst Stimmgabeln. *Arch. Ohreneilk.* **50**, 197–8.
STEPHENS, S. D. G. (1974). Some early British contributors to the development of Audiology. *Br. J. Audiol.* **8**, 125–9.
—— and ANDERSON, C. M. B. (1971). Experimental studies on the uncomfortable loudness level. *J. Speech Hearing Res.* **14**, 262–70.
—— BLEVGAD, B., and KROGH, H. J. (1977). The value of some suprathreshold auditory measures. *Scand. Audiol.* **6**, 213–21.
STEVENS, S. S. (1935). The relation of pitch to intensity. *J. acoust. Soc. Am.* **6**, 150–4.
—— and NEWMAN, E. B. (1934). The localization of pure tones. *Proc. Acad. Sci., Wash.* **22**, 668–72.
—— —— (1936). The localization of actual sources of sound. *Am. J. Psychol.* **48**, 297–306.
STRAUSS, P. and ALBERTY, K. (1974). Recruitment in Kalibrierten Weber Test noch Stapedektomie. *Lar. Rhinol. Otol. Grenzgeb.* **53**, 730–4.
SULLIVAN, J. A., GOTLIEB, C. C., and HODGES, W. E. (1947). Shift of bone conduction threshold on occlusion of the external ear canal. *Laryngoscope, St. Louis.* **57**, 690–703.
SUTER, A. H. and VON GIERKE, H. E. (1976). Evaluation and compensation of occupational hearing loss in the United States. In *L'Uomo e il Rumore* (ed. G. Rossi and M. Vigone) p. 360. Minerva Medica, Turin.
TARCHANOW, J. (1878) Das Telephon als Anzeiger der Nerven- und Muskelströme biem Menschen und den Thieren. *St. Petersburger med. Wschr.* **3**, 353–7.
TEAL, F. F. (1918). A new ear test for malingering. *Laryngoscope, St. Louis* **28**, 615.
THOMPSON, S. P. (1878). Phenomena of binaural audition. *Phil. Mag.* **6**, 383–91.
TONNDORF, J. (1958a). Harmonic distortion in cochlear models. *J. acoust. Soc. Am.* **30**, 929–37.
—— (1958b). Localization of aural harmonics along the basilar membrane of guinea pigs. *J. acoust. Soc. Am.* **30**, 938–43.
—— (1976). Bone conduction. In *Auditory system* (ed. W. D. Keidel and W. D. Neff) Vol. V/3, Chap. 2 [*Handbook of Sensory Physiology*]. Springer, Berlin.
—— CAMPBELL, R. A., BERNSTEIN, L., and RENEAU, J. P. (1966). Quantitive evaluation of bone conduction components in cats. *Acta oto-lar.* Suppl. **213**, 10–38.
TONNING, F. M. (1975). Auditory localization and its clinical application. *Audiology* **14**, 368–80.
TORTUAL, A. (1827). *Die Sinne des Menschen und die wechselnden Beziehungen ihres Physiologie und Organisation.* Lebens, Münster.
TREITEL, L. (1891). Ueber Diplacusis binauralis. *Arch. Ohrenheilk.* **32**, 215–24.

TROWBRIDGE, B. C. (1947). Correlations of hearing tests. *Archs Otolar.* **45**, 319–34.

TSCHIASSNY, K. (1946). Tuning fork tests, a historical review. *Ann. Otol. Rhinol. Lar.* **55**, 423–30.

UNGER, M. (1939). Objective measurements of hearing. *Archs Otolar.* **29**, 621–3.

URBANTSCHITSCH, V. (1881). Zur Lehre von der Schallempfindung. *Arch. ges. Physiol.* **24**, 574–95.

WALLACH, H. (1940). The role of head movements and vestibular and visual cues in sound localization. *J. exp. Psychol.* **27**, 339–68.

WALSH, E. G. (1957). An investigation of sound localization in patients with neurological abnormalities. *Brain* **80**, 222–50.

WARD, W. D., SELTERS, W., and GLORIG, A. (1961). Exploratory studies on temporary threshold shift from impulses. *J. acoust. Soc. Am.* **33**, 781–93.

WATSON, L. A. (1944). Certain fundamental principles in prescribing and fitting hearing aids. *Laryngoscope, St. Louis* **54**, 531–58.

WEBER, E. H. (1834). *De pulsu, resorptione, auditu et tactu.* In *De utilitate cochleae in organo auditus*, Chap. VI, pp. 25–44. Leipzig.

—— (1848). Ueber die Umstände durch welche man geleitet wird manche Empfindungen auf aüssere Objecte zu beziehen. *Ber. sächs. ges. Wiss.* **2**, 226–37.

WEGEL, R. L. and LANE, C. E. (1924). The auditory masking of one pure tone by another and its probable relation to the dynamics of the inner ear. *Physiol. Rev.* **23**, 266–85.

WHEATSTONE, C. (1827). Experiments in audition. *Q. J. Sci. Lit. Arts* 67–72.

WILLIAMS, H. L. (1952). *Ménière's disease*, p. 109. C. Thomas, Springfield.

DE WIT, C. A. P. and VAN DISHOECK, H. A. E. (1959). L'épreuve de Gellé quantitative au moyen du pneumophone. *Acta oto-lar.* **13**, 115–21.

VON WITTICH (1861). Ein Fall von Doppelhören au sich selbst beobachter. *Königsberg. med. Jahrb.* 3.

WOLF, O. (1871). Sprache und Ohr. Acustische, physiologische und pathologische Studien. Vieweg, Braunschweig.

—— (1873). Neue Untersuchung über Hörprüfung und Hörstörungen. *Arch. Augen heilk.* **3**, 35–55.

—— (1874). Neue Untersuchungen über Hörprüfung und Hörstörungen. *Arch. Augen heilk.* **4**, 125–61.

—— (1879). Die Hörprüfung mittelst der Sprache. *Z. Ohrenheilk.* **34**, 289–311.

WOLLASTON, W. H. (1820). On sounds inaudible by certain ears. *Phil. Trans. R. Soc.* **110**, 306–14.

WOOD, A. B. (1942). *A textbook of sound.* Bell, London.

YATES, A. L. (1933). Hearing tests: memorandum on the use of tuning forks. *J. Lar. Otol.* **48**, 89–94.

YOUNG, P. T. (1931). The role of head movements in auditory localization. *J. exp. Psychol.* **14**, 95–124.

YOUNG, R. W. (1957). Physical properties of noise and their specification. In *Handbook of noise control* (ed. C. M. Harris) Chap. 2, pp. 2–6. McGraw-Hill, New York.

ZURMÜHL, G. (1930). Abhängigkeit der Tonhöhenempfindung von der Lautstärke und ihre Beziehung zus Helmholtzschen Resonanztheorie des Hörens. *Z. Sinnesphysiol.* **61**, 40–86.

NOTE ADDED IN PROOF

S. D. G. Stephens has called the author's attention to the fact that the so-called Wheatstone–Bing phenomenon was first described by Koyter (or Coiter) in *De Auditus Instrumento* which was published in Groningen in 1572.

15 Clinical audiometry

S. D. G. STEPHENS

It may be argued that the function of clinical audiometry is to provide quantitative support for the qualitative findings derived from the basic clinical tests. As shown in the previous chapter there is an extensive variety of clinical tests using tuning forks and other simple equipment which can provide valuable information on a wide range of aspects of auditory function. Furthermore, the equipment is simple, cheap, and, in the right hands, very reliable.

What then are the benefits to be derived from clinical audiometry? By providing quantitative measures, in addition to some dubious scientific credibility to the results, it establishes a baseline for any changes, improvements or otherwise, which may occur as a result of the treatment or natural progression of the condition leading to auditory dysfunction. It is thus important to think of all audiometric tests particularly in terms of their quantitative rather than qualitative values, bearing in mind the various sources of variability which may account for certain differences.

From a qualitative point of view there are six questions which both the clinical assessment and clinical audiometry are required to answer:

1. Does the patient have some degree of auditory dysfunction?
2. Is this dysfunction real or non-organic?
3. Is any hearing loss conductive or sensorineural?
4. If sensorineural, is the lesion end-organ or neural?
5. If neural, is the lesion in the cochlear nerve or more rostrally sited?
6. If central, is the lesion in the brainstem, midbrain, or auditory cortex?

The more sceptical clinician may question the value of certain of these distinctions, arguing that he is more concerned with the pathological nature of the underlying disease rather than with its specific manifestations. However, despite the fact that various disorders may show themselves by lesions in different parts of the auditory system with, for example, measles resulting in middle ear or cochlear damage, vestibulocochlear Schwannomas affecting initially either the cochlea, cochlear nerve or brainstem, the definition of the site of lesion may help to limit the number of possibilities in the diagnostic quest.

This chapter will, therefore, be divided according to these six functions of clinical audiometry with a description and evaluation of the various tests which are generally considered to be of value in these circumstances.

DETERMINATION OF AUDITORY DYSFUNCTION

The majority of patients who seek attention, purporting to suffer from auditory dysfunction, do so because they feel that their auditory sensitivity is impaired. Others may have problems in discriminating speech under certain circumstances, such as in noise, others may have problems of directionalization, others with tinnitus, and yet others may complain of a variety of auditory distortions.

Auditory sensitivity is generally evaluated using one of two approaches, measuring the sensitivity of the ear to acoustically simple but cognitively meaningless sinusoidal stimulation as used in pure-tone audiometry or by measuring the sensitivity to acoustically complex and cognitively meaningful speech-like stimuli. Loss of auditory sensitivity particularly to the acoustically simple stimuli is almost invariably related to lesions in the middle ear, end-organ, or cochlear nerve, with it being exceptional for more rostrally placed disorders to cause a loss of sensitivity to pure-tone audiometry. A further possible way of detecting impaired sensitivity in the middle ear and cochlea may come with the work of Kemp (1978) on the resonances arising in the cochlea at low stimulus levels which cannot be detected in the presence of minor middle ear or end-organ dysfunction, although for very different reasons.

To return, however, to the most widely used audiometric measure, that of pure-tone audiometry, the reader is faced with an extensive literature on techniques to be used and conditions which may influence the results. Discussion of this dates back at least to Richardson (1879) who used Hughes' Audiometer which, however, produced stimuli which were far from being pure tones (Stephens 1979). He advocated an ascending threshold technique with the tester starting, after demonstrating the stimulus at a clearly audible level, with the no stimulus condition and increasing the intensity until the listener was able to hear the stimulus. Richardson also referred to a variety of factors such as the ambient noise level, the attention and comfort of the patient which could influence the obtained threshold level. These and other factors which may influence the outcome of any audiometric threshold determination are shown in Table 15.1.

The ways in which a number of these may influence the auditory threshold have been discussed elsewhere by Burns (1968), Robinson (1960), Hyde and Stephens (1979), and other studies to which the reader is referred for more detailed discussion.

It will be apparent that many of these factors may interact so that, for example, the comfort and conditions of the test room together with the attitude of the tester will influence the motivation of the subject. Likewise, the personality of the subject may influence his response criterion, the variability of the detection threshold and also learning effects (Stephens 1969, 1971).

Since the earliest reports by Richardson (1879) a variety of techniques for auditory threshold determination have been described generally following standard psychometric principles (e.g. Guilford 1954). Since 1947, when Békésy developed his semi-automatic audiometer, the use of this tracking procedure has become popular both in clinical and in industrial hearing

TABLE 15.1. *Sources of variance in audiometric testing*

Room	Noise levels	
	Temperature	
	Reverberation	
	Ventilation	
Equipment	Calibration	– frequency
		– intensity
		– standard used
	Stimulus	rise/fall times
	Distortion	
	Stimulus duration	
	Voltage stability	
	Intermittent faults	– leads etc.
	Earphone	– circumaural
		– Supra aural – hard cushion
		– soft cushion
		– insert type
		– maximum output levels
Tester	Attention	
	Response criteria	
	Motivation	
	Personality	– interpretation
		– expectancy bias
Test technique	Ascending/descending/hybrid	
	Stimulus duration	
	Manual/semi-automatic	
	Response indicating method adopted	
	Instructions	
	Interstimulus intervals	
Earphone/subject Interaction	Comfort	
	Leak	
	Standing waves	
Subject	Motivation	
	Comprehension of instructions	
	Judgemental criteria	
	Detection variance	
	Learning effect	
	Personality	
	Circadian effects	
	Attention	
	Comfort	
	Fatigue	
	Colds	
	Wax, TTS, etc.	
	Real fluctuations in hearing level	
Tester/subject Interaction		

measurement procedures. Other approaches have derived from the development of signal detection theory in psychophysics, and a logical extension of this recently has been the application of adaptive techniques. Such techniques are particularly suitable to on-line computer administered audiometry which should come to have an increasingly important role over the next decade or two.

Despite this, at the present time manual audiometry still remains the most extensively used in clinical practice. A variety of techniques have been used for this, and a recent study by Bassom (1974) has indicated that from the point of threshold sensitivity and of intrasubject variance, there is little to choose between a variety of these techniques. The approach most commonly used in the United States and also quite extensively in Europe is that advocated by Hughson and Westlake (1944). Like most approaches this follows a 50 per cent correct response criterion for determination of the threshold level. Also like several other approaches it brackets around the threshold but takes only points in increasing intensity as determinants of the 'true' threshold level, thus reducing the problem of 'false positive' responses commonly found with descending techniques.

Techniques such as that developed by Hughson and Westlake (1944) are essential in clinical audiometry which is generally based on audiometers with 5-dB steps. They allow a method-of-limits approach to be used and if necessary an extrapolation technique may be applied to determine a more precise threshold between the 5-dB steps. The Hughson–Westlake technique differs from method of limits technique in that, although the procedure brackets around the threshold, the actual determination is based on ascending responses alone rather than on a mean of ascending and descending responses.

Table 15.2 shows the median intrasubject variance found with this technique in two groups of experimentally naïve subjects, a group of 24 naval ratings and a group of 12 Cambridge housewives (Stephens 1969). Similar results have been found with self-recording or Békésy audiometry (Delany 1970) and which also show the smallest variance around 1000 Hz. This may be attributed to earphone leak effects which increase the variance at low frequencies, and critical aspects of earphone position at the higher frequencies with the nodes and antinodes of standing waves in the external acoustic meatus.

TABLE 15.2. *Median intrasubject threshold variance* (dB^2) *for two groups of subjects using the Hughson–Westlake technique. Group A,* $n=24$; *Group B* $n=12$. (From Stephens 1969)

	Frequency (Hz) 250	1000	4000	8000
Group A	7.6	5.1	7.1	23.7
Group B	8.5	4.8	8.3	14.6

Although giving similar results in terms of the intrasubject variance, manual and Békésy techniques differ in their absolute threshold sensitivity (Burns and Hinchcliffe 1957; Robinson and Whittle 1973). The latter study indicates that thresholds determined by Békésy audiometry are approximately 3 dB more sensitive than those found by manual audiometry.

In any threshold determination, if there is an interaural disparity in threshold sensitivity, masking is essential. Masking entails administering a noise to the non-test ear to ensure that the stimulus presented to the test ear is heard only when that ear is being tested. This is particularly important in the definition of conductive hearing losses and will be discussed in more length in that section.

Thresholds may be determined for speech stimuli as well as for pure tones. This is of considerable relevance in certain individuals such as those with brain tumours who find it difficult to respond to non-speech stimuli, and also in certain young patients with non-organic hearing loss. This latter group will be discussed further in the next section.

The materials used for the determination of speech thresholds differ in different countries and, with divergent materials there is some variation in sensitivity in addition to the problems which arise with regard to the calibration of speech material. All techniques are normally based, as with pure-tone thresholds, on a 50 per cent criterion, although certain patients with *severe* sensorineural hearing losses may never reach a 50 per cent discrimination score.

The materials most commonly used for the determination of speech thresholds are spondees or bisyllables (USA and Sweden), digits (Denmark), and monosyllables (UK and France). As with the determination of pure-tone thresholds, various techniques may be used, but in practice these seem to make little difference. The most sensitive thresholds are obtained with digits (highest redundancy) and the least sensitive with monosyllables (lowest redundancy).

Speech thresholds are important in that, in addition to patients who cannot or will not respond to pure-tone stimuli, others with cerebellopontine angle tumours or brainstem lesions may have normal thresholds for pure tones but grossly elevated thresholds for speech material. This is discussed further in the context of separating end-organ from neural disorders.

Other patients, while having normal thresholds and sensitivity to standard speech material may complain of poor discrimination of speech in difficult listening conditions such as in a background of noise or other voices. This may be related to subclinical end-organ damage in some cases (Evans 1979), but in many others may be related to central auditory dysfunction and an extension of the 'minimal brain damage' syndrome to adults. Such individuals will often then perform badly at sensitized or low redundancy speech measures (speech in noise, competing messages, etc.) which are commonly used in tests of central auditory function.

Other patients with disorders of central auditory function particularly at a brainstem level may show normal sensitivity but impaired directionalizational ability. This will arise from the fact that the brainstem is unable to integrate adequately the input from the two ears.

Certain individuals with mild 'subclinical' cochlear damage, such as Ménière's disorder in a remission phase, may clinically demonstrate this only by the presence of diplacusis binauralis. Although this is classically demonstrated using a tuning fork, valuable quantitative measures may be obtained using frequency matching procedures, most simply performed using an audiometer with two separate oscillators. It is in these cases, essential to monitor the output frequency of each channel using a frequency counter.

REAL OR NON-ORGANIC HEARING LOSS

The clinician often obtains useful clues as to whether or not a patient may have a non-organic hearing loss from informed observations, from inconsistencies in the anamnesis (or case history) and from his clinical examination of the patient. He should also be particularly alert to the possibility in certain patient groups—compensation cases, the military, teenage children.

The role of the audiometric investigations in such patients will be to support or confirm his suspicions and to give an indication as to the patient's true hearing sensitivity. Indeed approximately 50 per cent of patients with non-organic hearing loss have an abnormally elevated 'real' threshold which is then consciously or subconsciously further elevated. In some of these patients this non-organic 'overlay' may not have been suspected from the clinical observations and carefully performed audiometric tests may give valuable information in such cases.

Most of the basic clinical tests for non-organic hearing loss have been discussed in Chapter 9. In addition to the tuning fork tests (e.g. Teal and Stenger) and other approaches such as the Lombard effect, further clues may be derived from behaviour such as perfect understanding of speech when the patient is able to see the lips of the speaker and no discrimination or hearing whatsoever in the absence of such speech-reading (lip-reading). This is obviously impossible as only about 40 per cent of speech articulations are visible on the lips. Again with patients claiming a unilateral loss, useful pointers may be obtained from whispered questions posed while the 'good' ear is being examined with Siegle's speculum. In cases of a 'genuine' hearing loss the sound of the air emerging from the speculum should mask the 'good' ear so soft questions would only be heard in the 'deaf' ear.

From an audiometric standpoint, pure-tone audiometry may often indicate a flat bilateral sensorineural hearing loss of 60–70 dB as this corresponds well to the subject's most comfortable listening level. The audiometric threshold may show marked variability on repeated testing with differences of 20 dB or more between successive measures at the same frequency. As may be deduced from Table 15.2 this will be well outside the 99 per cent confidence interval normally expected, particularly in the speech frequencies.

Should a discrepancy be found between the two ears, a denial of the transcranial transmission effect can give further evidence of a non-organic lesion. Thus an unmasked right–left difference by air conduction cannot normally exceed 60 dB and by bone conduction rarely 10 dB. These unilateral losses are also very amenable to testing by the audiometric version of Stenger's (1900) test. The tuning-fork test has been described in some detail by Hinchcliffe and is based on the fact that when the same signal is presented simultaneously to the two ears and the subjective intensity in one ear exceeds that in the other ear by more than 10 dB, the sound is heard only as if it is in the 'louder' ear. Hence presenting the signal at 5 dB below the admitted threshold to the 'bad' ear of a patient and 5 dB above the threshold of the 'good' ear, if the difference between the two ears claimed by the subject is genuine, it will be heard in the 'good' ear. If the 'bad' ear threshold is in fact more sensitive than admitted, the patient will hear the sound only in his 'bad' ear and will deny hearing a signal even though one is present as a suprathreshold level in his 'good' ear. Then by further reducing the stimulus level in his 'bad' ear an approximate threshold may be determined by finding the highest intensity presented to the 'bad' ear at which the sound is claimed to be heard in the 'good' ear. At this level it may be taken that such an intensity is within 10 dB of the 'true' threshold provided that the threshold for the 'good' ear is genuine. Problems with this technique may be caused by diplacusis binauralis and other distortions which may be found when the patient is exaggerating co-existent cochlear damage in the 'bad' ear. In cases of diplacusis binauralis the intracranial fusion of the sound inputs will not occur in the normal way.

The test may be performed using most clinical audiometers which have two output channels from a single oscillator, and which can be switched on simultaneously. A non-synchronous onset can provide useful clues to the listener and may invalidate the results.

The Stenger test may also be performed using Békésy Audiometry (Cheesman and Stephens 1965; Watson and Voots 1964). Békésy audiometry may also be useful as an indicator test for non-organic hearing loss in patients with bilateral hearing losses, often showing the 'Type V' audiogram of Jerger and Herer (1961). In this 'Type V' audiogram, the threshold for the interrupted signal is plotted as less sensitive than that for the continuous signal, in contrast to the Jerger Type II–IV audiogram in which the converse occurs. The mechanism in this case seems to stem from an aspect of the temporal summation of loudness by which a suprathreshold interrupted tone is heard as less loud than a continuous tone. This is reflected in the differential aspects of the plotted most comfortable (Ventry, Woods, Rubin, and Hill 1971) and uncomfortable loudness level (Stephens and Anderson 1971) measures, in which the responses to interrupted signals occur at intensities about 5 dB greater than those to continuous signals.

Coles and Priede (1972) have claimed that about 60 per cent of their patients with non-organic hearing loss showed a Type V Békésy response. The author's experience with more sophisticated equipment, however, suggests that this may be a more common finding among such patients. However, even so this technique is useful only as an indicator of non-organic hearing loss and not as a measure of the real hearing level, and hence is of little value in those patients in whom a non-organic loss has already been demonstrated.

In a number of such patients, and particularly among adolescents, speech audiometry may be useful in defining the real threshold. In many patients, carefully performed speech audiometry may show essentially normal thresholds despite persistently elevated results with pure tones. This may be related to the difficulty for the patient to determine a fixed reference level with the continuously varying speech material particularly when the Fournier technique (Coles, Markides, and Priede 1973) is used. By means of this technique, which involves stimulus presentation at levels descending in large steps and ascending in small steps so as to confuse further the subject's idea of a reference level, reliable speech thresholds may often be obtained provided that the patient is prepared to respond at all. Such false non-responders may sometimes be detected by judicious use of the intercom system turned up to maximum level, as sometimes the patient is unable to prevent himself from softly whispering the words which he clearly hears at the level at which he feels the tester will not detect. Other suggestive evidence of non-organic hearing loss in speech audiometry may come from the response patterns in which the subject may, for example, respond accurately to every third word not responding at all to the intervening words, by always missing either the first or last phonemes from the target words, or by going from a 100 per cent correct detection level to a 0 per cent with an intensity change of only 5 dB.

More recently, electroacoustic impedance techniques based on acoustic reflex threshold (ART) measures have obtained some popularity in the detection of non-organic hearing loss and in estimating the 'true' threshold. The initial approach was based on the simple concept that it was impossible for a patient to have an acoustic reflex threshold at a level more sensitive than his subjective threshold. Thus if a patient gave a subjective threshold in one ear of 100 dB and his acoustic reflex threshold in that ear was 80 dB, the subjective threshold was obviously called into question.

A more sophisticated approach stems essentially from the work of Niemeyer and Sesterhenn (1974) who showed that while the ART for broad-band noise is approximately 15 dB more sensitive than that of a 1000-Hz tone when both are expressed in terms of SPL, this difference is reduced when cochlear pathology is present. These authors and other subsequent workers proposed ways of calculating the 'true' threshold from the pure tone. Wide band noise vs tone ART differences in these cases were proposed as a means of calculating the 'true' loss, but unfortunately the variance of these predictions is somewhat high. Johnsen, Osterhammel, Terkildsen, Osterhammel and Huis in't Velt (1976) have suggested that better predictions may be based on a consideration of the absolute level of the ART for a wide band noise alone, but this too exhibits considerable variability. More recently Sesterhenn and Breuninger (1977) have proposed a different method based on the potentiation of one tonal ART by the low level presentation of a tone at another frequency, and this may prove to be of value when more normative data are available. Other approaches such as the reflex relaxation index of Norris, Stelmachowicz, and Taylor (1974) and measures based on temporal summation of the ART have proved somewhat variable in this context. It should further be emphasized that such measures are only obtainable in fundamentally normally hearing subjects or in those with a non-organic overlay to an end-organ disorder.

With the advent of the averaging computer in the audiology department auditory electrophysiological measures have been widely applied to the detection of non-organic hearing loss and to the determination of the 'true' thresholds in such patients. These measures have been extensively described elsewhere in this book (Chapters 26 and 40) and most have been applied to this context at one time or another. Of all the measures, that which has best stood the test of time in non-organic hearing loss is the slow vertex response. This measure has the advantages of being a large voltage response (approximately 30 μV), frequency specific, and derived from the rostral end of the auditory pathway. Even in English legal practice it has come to be regarded as an effective indication of the patient's 'true' level of auditory function, although it presumably cannot incorporate the cognitive aspects of the stimulus in the same way as the contingent negative variation (CNV) based measures might. However, the latter have not yet been applied in this context.

Many studies have shown that in co-operative adult subjects the audiometric threshold determined by means of the slow vertex response approximates to ± 10 dB of the subjective threshold. Use of this technique in patients with suspected or proven non-organic hearing loss is usually based on the premise that this holds true for such patients as well.

CONDUCTIVE VERSUS SENSORINEURAL HEARING LOSS

The qualitative decision as to whether a patient has a conductive or sensorineural hearing loss is generally made by the clinician on the basis of his otoscopic examination and tuning-fork tests. In patients with 'pure' conductive or sensorineural hearing loss such a decision really requires little audiometric confirmation. In patients with mixed hearing losses, however, it may be useful to determine the relative sensorineural and conductive components so as to derive some estimation of the maximum benefit which could result from surgical intervention or the amplification which might be needed in prosthetic (hearing aid) management of the patient. In addition electroacoustic impedance measures may provide some evidence as to the nature of the underlying lesion.

Some of the early diagnostic audiometric tests such as the intensity difference limens and the alternate binaural loudness balance were developed basically to differentiate between conductive and 'sensorineural' (i.e. end-organ) hearing loss, although this function disappeared with the advent of better calibrated air and bone conduction measures and with electroacoustic impedance measuring devices. It is important, however, to remember this historical origin of these tests in any consideration of their shortcomings in the differentiation of end-organ and neural disorders.

Bone conduction audiometry has been available since before the Second World War (e.g. Bárány, 1938) but one of its major problems for many years stemmed from the problems entailed in the calibration of the output. This difficulty has in the past been overcome by the development of adequate artificial mastoids (see Chapter 8) but still there is controversy as to the basic units of calibration, whether the basic reference should be in terms of acceleration or of force. Furthermore, Lightfoot and Hoare (1979) have recently shown significant discrepancies between different vibrators calibrated on different devices.

In addition there are considerable methodological problems with bone-conduction audiometry. Mastoid placement of the vibrator can result in considerable intrasubject variance problems on repeated testing. It also has the disadvantage of giving the clinician or tester a false sense of laterality. Thus forehead placement of the vibrator is to be recommended partly on the grounds of the lower variance involved and partly on the basis that it will ensure that the tester masks the non-test ear. Because of the transcranial transmission characteristics of bone conducted sound, which in certain patients with asymmetrical skulls may be more intense in the ear furthest from the vibrator, an unmasked bone-conduction measure is at best valueless.* It is to be hoped, however, that with developments and standardization of calibration techniques and the refinement of bone-conduction vibrators over the next few years, the technique will come to have the value which many of its users assume it has at present.

The importance of adequate masking in such measures cannot be emphasized too much. In patients with mixed and conductive hearing losses the masking problem is so great that it cannot be performed on an arbitrary *ad hoc* basis with a fixed level of masking presented to the non-test ear which may itself have a conductive problem of uncertain extent. The masking must be performed carefully at ascending masking levels to attain the true masking 'plateau' (e.g. Coles and Priede 1970) shown in Fig. 15.1, at which the test ear is being tested without undue central or cross-over masking effects. It is far more valuable to perform properly masked bone-conduction measures at one or two frequencies than to delude oneself with hurriedly or arbitrarily derived measures on a wide frequency range. If one frequency is to be used, 500 or 1000 Hz would seem most relevant; if two frequencies are to be used 500 and 2000 Hz are probably the most valuable. Again there is the further danger of false vibrotactile thresholds which may give the impression of a conductive hearing disorder in patients with severe sensorineural hearing loss. An example of the vibrotactile thresholds for such a patient is shown in Fig. 15.2. From this and from more extensive investigations (e.g. Verrillo 1975) it may be safely assumed that bone-conduction

* It may be argued that a B C threshold in cases with no air–bone gap is a valid measure. This may be so but it is the author's practice to eschew B C audiometry if the fork tests (especially the Bing test) and impedance testing indicate that an air–bone gap is improbable.

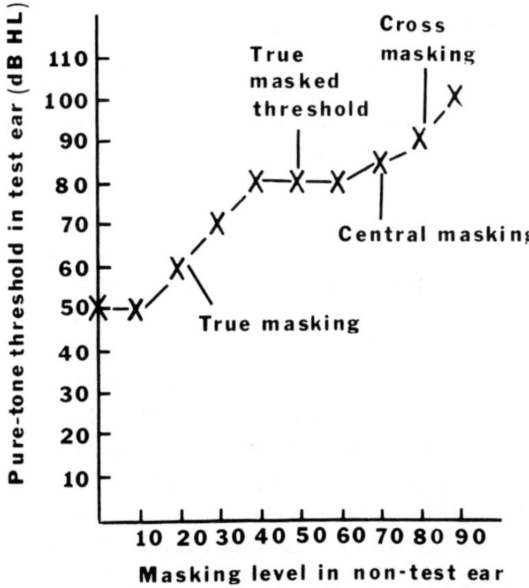

Fig. 15.1. Masking chart indicating plateau of effective masking.

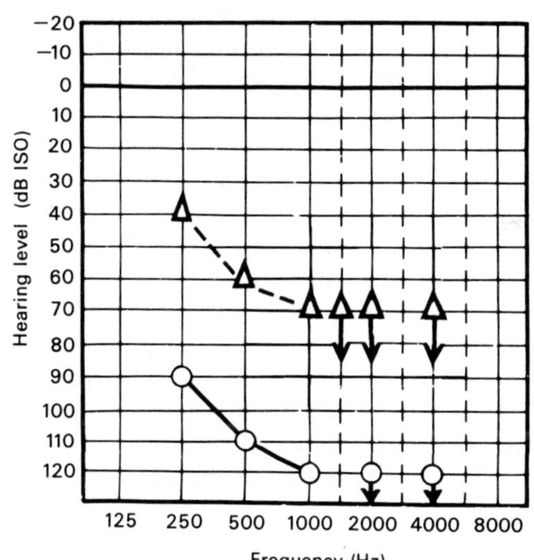

Fig. 15.2. Vibrotactile thresholds giving a false air-bone gap in a patient with a profound sensorineural hearing loss. o——o Air conduction thresholds. △——△ Bone conduction thresholds.

thresholds measurable above 1500 Hz may have more credibility than those obtained below that frequency.

Because of the problems of masking bone conduction, Rainville (1955) and Jerger and Tillman (1960) have in the past developed reverse masking-type tests known as the Rainville test and the SAL (sensorineural acuity level) test respectively. They essentially entail presenting an air conduction stimulus to the test ear and a bone-conduction masker to the forehead and then measuring the degree of threshold shift induced by such a masker. The work of Goldstein, Hayes, and Peterson (1962) and others has shown that in addition to being more complicated than traditional bone-conduction testing these tests have no real advantage in overcoming masking problems, and consequently have little or no role in current audiological practice.

The tests which have, on the other hand, revolutionized modern audiological practice in the evaluation of middle-ear function and disorders are those based on acoustic or electro-acoustic measures. The development of modern techniques in this field stems essentially from the work of Metz (1946) who studied not only the passive measures of the changes in middle-ear impedance (or its reciprocal, admittance) as a function of the pressure in the sealed external acoustic meatus, but also the dynamic changes resulting from a contraction of the stapedius muscle. From the standpoint of the recognition and evaluation of middle-ear disorders, most information may be derived from passive measures with the dynamic measures merely having a binary value in most cases. Thus the acoustic stapedius reflex contraction is either present or absent, it being absent when there is a significant conductive hearing loss. The principal exception to this 'binary' effect may occur in early otosclerosis in which, testing with a probe tone of 220 Hz, acoustical stimulation may result in an increase in admittance at the onset and offset of the stimulus rather than the decrease which characteristically occurs in normal ears and in those with end-organ damage alone.

Among the passive measures two important elements may be derived. These are the middle-ear pressure measure and the compliance or gradient measure. The former is indicated by the fact that admittance is greatest when the pressure in the occluded external acoustic meatus is equal to that of the middle ear. Any abnormalities in this middle-ear pressure are almost invariable in the direction of reduced pressure caused by obstruction of the Eustachian tube and the absorption of oxygen from the air in the middle-ear cleft. A reported example of increased middle-ear pressure occurs during the positive pressure inflation of the lungs in anaesthesia, particularly with the use of nitrous oxide anaesthesia.

If there is a negative middle-ear pressure the function of the Eustachian tube may be further tested by instructing the patient to swallow and by observing whether the middle-ear pressure tends to normalize. This may be followed by repeated swallowing. If the admittance pattern is essentially normal but there is a negative pressure the disorder may generally be attributed to Eustachian tube dysfunction and a cause for this must be sought by other means.

The admittance and gradient measures are two which are often considered together and which involve a comparison between the admittance at the pressure which resulted in maximum admittance and the admittance at +200 mm H_2O in the former case, and at ±50 mm H_2O relative to the peak in the case of gradient. The admittance/compliance measure is at present the most extensively used, but Brooks (1979) and others have argued recently in favour of the gradient measure in the differentiation of abnormal middle-ear conditions.

A low gradient or admittance with a normal middle-ear pressure may be suggestive of fibrosis in the middle ear secondary to otitis media or of otosclerosis. Unfortunately the admittance may vary considerably from case to case in otosclerosis with many, if not most, patients showing results within the normal range. Morrison (1979) has presented evidence that this may be related to the severity of the otosclerosis, patients with severe thickening of the footplate having lower admittance than those with less thickening. Whether this relates to the state of the footplate or to changes occurring in the fibrous structure of the middle layer of the tympanic membrane is debatable. Lutman (1979) has argued that most significant changes in admittance stem from factors involving the tympanic membrane. Thus in osteogenesis imperfecta for example, although in most patients the lesion involved stapedial fixation, the admittance found (Carruth, Lutman, and Stephens 1978) often shows a marked increase owing to thinning of the tympanic membrane.

Reduced admittance is also found in seromucous otitis media, but in this case is associated with reduced middle-ear pressure which may be as low as −400 mm H_2O below atmospheric pressure. This flat negative pressure curve is regarded as the classical result found in this condition often popularly known as 'glue ear'. In such cases the oxygen *and* the nitrogen of the middle-ear cleft have been largely absorbed.

Increased admittance occurs primarily in patients with healed perforations in which the epithelial lining of the middle ear has grown together with the stratified squamous epithelium of the outer ear, but with little fibrous tissue between them. As the admittance related to the tympanic membrane predominates in all measures, when this condition occurs little else may be detected. As mentioned earlier, increased admittance also occurs with the thin tympanic membrane of osteogenesis imperfecta and may also occur in cases of ossicular discontinuity, although the extent to which it occurs in such cases is somewhat debatable.

Thus in the audiological evaluation and determination of middle-ear disorders the two tests which are most commonly used are bone conduction audiometry and electroacoustic impedance measures. The extent to which these 'provide' reliable information which cannot be gleaned from a combination of careful otoscopy and intelligently performed tuning-fork tests remains controversial.

END-ORGAN VERSUS NEURAL DISORDERS

Much of the post Second World War diagnostic audiology has been plagued by the game known as 'hunt the eighth nerve tumour'. This has led to a plethora of tests being devised in an attempt to differentiate between end-organ and cochlear nerve lesions, when in their early stages many cochlear nerve lesions arising from vestibulocochlear nerve Schwannomas present with predominantly end-organ type findings.

As generally described, the patient with an end-organ disorder has recruitment (i.e. an abnormally rapid growth of loudness), an increased sensitivity to increments in the intensity of a stimulus, shows little or no abnormal adaptation and has relatively good speech discrimination, although this falls off with increasing severity of the hearing loss. By the same definition, the patient with a neural disorder has no recruitment or even derecruitment or loudness reversal (an abnormally slow growth of loudness with increasing stimulus intensity), poor discrimination of changes in intensity, marked abnormal adaptation, and speech discrimination disproportionately poor as compared with his threshold. Unfortunately among patients with end-organ disorders and those with cochlear nerve lesions there are often exceptions to these generalities and inconsistencies between them. Furthermore, such inconsistencies frequently occur in patients with Ménière's disorder and in those with vestibulocochlear Schwannomas, the two groups which the audiologist is most often called on to differentiate.

It must also be remembered that the prevalence of end-organ disorders among the hearing impaired population is considerably higher than the prevalence of neural disorders. Which way then does the investigative audiologist turn?

The only reasonable approach in this context must be one which uses a range of tests measuring a variety of these parameters supplemented where necessary by electrophysiological tests. In addition the clinician will base his evaluation of the patient on anamnestic, radiological, biochemical, and other considerations as he is concerned with the diagnosis and treatment of the specific underlying pathology rather than with the niceties of whether or not it is resulting in a neural or an end-organ lesion.

It is essential, however, to consider which tests within the existing range are most useful, at least to provide some diagnostic guide within the limitations alluded to earlier. It is important that any diagnostic test battery should concentrate on one test from each of several of the groups of psychophysical differences between end-organ and neural dysfunction rather than concentrating all the tests in one group. Thus it is important to use measures of recruitment, abnormal adaptation and perhaps discrimination measures rather than have several tests of recruitment or abnormal adaptation alone.

Recruitment testing dates back to the monaural loudness balance (MLB) techniques used by Pohlman and Kranz (1924) and refined by Reger (1936) as a clinical test and to the alternate binaural loudness balance (ABLB) test developed earlier by Fowler (1928a, 1936). Both measures involve the comparison of the loudness at different suprathreshold levels in a damaged ear with either a frequency at which the hearing is normal in the same ear or the same frequency in the normally functioning opposite ear. The former has the advantage that it may be used in patients with a symmetrical bilateral high-frequency hearing loss but has the disadvantages that it requires an audiometer with two independent oscillators. It is also found to be a difficult task to perform by many patients, this resulting in a fall in its reliability. The ABLB is one of the most popular of the tests of recruitment commonly used but has the disadvantage that it can normally be applied only to cases of unilateral hearing loss with essentially normal hearing in the opposite ear. It has the further disadvantage that the results may be complicated by diplacusis binauralis and other dysacuses.

Both measures suffer further from the problems of short-term memory effects which may be considerable in elderly patients. Furthermore most of their recent advocates from a diagnostic standpoint (e.g. Coles 1972) emphasize that the results obtained are valuable only when there is 'complete recruitment', i.e. when a stimulus at a given sound pressure level (SPL) in the test ear frequency is reported as being equally loud as the comparison stimulus in the normally hearing ear at the same SPL. Various degrees of 'incomplete' recruitment may be found in neural dysfunction. Examples of the different patterns of results are shown in Fig. 15.3.

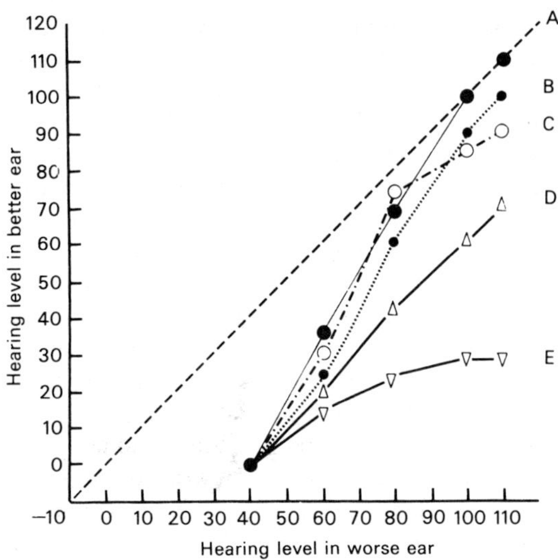

Fig. 15.3. Loudness balance chart indicating main patterns of results. A—Complete recruitment. B—Incomplete recruitment. C—Derecruitment. D—No recruitment. E—Loudness reversal.

Watson in 1944 introduced the concepts of the most comfortable loudness level (MCL) and uncomfortable loudness level (ULL) in the context of hearing aid fitting and these were subsequently applied by Bangs and Mullins (1953) and others, to the evaluation of recruitment. By these means, with which the subject is required to indicate his most comfortable listening level in the former and the lowest level at which the stimulus becomes uncomfortably loud in the latter, two equal loudness contours otherwise obtainable by the MLB technique may be simply derived. Stephens,

Blegvad, and Krogh (1977) have shown that both the intra- and intersubject variance of the MCL are too high for it to be a useful absolute measure, although some helpful information may be obtained by a comparison of the MCL contour with the threshold contour, both being derived by means of a self-recording audiometer.

The ULL, sometimes known as the loudness discomfort level (LDL) or, more accurately, as the threshold of uncomfortable loudness (TUL) has lower intrasubject variance although the intersubject variance measure may be biased by such factors as noise experience and personality (Stephens and Anderson 1971). This can, however, in inter-ear and frequency comparisons within the same subject provide evidence of complete recruitment and has the great advantage of requiring only a simple audiometer for its determination, albeit one with a high maximum output.

A number of other measures, better referred to as tests of intensity discrimination have been alluded to as measures of recruitment, but Fernandes (1978) has shown little relationship between these and 'true' recruitment measures. Evans (1975) has related frequency discrimination measures and psychophysical tuning curves to recruitment but there is as yet a dearth of material on the results of such measures in neural disorders.

Of more established value as a measure of or related to recruitment is the acoustic reflex threshold as determined by electroacoustic impedance meters or bridges. Again a comparison between such measures in the two ears and a consideration of their level in relation to the hearing loss can provide valuable information in the differentiation between end-organ and neural disorders. In many of the latter, the acoustic reflex threshold may be grossly elevated or absent. In addition, in certain of those patients with neural disorders and reasonably normal reflex thresholds, marked decay of the reflex may be found when the stimulus is presented at 10 dB above the acoustic reflex threshold. This will be discussed further below.

Of all audiometric tests those of abnormal adaptation probably have the most synonyms (e.g. functional exhaustibility, tone decay, temporary threshold drift). Although dating back to the work of Gradenigo (1893), the approaches currently used stem from the work of Reger and Kos (1952), Carhart (1958) and Anderson, Barr, and Wedenberg (1970). These were the pioneers of the measures of abnormal adaptation using Békésy audiometry, manual audiometry and acoustic reflex decay respectively.

As some degree of abnormal adaptation may occur in end-organ disorders, in the performance of such tests a balance must be struck between high sensitivity in which there will be few false-negative responses but many false-positive responses, and reliability in which there will be few false-positives but rather more false-negatives. In this context it is valuable to use a high-sensitivity test as a screening measure, and a less-sensitive test to evaluate further those patients showing abnormal adaptation with the former.

Most studies (e.g. Stephens and Hinchcliffe 1968) have shown the Carhart type tests of abnormal adaptation using a manual audiometer, in which the stimulus level is increased in 5-dB steps when the patient no longer hears the stimulus, to be the most sensitive measures of abnormal adaptation. Furthermore, the sensitivity increases with increasing frequency. These authors also suggested that little is to be gained from the standpoint of differential diagnosis by presenting the stimulus for 60 s as opposed to 30 s. Subsequently Olsen and Noffsinger (1974) have advocated starting the test at 20 dB sensation level.

Thus a reasonable approach to use is to present a 4000-Hz stimulus at 20-dB sensation level and to determine the intensity level at which the patient can hear the tone for 30 s. If there is more than 10 dB adaptation from this level, the procedure is repeated at 2000 Hz and also with fixed frequency Békésy audiometry; 4000 Hz rather than 8000 Hz is used as the stimulus because with the latter the number of false-positive responses (i.e. abnormal adaptation) found with end-organ lesions is unacceptably high. Care, however, has to be taken in interpretation of the results in the presence of contralateral masking which Snashall (1974) and others have shown to increase the degree of abnormal adaptation in patients with end-organ lesions.

For the more definitive measure, following the example of Reger (1965), fixed-frequency Békésy audiometry is used rather than the sweep frequency approach advocated by Jerger (1960a). Palva, Karja, and Palva (1970) however, have suggested that the sensitivity of the latter may be enhanced by reverse frequency sweep, i.e. going from high frequencies to low with the continuous stimulus followed by the reverse with the interrupted signal.

In the past decade a valuable addition to the abnormal adaptation test battery has come with the measure of acoustic reflex decay (Anderson *et al.* 1970). In this the stimulus is presented at 10 dB above the acoustic reflex threshold and the degree of adaptation measured over 10 s. It has been argued that patients with vestibulocochlear Schwannomas show adaptation of 50 per cent of the onset level within 6 s. Again, however, some false positive responses occur in patients with Ménière's disorder. The test stimulus furthermore must be 500 Hz, 1000 Hz, or wideband noise (Cleaver and Stephens 1977) as when higher frequencies are used normally hearing patients and those with end-organ disorders show significant adaptation.

Thus in the test battery for abnormal adaptation it may be argued that there is a quick and simple screening measure in the use of the Olsen and Noffsinger (1974) technique with the stimulus presented at 20 dB sensation level at 4000 Hz for 30 s. If no abnormal adaptation is found there, almost invariably it may be assumed that no abnormal adaptation will be found in the other threshold-type measures. Should there be abnormal adaptation use the same procedure at 2000 Hz following which a fixed-frequency Békésy approach should be used. In addition, so much value may be derived from the acoustic reflex measures and little additional time is spent by the performance of the acoustic reflex decay test in addition to the standard measures. This should be performed initially at 1000 Hz, or with wide-band noise depending upon whether or not the tonal reflex thresholds are obtainable. It must, however, be borne in mind that some patients show abnormal adaptation to the acoustic reflex stimulus and not to a threshold test and that the converse may also occur. Furthermore, as a word of caution, the author has known one or two cases with proven neural lesion which have shown abnormal adaptation only to sweep-frequency Békésy testing and not to any of the other tests which are normally regarded as being more sensitive.

Tests of intensity discrimination, usually under the title of tests of recruitment, have been advocated in the context of diagnostic audiometry for a number of years. These may entail the detection of intensity modulation (Lüscher–Zwislocki test, 1951; SISI test, Jerger, Shedd, and Harford 1959) or a paired comparison of two stimuli of different intensity (Denes and Naunton 1950). In addition tests dependent on the rate of increase in detectibility at threshold level have been described by Békésy (1947) and by Barr-Hamilton, Tempest, and Bryan (1971). Despite manipulation of the stimulus parameters used in these tests by various subsequent authors, none of these has proven particularly effective at differentiating between end-organ and neural lesions, and they are not currently used for this purpose in most major audiological centres.

The value of speech discrimination testing in this context is also controversial. Classically very poor speech discrimination is found in neural disorders but this is by no means invariable. Conversely, although most patients with end-organ disorders show speech discrimination falling off steadily with increasing hearing loss above a speech reception threshold (SRT) of 30 dB (e.g. Hood and Poole 1971), some patients with Ménière's disorder may show disproportionately poor speech discrimination.

Many problems arise from differences in the material and methodology used for the determination of speech discrimination measures in different centres. Usually phonetically balanced (PB) or isophonemic tests are used for such measures, although the quality and type of recording may vary considerably both within and between countries. Thus in certain places the discrimination score is determined at an arbitrary intensity level above the SRT, in others at the most comfortable listening level, and in others at the point of maximal discrimination on a full discrimination curve. Frequently these points differ and hence significant differences may occur in the derived discrimination score particularly in patients with sensorineural hearing loss.

If a speech audiometric procedure is to be used for diagnostic purposes it is most valuable to plot the entire discrimination curve based on, for example, ten-word lists scored by phonemes (Boothroyd 1968) and then to present two or more extra lists at the point of optimal discrimination derived from this procedure. This approach has the advantage that three aspects of reported differences between end-organ and neural disorders may be derived; (i) the difference between the SRT and the predicted from the pure-tone audiogram; (ii) the optimal or maximal discrimination score; and (iii) the narrowed dynamic range of high discrimination scores (Coles *et al.* 1973).

In this and other speech discrimination measures the importance of adequate masking must be borne in mind (e.g. Coles *et al.* 1973) but obvious errors derived from inadequate masking may be more easily detected when the complete discrimination curve is plotted than when just one arbitrary point is measured.

This procedure obviously takes a finite amount of test time and the cost–benefit ratio in this context is far from clear. A number of reports using this procedure in patients suspected of having or proven to have eighth nerve tumours have been far from unanimous in their results.

It is the author's contention, therefore, that in audiometric screening for cochlear nerve lesions the two most helpful measures are based on the acoustic reflex determinations, including reflex decay, and sensitive tests of abnormal adaptation alluded to earlier. These should be coupled with radiological investigations of the internal acoustic meati and evaluation of vestibular function. If indications of possible neural dysfunction are derived from these measures, electrophysiological tests are then indicated. Beagley (Chapter 32) has discussed these aspects, and here one can but emphasize the importance of taking an integrated look at a combination of electrocochleographic and brainstem measures in order to obtain the most reliable results, bearing in mind the shape and polarity of the cochlear nerve waveform, the behaviour of the summating potential, the relationship between the cochlear microphonic and the action potential, and the latency difference between the cochlear nerve action potential and the upper brainstem waves.

COCHLEAR NERVE VERSUS BRAINSTEM DISORDERS

This differentiation is notoriously difficult to make in patients with a degree of sensorineural hearing loss, as any distorted input from the cochlear nerve will impair aspects of brainstem function such as directionalization (e.g. Nordlund 1964) and masking level differences (e.g. Olsen, Noffsinger, and Carhart 1976). Therefore, further consideration in this section will be restricted to those patients showing essentially normal thresholds to pure-tone audiometry. In patients with a hearing loss and suspected of central auditory dysfunction a very carefully performed array of electrophysiological measures in the hands of an experienced interpreter of such results is essential.

For the normally hearing patient three approaches may be made to achieve this differentiation; behavioural or subjective testing, acoustic reflex-based measures, and electrophysiological studies. The behavioural measures may be further subdivided into those 'classical' measures used in the investigation of peripheral disorders and to those specifically developed to investigate the central auditory pathways. Again, as was argued in the discussion of neural and end-organ disorders, it is essential that the results of these types of tests be considered in relation to each other.

Further information may be derived from an investigation of related disorders of equilibrium which will show parallelism in the case of eighth nerve lesions but divergence in central disorders related to the different pathways followed within the central nervous system. The range of these various investigations has been discussed elsewhere (e.g. Stephens 1976a) and the interrelationships between the different measures investigated by Stephens and Thornton (1976).

For the clinician concerned essentially with complaints of disorders of hearing and balance, what is important is to determine which of these various investigations might be worthwhile to perform as screening measures for central lesions. What is needed is an approach which is simple, reliable and not excessively time consuming. Unfortunately there is some incompatability between these demands with regard to techniques currently available and a battery approach is probably still necessary.

Of the 'standard' tests of peripheral function, a measure described as sensitive to brainstem disorders by Reger (1965), Eichel, Hedgecock, and Williams (1966) and others is that of abnormal adaptation at threshold or 'tone decay'. Bilateral abnormal adaptation in the presence of normal hearing is certainly suspicious of a pontine disorder. Unfortunately Stephens and Thornton (1976) and others have found that many patients with brainstem disorders do not have abnormal adaptation.

Related to this measure is the adaptation of the acoustic reflex (Anderson *et al.* 1970) which when present bilaterally may certainly be suspicious of a brainstem disorder, but again this is by no means a universal finding in such lesions. Examination of the pattern of acoustic reflexes in the presence of normal peripheral auditory function can be most helpful when both ipsilateral and contralateral stimulation is taken into account. Thus, for example with midline pontine lesions, the contralateral reflex may be abolished while the ipsilateral reflexes remain normal. This is certainly a useful measure in the investigation of lower brainstem lesions, but obviously as the basic reflex pathway does not involve structures rostral to the olivary complex, it will be insensitive to more central lesions.

Among the more specific tests designed to test central auditory function, encouraging results have been obtained with certain measures involving binaural interaction and also with temporal summation testing (Stephens 1976b). This last, in a variety of central lesions, shows an abnormally steep function, as opposed to the flatter functions found by many workers in end-organ disorders. Like abnormal adaptation, this phenomenon is not found in all patients with central lesions, but when present it is indicative of central dysfunction. This dysfunction may, however, be located in a variety of areas of the central auditory pathways from the lower brainstem of the cortex.

A variety of binaural interactive tests have been described ranging from central masking, masking level differences (MLD), and lateralization or directionalization. These all involve testing of the interactive mechanism at the superior olive, inferior colliculus, and other levels. Evidence from Goldstein and Stephens (1975) suggests that there are probably several distinct mechanisms involved here so that it is difficult to advocate one test at the expense of others. From the point of view of simplicity for the listener an

MLD measure provides an easily understood test, and has given useful diagnostic information (Olsen *et al.* 1976; Quaranta, Cassano, and Cervellera 1978). The simplified lateralization test advocated by Groen (the Groen stethoscope) (1969) has not unfortunately stood the test of time.

Probably the most widely used measure of brainstem function involves the use of brainstem evoked response measures (BSER) developed initially by Sohmer and Feinmesser (1967). These responses are derived from a variety of centres within the brainstem and are discussed elsewhere in this book (Chapter 32). The disadvantage of this technique is that it measures only the transient onset responses rather than those to sustained stimulation. It is possible, however, to measure some aspects of binaural summation and interaction with this measure (e.g. Blegvad 1975) and often the general results relate well to the findings of behavioural and other tests (Stephens and Thornton 1976).

The other major advantage of the BSER is that it is very sensitive to the increased conduction times found in demyelinating disease (e.g. Thornton and Hawkes 1976) and may be useful as a screening measure for this condition.

CORTICAL DISORDERS

Whereas the evaluation of brainstem function is difficult and remains a very nebulous area, that of dysfunction of the auditory cortex is even more obscure. Most of the tests traditionally used have been based on the findings of Bocca and his co-workers (Bocca, Calearo, and Cassimari 1954) that low redundancy speech material presented to the left ear is poorly discriminated when there is a lesion of the right primary auditory cortex, and material presented to the right ear is poorly discriminated with left cortex lesions.

A variety of techniques have been used to reduce the redundancy of the speech material (e.g. Stephens 1976a) including filtering, time compressing, presenting in the presence of ipsilateral masking noise, etc. In general the findings with such material support the contentions of the Italian workers but the interrelationships between the results obtained with different tests of this nature remain somewhat obscure (Davis and Stephens 1978). In addition, a variety of non-auditory variables such as the intelligence, personality and linguistic background of the subjects can influence the outcome of many of these tests (Davis, Kastelanski, and Stephens 1976; Bergman, Hirsch, and Najenson 1977).

Given this problem with speech material in the evaluation of cortical function, it behoves us to examine the possibilities of non-speech tests. A variety of techniques have been used in this context ranging from the alternate binaural loudness balance (Jerger 1960b) to rhythm perception to temporal summation (Baru and Karaseva 1972). In all cases the rationale has been that the performance will be impaired in the ear contralateral to the damaged cortex. Little consideration has been given, however, to the differential functions of the right and left auditory cortices being dominant for different aspects of auditory perception, although indeed this may be a second-order effect.

Thus at present there is little reason to advocate the use of non-speech tests in preference to speech material in this context and it is the author's experience that many patients with cortical disorders are able to perform adequately at tests involving speech material but find it difficult to grasp the performance of certain non-speech tests.

Among the speech tests the most simple and robust at the present time would seem to be the staggered spondaic word test (Katz 1962) and ipsilaterally masked speech material. In addition, however, evidence from Lynn and Gilroy (1977) and from Bergman *et al.* (1977) emphasize the importance of the use of competing sentence material. Such test material can test the integrity of the parietal lobe and the corpus callosum pathways linking the non-dominant cortex to the dominant. In such lesions the competing material presented to the ear opposite to the non-dominant cortex is poorly discriminated.

Electrophysiological tests such as the middle latency responses (Mendel and Goldstein 1969) and the slow vertex response have been used in various patients with cortical lesions but most of the evidence of their value in this respect has been far from clear. A recent report, however, by Parving, Larsen, Larsen, Salomon and Elberling (1980) indicates that both these sets of responses may be essentially normal in a patient with bilateral temporal lobe lesions. In view of the controversial nature of these results, more studies are needed in such patients applying the modern techniques used by Parving *et al.* (1980).

The importance of that study stems not so much from electrophysiological tests used but from the quality of the blood flow studies to evaluate the precise site of lesion in the patient concerned. As such an approach becomes more extensively applied in patients to whom various audiometric tests of central auditory function are administered we should acquire a better understanding of this function and the relative value of the different tests.

REFERENCES

ANDERSON, H., BARR, B., and WEDENBERG, E. (1970). The early detection of acoustic tumours by the stapedius reflex test. In *Sensorineural hearing loss* (ed. G. E. W. Wolstenholme and J. Knight) pp. 275–94. Churchill, London.

BANGS, J. L. and MULLINS, C. J. (1953). Recruitment testing and its implications. *Archs Otolar.* **58**, 582–92.

BÁRÁNY, E. (1938). A contribution to the physiology of bone conduction. *Acta oto-lar.* Suppl. 26.

BARR-HAMILITON, R. M., TEMPEST, W., and BRYAN, M. E. (1971). The differential detectability index: a new monaural test for the locus of hearing disorders. *Sound* **5**, 2–6.

BARU, A. V. and KARASEVA, T. A. (1972). *The brain and hearing*. Consultants Bureau. New York.

BASSOM, G. (1974). Methodology of measurement of pure-tone thresholds. MSc Thesis, University of Southampton.

Békésy, G. von (1947). A new audiometer. *Acta oto-lar.* **35**, 411–22.

Bergman, M., Hirsch, S., and Najenson, T. (1977). Tests of auditory perception in the assessment and management of patients with cerebral cranial injury. *Scand. J. rehab. Med.* **9**, 173–7.

Blegvad, B. (1975). Binaural summation of surface recorded electrocochleographic responses. *Scand. Audiol.* **4**, 233–5.

Bocca, E., Calearo, C., and Cassimari, V. (1954). A new method for testing hearing in temporal lobe tumours. *Acta oto-lar.* **44**, 219–21.

Boothroyd, A. (1968). Developments in speech audiometry. *Sound* **2**, 3–11.

Brooks, D. N. (1979). Evaluation and clinical applications of impedance measurement. Medical Research Council Proceedings MRC 79/17, London.

Burns, W. (1968). *Noise and Man.* Murray, London.

—— and Hinchcliffe, R. (1957). A comparison of auditory threshold as measured by pure tone and by Békésy audiometry. *J. acoust. Soc. Am.* **29**, 1274–7.

Carhart, R. (1958). Clinical determination of abnormal auditory adaptation. *Archs Otolar.* **65**, 32–9.

Carruth, J. A. S., Lutman, M. E., and Stephens, S. D. G. (1978). An audiological investigation of osteogenesis imperfecta. *J. Lar. Otol.* **92**, 853–60.

Cheesman, A. D. and Stephens, S. D. G. (1965). A new method for the detection of functional hearing loss. *Charing Cross Hosp. Gaz.* Sci. Suppl. **3**, 7–12.

Cleaver, V. C. G. and Stephens, S. D. G. (1977). Observations on the clinical use of broad-band noise as an acoustic reflex stimulus. *Br. J. Audiol.* **11**, 22–4.

Coles, R. R. A. (1972). Can present day audiology really help in diagnosis?—An otologists question. *J. Lar. Otol.* **86**, 191–224.

—— and Priede, V. M. (1970). On the misdiagnosis resulting from incorrect use of masking. *J. Lar. Otol.* **84**, 41–63.

—— —— (1972). Non-organic overlay in noise induced hearing loss. *Proc. R. Soc. Med.* **64**, 194–9.

—— Markides, A., and Priede, V. M. (1973). Uses and abuses of speech audiometry. In *Disorders of auditory function* (ed. W. Taylor) pp. 181–202. Academic Press, London.

Davis, R. J. and Stephens, S. D. G. (1978). Low redundancy speech tests—an evaluation. ISVR Technical Memorandum No. 577, University of Southampton.

—— Kastelanski, W., and Stephens, S. D. G. (1976). Some factors influencing the results of speech tests of central auditory function. *Scand. Audiol.* **5**, 179–86.

Delany, M. E. (1970). On the stability of auditory threshold. National Physical Laboratory Aero Report AC44.

Denes, P. and Naunton, R. E. (1950). The clinical detection of auditory recruitment. *J. Lar. Otol.* **64**, 375–98.

Eichel, B. S., Hedgecock, L. D., and Williams, H. L. (1966). A review of the literature on the audiologic aspects of neuro-otologic diagnoses. *Laryngoscope, St. Louis* **76**, 1–29.

Evans, E. F. (1975). The sharpening of cochlear frequency selectivity in the normal and abnormal cochlea. *Audiology* **14**, 419–42.

—— (1979). Pathophysiology of cochlear hearing loss. Paper presented to Royal Society of Medicine, 2 February 1979.

Fernandes, M. (1978). JND measurements of intensity as reflected in a damaged cochlea. Progress Report, University of Southampton.

Fowler, E. P. (1928). Marked deafened areas in normal ears. *Archs Otolar.* **8**, 151–5.

—— (1936). A method for the early detection of otosclerosis; a study of sounds well above threshold. *Archs Otolar.* **24**, 731–41.

Goldstein, D. P. and Stephens, S. D. G. (1975). Masking level difference: a measurement of auditory processing capability. *Audiology* **14**, 354–67.

—— Hayes, C. S., and Peterson, J. L. (1962). A comparison of bone conduction thresholds by conventional and Rainville methods. *J. Speech Hear. Res.* **5**, 244–55.

Gradenigo, G. (1893). On the clinical signs of affectations of the auditory nerve. *Archs Otolar.* **22**, 213–15.

Groen, J. J. (1969). Diagnostic value of lateralization ability for dichotic time differences. *Acta oto-lar.* **67**, 326–32.

Guildford, J. P. (1954). *Psychometric methods.* McGraw-Hill, New York.

Hood, J. D. and Poole, J. (1971). Speech audiometry in conductive and sensorineural hearing loss. *Sound* **5**, 30–8.

Hughson, W. and Westlake, H. (1944). Manual for program outline for rehabilitation of aural casualties both military and civilian. American Academy of Ophthalmologists and Otologists, Rochester.

Hyde, M. L. and Stephens, S. D. G. (1979). Psychoacoustical experimentation. In *Auditory investigation: the scientific and technological basis* (ed. H. A. Beagley) pp. 526–51. Oxford University Press.

Jerger, J. (1960a). Békésy audiometry in analysis of auditory disorders. *J. Speech Hear. Res.* **3**, 275–87.

—— (1960b). Observations on auditory behaviour in lesions of the central auditory pathways. *Archs Otolar.* **71**, 797–806.

—— and Herer, G. (1961). Unexpected dividend in Békésy audiometry *J. Speech Hear. Disord.* **26**, 390–1.

—— and Tillman, T. (1960). A new method for the clinical determination of sensorineural acuity level (SAL). *Archs Otolar.* **71**, 948–53.

—— Shedd, J., and Harford, E. (1959). On the detection of extremely small changes in sound intensity. *Archs Otolar.* **69**, 200–11.

Johnsen, N. J. Osterhammel, D., Terkildsen, K., Osterhammel, P., and Huis in't Veld, F. (1976). The white noise middle ear muscle reflex threshold in patients with sensorineural hearing impairment. *Scand. Audiol.* **5**, 131–5.

Katz, J. (1962). The use of staggered spondaic words for assessing the integrity of the central auditory nervous system. *J. aud. Res.* **2**, 327–37.

Kemp, D. T. (1978). Stimulated acoustic emissions from within the human auditory system. *J. acoust. Soc. Am.* **64**, 1386–91.

Lightfoot, G. R. and Hoare, N. (1979). Investigations into bone conduction calibration. *Clin. Otolar.* **4**, 234.

Lüscher, E. and Zwislocki, J. (1951). Comparison of various methods employed in the determination of the recruitment phenomenon. *J. Lar. Otol.* **65**, 187–95.

Lutman, M. E. (1979). Techniques for middle ear measurements. Medical Research Council Proceedings MRC 79/17, London.

Lynn, G. E. and Gilroy, J. (1977). Evaluation of central auditory function in patients with neurological disorders. In *Central auditory dysfunction* (ed. R. W. Kieth) pp. 177–221. Grune and Stratton, New York.

Mendel, M. and Goldstein, R. (1969). Stability of the early components of the averaged electroencephalographic response. *J. Speech Hear. Res.* **12**, 344–50.

METZ, O. (1946). The acoustic impedance measured on normal and pathological ears. *Acta oto-lar.* Suppl. 63.

MORRISON, A. (1979). The impedance bridge in clinical otology with particular reference to diagnosis and assessment. Medical Research Council Proceedings MRC 79/17, London.

NIEMEYER, W. and SESTERHENN, G. (1974). Calculation of the hearing threshold from the stapedius reflex threshold for different sound stimuli. *Audiology* **13**, 421–7.

NORDLUND, B. (1964). Directional audiometry. *Acta oto-lar.* **57**, 1–18.

NORRIS, T. W., STELMACHOWICZ, P., and TAYLOR, D. (1974). Acoustic reflex relaxation to identify sensorineural hearing impairment. *Archs Otolar.* **99**, 194–7.

OLSEN, W. O. and NOFFSINGER, D. (1974). Comparison of one new and three old tests of auditory adaptation. *Archs Otolar.* **99**, 94–9.

——, —— and CARHART, R. (1976). Masking level differences encountered in clinical populations. *Audiology* **15**, 287–301.

PALVA, T., KARJA, J., and PALVA, A. (1970). Forward vs reversed Békésy tracings. *Archs Otolar.* **87**, 449–52.

PARVING, A., LASSEN, N. A., LARSEN, B., SALOMON, G., and ELBERLING, C. (1980). Auditory evoked responses in a case of bilateral temporal lobe lesion with auditory agnosia. *Scand. Audiol.* **9**, 161–7.

POHLMAN, A. G. and KRANZ, F. W. (1924). Binaural minimum audition in a subject with ranges of deficient acuity. *Proc. Soc. Exp. Biol. Med.* **21**, 335–7.

QUARANTA, A., CASSANO, P., and CERVELLERA, G. (1978). Clinical value of the tonal masking level difference. *Audiology* **17**, 232–8.

RAINVILLE, M. J. (1955). Nouvelle méthode d'assourdissement pour le relevé des courbes de conduction osseuse. *J. fr. Oto-rhino-lar.* **4**, 851–8.

REGER, S. N. (1936). Differences in loudness response of normal and hard-of-hearing ears at intensity levels slightly above threshold. *Ann. Otol. Rhinol.* **45**, 1029–39.

—— (1965). Pure-tone audiometry. In *Audiometry, principles, and practices* (ed. A. Glorig) pp. 108–50. Williams and Wilkins, Baltimore.

—— and KOS, C. M. (1952). Clinical measurements and implications of recruitment. *Ann. Otol. Rhinol.* **61**, 810–23.

RICHARDSON, B. W. (1879). Some researches with Professor Hughes' new instrument for the measurement of hearing; the audiometer. *Proc. R. Soc.* **29**, 65–70.

ROBINSON, D. W. (1960). Variability in the realization of the audiometric zero. *Ann. Occup. Hyg.* **2**, 107–26.

—— and WHITTLE, L. S. (1973). A comparison of self-recording and manual audiometry. *J. Sound. Vib.* **26**, 41–62.

SESTERHENN, G. and BREUNINGER, H. (1977). Determination of hearing threshold for single frequencies from the acoustic reflex. *Audiology* **16**, 201–14.

SNASHALL, S. E. (1974). The effect of contralateral masking on tests of auditory adaptation at threshold. *Scand. Audiol.* **3**, 159–69.

SOHMER, H. and FEINMESSER, M. (1967). Cochlear action potentials recorded from the external ear in man. *Ann. Otol. Rhinol.* **76**, 427–35.

STENGER, S. (1900). Ein Versuch zur objektiven Feststellung einseitiger Taubheit, bezw. Schwerhörigkeit mittelst Stimmgabeln. *Arch. Ohrenheilk.* **50**, 197–8.

STEPHENS, S. D. G. (1969). Auditory threshold variance, signal detection theory and personality. *Int. Audiol.* **8**, 131–7.

—— (1971). Some individual factors influencing audiometric performance. In *Occupational hearing loss* (ed. D. W. Robinson) pp. 109–20. Academic Press, London.

—— (1976a). Application of psychoacoustics to central auditory dysfunction. In *Scientific foundations of otolaryngology* (ed. R. Hinchcliffe and D. Harrison) pp. 352–61. Heinemann, London.

—— (1976b) Auditory temporal summation in patients with central nervous system lesions. In *Disorders of auditory function II* (ed. S. D. G. Stephens) pp. 231–41. Academic Press, London.

—— (1979). David Edward Hughes and his audiometer. *J. Lar. Otol.* **93**, 1–6.

—— and ANDERSON, C. M. B. (1971). Experimental studies on the uncomfortable loudness level. *J. Speech Hear. Res.* **14**, 262–70.

—— and HINCHCLIFFE, R. (1968). Studies on temporary threshold drift. *Int. Audiol.* **7**, 267–79.

—— and THORNTON, A. R. D. (1976). Subjective and electrophysiologic tests in brain-stem lesions. *Archs Otolar.* **102**, 608–13.

—— BLEGVAD, B., and KROGH, H. J. (1977). The value of some suprathreshold auditory measures. *Scand. Audiol.* **6**, 213–21.

THORNTON, A. R. D. and HAWKES, C. H. (1976). Neurological applications of surface recorded electrocochleography. *J. Neurol. Neurosurg. Psychiat.* **39**, 586–92.

VENTRY, I. M., WOODS, R. W., RUBIN, M., and HILL, W. (1971). Most comfortable loudness level for pure tones, noise and speech. *J. acoust. Soc. Am.* **49**, 1805–13.

VERRILLO, R. T. (1975). Cutaneous sensation. In *Experimental sensory psychology* (ed. B. Scharf), pp. 151–84. Scott Foresman, Glenview, Ill.

WATSON J. E. and VOOTS, R. (1964). A report on the use of the Békésy audiometer in the performance of the Stenger test. *J. Speech Hear. Disord.* **29**, 36–46.

WATSON, L. A. (1944). Certain fundamental principles in prescribing and fitting hearing aids. *Laryngoscope, St. Louis* **54**, 531–58.

16 Speech audiometry

J. D. HOOD

There now exists a substantial body of evidence to suggest that in all the higher vertebrates, and indeed many primitive animals, the auditory characteristics of each species have evolved in ways most suited to the animals' individual requirements. At times these take on a remarkable specificity. In Man these characteristics are uniquely suited to the reception of speech sounds so much so that there can be little doubt that speech communication has been their prime evolutionary objective. This fact is often overlooked in our present preoccupation with pure tones which, although providing a simple and convenient means for applying graded auditory stimuli, can in no way be considered either physiologically or teleologically appropriate. It has, therefore, been argued that more attention should be given to speech or speech-like stimuli in the development of audiological test procedures.

Unfortunately it cannot be claimed that speech audiometry has as yet attained anything approaching the precision of pure-tone audiometry. Nevertheless, it can provide valuable information in assessing a deaf person's social disability, in the prescription of hearing aids and in diagnosis. According to Lyregaard, Robinson, and Hinchcliffe (1976) in a comprehensive review of the subject the first systematic use of recorded speech for clinical purposes was by Oscar Wolf as long ago as 1874. It was, however, the impetus of the communication engineers, particularly during the Second World War, that led to the development of formally structured test procedures for the rating of the quality of communications systems which in turn were subsequently applied to audiology retaining much of the terminology. Prominent among these were the word lists compiled by the Psycho-acoustic laboratory at Harvard which have exerted a persisting influence to this day. The Harvard PB50 word lists were based upon the following criteria (Egan 1944).

1. Monosyllabic structure of words.
2. Equal average difficulty of lists.
3. Equal range of difficulty of lists.
4. Equal phonetic composition of lists.
5. A composition representative of American/English speech.
6. Words in common use.

Similar lists have since been compiled by Peterson and Lehiste (1962); Tillman, Carhart, and Wilber (1963); Tillman and Carhart (1966); and Boothroyd (1967).

While in theory lists of this kind would appear to present the ideal, many of the criteria are heavily dependent upon the voice production of the speaker which can vary substantially from one person to another and even at different times, with the same speaker (Brandy 1966). For this reason it is impractical to use live voice presentation in speech audiometry since it imposes an unacceptable element of variability. The same element of variability is, of course, present when speech is recorded but subsequent validatory tests make it possible to reject those recordings which depart markedly from the norm. In addition, as will be shown later, it is possible to manipulate the recorded material in such a way as to gain greater uniformity of the individual word lists and thus enhance the confidence limits of the tests. Nevertheless, as Kreul, Bell, and Nixon (1969) point out, only the material as recorded by a particular individual constitutes the characteristics of a speech intelligibility test. Sentence material is little used in speech audiometry because the tests become particularly time consuming. According to Fletcher (1929), however, a consistent relationship exists between sentence intelligibility and word articulation. This relationship is exemplified by the two curves shown to the left of Fig. 16.1. Because of the contextual content of sentences it will be seen that sentence intelligibility rises much more steeply than word articulation. The relationship between the two indicates that a person attaining only a 40 per cent word articulation score would, nevertheless, perceive 90 per cent of the content of sentences and therefore experience very little difficulty with normal conversation.

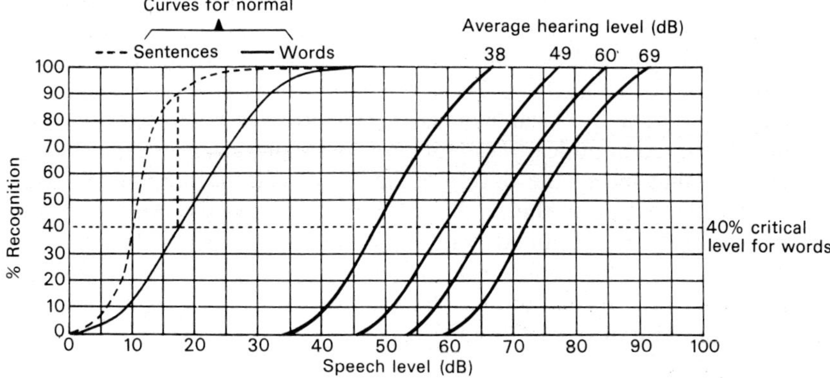

Fig. 16.1. Typical articulation curves in conductive hearing loss.

SPEECH DISCRIMINATION IN CONDUCTIVE AND COCHLEAR DEAFNESS

A deaf patient's ability to understand amplified speech can differ considerably according to the underlying pathology of the deafness. By way of example the data presented in the following have been derived from 30 subjects with conductive deafness due mostly to otosclerosis and 43 subjects with cochlear deafness caused by Ménière's disease (Hood and Poole 1971).

The test procedure followed that described in an MRC special report *Hearing aids and audiometers* No. 261, (1947) HMSO. The subject sat with the test ear against a rubber ring attached at a fixed distance to a loudspeaker. Recorded lists of phonetically balanced words (derived from the Harvard PB50 lists) with 25 words in each, were played at a number of intensity levels and the percentage number of words correctly perceived scored at each level. The non-test ear was excluded by appropriate levels of wide band noise. Typical results are shown in Fig. 16.1, the zero reference level being the intensity at which a normal hearing subject could detect the sound of 50 per cent of the words without understanding them, the so-called speech detection threshold (SDT). To the left is the speech audiogram for normal subjects, while to the right are shown the average curves for conductive hearing losses grouped at approximately 10 dB intervals on the basis of their individual average hearing levels at 500, 1000, and 2000 Hz. The curves follow the same course as the normal curve but are displaced to the right of it as a result of the hearing loss. Their displacement at the 50 per cent level is usually referred to as the speech reception threshold (SRT) which, in this instance, bears a linear, though not quite one-to-one, relationship with the pure-tone hearing loss. The curves exemplify the excellent speech discrimination abilities of these patients. Given sufficient amplification their response matches that of normal subjects. This is in marked contrast to the curves from the patients with Ménière's disease. The striking feature of the curves in this group was their variability. This is illustrated in Fig. 16.2 which

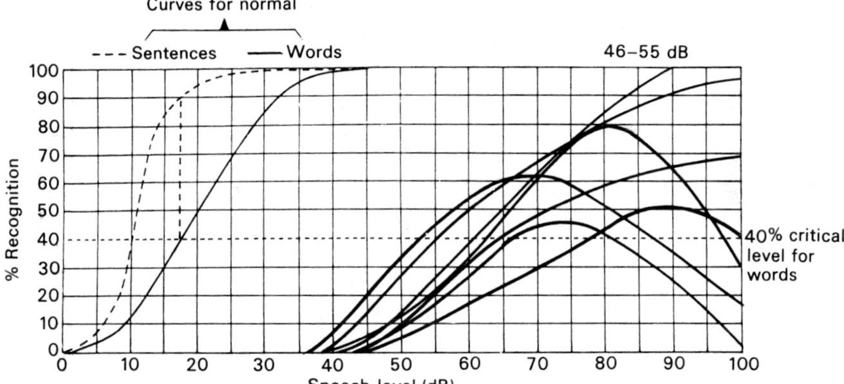

Fig. 16.2. Articulation curves from seven patients with Ménière's disease and comparable pure-tone hearing loss.

shows by way of example, a selection of the speech curves from the 17 comprising the group with average hearing levels of 46 to 55 dB. The marked variation in these curves, all from subjects with only slight differences in their hearing levels, is typical of Ménière's disease and of 'cochlear' deafness in general. Since these are subjects with almost identical pathologies and hearing levels it follows that other factors must be involved to account for this variability. Interestingly, normal hearing subjects presented with speech distorted in a manner which simulates recruitment in cochlear deafness, exhibit a strikingly similar diversity of speech audiograms. This is probably true of any system which debases intelligibility and it seems likely that the factor common to both is the individual's speech redundancy factor. Normal speech contains a considerable element of redundant information but this redundancy will, in part at any rate, be a reflection of any particular individual's power of perception. If this be high then speech can be appreciably distorted without loss of discrimination, if it be low then the vital information content of speech will be eroded and discrimination will be lost. These curves highlight the fallacy of the practice adopted by some audiologists in which a single score is obtained at one level only, usually a sensation level of 30 or 40 dB above the speech detection threshold. In these cases a test of this kind could produce a score well below the subject's maximum discrimination score besides providing little information of value about the subject's toleration of amplification.

One obvious explanation for the poor speech discrimination in the Ménière's group is, of course, the presence of loudness recruitment though clearly other contributing factors may also be involved. Since the degree of recruitment increases with hearing loss it is to be expected that speech discrimination will be similarly affected. In Fig. 16.3 are shown the group average speech curves for Ménière's disease together with the recruitment curves which would be associated with their respective 'hearing levels'. The normality of the curve for the 31 dB group suggests that speech discrimination remains unimpaired until recruitment exceeds the level shown. Thereafter, with increasing hearing loss and a concomitant increase in recruitment angle, speech discrimination becomes progressively more impaired. This implies that below a deafness of 31 dB the distortion introduced by recruitment removes only the speech redundancy leaving sufficient information content for full intelligibility. The matter is illustrated schematically in Fig. 16.4. The lower horizontal is taken to represent the minimal information content of speech essential for 100 per cent intelligibility; the area above, the redundant information normally present. The diagonal line represents the manner in which the information content is progressively eliminated as a result of recruitment associated with the hearing loss. It crosses the minimal line at a point corresponding to a deafness of 31 dB. With deafness up to 31 dB, therefore, despite the presence of loudness recruitment, speech discrimination will remain unimpaired. Thereafter, with greater degrees of recruitment associated with more severe hearing losses the essential information content is progressively eroded until at the extreme end of the scale the distortion is so great that intelligibility approaches zero. It is of some interest that the critical level of 31 dB is in good accord with Evans' (1975) recent electrophysiological studies of the toxic affects of certain drugs upon the cochlea. Apparently the effective bandwidth of the tuning curves in the cat is maintained relatively unchanged until the threshold at the critical frequency is elevated some 30–40 dB when thereafter it rapidly increases. This would suggest a widening of the critical frequency band with

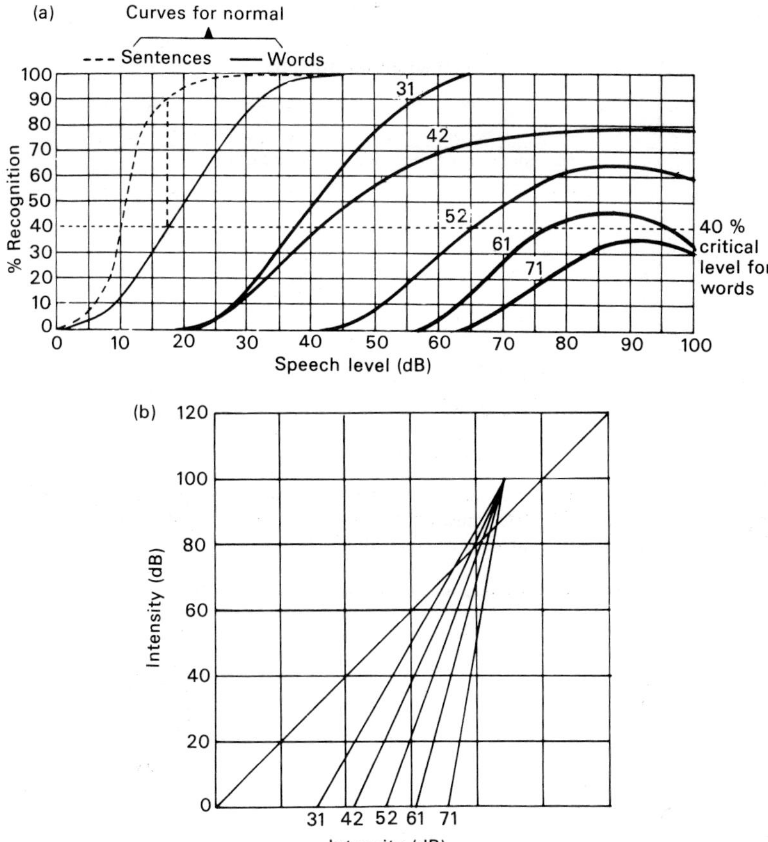

Fig. 16.3. (a). Average articulation curves for varying degrees of pure tone loss in patients with Ménière's disease. The curves shown in (b) indicate the recruitment to be expected at each hearing level.

progressive loss of discriminative ability. In Fig. 16.5 the maximum discrimination scores derived from the data given in Fig. 16.3 have been plotted against the corresponding pure-tone hearing losses. The result is an astonishingly linear relationship which with extrapolation crosses the zero at a hearing loss of about 90 dB. By an odd coincidence the relationship is identical to the scale of percentage disability proposed by the USA Committee on Conservation of Hearing (Lierle 1959) shown to the right of the figure. Needless to say this is a generalization and bearing in mind the variability in speech audiograms for given pure tone losses it is to be expected that certain patients in this category might conceivably exhibit minimal speech discrimination. It is, however, unlikely to be of any practical use.

In terms of the differential diagnosis of conductive and sensorineural

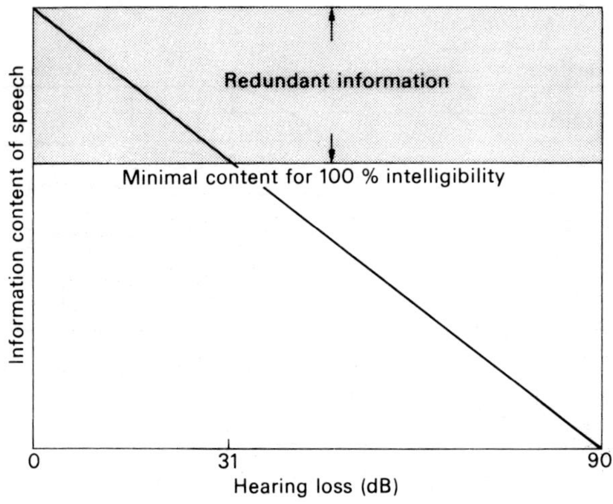

Fig. 16.4. The shaded area represents redundant information in speech. The straight line curve indicates how the information content of speech is progressively eroded by distortion associated with cochlear deafness.

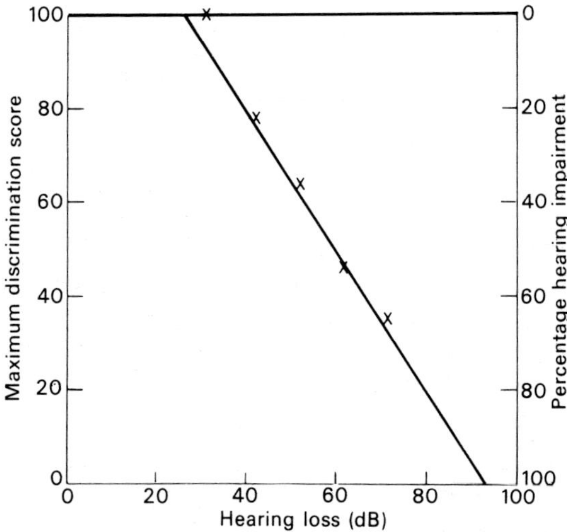

Fig. 16.5. Maximum discrimination scores derived from data given in Fig. 16.3 plotted against hearing loss. Curve relates to Unites States percentage scale of disability.

deafness, information of this kind adds little of value to the conventional air and bone conduction tests. Speech audiometry, however, can be of particular value in the differential diagnosis of cochlear and nerve fibre lesions since the latter invariably exhibit poorer speech discrimination than the former. To make this differentiation of course, requires some knowledge of the distribution of the speech audiograms in cochlear lesions. Thus the shaded areas in Fig. 16.6 indicate the limits of the speech audiograms for particular

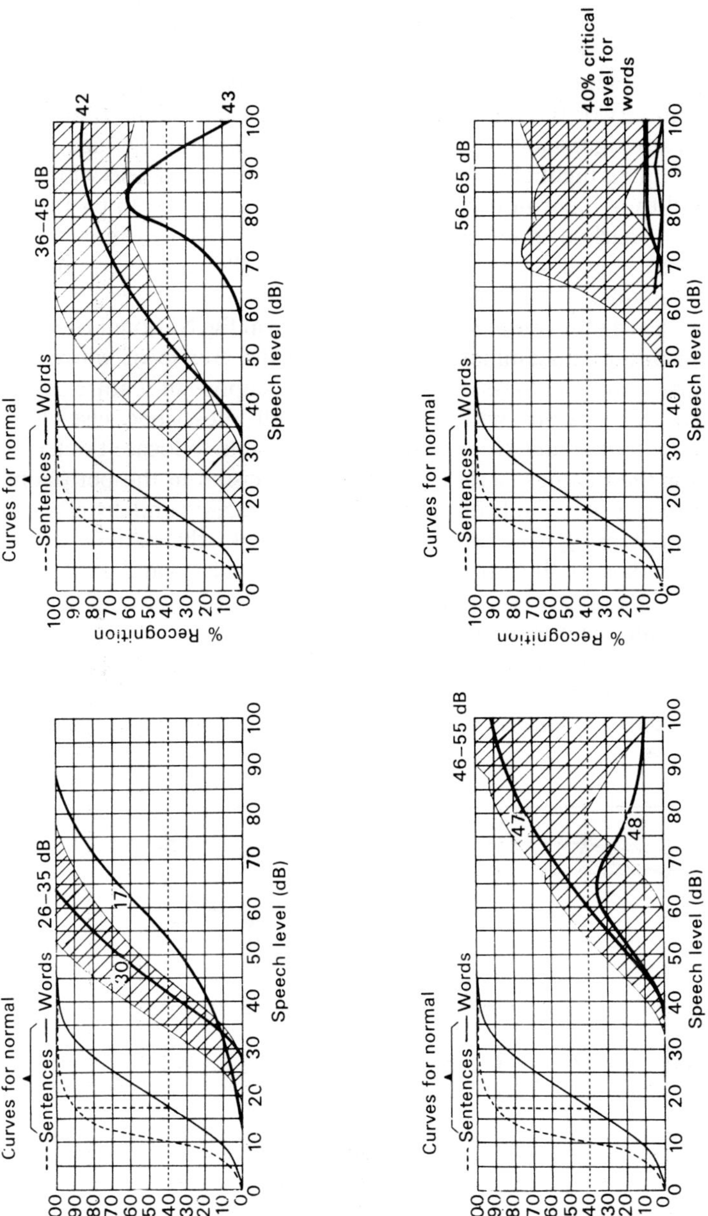

Fig. 16.6. Shaded areas indicate limits of speech audiograms for particular degrees of hearing loss in 43 patients with Ménière's disease. Full line curves are from patients with confirmed tumours of the eighth nerve.

degrees of hearing loss in the 43 cases of Ménière's disease. The full line curves are all from patients with confirmed tumours of the eighth nerve. Those falling within the shaded areas are equivocal, those falling without, are self-evident. Coles (1972) adopting similar techniques, compared the maximum discrimination scores in two groups of patients with cochlear lesions and tumours of the eighth nerve respectively and found a marked and diagnostically significant separation when related to the average pure-tone thresholds. This highlights the diagnostic value of speech tests which on the whole tend to be neuro-otological rather than otological. In particular they can reveal marked abnormalities where the results of other audiological tests are either negative or equivocal. The following, by no means unique case, provides a particularly good example.

The patient, a girl of seventeen, was an in-patient at the National Hospital during an episode of disseminated sclerosis, in the course of which she developed vertigo and deafness of the left ear. An important feature of this case was that, for reasons which have been fully described elsewhere (Citron, Dix, Hallpike, and Hood 1963) it was possible to locate the lesion responsible for the deafness with considerable precision in the peripheral portion of the nerve at a point central to the spiral ganglion and distal to the cochlear nuclei. During the course of the four weeks the patient was in hospital, the deafness of the left ear completely disappeared and during this time it was possible to carry out at regular intervals, pure-tone audiograms, speech audiograms, and tests of the loudness function.

In Fig. 16.7 is shown the rapid recovery of the pure-tone threshold from almost total loss of hearing on the first day of testing to normal threshold on the fourteenth day. Loudness balance tests were begun on the seventh day

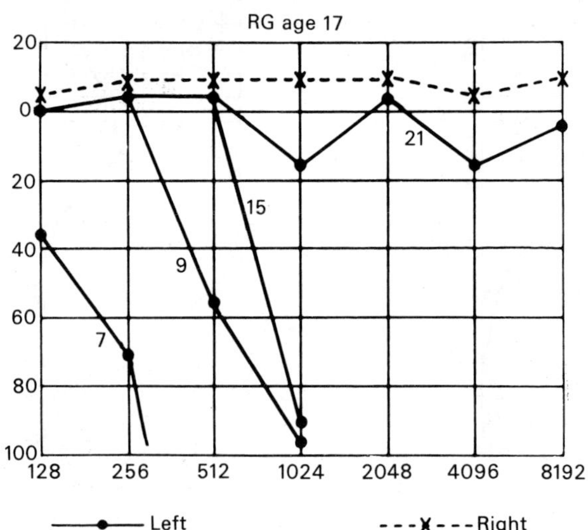

Fig. 16.7. Recovery of pure-tone threshold found to occur on successive dates as shown in a patient with multiple sclerosis.

and repeated at regular intervals in the following three weeks. The results of some of these tests are shown in Fig. 16.8 together with the corresponding pure-tone audiograms. At these times of testing it will be seen that complete

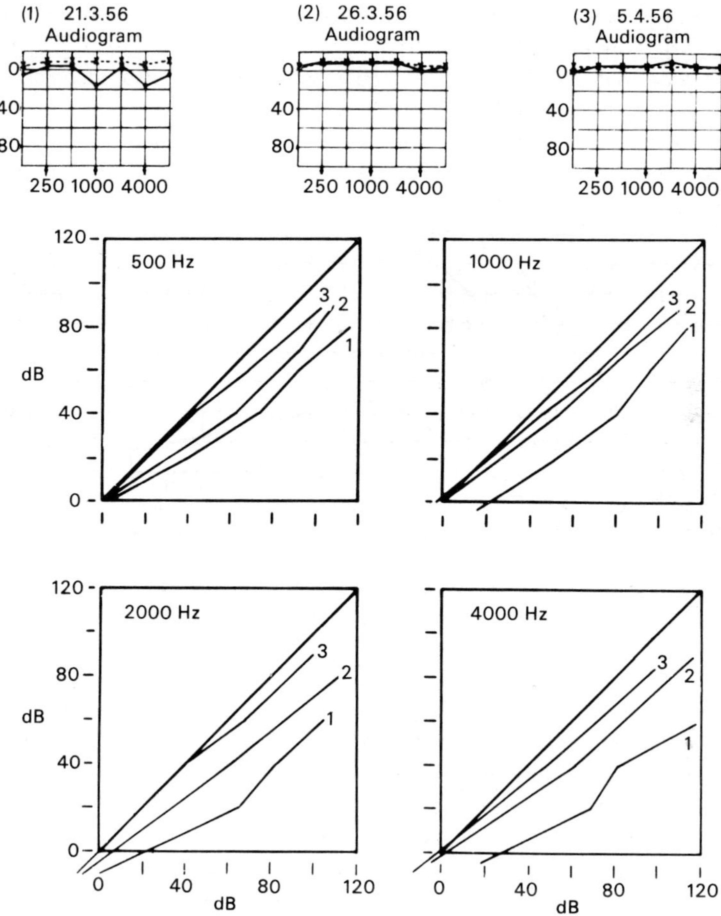

Fig. 16.8. Results of loudness balance tests on three successive occasions in patients with multiple sclerosis.

recovery of the pure-tone threshold had occurred; nevertheless, the loudness balance tests reveal a marked abnormality of the loudness function, the subsequent recovery of which is shown by the three curves at each frequency. Speech audiograms carried out on the same three occasions are shown in Fig. 16.9 and it will be seen that a close correlation exists between the results of the two procedures. Thus in the results of both tests, curves number 1 both show very marked abnormalities, while curves number 3 show an almost complete return to normality.

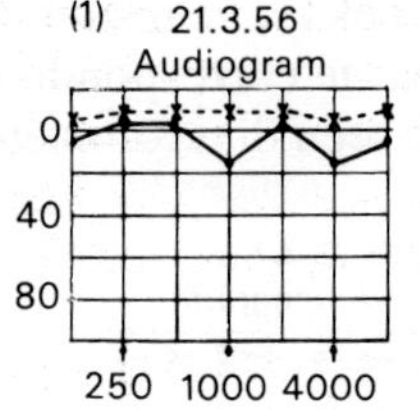

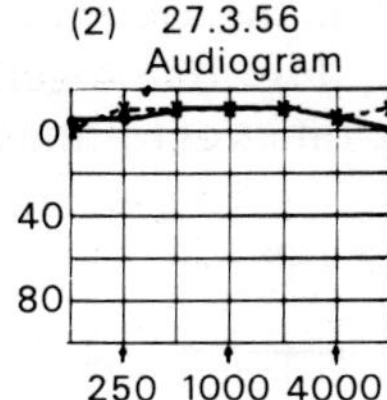

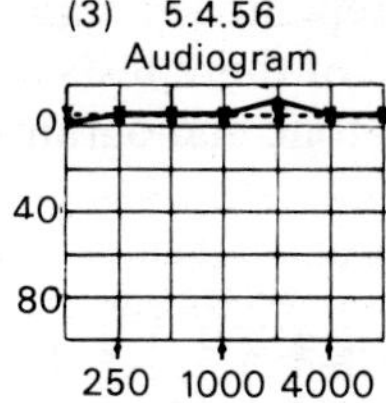

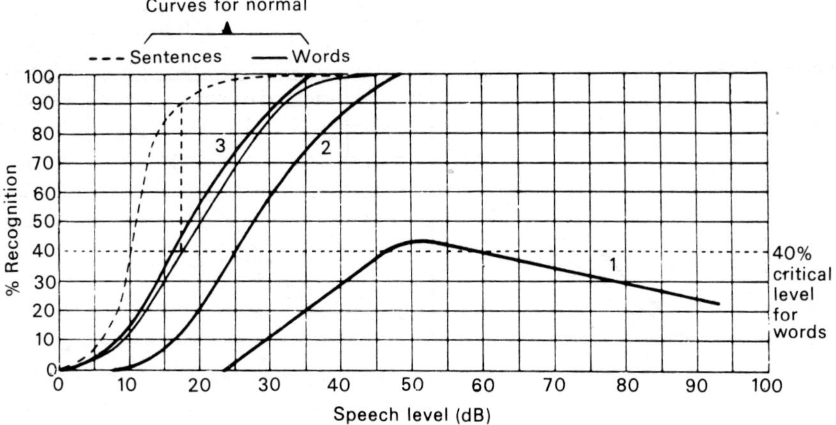

Fig. 16.9. Speech audiograms obtained on three successive occasions (see Fig. 16.8).

This and similar cases we have encountered at The National Hospital exemplify the seeming irrelevance of the pure-tone threshold to speech discrimination ability in 'neural' lesions and it is becoming increasingly clear that marked derangements of the central pathways subserving speech perception can occur in the presence of normal or near-normal auditory pure-tone thresholds. In the case of more subtle derangements further refinements of the testing procedure are called for and will be dealt with in the following section.

SPEECH TESTS IN CENTRAL DEAFNESS

Upon the hypothesis that patients with lesions of the central auditory pathways need all the available information contained in speech to ensure full intelligibility, Bocca and colleagues (Bocca, Calearo, and Cassinari, 1954; Bocca, Calearo, Cassinari, and Migliavacca 1955) reasoned that by eliminating those elements which to a normal person would be considered redundant, derangements of speech perception should be made apparent. Bocca adopted the expedient of using filtered speech for this purpose and showed that in temporal-lobe lesions speech perception at the contralateral ear was significantly worse than at the ipsilateral ear. Subsequently the sensitization of speech has been advocated by a variety of other methods such as time compression or accelerated speech (Calearo and Lazzaroni 1957), periodic interruption (Bocca, Calearo, and Cassinari 1957), oscillating speech from one ear to the other (Hennebert 1955; Bocca *et al.* 1957), high-intensity speech (Greiner and Lafon 1957), and the re-synthesis of the two semispectra of the message delivered to each ear simultaneously (Matzker 1957).

Morales, Garcia, and Poole (1972) adopted the simple expedient of removing redundancy by introducing white noise at two arbitrary signal to noise ratios defined as 0 dB and 5 dB respectively, both of which produced a significant debasement of intelligibility to normal hearing persons. Their results on a series of patients with temporal lobe lesions are shown in Table 16.1. It will be seen that although no systematic differences are apparent at the two ears with unmasked speech, substantially reduced scores appear at the contralateral ear relative to the ipsilateral ear at both signal-to-noise ratios.

TABLE 16.1. *Temporal lobe lesions.* (*Reproduced by the permission of the editor*, Acta Otolaryngologica)

	% Scores for normal speech		% Scores for masked speech			
			S/N ratio 0 dB		S/N ratio +5 dB	
Diagnosis	Ip.	Con.	Ip.	Con.	Ip.	Con.
1. Left temporo-occipital astrocytoma, grade III	96	88	32	4	60	40
2. Left parietotemporal astrocytoma	100	88	36	16	68	56
3. Right temporal lobe haematoma	92	92	48	20	76	48
4. Left parietotemporal astrocytoma, grade III	92	92	36	24	68	48
5. Left temporo-occipital astrocytoma, grade IV	100	96	44	44	72	56
6. Right parietotemporal astrocytoma, grade III	88	84	40	20	76	52
7. Right parietotemporal metastatic epidermoid carcinoma	96	80	40	16	56	36
8. Left temporal astrocytoma, grade III	84	84	16	20	36	48
9. Left temporal cholesteatoma	88	80	36	24	64	44
10. Right temporal lobe haematoma	92	84	44	12	72	32

Morales Garcia, and Poole carried out a further study upon 15 patients with brain-stem lesions in 14 of whom, hearing levels were within normal limits. Their results are displayed in Fig. 16.10 which shows by way of comparison the effect of various signal-to-noise ratios upon speech discrimination in 21 normal subjects. The full-line curves in both scattergrams are derived from the normal subjects and it will be seen that in the case of the

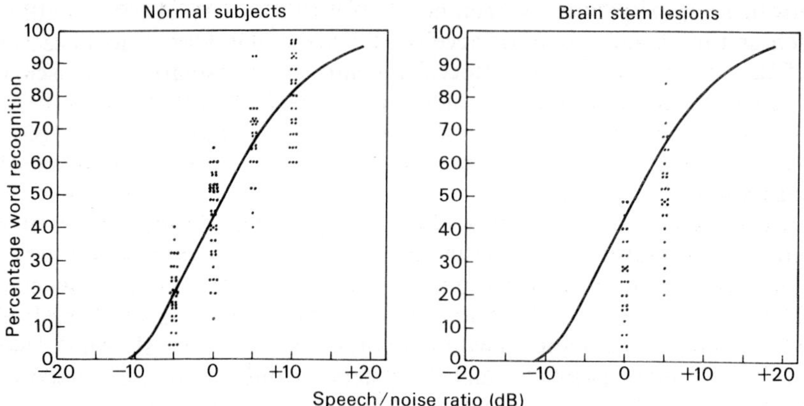

Fig. 16.10. Results of masked speech tests at various signal-to-noise ratios in 14 normal subjects and 15 patients with brain stem lesions. (Reproduced by permission of the editor, *Acta Otolaryngologica*.)

brain-stem lesions the scores are displaced below the curve revealing consistently poorer speech discrimination.

Unfortunately the scatter of the results and the overlap with the normal group is such that it would be difficult to apply this test with any particularly meaningful diagnostic criteria. Nevertheless, the results are important in their demonstration of subtle derangements of the brain-stem pathways subserving speech perception in patients with normal pure-tone thresholds and in whom no other auditory abnormality could be detected.

SPEECH AUDIOMETRY IN THE DETECTION OF NON-ORGANIC HEARING LOSS

Although a variety of strategems involving pure-tone testing have been advocated in the past for the investigation of functional hearing loss it has long been recognized that speech tests of one kind or another can provide a valuable indication of inconsistent response behaviour. One of the earliest and best known is the Doerfler–Stewart test (1946) designed to detect the presence of binaural non-organic hearing loss. This test is based upon the presumption that in the presence of a masking noise the patient with non-organic hearing loss fails to identify words at a level some 10 or 15 dB lower than would normally be expected. In a modified form of the Stenger test (Taylor 1949) speech is delivered at varying intensities to the two ears and it is the examiners' endeavour to confine the stimulus to the 'deaf' ear while persuading the subject that it is being applied to its opposite.

The test calls for particular skill if the examiner is not to be as confused as the patient. However, provided the patient admits to some degree of hearing it is rare, as Carhart (1952) has pointed out, for a conventional speech test not to reveal bizarre responses wholly at odds with his pure-tone audiogram. Two fairly typical examples drawn from a group of ex-servicemen all of whom were in receipt of pensions for war injuries, are shown in Fig. 16.11. The first, a man of 46, suffered bilateral deafness when a mine exploded close by him in 1944. His pure-tone thresholds were particularly variable and the best hearing he would admit to is shown in the audiogram. The speech audiogram, however, is completely at variance with this degree of deafness. The speech reception thresholds at the two ears were only of the order of 60 and 70 dB and, furthermore, discrimination scores in excess of 80 per cent are completely out of character with a deafness of this severity. This patient was certainly deaf, but in all probability the deafness did not exceed 60 dB at the main speech frequencies.

The second patient, again an ex-service man, had a 25-year history of bilateral otitis externa. The best hearing he admitted to is shown in Fig. 16.11(b). The speech audiogram at the right ear on the other hand, takes an unnaturally shallow course with a speech reception threshold of 35 dB. There is a more profound loss at the left ear. On the basis of these findings it is highly likely that in effect he had a trivial loss at the right ear and a moderate to severe loss at the left.

CONFIDENCE LIMITS OF SPEECH MATERIAL

Despite the fact that speech audiometry in one form or another is now widely used, there exists at the present time, no clear consensus of opinion on the choice of material or the method of administration of the tests. In particular, although certain reference levels such as the speech detection threshold and the speech reception threshold are in general use any form of international standardization is conspicuously lacking. Furthermore, it will be clear from the foregoing that there is scope for further refinements in respect of the test material itself with a view to improving the confidence limits and hence the reliability of speech tests. With these aims in view Hood and Poole (1977) carried out validatory tests upon twenty MRC lists re-recorded by a professional announcer. The lists were compiled from the Harvard PB50 lists and typical examples are given in Table 16.2.

Forty-five normal hearing subjects took part in tests carried out free-field. Each list was tested six times at each of one of six sensation levels, 10, 15, 20, 25, 30, and 35 dB. In this way each list was tested 36 times in all, the order and level of presentation being systematically varied to ensure identical conditions for each. Some comment is called for first on the sensation level itself.

Hood and Poole took as their reference level the SDT, the level at which 50 per cent of the words could be heard without being understood. In Fig. 16.12 are shown a typical selection of curves relating the number of speech sounds heard to intensity expressed in arbitrary levels. The lists in fact comprised 30 words, the first five in each being discarded in subsequent articulation tests. A score of 15, therefore, represents the 50 per cent detectability level. It will be seen that they are all of the same form and that detectability rises at a rate of about two words per dB. This means that once

TABLE 16.2. *95% confidence limits (two standard deviations)*

List	Sensation Levels re SDT						
	10 dB	15 dB	20 dB	25 dB	30 dB	35 dB	Overall
(1)3/1 m1	21.4%	22.8%	16.2%	12.8%	13.6%	9.2%	16.8%
(2)3/1 m2	11.4	20.2	15.0	12.0	9.2	5.4	13.0
(3)3/2 m1	12.6	9.0	11.4	14.6	9.8	7.2	11.0
(4)3/2 m2	13.4	9.0	11.0	10.8	10.4	4.0	10.2
(5)3/3 m1	9.0	26.8	13.4	18.8	7.6	10.4	15.8
(6)3/3 m2	9.8	24.8	15.8	7.6	6.0	4.0	13.4
(7)3/4 m1	12.2	20.2	21.0	10.8	8.6	4.6	14.2
(8)3/4 m2	10.0	9.8	16.0	12.8	13.0	12.8	12.6
(9)3/5 m1	6.6	21.0	7.6	17.8	10.8	4.6	12.8
(10)3/5 m2	24.8	12.0	7.2	10.4	11.0	13.4	14.2
(11)3/6 m1	7.6	22.4	15.0	9.8	6.2	9.2	13.0
(12)3/6 m2	15.8	12.0	11.0	18.4	13.6	11.0	13.8
(13)3/7 m1	13.6	4.6	12.0	24.2	18.8	4.0	14.8
(14)3/7 m2	11.0	13.0	14.4	18.4	12.0	7.2	13.2
(15)3/8 m1	17.2	17.2	15.0	22.4	7.6	7.6	15.4
(16)3/8 m2	8.6	23.0	21.8	10.8	7.6	16.2	15.8
(17)3/9 m1	10.0	10.8	32.8	18.2	11.0	7.2	17.4
(18)3/9 m2	6.0	15.6	19.4	16.4	5.4	10.8	13.4
(19)3/10 m1	13.8	31.4	26.2	13.8	10.8	11.0	19.6
(20)3/10 m2	12.2	6.6	12.8	12.0	16.6	6.0	11.6
Means	12.4	16.6	15.8	14.6	10.5	8.3	14.1

a score is obtained at the first trial the 50 per cent level can easily be predicted and confirmed by subsequent testing. In practice this proved to be a simple and rapid procedure with an accuracy of ±1 dB. Kreul *et al.* (1969) urge that 'test standards be based on listener responses to the recorded lists'. As will be shown later, the SDT in the normal varies little with hearing level and this fact, coupled with its ease of determination commends it as an acceptable standard upon which all recorded speech material could be based.

The raw data from the lists referred to this level are presented in Fig. 16.13. Each point represents the articulation score of a subject at a particular sensation level. The crosses are the mean values and through these have been inscribed by hand the curve of best fit. The 95 per cent confidence limits are shown in Table 16.4. It is clearly apparent that first there is an appreciable scatter of the data, and second that the curves differ from each other both in respect of slope and displacement. This results in part from chance factors such as the speaker's intonation, his level of vocalization and so forth occurring during the actual recording and is further exemplified by the regression curves derived from the linear portion of the curves shown to the left of Fig. 16.14. In an attempt to realign the curves, the departures of the individual curves from the mean at the centre of the curves were measured

Fig. 16.11. (a) and (b). Pure-tone and speech audiograms in non-organic hearing loss.

(a)

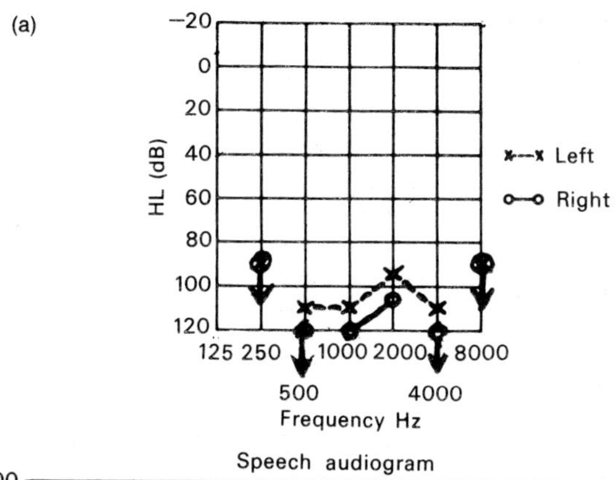
−20
0
20
40
60
80
100
120
HL (dB)
125 250 1000 2000 8000
500 4000
Frequency Hz
Left
Right

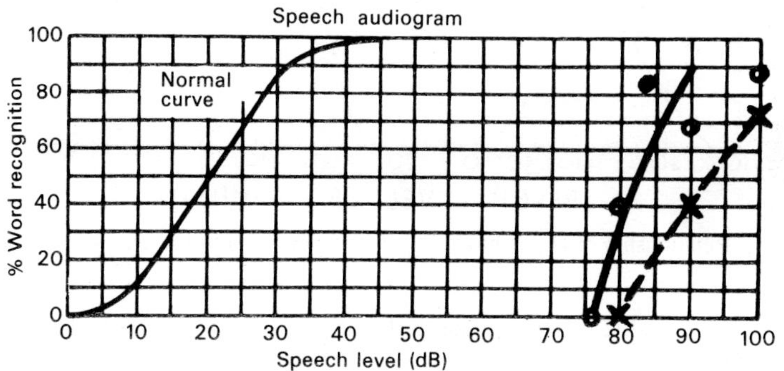
Speech audiogram
100
80
60
40
20
0
% Word recognition
Normal curve
0 10 20 30 40 50 60 70 80 90 100
Speech level (dB)

(b)

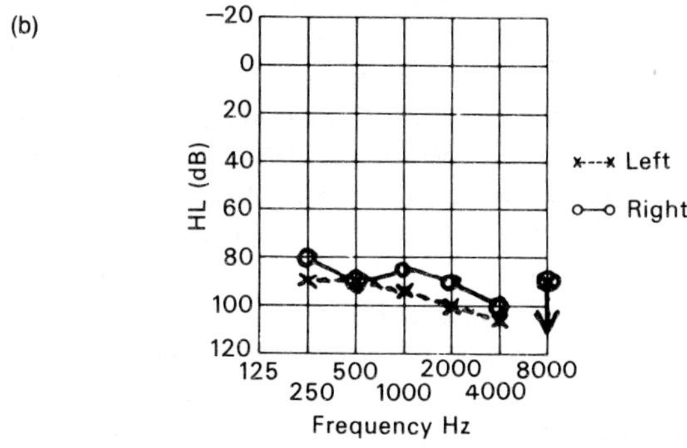
−20
0
20
40
60
80
100
120
HL (dB)
125 500 2000 8000
250 1000 4000
Frequency Hz
Left
Right

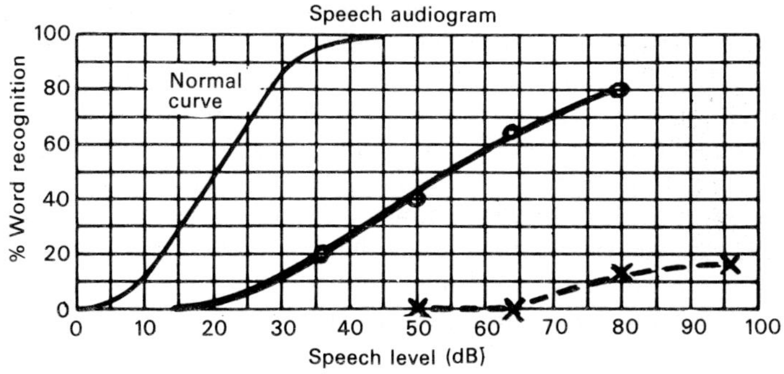
Speech audiogram
100
80
60
40
20
0
% Word recognition
Normal curve
0 10 20 30 40 50 60 70 80 90 100
Speech level (dB)

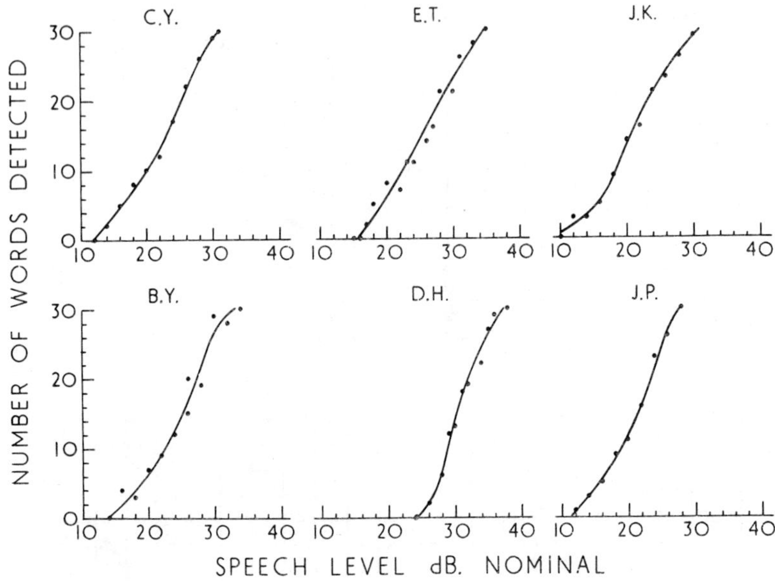

Fig. 16.12. Relationship of words heard (but not understood) to intensity level.

and from these values it was possible to compute that intensity adjustment which would either bring the curves into virtually complete correspondence in the case of curves with the same slope as the mean or cross each other at the 17.5 dB sensation level in the case of those with differing slopes. The result of this operation is shown to the right of Fig. 16.14.

Five of the lists departed markedly from the rest in respect of slope and if this, as is to be anticipated, has any appreciable bearing upon the identity of the lists, then the removal of these five lists should bring about a further improvement. The result of this procedure is shown by the hatched area.

In order to establish the effect of these adjustments upon the confidence limits of the material, data were taken from 16 subjects who were tested with all 20 lists and plotted as individual speech audiograms. Two typical examples are shown in the upper curves of Fig. 16.15.

The 95 per cent confidence limits are shown as the uncorrected values given in column 1, Table 16.4. These data may now be taken as a base line from which improvements resulting from these various manipulations can be measured, as shown in columns 2 and 3. Thus it will be seen that adjusting all 20 lists to coincidence improves the confidence limits overall from ±16.2 to ±13.6 per cent while additionally eliminating the five rogue lists brings further useful improvement to ±12.7 per cent. The effect on the two examples given in Fig. 16.15 is shown in the lower curves. This exercise, therefore, has clearly demonstrated that an approach of this kind can appreciably improve the confidence limits of speech material. Clearly, further refinements might be obtained using more rigid criteria for the

TABLE 16.3.

A	now		quite		sat		sail	
B	jack		bed		feet		take	
C	slit		near		head		right	
D	last		run		bright		bore	
E	town		wall		thought		tea	
1	fin		strife		share		most	
2	cloak		bar		axe		cry	
3	shed		bask		thorn		doubt	
4	doom		rise		thine		goat	
5	rut		fern		thaw		dip	
6	hatch		pan		fade		probe	
7	rack		fraud		lip		punch	
8	pearl		death		loud		pond	
9	bush		rat		lunge		sprig	
10	float		slip		rose		flat	
11	bath		creed		chill		tab	
12	sage		deed		sieve		feel	
13	test		end		his		arc	
14	tick		crash		chain		mouse	
15	pinch		heap		cub		kit	
16	blonde		pest		sack		rice	
17	starve		hunt		claw		crutch	
18	slap		ford		grey		net	
19	scab		wheat		waste		arm	
20	new		hid		hide		wood	
21	peck		not		crab		beam	
22	bus		such		chaff		code	
23	hiss		bride		lynch		snow	
24	kite		fuss		trod		prod	
25	course		pile		art		shop	

selection of slopes but on present evidence it seems likely that this would follow a law of diminishing returns. In consequence the impression is that in the final analysis the established limits must largely if not exclusively, reflect the intersubject redundancy factor referred to earlier as well as intrasubject variability concerned with such matters as attention, motivation, and vigilance upon which we can exert very little control.

Needless to say, further improvements can be obtained using phonemic analysis, i.e. scoring each correct consonant or vowel irrespective of whether the whole word was heard correctly. Applied in this way to the 16 subjects referred to in Table 16.4 the confidence limit of ±12.7 per cent for words is further reduced to ±9.5 per cent for phonemes. On present evidence it seems likely that in considering the reliability of speech audiometry a figure of this order is approaching the ultimate that can be expected. In effect this means that if speech material of this kind is used, say, to assess the effectiveness of different hearing aids using only a single list for each,

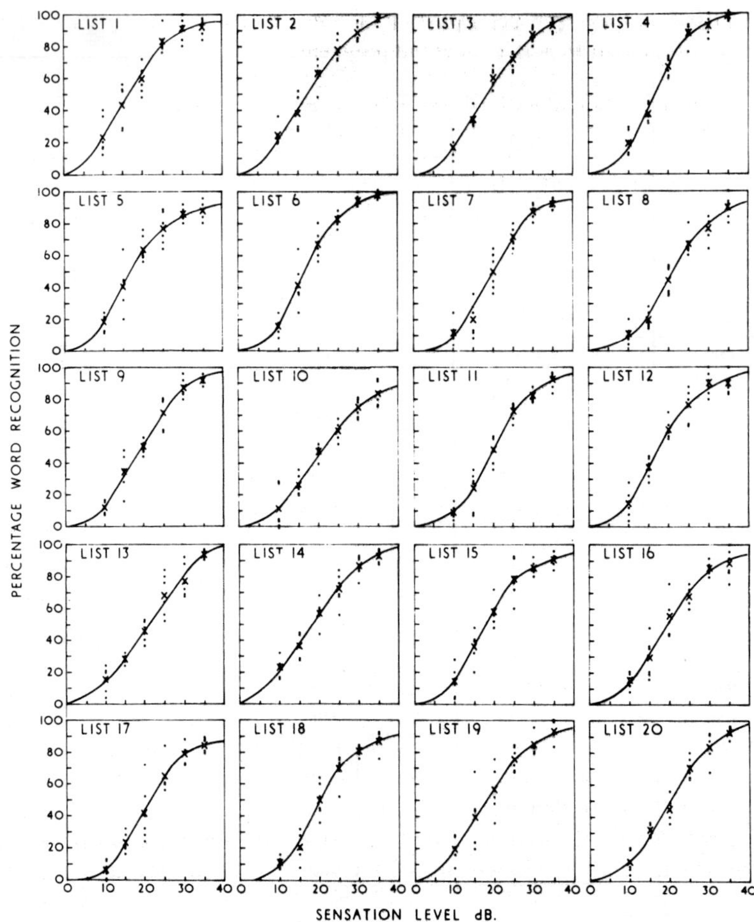

Fig. 16.13. Raw data, 20 lists (see text).

then for there to be a 95 per cent probability that one aid was better than another the scores would need to differ by 19 per cent.

SPEECH DETECTION THRESHOLD, SPEECH RECEPTION THRESHOLD, AND HEARING LEVEL

A number of earlier studies, Carhart (1952), Gjaevenes (1969) and Jerger and Jerger (1976) have shown what appears to be a remarkably good correlation between the speech reception threshold and pure-tone hearing level averaged over the main speech frequencies. Carhart in particular demonstrates a striking one-to-one relationship. If this is in fact so then of course, the SRT can be presumed to provide a very satisfactory prediction of HL for pure-tones and vice versa. However, a little thought will show that this cannot be accepted as a generalization. Thus if we turn to Figs 16.3 and

TABLE 16.4. *Improvement in 95% confidence limits following adjustment of lists*

Subject	95% Confidence Limits (SD × 2) 20 Lists Unadjusted	Adjusted	15 Lists Adjusted
HO	±18.6%	±14.7%	±14.3%
JA	22.1	20.3	20.6
BY	21.6	16.6	14.8
KM	18.5	11.9	11.6
SH	11.6	12.5	11.9
SK	14.9	13.1	12.8
CY	12.0	10.5	8.9
LS	19.6	17.6	16.5
SA	15.1	11.3	9.7
LC	14.6	15.2	16.3
SG	17.2	13.2	14.0
FK	13.7	15.8	14.3
JA	14.3	10.9	10.1
MR	20.0	14.6	12.8
DL	11.6	9.2	7.1
PD	13.4	10.3	7.0
Means	16.2%	13.6%	12.7%

16.5 it is obvious that in the case of Ménière's disease, as the hearing level increases the maximum discrimination score falls, with a marked change in the form of the curve so that SRT increases disproportionately with HL and with maximum discrimination scores less than 50 per cent a conventional SRT cannot of course, be established. Jerger, recognizing this difficulty, measured the SRT at the 50 per cent level on patients with maximum discrimination scores greater than 70 per cent and at the 25 per cent level on patients with maximum scores less than 70 per cent excluding altogether from his study all patients with maximum scores less than 31 per cent. Even so, Jerger's own data clearly indicates that in sensorineural deafness, as the maximum discrimination score falls, the discrepancy between SRT and HL increases quite strikingly.

With these considerations in mind it is of interest to consider the relationship of HL to SRT in the case of normal hearing subjects. This is shown in Fig. 16.16 (Hood and Poole 1977). In the absence of any standard physical measure of speech level the SRTs are expressed in arbitrary units. It is clear from the scattergram that within the range of HLs that can be considered to encompass normal hearing SRT does not increase in direct proportion to hearing level, indeed in this instance according to the regression curve an increase of 4 dB in hearing level raises the SRT by only 1 dB on average.

The comparable relationship established between HL and SDT is shown in Fig. 16.17. Once again the surprising finding is that a fourfold change in HL brings about only a onefold change in SDT.

These apparently paradoxical findings conflict with the general expecta-

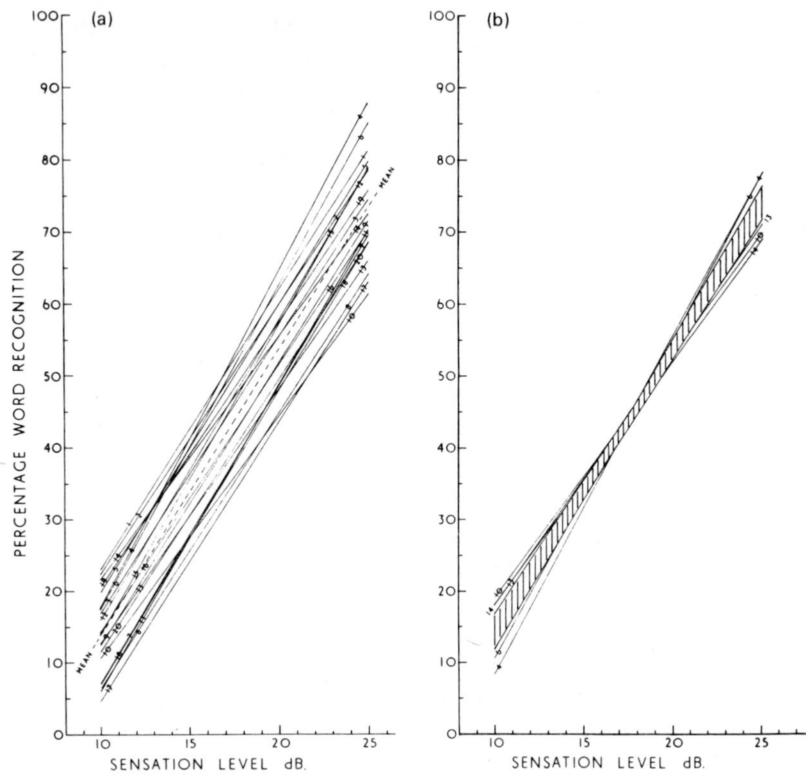

Fig. 16.14. (a). Regression curves of individual lists. (b) Curves adjusted to coincidence, shaded portion excludes five 'rogue' lists. From practical considerations adjustments were made to the nearest 0.5 dB.

tion implicit in the studies on deaf subjects referred to earlier that our ability to hear and understand speech should correlate closely with hearing level. One explanation that comes to mind at least to account for the HL/SRT relationship concerns the amount of redundant information present in normal speech. From an evolutionary point of view, this would seem to provide the essential reserve, which is vital for the maintenance of speech communication throughout life, when the information content of speech is progressively eroded by the changes in hearing level accompanying old age. The redundancy factor is, however, by no means constant from one individual to another, and furthermore, there is abundant evidence that it is plastic since it is well known that a deaf subject provided with a hearing aid for the first time can, with persistence, effect marked improvements in his speech discrimination.

If these considerations apply to deafness they apply equally well to hearing levels within the normal range. The pure-tone threshold is in many respects an unphysiological measurement of hearing because under no

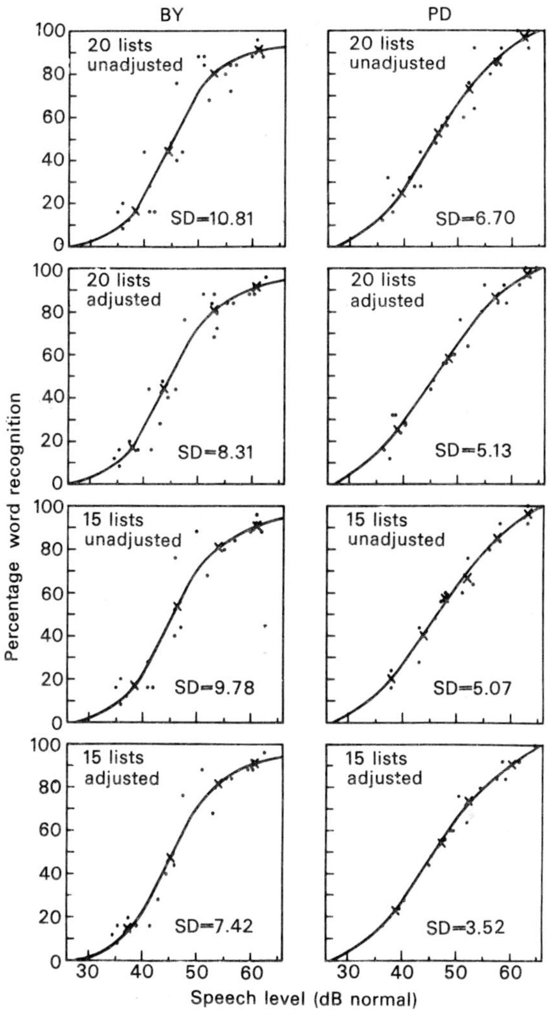

Fig. 16.15. Effects of intensity adjustments and rejection of 'rogue' lists in two subjects.

natural circumstances are we required to perceive pure tones at liminal levels. By and large we are accustomed to using our hearing for the reception of speech and to this end it can be argued that we subconsciously utilize our available hearing to the best of our ability and if our hearing is somewhat less acute than that of our better hearing peers then we compensate by acquiring better discriminative abilities.

In this event, SRT will, to an appreciable extent, be independent of HL. The relationship between hearing level and SDT might, however, appear more problematical. Nevertheless, it is worth recalling that the SDT is in no sense a liminal threshold as is the pure-tone threshold, indeed at this level

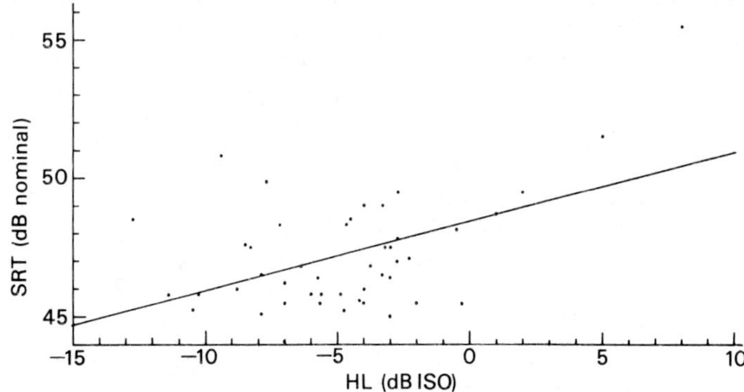

Fig. 16.16. Relationship between speech reception threshold and hearing level.

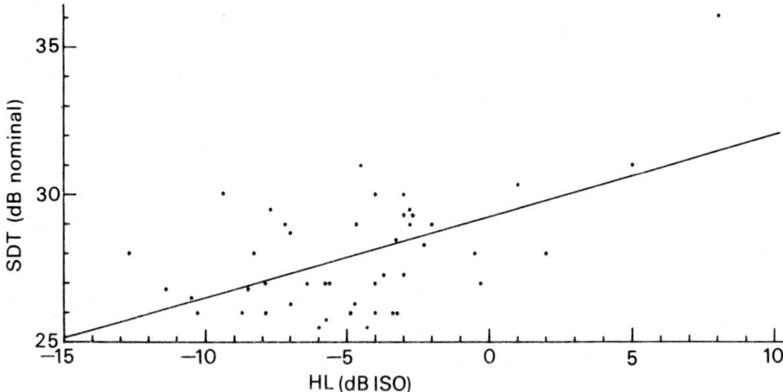

Fig. 16.17. Relationship between speech detection threshold and hearing level.

many of the louder speech sounds are heard well above the threshold, in addition, it can be argued that while we are not attuned to the detection of pure tones at threshold levels, the detection of speech sounds with their distinctive spectra at all levels is a familiar every day occurrence and on this account the neural information at the level of the central auditory pathways may well be processed quite differently.

In fact there is good psychophysical evidence for this notion. Thus Kay and Matthews (1972) have clearly demonstrated the existence of certain channels selectively tuned to frequency modulation which they maintain are the substrata of auditory speech analysis. In this connection it is worth recalling that marked speech discrimination derangements can be demonstrated in patients with central auditory lesions, in whom the pure-tone thresholds are within normal limits.

This is an area about which we presently know very little and clearly more research is needed. In the past we have perhaps taken too simplistic a view of speech perception. Certainly hearing loss degrades speech perception but the relationship might not be quite so straightforward as has implictly been assumed, in particular the question of redundancy needs to be considered in more detail. Thus, Gat and Keith (1978) have shown that whereas native and non-native subjects both performed comparably to speech tests in the quiet the non-native subjects performed significantly worse in the presence of noise. The obvious interpretation of these findings is that the limited linguistic experience of the non-native subjects imposed a low redundancy factor so that in the presence of noise, information vital to intelligibility was quickly eroded. This, however, is only a question of degree; similar, if smaller, differences might well be evident between say, the recluse and the gossip.

At present we have no means of quantifying this aspect yet it must exert an important unknown influence upon any subject's responses to speech tests and in consequence set a limit to their diagnostic reliability.

A promising new development involving synthesized speech in which much of the redundant information can be removed has been outlined elsewhere (Fourcin 1979). Coupled with new interactive testing techniques this might well surmount the problem of redundancy and bring to speech tests the precision they presently lack.

REFERENCES

Bocca, E., Calearo, C., and Cassinari, V. (1954). A new method for testing hearing in temporal lobe tumours. *Acta oto-lar.* **44**, 219–21.

—— —— and —— (1957). La surdité corticale. *Rev. Lar. Otol. Rhinol.* **78**, 777.

—— —— —— and Migliavacca, F. (1955). Testing 'cortical' hearing in temporal lobe tumours. *Acta oto-lar.* **45**, 289–304.

Boothroyd, A. (1967). The discrimination by partially hearing children of frequency distorted speech. *Int. Audiol.* **6**, 136–45.

Brandy, W. T. (1966). Reliability of voice tests of speech discrimination. *J. Speech Hear. Res.* **9**, 461–5.

Calearo, C. and Lazzaroni, A. (1957). Speech intelligibility in relation to the speed of the message. *Laryngoscope, St. Louis* **67**, 410.

Carhart, R. (1952). Speech audiometry in clinical evaluation. *Acta oto-lar.* **41**, 18–42.

Citron, L., Dix, M. R., Hallpike, C. S., and Hood, J. D. (1963). A recent clinico-pathological study of cochlear nerve degeneration resulting from tumour pressure and disseminated sclerosis, with particular reference to the finding of normal threshold sensitivity for pure tones. *Acta oto-lar.* **56**, 330–7.

Coles, R. R. A. (1972). Can present day audiology really help in diagnosis? An otologist's question. *J. Lar. Otol.* **86**, 191–224.

Doerfler, L. G. and Stewart, K. (1946). Malingering and psychogenic deafness. *J. Speech Dis.* **11**, 181–6.

Egan, J. P. (1944). Articulation testing methods II. OSRD Report No. 3802. Psychoacoustic Laboratory, Harvard University, Cambridge, Mass.

Evans, E. F. (1975). Normal and abnormal functioning of the cochlear nerve. In *Sound reception in mammals* (eds. R. J. Bench, A. Pye, and J. D. Pye) pp. 133–65. Zoological Society: Academic Press, London.

Fletcher, H. (1929). *Speech and hearing.* Macmillan, London.

Fourcin, A. J. (1979). Speech pattern audiometry. In *Auditory investigation: the scientific and technological basis* (ed. H. A. Beagley) pp. 170–208. Oxford University Press.

GAT, I. B. and KEITH, R. W. (1978). An effect of linguistic experience. *Audiology* **17**, 339–45.

GJAEVENES, K. (1969). Estimating speech reception thresholds from pure tone hearing loss. *J. Audit. Res.* **9**, 139–44.

GREINER, G. F. and LAFON, J. C. (1957). La distorsion spatiale du test phonétique dans les dyslexies sans surdités tonales et son utlisation dans le dépistage des surdités corticales. *Annls Oto-lar.* **74**, 400–10.

HENNEBERT, D. (1955). L'intégration de la perception auditive et l'audition alternante. *Acta otor-rhino-lar. Belg.* **9**, 344–6.

HOOD, J. D. and POOLE, J. P. (1971). Speech audiometry in conductive and sensori-neural hearing loss. *Sound* **5**, 30–8.

—— —— (1977). Improving the reliability of speech audiometry. *Br. J. Audiol.* **11**, 93–101.

JERGER, S. and JERGER, J. (1976). Estimating speech threshold from the PI–PB function. *Archs Otolar.* **102**, 487–96.

KAY, R. H. and MATTHEWS, D. R. (1972). On the existence in human auditory pathways of channels selectively tuned to the modulation present in frequency–modulated tones. *J. Physiol., Lond.* **225**, 657–77.

KREUL, J. E., BELL, D. W., and NIXON, J. C. (1969). Factors affecting speech discrimination test difficulty. *J. Speech Hear. Res.* **12**, 281–7.

LIERLE, D. M. (1959). Report of the Committee on Conservation of Hearing. *Trans. Am. Acad. Ophthal. Otolar.* **63**, 236–8.

LYREGAARD, P. E., ROBINSON, D. W., and HINCHCLIFFE, R. (1976). A feasibility study of diagnostic speech audiometry. NPL Acoustics Report Ac 73.

MATZKER, J. (1957). Ein neuer Weg zur otolgischen Diagnostik zerebraier Erkrankungen. Der binaural Test bei raumverengenden endokraniellen. *Prozessen Z. Lar. Rhinol. Otol.* **36**, 177–89.

PETERSON, G. E. and LEHISTE, I. (1962). Revised C.N.C. Lists for auditory tests. *J. Speech Hear. Dis.* **27**, 62–70.

TAYLOR, G. J. (1949). An experimental study of tests for the detection of auditory malingering. *J. Speech Hear. Dis.* **14**, 119–30.

TILLMAN, T. W. and CARHART, R. (1966). An expanded test for speech discrimination utilizing CNC monosyllabic words (North-western University Auditory Test No. 6). Technical Report SAM-TR-66-55. USAF School of Aerospace Medicine, Aerospace Medical Division (AFSC), Brooks Air Force Base, Texas.

—— —— and WILBER, L. (1963). A test for speech discrimination composed of C.N.C. monosyllabic words (N. U. auditory test No. 4). Technical Report No. SAM-TDR-62-135. USAF, School of Aerospace Medicine.

WOLF, O. (1874). New investigations on the methods of examination and derangements of hearing. *Archs Ophthal. Otol.* **4**, 67–86.

17 Diagnosis of acoustic neuroma

W. P. R. GIBSON

There are clearly two stages of progression of an acoustic neuroma—the otological period and the neurological period. As the tumour slowly enlarges the patient first enters the otological period and suffers from symptoms such as auditory loss or dysfunction, tinnitus, or imbalance; then, after a variable period, the tumour becomes large enough to cause neurological symptoms. Although an acoustic neuroma is a benign tumour histologically, once it enters the neurological stages its course is far from benign. Cushing (1917) has described the sequence of events as follows: suboccipital discomfort, instability of cerebellar origin, evidence of impairment of adjacent cranial nerves, raised intracranial pressure, and finally dysarthria, dysphasia and decerebrate attacks with respiratory failure causing death. The exact order of occurrence is debatable but the important feature is that the tumour runs a slowly progressive course which ends in death unless the appropriate treatment is forthcoming.

In days bygone, the slow course of the tumour coupled with the appallingly high surgical mortality (Tooth (1912) quotes a mortality of 75 per cent with most survivors being severely disabled) forced physicians to advise leaving surgery until the patient was already becoming handicapped, and for surgeons to only undertake partial tumour removal. This situation has altered dramatically owing to both improved surgical and anaesthetic techniques and to new operative aids such as the operating microscope. Today the surgical removal of small* acoustic neuromas has a negligible mortality. House (1978) reported no deaths amongst the last 300 tumours he has excised. The additional bonus for the patient is that the postoperative disability is slight. It is usually possible to preserve the facial nerve and it is possible, in some instances, even to preserve hearing. The patient now has everything to gain from early diagnosis and surgery: nothing can be offered by delaying diagnosis and surgery except a miserable existence with a deformed face, or worse, chronic ataxia, dementia, or even death.

The onus is on the otologist to detect acoustic neuromas at an early stage. In many respects this is an impossible and daunting task. Otologists see hundreds of patients every year with unilateral cochlear dysfunction and yet only a handful have an early acoustic neuroma. It is quite impossible to submit every patient to the full range of tests necessary to detect the tumour as this would lead to the otologist spending a disproportionate time searching for rare tumours and neglect other important duties. This chapter will

* In the classification of size, a large tumour is over 3.5 cm in diameter, a medium tumour is under 3.5 cm in diameter but not confined to the internal acoustic meatus, and a small tumour lies entirely within the internal acoustic meatus.

try to present a reasoned approach to early diagnosis of acoustic neuromas which starts by treating all patients as suspects and gradually selects, according to the test results, so that only the highly probable cases are actually subjected to the more unpleasant procedures such as cysternography or angiography.

The investigations that are outlined serve equally well to detect the less common tumours of the cerebellopontine angle. At the end of the chapter, the differential diagnosis will be mentioned.

THE HISTORY

In the vast majority of patients the first symptoms of an acoustic neuroma are either auditory or vestibular dysfunction (Table 17.1). In many cases the patient notices these symptoms but does not consider them serious enough to merit the advice of a physician, and present much later in neurological clinics complaining of headaches, blurring of vision, ataxia, or trigeminal symptoms.

The period between the first otological symptoms and the development of neurological symptoms is extremely variable, from only six months to many years, but is generally around two years. Clinically it appears that the progression is often very rapid in younger patients and much slower in the elderly.

TABLE 17.1. *Unilateral acoustic neuromas – presenting symptoms in 123 cases. (Reproduced from Morrison (1975) by permission)*

Symptom	Primary complaint (%)	Secondary complaint (%)
Deafness/tinnitus	60	15.5
Unsteadiness	7	30
Headache	15.5	14
Vth nerve symptoms	7	14.5
Failing vision	2.9	12.6
Earache	4.2	4.2
True vertigo	3.4	2.9
Drowsiness and vomiting	–	3.4
Altered taste	–	2.9

The first and most important feature of the history which should raise suspicion is when the symptoms are unilateral. Bilateral tumours occur in 8 per cent of affected patients but are usually associated with obvious neurofibromatosis.

The otological symptoms can be classified into three main groups:

Audiological symptoms

The most usual auditory symptom is hearing loss, but as most of these tumours, despite their common name, arise from the myelin sheath of the vestibular nerve, it is not surprising to find reports of patients with early tumours who suffer from little or no auditory dysfunction. Logically, one may deduce that 100 per cent of tumours have no cochlear symptoms initially and that auditory symptoms only arise when the tumour reaches sufficient size to compress the cochlear nerve or interfere with its blood supply. Apart from loss of hearing acuity, patients may complain of loss of speech discrimination or difficulties in locating the source of sounds. A common early symptom is difficulty using a telephone in the affected ear. Tinnitus can be noticed by the patient before he notices any change in his hearing. The tinnitus is generally a high-pitched broad-band noise rather than a pure tone. It is rarely pulsatile.

In the early stages of tumour growth, the hearing can fluctuate owing to vascular factors. The author can recall one patient whose hearing actually improved during a glycerol dehydration test. About 10 per cent of patients who complain of a sudden hearing loss are found to have an acoustic neuroma and conversely about 20 per cent of patients with acoustic neuromas complain of a sudden loss of hearing during the course of the disorder (Morrison 1975). Often the hearing seems to recover partially and the unwary clinician can fail to detect the tumour. All patients with sudden hearing losses should be carefully investigated.

Vestibular symptoms

It seems probable that the vestibular nerve is affected before the cochlear nerve, but despite this vestibular symptoms are less common than auditory symptoms. The loss of vestibular function is usually insidious and most patients only experience slight difficulties of balance whenever their ability to see is poor. For instance, they may complain of veering towards the affected side whenever they are walking in a dimly lit street.

The incidence of rotational attacks of vertigo is only around 4 per cent so that differential diagnosis from Ménière's disorder can usually be reached on this symptom alone (Ozsahinoglu and Harrison 1974). Positional vertigo associated with rapid movements of the head usually from one side to the other or on turning corners fast when walking occurs in about 33 per cent of patients (Ozsahinoglu and Harrison 1974). As the tumour enlarges it begins to interfere with cerebellar function and abnormalities of stance and gait occur.

Other symptoms

Suboccipital discomfort is rare during the early stages (King, Gibson, and Morrison 1976) but on careful questioning, nearly 33 per cent of patients do complain of some discomfort in or around the affected ear. The probable mechanism is the comparative vulnerability of the small diameter fibres which travel with the facial nerve and are later distributed along the vagus nerve as the post-auricular cutaneous nerve (Arnold's nerve). Paralysis of the larger motor fibres of the facial nerve occurs only with very large tumours.

Rarely patients present with a disturbance of taste on the anterior two-thirds of the ipsilateral side of the tongue. These fibres travel with the facial nerve before passing along the chorda tympani nerve.

Headache is a common symptom even in early tumours but as it occurs in many other conditions, it is rarely sufficient to raise suspicion. The other symptoms such as fifth nerve involvement, failing vision, and drowsiness and vomiting are only encountered in fairly large tumours.

THE EXAMINATION

The usual otological examination should be performed and in addition there are a number of simple neurological signs which should be sought whenever an acoustic neuroma is suspected. These neurological signs often appear long before the patient notices any neurological symptoms.

Papilloedma

The presence of papilloedema indicates a large tumour. Papilloedema has to be marked before the patient has any visual impairment, and then often only a slight peripheral haziness of vision is noted. About 15 per cent of patients first present after they have developed papilloedema as they may have only previously had only minor aural symptoms which they have ignored.

Ocular muscle palsies

Paralysis of the eye muscles is a very late sign. Large tumours can cause an ipsilateral VI paralysis.

Nystagmus

The subject of nystagmus is discussed in greater detail later in this chapter under the heading of electronystagmography. Nevertheless, nystagmus can be observed in many cases by simple naked-eye examination. Unless the tumour is large enough to compress the brainstem and cerebellum, the nystagmus is increased in amplitude or only becomes apparent when the patient is unable to fixate his gaze. It is important, therefore, to examine the patient's eyes using Frenzel's glasses. Under these circumstances, nystagmus can be observed in 60 per cent of medium sized tumours and in 33 per cent of the small tumours (Morrison 1975).

Trigeminal nerve dysfunction

Facial numbness or facial pain is generally only experienced by patients with large tumours. Nevertheless, 80 per cent of patients with tumours have diminished corneal sensation on the affected side. The concept of the 'corneal reflex' should be abandoned as it suggests dabbing the cotton wool directly onto the cornea and looking to see if the patient blinks. The cotton wool should gently approach the cornea from the side and the patient is asked to describe his subjective sensation.

Facial nerve dysfunction

Obvious motor nerve involvement is a late sign as the large motor fibres are surprisingly resistant to compression by tumour enlargement within the internal acoustic meatus. Slight dysfunction of the nerve may occur more commonly but can only be detected by measuring the velocity of nerve condition. Pulec and House (1964) measured the timing of the blink reaction using high-speed cinephotography. Nine out of 11 patients with proven tumours had a blink delayed by more than 4 milliseconds on the affected side compared with the unaffected side. The two with no delay had small tumours. Krott, Peremba, and Busse (1969) have reported similar increased latencies using electromyographic studies in 19 out of 28 patients with proven tumours.

Disorders of taste are often detected in small tumours. The disturbance is best measured using electrogustometry. This enables one to measure the threshold of taste for an electric current in milliamperes. A difference of over 10 mA is considered significant. Morrison (1975) found a disturbance of taste in 50 per cent of small tumours. (Table 17.2).

TABLE 17.2. *The incidence of altered taste as measured by electrogustometry (71 cases). (Reproduced from Morrison (1975) by permission)*

Tumour size	Altered taste threshold(%)†
Large (35)	86
Medium (30)	53
Small (6)	50

† Electrogustometric threshold difference of 10μA or greater.

Lacrymation

Diminished lacrymation on the affected side may occur in early tumours as the small secretomotor parasympathetic fibres travel with the facial nerve through the internal acoustic meatus. A third of small tumours cause decreased tearing on the affected side (Table 17.3).

TABLE 17.3. *The incidence of diminished lacrymation as measured by Schirmer's test (71 cases). (Reproduced from Morrison (1975) by permission)*

Tumour size	Diminished lacrymation(%)†
Large (35)	77
Medium (30)	47
Small (6)	33

† Schirmer's test difference of 5 mm or greater.

Loss of sensation

Loss of sensation within the tragus of the affected ear has been described by Hiltseberger and House (1964). The sensory fibres concerned are thought to arise from the facial nerve and later to pass to the vagus and then to the posterior meatal wall and tragus. This is the so-called 'zone of Ramsay Hunt'.

Other cranial nerve dysfunctions

Loss of function of the ninth, tenth, eleventh, and twelfth cranial nerves occurs as the tumour extends inferiorly towards the foramen magnum drawing these cranial nerves around its lower pole. Loss of function of these nerves always indicates a very large acoustic neuroma although these signs appear earlier in other cerebellopontine angle tumours when the pathological condition is not benign.

Local pain

Almost 33 per cent of patients complain of a deep-seated pain within the affected ear (Morrison 1975). This symptom can occur even with small tumours. It is possibly due to pressure effects upon the dural lining of the internal acoustic meatus. Tomography should be carried out on all patients with unexplained otalgia.

Abnormal stance and gait

Although the loss of vestibular function is usually insidious, the patient may have abnormalities of gait and stance. In early cases, the gait is usually normal but there can be abnormal posture when the patient closes his eyes. Patients with acoustic neuromas often complain thet they have difficulty walking in the dark. Often they veer towards the affected side. Gross difficulties of gait and stance occur when a large tumour interferes with cerebellar function.

Cerebellar dysfunction

The presence of cerebellar dysfunction indicates that the tumour has extended backwards to affect the middle cerebellar peduncle and the flocculus. Minor degrees of cerebellar dysfunction can often be most easily detected by characteristic changes of the electronystagmogram. These changes are discussed later in this chapter.

THE INVESTIGATIONS

The vigour with which the clinician pursues the investigations should depend on the likelihood of the patient having an acoustic neuroma. Nevertheless, early diagnosis does depend on a high suspicion index and it is only reasonable to abandon the diagnosis after *several* investigations have proved negative. Table 17.4 illustrates the author's approach, beginning with simple investigations for *all* patients presenting with auditory dysfunction and proceeding to the next stage of investigation whenever the results are in the least suspicious.

TABLE 17.4. *A flow chart for the investigation of suspected cases of acoustic neuroma*

Pure-tone audiogram (± loudness discomfort level)
Impedence audiometry – tympanometry
– acoustic reflex thresholds
– acoustic reflex adaptation
Radiography of the mastoid and IAM
Serology

↓

Adaptation tests
Alternate loudness balance test
Speech audiogram
(Békésy audiogram and SISI test)
Caloric tests and electronystagmography
Tomography of IAM

↓

Electric response audiometry (ECochG and BSER)
Computerized axial tomography

↓

CAT scan with oxygen cysternography
(Air encephalography and vertebral arteriography)

↓

Surgical exploration

Audiometric investigation

The classic audiometric findings on testing an acoustic neuroma patient are a unilateral hearing loss, absence of recruitment, abnormal adaptation, and poor speech discrimination. If a clinician relies on finding all these classic signs before reaching his diagnosis he will be disappointed. Virtually all tumours have some atypical audiological features and the percentage of atypical features is increased if the tumour is small.

Pure-tone threshold audiometry (PTTA)

This is the most commonly available audiometric test which measures the hearing threshold for pure-tone bursts delivered through an earphone (air conduction) or by a vibrator placed on the skull (bone conduction). Most acoustic neuromas cause some hearing loss although there are an increasing number of reports of tumours reaching fairly large proportions without significantly affecting the PTTA (e.g. Jerger 1973). Occasionally a long-standing auditory disorder may obscure the hearing alteration due to the tumour and the clinician can easily be misled.

When the PTTA is affected, inspection of the air and bone thresholds reveals a sensorineural hearing loss. Johnson (1977) reported the audiometric patterns encountered on testing 425 patients with surgically proven tumours (Table 17.5). Morrison (1975) provided similar figures after testing a smaller series. Although a high tone loss occurs most commonly, this cannot be considered diagnostic as this particular audiometric pattern occurs in many other auditory disorders, such as presbyacusis.

TABLE 17.5. *The pattern of the pure-tone audiogram in 425 cases. (Reproduced from Johnson (1977) by permission)*

Type of loss	%
High-tone loss	66
Flat loss	13
Trough-shaped loss	12
Low-tone loss	9

The loudness discomfort level (LDL)

The LDL is a simple test for recruitment and is mentioned at this time because it can be easily performed after the PTTA. It only takes a few minutes to accomplish and it has the advantage of being a monaural test of recruitment. Patients with a recruiting hearing loss usually have a LDL within 10 dB of the unaffected ear. A raised LDL indicates either a conductive or a non-recruiting hearing loss. The subjective nature of the test limits its exactness but nevertheless it does provide a useful screening procedure, especially if impedance audiometry is not available.

Alternate binaural loudness balance (ABLB)

This test compares the growth of loudness between the affected and the non-affected ear. Some pitfalls are avoided by using the more normal ear as the reference ear (Hood 1977a). Table 17.6 shows the results of the ALBL in a series of 104 patients examined by the author.

TABLE 17.6. *The alternate loudness balance test for recruitment in 104 cases*

Tumour size	Absent recruitment(%)
Large (42)	81
Medium (50)	58
Small (12)	50

Johnson (1977) found similar results although he did not relate them to tumour size. He reported that only 50 per cent of his patients had complete absence of recruitment and 23 per cent had complete recruitment. Many of his cases were small or medium-sized tumours.

Short increment sensitivity test (SISI)

Low SISI scores (0–30 per cent) are said to be typical of a neural hearing loss. There are, however, several difficulties encountered on applying the test. Some patients give a high SISI score at one frequency and a low SISI score at another frequency. Johnson (1977) gave several examples; one patient had a SISI score of 0 per cent at 1 kHz and a SISI score of 100 per cent at 2 kHz. In other patients the hearing loss is so severe that the test can only be applied at certain frequencies if at all. Sometimes abnormal auditory adaptation accounts for a high score initially and then the patient reports that he no longer hears the carrier tone. Johnson (1977) has reported the results of the SISI test in 362 patients with surgically-proven tumours (Table 17.7). He concludes that the test had little use for the diagnosis of early acoustic neuromas and has abandoned it as a routine test.

TABLE 17.7. *The SISI test in 362 cases. (Reproduced from Johnson (1977) by permission)*

SISI score(%)	%
0 – 30	38
35 – 65	11
70 – 100	34

Tests of abnormal auditory adaptation

Acoustic neuromas classically exhibit temporary threshold drift. The hearing of the patient deteriorates with prolonged exposure to sound and the sound intensity appears to fade. This phenomenon has been called 'tone decay' but this is misleading as it is the intensity which appears to decrease and not the frequency. There are several different tests of abnormal adaptation which can be measured both at near-hearing threshold levels as well as at higher suprathreshold levels. Only three methods which involve the use of the pure-tone audiometer will be mentioned.

THE MODIFIED CAHART PROCEDURE

This test measures the alteration of hearing which occurs at near threshold levels. Pure tones at 250, 1000, or 4000 Hz are presented continuously at 5 dB SL and the intensity is raised 5 dB each time the patient no longer hears the sound. Over 20 dB adaptation is under three minutes at frequencies below 2 kHz is suggestive of a neural lesion. A small amount of adaptation of higher frequencies commonly occurs in purely sensory lesions.

Analysis of this test performed on 104 patients with acoustic neuromas and seen by the author revealed that the typical abnormal adaptation only occurred in half of the small tumours (Table 17.8).

GREEN'S MODIFIED TONE-DECAY TEST

Johnson (1977) used Green's modification of Cahart's test (Green 1963). This test measures the adaptation occurring within one minute and the patient is asked to pay particular attention to any changes in the tone of the

TABLE 17.8. *The modified Cahart test for adaptation in 104 cases (1 kHz)*

Tumour size	Over 20 dB adaptation(%)	Less than 20 dB(%)
Large (42)	83	17
Medium (50)	62	38
Small (12)	50	50

stimulus. He found marked adaptation at one or more frequencies in 40 per cent of patients and moderate adaptation in 38 per cent (304 patients were tested).

JERGER'S SUPRATHRESHOLD TEST FOR ABNORMAL AUDITORY ADAPTATION

Jerger and Jerger (1975) suggested a method of using the pure-tone audiometer to measure suprathreshold adaptation. A pure tone (500, 1000, or 2000 Hz) is presented continuously at 110 dB SPL. If the patient ceases to hear the sound within 60 seconds, the test is regarded as positive. Jerger and Jerger (1975) found that only 4 per cent of patients with known neural lesions escaped diagnosis. Unfortunately, the test does provide a large number of false-positives and 45 per cent of patients with purely sensory conditions gave positive results. This test is useful only as a quick screening method. The more reliable methods of measuring suprathreshold adaptation involve the Békésy audiometer and impedance measurements.

Békésy audiometry

This can be used either for sweep frequency testing or for fixed frequency testing.

SWEEP FREQUENCY TESTING

This was performed on 363 patients with surgically proven tumours by Johnson (1977). He found it difficult to analyse the results exactly as many of the traces did not fit into the four groups described by Jerger (1960). He concluded that the size of the gap (i.e. the threshold for continuous tones and the threshold for pulsed tones) between the pulsed and continuous traces was more important than the frequency at which the gap occurred. The results of testing are shown in Table 17.9.

TABLE 17.9. *Békésy audiometry results in 363 cases. (Reproduced from Johnson (1977) by permission)*

Békésy Type	%
I	8
II	35
III	35
IV	22

Johnson (1977) reported that the number of type III and type IV Békésy traces was 10 per cent less than in his previous series (1968, 1970). This he attributed to the larger number of smaller tumours in the most recent series.

FIXED FREQUENCY TESTING

This involves using the Békésy audiometer to measure adaptation at predetermined frequencies (usually 500 or 1000 Hz). If the continuous tracing falls more than 40 dB below the pulsed tracing, indicating a raised continuous-tone threshold, the presence of a retrocochlear tumour is likely. The test is a sophisticated means of measuring abnormal adaptation but there are no reported series showing that it is any more sensitive than the modified Cahart test or Green's MTTD procedure.

Fixed-frequency Békésy testing can also be used to measure supra-threshold adaptation by asking the patient to maintain the intensity at either the most comfortable loudness level or at the loudness discomfort (uncomfortable) loudness level.

Speech audiometry

Many authorities believe that speech audiometry is one of the best means of detecting early acoustic neuromas. The typical finding is a far worse speech discrimination than the pure-tone audiogram would suggest.

Analysis of 94 patients seen by the author showed poor maximum discrimination scores (less than 60 per cent) in a high proportion of small tumours as well as in the larger tumours (Table 17.10).

TABLE 17.10. *Speech audiometry results in 94 cases*

Tumour size	Poor speech discrimination(%)†
Large (36)	88
Medium (46)	80
Small (12)	75

† Maximum score less than 60 per cent.

Johnson (1977) has tested 425 patients and reports that there were a number of patients with only slight or moderate pure-tone hearing losses who had considerable difficulty distinguishing speech sounds. 72 per cent of his patients had maximum speech discrimination scores of less than 60 per cent. He did report, however, that 120 patients (20 per cent) had speech discrimination scores of over 80 per cent. Speech audiometry does reveal more smaller tumours than pure-tone audiometric tests (loudness balance or adaptation) but a significant number of patients with purely cochlear disorders also give low speech-discrimination scores.

Impedance audiometry

Johnson (1977) concluded that impedance audiometry provides the single most positive test for the diagnosis of acoustic neuromas, although he does mention that electric response audiometry had not been included in his test battery. The diagnosis depends on the absence or elevation of the acoustic reflex threshold and on abnormal adaptation of the reflex. The major drawback of using the impedance audiometer is that the patient must have normal middle-ear mechanisms. This can be determined simply by tympanometry before the acoustic reflex tests are undertaken. Patients with conductive losses on pure-tone threshold audiometry must also be excluded.

The acoustic reflex threshold (ART) test for recruitment

Metz (1952) first described the use of the ART to assess recruitment. In normal hearing subjects, the stapedius muscle first begins to contract reflexly (ART) at about 75 dB above the threshold of hearing for that sound (Chiveralls, FitzSimons, Beck, and Kernohan 1976). A patient with a recruiting (sensory) hearing loss has a smaller gap between the ART threshold and his hearing threshold and often there is little difference between the ART in recruiting ears and normal ears. Patients with acoustic neuromas have much higher ART when the sound is presented to the affected ear and often the acoustic reflex cannot be obtained even at the maximum output of the audiometer. Chiveralls *et al.* (1976) suggested that a sensitive method of diagnosing an acoustic neuroma is to compare the ART of the two ears. A difference of over 20 dB between the ears is highly sensitive of a neural lesion providing a conductive pathological condition has been properly excluded. The author has analysed 102 acoustic neuroma cases according to the ART difference (Table 17.11) and finds that even in the small tumours, the test is over 70 per cent positive. The test is even more sensitive (90 per cent positive) if a criterion difference of 15 dB is accepted, but this does increase the number of false positive diagnoses appreciably.

TABLE 17.11. *The acoustic reflex threshold in 102 cases*

Tumour size	Absent reflexes or at least 20 dB differences(%)†	15 dB difference(%)†
Large (41)	88	12
Medium (50)	76	16
Small (11)	73	18

† Relates to the difference between the ART in the normal and in the affected ear at frequencies 500 Hz to 2 kHz.

The acoustic reflex test for adaptation

Anderson, Barr, and Wedenberg (1970) studied 17 patients with verified acoustic neuromas. In seven patients the acoustic reflex was not obtainable on stimulating the affected ear and the diagnosis could be suspected on the basis of a raised ART. In the remaining ten patients, the acoustic reflex showed abnormal adaptation and the maximum amplitude of the reflex contraction halved within five seconds. Chiveralls *et al.* (1976) investigated the acoustic reflex adaptation in a group of normal subjects and a group of patients with cochlear hearing defects and found no subject showed abnormal adaptation at 500 Hz but that 50 per cent adaptation within five seconds occurred with increasing probability as the stimulus frequency was raised (Table 17.12).

TABLE 17.12. *Acoustic reflex adaptation in normal subjects and patients with sensory hearing loss. (Reproduced from Chiveralls* et al. *(1976) by permission)*

	50% decrement times (s)			
Frequency (Hz)	500	1k	2k	4k
Normal ears				
Mean	no decay	32.0	14.5	7.4
SD	—	6.5	5.0	2.1
Range		12.5–60	2.3–34	1.5–12.5
(*N*) ears	106	106	107	101
Ears with sensory loss				
Mean	no decay	18.1	10.2	5.5
SD	—	12.9	8.3	4.9
Range	—	0.5–52	0.5–34.5	0.5–17.5
(*N*) ears	58	58	59	39

The author has never encountered a patient who had abnormal adaptation of the acoustic reflex at 500 Hz except patients with tumours of the eighth nerve. Abnormal adaptation at 1 kHz is very common in acoustic neuroma patients but unfortunately is often seen in patients with purely cochlear disorders. There does not appear to be any diagnostic significance when abnormal adaptation of the acoustic reflex is found at 2, 3, and 4 kHz. The author's findings in a small series are shown in Table 17.13.

TABLE 17.13. *Acoustic reflex adaptation in 40 cases of known acoustic neuroma which provided a clear acoustic reflex*

Number of affected ears	Over 50% decrement within 5 seconds (%)	
	500 Hz	1 kHz
40	62	90

Sheehy and Inzer (1976) have analysed the results of acoustic reflex tests and reported that the test was positive (either raised threshold or presence of abnornal adaptation) in 88 per cent of patients with acoustic neuromas. Similar results were mentioned by Johnson (1977). Impedance audiometry is a quick and simple test to perform and it should be used routinely on all patients presenting with hearing problems.

Electric response audiometry

Electric response audiometry (ERA) involves recording the bio-electric activity from various parts of the auditory system. The two most useful methods of ERA for the diagnosis of acoustic neuroma appear to be transtympanic electrocochleography (ECochG) and the acoustic brainstem electrical response (BSER).

ELECTROCOCHLEOGRAPHY

This test records the electrical activity of the cochlea and primary eighth nerve fibres. There are usually characteristic features whenever an acoustic neuroma is present; these include (i) preservation of the cochlear microphonic (CM), (ii) distortion of the action potential/summating potential (AP/SP) complex, and (iii) presence of the AP at stimulus intensities which cannot be heard by the patient.

Morrison, Gibson, and Beagley (1976) have used ECochG to investigate patients with acoustic neuromas. The test was judged positive in 91 per cent of cases (Table 17.14). The distortion of the AP/SP deserves special mention. It is due to a DC component which can only be recorded when the bandpass of the recording amplifiers admits DC potentials; if a 250 Hz low-cut filter is used the AP/SP complex appears to be normal. The usual effect is a broadening of the AP/SP complex. This is more obvious in the laterally placed tumours and it is especially marked in neurofibromatosis. The abnormal DC component is non-adaptive at fast interstimulus intervals. It can be distinguished from the SP as it has a definite onset latency (0.7–0.9 milliseconds after the stimulus onset); it is more marked at higher audiometric frequencies such as 8 kHz and it does not show such a clear relation to the stimulus duration as the SP. A possible explanation for its presence in ECochG recordings from ears with acoustic neuromas is that it represents the summation of monophasic unit AP (rather than the normal diphasic unit AP (Beagley, Legouix, Teas, and Remond (1977)). These monophasic potentials may occur with poor synchrony with each unit firing irregularly so that adaptation is not evident.

TABLE 17.14. *The ECochG in 64 acoustic neuromas*

Size of tumour	Wide SP/AP(%)	Large CM(%)	Threshold exceeded(%)	Report positive(%)
Small (10)	90	78	30	80
Medium (24)†	73	83	6	78
Large (30)†	78	89	40	100

† Two medium and three large tumours provided no AP/SP waveform.
Wide SP/AP complex refers to over 3 ms widening of the complex using 110 dB HL click stimulus.
Large CM is over 5μV p/p at 110 dB HL (Click stimulus).
Threshold exceeded means ECochG threshold is 20 dB or more sensitive than the patient's hearing threshold.

In some recordings from ears affected by acoustic neuromas, the SP is large. This may be due to vascular effects. Another common finding was the presence of large cochlear microphonics in the affected ear. Often the CM appeared larger than in the normal ear; this finding is difficult to explain on physiological grounds.

When the tumour is more medially placed, the AP/SP complex is often normal but often the AP threshold is lower than the patient's hearing threshold showing that the peripheral auditory mechanism is comparatively intact and the neural pathway has been deranged at a higher level. If the patient has good hearing, this point is difficult to establish and it is wise to combine the ECochG with the brainstem electric responses.

BRAINSTEM ELECTRICAL RESPONSES (BSER)

The BSER are an interesting series of potentials derived from the eighth nerve (Wave I), from the region of the cochlear nucleus (Wave II), from the region of the superior olivary complex (Wave III), and from the region of the inferior colliculus (Wave IV, Wave V). Selters and Brackmann (1977) used the BSER as a diagnostic test for a series of 100 patients, 36 with acoustic neuromas and 10 with other tumours of the cerebropontine angle. In 46 per cent of the tumour group, the Wave V was poorly formed or unidentifiable. When present the Wave V was delayed in comparison with the normal ear. They used an 83 dB HL click stimulus and restricted the test to patients with pure-tone thresholds which were better than 75 dB average for the frequencies 2, 4, and 8 kHz. A correction factor had to be applied whenever the hearing threshold of the two ears differed by more than 50 dB. The test was deemed positive whenever the latency of the Wave V between the affected ear and the normal ear differed by 0.2 ms (0–50 dB), 0.3 ms (50–65 dB), and 0.4 ms (65–75 dB). Using these criteria Selters and Brackmann (1977) successfully identified 96 per cent of the tumour group and only reached the wrong diagnosis in 12 per cent of the control group (false-positive).

Selters and Brackmann (1977) also noted that whenever there was a marked delay between the Wave III and the Wave V peaks, a large tumour compressing the brainstem was present. They hoped that this finding would prove helpful in estimating the size of an acoustic neuroma.

The BSER does appear to be a very powerful tool for the diagnosis of acoustic neuroma. There are some problems. The test is not applicable to patients with hearing losses of over 75 dB. If there is a conductive element to the hearing loss, then latency measurements are hazardous. Measurement of the Wave I–Wave V latency is more accurate than relying on the Wave V latency measurement alone. It seems probable that there is still a place for transtympanic ECochG and that the best use of ERA for diagnosis of acoustic neuromas will involve the combination of both BSER and ECochG. These tests theoretically sandwich the tumour between them.

Vestibular investigation

In theory, an acoustic neuroma should initially affect the vestibular nerve. It arises most commonly from the myelin sheath around the inferior vestibular nerve and its correct title should be, perhaps, a vestibular nerve Schwannoma. In fact, the vestibular disturbance caused by acoustic neuromas is slight and insiduous and there is difficulty in many cases in demonstrating any vestibular damage. This may be because the tests of vestibular function are crude when compared with audiometric tests.

The vestibular system can be investigated by examination of the stance and gait and by investigation of nystagmus. Stance and gait are usually assessed by the Romberg test (in which the patient stands to attention with his eyes closed), the Unterberger test (in which the patient marches on the spot with his eyes closed and his arms outstretched), and by asking him to walk a straight line with his eyes open and then closed. Patients with recent vestibular lesions tend to become unstable when they close their eyes and to veer in the direction of the affected ear. If the lesion occurs more gradually then central compensation occurs and the patient may perform these simple tests without fault. Once the tumour becomes very large, cerebellar function may fail and gross abnormalities of gait and stance are obvious even when the patient keeps his eyes open.

The tests for nystagmus may be classified into a search for spontaneous nystagmus and the observation of the characteristics of induced nystagmus. Spontaneous nystagmus is more evident, in the case of a peripheral vestibular lesion, when the patient abolishes optic fixation (shuts his eyes or is examined in darkness) or wears Frenzel's glasses which prevents fixation. The most useful means of searching for nystagmus involves the technique of electronystagmography.

ELECTRONYSTAGMOGRAPHY (ENG)

The advantages of ENG compared to merely observing the patient's eyes include: permanent recording of any nystagmus which allows for detailed analytical study, the opportunity to record nystagmus with the eyes closed or in darkness, and the identification of nystagmus not readily apparent on simple examination with the naked eye.

The corneoretinal potential provides the basic mechanism of ENG. It is an electrical dipole which exists between the positively-charged cornea and the more negatively charged retina. Small movements of the eyes can be detected from changes in the corneoretinal potential as measured from electrodes attached to the skin around the eye. The corneoretinal potential varies from person to person and is affected by changes in visual acuity and illumination. Nevertheless, it does provide a very useful clinical method of recording nystagmus.

The ENG may be used to search for spontaneous nystagmus. The incidence of spontaneous nystagmus in acoustic neuroma is surprisingly high and depends on the size of the tumour (Table 17.15).

TABLE 17.15. *The incidence of spontaneous nystagmus as detected using Frenzel's glasses or ENG. (Reproduced from Morrison (1976) with permission)*

Tumour size	Percentage having nystagmus
Large (35)	86
Medium (30)	60
Small (6)	33

The character of the spontaneous nystagmus is a useful clue to the size and position of the tumour. The nystagmus alters as the tumour enlarges to involve progressively the vestibular nuclei, cerebellum (first unilaterally and then bilaterally), and the upper brainstem.

Small tumours

These tumours only affect the vestibular nerve. The nystagmus is not marked because of the gradual nature of the damage to the nerve which allows central compensation to occur. The nystagmus is increased by abolishing optic fixation (closing the eyes or testing in darkness). The nystagmus has a characteristic saw-toothed appearance on the ENG record, usually has its fast component directed towards the normal ear, and is most marked when the patient looks in this direction (centrifugal vestibular nystagmus). In its mildest form, the spontaneous nystagmus is only evident on ENG recordings made in darkness or when the eyes are closed; and is only evident when the patient gazes away from the affected ear (first degree nystagmus only evident without optic fixation). In other more severe cases the nystagmus may be just visible with the patient fixing his gaze and becomes more obvious on abolishing optic fixation (first degree with optic fixation—second or third degree without optic fixation). By definition, nystagmus is first degree when it is only evident in one field of gaze, i.e. looking to the left, second degree if it is evident with the eyes looking ahead as well as looking to one side; and third degree when it is present in all three fields of gaze, i.e. even on looking to the opposite side.

Occasionally centripetal nystagmus is encountered on testing small tumours. This is a nystagmus which has its fast component directed towards the midline on lateral gaze. It is caused by a pathological drift of the eyes outwards and the compensatory bias as the eyes quickly try and compensate for this drift. Centripetal nystagmus is seen in a widespread field of disorders ranging from peripheral vestibular disorders to cerebellar and brainstem disorders (Leech, Gresty, Hess, and Rudge 1977).

Tumours affecting the vestibular nuclei

Larger tumours which affect the vestibular nuclei within the brainstem usually cause spontaneous vestibular nystagmus which is evident in the presence of optic fixation. It is most evident in the field of gaze directed away from the affected side. The difference between this nystagmus and nystagmus due to a purely vestibular nerve lesion may be apparent when optic fixation is abolished. The nystagmus may decrease or disappear on closing the eyes. In darkness, the nystagmus alters little from the amplitude of the nystagmus recorded with optic fixation but the velocity of the slow component may be decreased.

Tumours affecting the cerebellum

These produce nystagmus which is directed towards the affected ear and most apparent when the patient looks in this direction. The nystagmus is usually less apparent on eye closure or in darkness, and it is caused by compression of the infneor cerebellar lobes, especially the flocculonodular lobe. The recorded nystagmus may comprise both cerebellar nystagmus and nystagmus due to vestibular nerve damage—a coarse nystagmus on gaze towards the affected side and a finer nystagmus on opposite gaze.

Very large tumours may affect the function of both sides of the cerebellum due to contra-coup damage, the cerebellum being squashed into the opposite side of the skull. This causes a bidirectional coarse cerebellar nystagmus (Bruyn's nystagmus). Enlargement of the tumour in a superomedial direction compresses the upper brainstem and may cause an upbeating vertical nystagmus.

The bithermal caloric tests

The earliest reports suggested that the caloric responses of the affected ear were abnormal in 100 per cent of acoustic neuromas (Cawthorne, Dix, and Hood 1969), but these reports were based on the findings only in large tumours. Undoubtedly normal caloric responses can be encountered on testing smaller tumours, and the use of a physiologically incorrect test procedure may further obscure the presence of abnormalities in other cases. These results have led to some disillusionment with the bithermal caloric test as a method of detecting early acoustic neuromas (Brackman, personal communication).

Consider the physiology of caloric induced nystagmus. The amplitude of the nystagmus is related to the degree of cupula deflection and the time course of the nystagmus depends on the elastic mechanism of the cupula. Fig. 17.1 shows a diagram of the time course of mechanical deflection of the cupula (C). The normal neural response (A) follows the same time course and the neural activity becomes sufficient after about 40–50 seconds for the induced nystagmus to be evident in the presence of optic fixation. In the case of reduced neural transmission (B) resulting from an acoustic neuroma the amplitude of the induced nystagmus never becomes great enough to be visible in the presence of optic fixation but its time course remains unaltered.

The bithermal caloric test can be performed most simply by merely observing the duration of the induced nystagmus in the presence of optic fixation. Unfortunately some subjects show such marked central suppression of nystagmus (especially common in neurotic subjects) that it is difficult

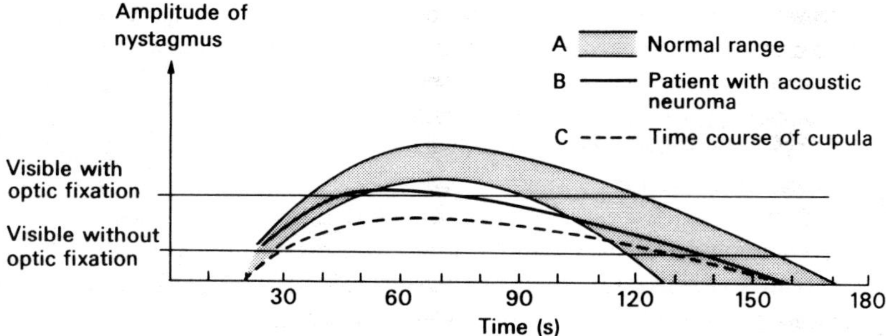

Fig. 17.1. The interrupted line (C) represents the time course of the cupular deflection. The neural response as indicated by the nystagmus follows this time course. The lines containing the dots (A) shows the amplitude (arbitrary units) and the duration of the induced nystagmus in a group of 20 normal subject (± 2SD) tested by WPRG. The thick line (B) shows the response obtained from a patient with a 2 cm acoustic neuroma; note that the duration is unaffected but that the amplitude is reduced.

to see any nystagmus during optic fixation. This has led some workers using either Frenzel's glasses or ENG with eyes closed to enhance the induced nystagmus. If these latter measures are undertaken, duration measures are no longer valid for detecting vestibular nerve lesions as the end points without optic fixation tend to crowd together whether the nerve is damaged or not (see Fig. 17.1). Amplitude measurements with ENG can also pose difficulties. Generally, the velocity of the slow component is used for measurements but the testing cannot be done with the patient's eyes closed as it is not possible to calibrate the eye movements. The corneoretinal potential changes when the eyes are closed or put in darkness and at least ten minutes must lapse before stable potentials can be recorded. The major problem facing testing with eyes closed is that the eyes may roll upwards under the closed lids (Bell's phenomena) or drift in the direction of the slow component; both these eye movements suppress the induced nystagmus and unless four-channel D.C. recordings are available, these eye movements remain undetected. Probably the safest method of detecting minor neural abnormalities remains simply measuring the duration during optic fixation (Hood 1977b).

The results of bithermal caloric testing are shown in Table 17.16. A difference of over 15 seconds between the duration of the nystagmus (with

TABLE 17.16. *The results of bithermal caloric testing in 108 acoustic neuromas*

Tumour size	Absent(%)	Abnormal(%)	Normal(%)
Large (46)	83	15	2
Medium (50)	52	32	16
Small (12)	17	58	25

optic fixation) in the affected and non-affected ear was accepted as an abnormal response. It can be seen that the properly performed caloric test is useful as it is positive in 75 per cent of small tumours.

Radiographic investigation

PLAIN RADIOGRAPHY

Conventional radiography of the internal acoustic meatuses (IAM) includes Townes, Stenvers, and transorbital views but these views only demonstrate extensive destruction and are unable to show the minor IAM changes associated with the majority of tumours. Tomography and polytomography of the IAM should be undertaken. The 90 per cent normal range of dimensions of the IAM has been described by Valvassori (1969) and these provide the basis for diagnosis:

1. The vertical (height) range extends from 2–9 mm. The difference between the heights of the two meatuses does not exceed 1 mm. Problems can arise when the petrous apex is extensively pneumatized but this feature can usually be identified with good quality radiography.
2. The length of the posterior wall ranges from 4–11 mm. The difference between the length of the two meatuses does not exceed 3 mm.
3. The crista falciformis lies at, or just above, the midpoint of the vertical height and does not vary by more than 1 mm between the two meatuses.
4. The thickness of the meatal roof ranges from 3.5–7 mm and does not vary by more than 2 mm between the two sides.

Table 17.17 shows the tomographic findings in a series of 71 acoustic neuromas. The percentage of smaller tumours with abnormal radiographic features is higher than the percentage of large tumours. In part this reflects the initial method of diagnosis as many of the smaller tumours were found because of the radiographic changes, and in part this shows that some tumours can arise medially outside the IAM so that they reach a large size without causing any symptoms.

TABLE 17.17. *The radiological (tomography) findings in 71 acoustic neuromas. (Reproduced from Morrison (1975) by permission)*

Tumour size	Definitely abnormal(%)†	Suspicious(%)†
Large (35)	66	74
Medium (30)	73	83
Small (6)	83	100

† Definitely abnormal relates to a 2 mm difference in height between the IAM. Suspicious relates to less definite radiological changes, the figures include the definite cases.

COMPUTERIZED AXIAL TOMOGRAPH (CAT SCANNING)

The CAT scan has revolutionized neurology and has largely replaced the more invasive radiological techniques. All patients suspected of having an acoustic neuroma must have a CAT scan before any negative or positive contrast cisternomeatography is undertaken. These latter procedures are dangerous in the presence of a large tumour as coning can occur. Coning is compression of the brainstem and cerebellum into the foramen magnum causing death. It is caused by increased intracranial pressure.

The CAT scan will always detect tumours with a diameter of over 3 cm outside the porus, providing the scan is enhanced (e.g. using Conray ®). Cystic tumours can be overlooked by CAT scanning even when they are large if no contrast agent is used, and very cystic tumours can still pose problems even with enhancement. Often the tumour is much larger at surgery than expected. The smallest tumour seen by the author, which was detected by CAT scanning was 1 cm in diameter. Tumours entirely confined to the IAM cannot be detected with present-day techniques. CAT scans give other useful information as well, e.g. the presence or absence of hydrocephalus.

NEGATIVE-CONTRAST CISTERNOGRAPHY (PNEUMOENCEPHALOGRAPHY)

This test has largely been replaced by the CAT scan. It is performed under general anaesthesia using tomography (Morris and Wylie 1974). Tumours from 2–4 cm diameter can be readily identified and some useful information about the state of the brainstem and ventricular systems is also gained. The test is dangerous in the presence of raised intracranial pressure sufficient to cause papilloedema.

VERTEBRAL ARTERIOGRAPHY

The internal acoustic vascular complex is rarely visible using arteriography (Smaltino, Bernini, and Elefante 1971) and vertebral arteriography has no place in the diagnosis of small acoustic neuromas. It has some use in larger tumour cases when there is associated papilloedema as the risk of coning is avoided. Nevertheless, there are dangers due to embolization. The test has largely been superseded by the CAT scan although many authorities believe that it gives a better estimate of tumour size and helps to determine the relationship of the tumour to vital vessels before surgery is undertaken.

POSITIVE-CONTRAST MEATOCISTERNOGRAPHY

Although this test remains a reliable means of detecting small acoustic neuromas, there are drawbacks as the patient must be admitted to hospital as there can be a distressing headache which may last several days. The test can be performed adequately using simple sedation and local anaesthesia. It must not be undertaken unless the CAT scan is negative and the presence of papilloedema has been excluded.

The incidence of complications can be greatly reduced by using small quantities of contrast medium (1–1.5 ml) (House 1966) and not allowing the contrast medium to stray above the tentorium. The normal meatus should fill with contrast medium up to the fundus and the outlines of the acousticofacial bundle are usually identifiable. Occasionally it is possible to see the position of the anterior inferior cerebellar artery.

When an acoustic neuroma is present, three different pictures emerge depending on the size of the tumour. (i) If the tumour is small and exactly fits the fundus of the IAM, contrast medium does not flow past it but ends as a medially-concave, curved surface. (ii) If the tumour fills with the IAM without extending into the cerebropontine angle, the contrast medium fails to enter the IAM and stops at its medial pole. (iii) If the tumour extends into the cerebropontine angle, then the appearances are either: (a) a well-circumscribed tumour surrounded by contrast medium with clear separation from the brainstem, or (b) an incompletely circumscribed tumour which must be assumed to be in contact with the brainstem.

Strange filling defects can arise which make the clinician suspicious. For instance the contrast medium may not penetrate the IAM beyond its lateral two-thirds and ends in a laterally-concave, curved surface. If the meatus is very narrow, then the cause is usually fairly evident, but if the meatus is wide, then suspicion must remain and the patient has to undergo a further myelogram after one year.

CAT SCANNING WITH OXYGEN MEATOCISTERNOGRAPHY

The CAT scan has proved a disappointment for the detection of small tumours despite the use of enhancement techniques and cannot yet provide a diagnosis for intrameatal tumours. Nevertheless, there is considerable optimism that a new technique involving the intrathecal injection of a few millilitres of oxygen and the use of the CT scanning will provide an even better method of detecting these tumours than positive contrast techniques. The advantage from the patient's viewpoint is that the headache is considerably less using oxygen and rarely lasts for longer than 24 hours.

The diagnostic criteria involved are similar to those used for assessing positive contrast studies but it is hoped that oxygen will flow more easily into the meatus and so reduce the number of equivocal findings.

Other investigations

CEREBROSPINAL FLUID (CSF) EXAMINATION

The CSF protein level is only raised consistently in large tumours. There is no justification in admitting a patient for lumbar puncture alone but the CSF can easily be collected during positive- and negative-contrast meatocisternography. Apart from protein levels, glucose and full serological testing should be requested. The incidence of abnormal CSF protein levels is shown in Table 17.18.

TECHNETIUM BRAIN SCANNING

Radioactive brainscans will only demonstrate large tumours of over 3.5 cm diameter. Their use has been entirely replaced by CAT scanning.

TABLE 17.18. *The CSF protein in 71 acoustic neuromas. (Reproduced from Morrison (1975) by permission)*

Tumour size	Normal(%)	CSF protein level (mg%)	
		40–100(%)	100–500(%)
Large (35)	8	20	72
Medium (30)	34	43	23
Small (6)	83	17	0

DIFFERENTIAL DIAGNOSIS OF ACOUSTIC NEUROMA

Of tumours within the cerebropontine angle 90 per cent are acoustic neuromas. Other pathological conditions include meningiomas, gliomas, secondary carcinoma, neuromas of the V, VII, IX, and X cranial nerves, cholesteatomas, arachnoid cysts, ectasias of the basilar artery, etc. The ectactic basilar artery is best left surgically unexplored. It can usually be identified on positive-contrast cisternomeatography as the contrast medium appears to pulsate in and out of the IAM (Gibson and Wallace 1975).

Neurofibromatosis has a different histological picture to the vestibular Schwannona (*syn.* acoustic neuroma) as the tumour appears to invade the nerve itself. Often the patient has cutaneous neurofibromatosis and *café au lait* skin pigmentation. There may be multiple intracranial neurofibromas, bilateral eighth nerve involvement is common and there are often meningiomas present as well.

Multiple sclerosis may provide a retrocochlear audiological picture but invariably the hearing loss recovers within a few weeks. The brainstem electrical responses are particularly valuable for detecting small placques of demyelination which affect the auditory tracts without causing any hearing loss (Robinson and Rudge 1977).

The commonest cause for extensive negative investigation is when the clinician is faced with a patient with a unilateral hearing loss and equivocal findings on tomography. In the author's series, the commonest condition under these circumstances was Ménière's disorder. Normally, the typical history and the audiological picture showing recruitment or over recruitment and absent adaptation was sufficient evidence to refrain from cisternomeatography. The electrocochleogram (E Coch G) may yield a wide SP/A P complex but the CM is usually small. The widening in Ménière's disorder is due to a relative enhancement of the SP (summating potential). the BSER have normal Wave V latencies.

Idiopathic sudden hearing loss can cause difficulties as it may have a retrocochlear audiological picture. It is known that 10 per cent of these cases do have an acoustic neuroma present so extensive investigation may be required. Even recovery of hearing does not guarantee the absence of a tumour as some tumours can cause intermittent vascular effects. The ECochG can be helpful (Graham, Ramsden, Moffat, and Gibson 1978), but in cases of doubt cisternomeatography should be performed.

Syphilis can affect the ear and cause retrocochlear audiological hearing loss. The patients may also have difficulties with their vision and clouding of the cornea. Positive serology can be difficult to obtain and the fluorescent treponemal antibodies (FTA-abs) test may be the single positive feature (Ramsden, Moffat, and Gibson 1977). Sometimes the diagnosis is only reached with certainty after CSF examination.

Many other pathological conditions can mimick the presence of an acoustic neuroma. The author has encountered congenital CNS malformations, noise-induced hearing loss, otosclerosis, and carcinoma of the post-natal space, as well as several cases which remained undiagnosed.

CONCLUSIONS

An acoustic neuroma is a rare cause of a unilateral auditory dysfunction but its early detection by the otologist has great beneficial consequences for the patient. The usual methods of investigation have been reviewed and it has been found that the classic descriptions apply only to large tumours and new diagnostic criteria are necessary to diagnose small tumours.

In small tumours, the hearing loss may only be slight. Over 50 per cent of cases show recruitment with no abnormal auditory adaptation. The bithermal caloric tests are absent in under 25 per cent. The investigations which provide the best means for diagnosis are speech audiometry, acoustic reflex tests, electric response audiometry, and tomography of the IAM. Only the CAT scan for larger tumours, and cisternomeatography for small tumours provide definitive diagnosis.

ACKNOWLEDGEMENT

Nearly all the patients with acoustic neuromas seen by the author were under the care of Mr Andrew Morrison, senior consultant surgeon at The London Hospital, and many of the figures are based on his work. The author owes a great deal to his teaching and kindness.

REFERENCES

ANDERSON, H., BARR, B., and WEDENBERG, E. (1970). Early diagnosis of VIIIth tumours by acoustic reflex tests. *Acta oto-lar.* Suppl. **263**, 232–7.

BEAGLEY, H. A., LEGOUIX, J. P., TEAS, D. C., and REMOND, M. C. (1977). Changes in E Coch G in acoustic neuroma; some experimental findings. *Clin. Otolar.* **2**, 213–19.

CAWTHORNE, T., DIX, M. R., and HOOD, J. D. (1969). Vestibular syndromes and vertigo. In *Handbook of clinical neurology* (ed. P. J. Vinken, G. W. Bruyn). North-Holland, Amsterdam.

CHIVERALLS, K., FITZSIMONS, R., BECK, G. B., and KERNOHAN, H. (1976). The diagnostic significance of the stapedius reflex. *Br. J. Audiol.* **10**, 122–8.

CUSHING, H. (1917). *Tumours of the nervus acusticus and the syndrome of the cerebellopontine angle.* Saunders, Philadelphia.

Gibson, W. P. R. and Wallace, D. (1975). Basilar artery ectasia (an unusual cause of a cerebellopontine angle lesion and hemifacial spasm). *J. Lar. Otol.* **91**, 679–96.

Graham, J. M., Ramsden, R. T., Moffat, D. A., and Gibson, W. P. R. (1978) Sudden sensorineural hearing loss: electrocochleographic findings in 70 patients. *J. Lar. Otol.* **92**, 581–9.

Green, D. S. (1963). The modified tone decay test (MTDT) as a screening procedure for eighth nerve lesions. *J. Speech. Hear Disord.* **28**, 31–6.

Hitselberger, W. E. and House, W. F. (1964). Other cranial nerves and cerebellar signs. *Archs Otolar.* **80**, 693–7.

Hood, J. D. (1977a). Loudness balance procedures for the measurement of recruitment. *Audiology* **16**, 215–28.

—— (1977b). Whither vestibular tests? (Editorial). *Proc. R. Soc. Med.* **70**, 875–8.

House, W. F. (1966). Evaluation of transtemporal removal of acoustic neuromas. *Archs Otolar.* **84**, 255–65.

—— (1978). Translabyrinthine acoustic tumor removal. Paper read at the seminar on Diagnosis and Management of Acoustic Neuromas and Skull Base Tumours, 28 Feb.–3 March, Ear Research Institute, Los Angeles.

Jerger, J. (1960). Békésy audiometry in analysis of auditory disorders. *J. Speech Hear. Res.* **3**, 275–87.

—— (ed.) (1973). Diagnostic audiometry. In *Modern developments in audiology*. 3. Academic Press, New York.

—— and Jerger, S. (1975). Simplified tone decay test. *Archs Otolar.* **101**, 403–7.

Johnson, E. W. (1968). Auditory findings in 200 cases of acoustic neuromas. *Archs Otolar.* **88**, 598–603.

—— (1970). Auditory test results in 268 cases of confirmed retrocochlear lesions. *J. Int. Audiol.* **9**, 15–19.

—— (1977). Auditory test results in 500 cases of acoustic neuroma. *Archs Otolar.* **103**, 152–8.

King, T. T., Gibson, W. P. R., and Morrison, A. W. (1976). Tumours of the eighth cranial nerve. *Br. J. hosp. Med.* **16**, 259–72.

Krott, H. M., Peremba, M., and Busse, M. (1969). Mesure de la latence du nerf facial dans les neurinomes acoustiques. *Dt. Z. NervHeilk.* **195**, 344–55.

Leech, J., Gresty, M., Hess, K., and Rudge, P. (1977). Gaze failure, drifting eye movements and centripetal nystagmus in cerebellar disease. *Br. J. Ophthalm.* **61**, 774–81.

Metz, O. (1952). Threshold of reflex contractions of muscles of the middle ear and recruitment of loudness. *Archs Otolar.* **55**, 536–43.

Morris, L. and Wylie, I. G. (1974). A combined technique for investigation of the cerebello-pontine angle cistern and internal auditory canal. *Am. J. Roentg.* **122**, 560–70.

Morrison, A. W. (1975). *Management of sensorineural deafness*. Butterworths, London.

—— Gibson, W. P. R., and Beagley H. A. (1976). Transtympanic electrocochleography in the diagnosis of retrocochlear tumours. *Clin. Otolar.* **1**, 153–67.

Ozsahinoglu, C. and Harrison, M. S. (1974). The symptoms of neuro fibroma of the 8th nerve. *Br. J. Audiol.* **8**, 61–5.

Pulec, J. L. and House, W. F. (1964). Facial nerve involvement and testing in acoustic neuromas. *Archs Otolar.* **80**, 685–92.

Ramsden, R. T., Moffat, D. A., and Gibson, W. P. R. (1977). Transtympanic electrocochleography in patients with syphilis and hearing loss. *Annls Otol.* **86**, 827–34.

ROBINSON, K. and RUDGE, P. (1977). Abnormalities of the auditory evoked potentials in patients with multiple sclerosis. *Brain* **100**, 19–40.

SELTERS, W. A. and BRACKMANN, D. E. (1977). Acoustic tumour detection with brainstem electric response audiometry. *Archs Otolar.* **103**, 181–7.

SHEEHY, J. L. and INZER, B. E. (1976). Acoustic reflex test in neuro-otologic diagnosis. *Archs Otolar.* **102**, 647–53.

SMALTINO, F., BERNINI, F. P., and ELEFANTE, R. (1971). Normal and pathological findings of the angiographic examination of the internal auditory artery. *Neuroradiology* **2**, 216–22.

TOOTH, H. H. (1912). Some observations on the growth and survival period of intracranial tumours based on the records of 500 cases with special reference to the pathology of glioma. *Brain* **35**, 61–108.

VALVASSORI, G. E. (1969). The abnormal internal auditory canal: the diagnosis of acoustic neuroma. *Radiology* **29**, 449–59.

18 The role of drugs in audiological medicine

R. HINCHCLIFFE

In his *English Physitian*, Culpeper (1652) claimed a therapeutic value for certain plants in disorders of hearing. For example, the juice of the sow thistle 'boiled or thoroughly heated in a little Oyl of Bitter Almonds in the Pill of a Pomegranate, and dropped into the Ears, is a sure Remedy for Deafness, singings, etc.' 'The distilled Water of the green Husks (of the Walnut tree) being ripe, when they are shelled from the Nuts, being drunk with a little Vinegar, . . . wonderfully helpeth Deafness, the Noise and other pains in the ears.'

Unfortunately none of Culpeper's remedies was subject to an experimental comparative study* so we do not know whether or not these are of any value. The same criticism, however, applies to many other remedies for disorders of hearing which have emerged since, and are still emerging. Thus much of what will be mentioned in this chapter will inevitably be at the anecdotal level.

It will be convenient to group treatments according to the anatomical site of the disorder.

EXTERNAL EAR

Cerumen

In the general rural population, 23 per cent of men and 13 per cent of women have one or both external acoustic meatuses occluded by wax (Hinchcliffe 1961). Moreover, impacted ear wax may produce an overall hearing loss of 40 dB HL (Saltzman 1949). However, recent studies indicate that, in the past, the surdogenic properties of cerumen have perhaps been overstressed (Robinson, Shipton, and Hinchcliffe 1979). Nevertheless, there is a need to remove cerumen not only for inspection of the meatus and ear drum but also to ensure the validity of tests of acoustic function. In the general rural population, a wax curette alone can remove the cerumen in half the cases and syringing alone can remove it in one-third of the cases. There is a residuum of cases where a cerumenolytic agent is required as an adjunct to syringing.

In addition to the traditional cerumenolytics olive oil and sodium bicarbonate ear drops, a number of special preparations have been marketed. Fraser (1970) reported both an *in vitro* and in *in vivo* study of preparations of *p*-dichlorobenzene with turpentine oil, olive oil, sodium bicarbonate, triethanolamine polypeptide oleate-condensate, and sodium dioctyl sulpho-

* Reasons for referring to what have previously been called, for example, randomized control trials, as experimental comparative studies were set out in Hinchcliffe (1979).

succinate in both an oil and a water base. Only the two water-based preparations (sodium bicarbonate and a dioctyl) produced complete disintegration of the cerumen *in vitro*. Elderly patients with bilateral impacted hard wax were used for the *in vivo* experimental comparative study. The dichlorobenzene–turpentine preparation was found to be significantly more effective than both dioctyl preparations and the sodium bicarbonate solution. A statistically significant difference between the dichlorobenzene–turpentine preparation and either the olive oil or the triethanolamine preparation could not be demonstrated. In a previous experimental comparative study of a dichlorobenzene–turpentine preparation, hydrogen peroxide aural drops, olive oil, and sodium bicarbonate solution, only olive oil was found to be significantly better than no treatment at all (Hinchcliffe 1955). It would thus appear that olive oil is the cerumenolytic of choice, particularly as it is also bland and inexpensive.

Otitis externa

Unlike otitis media, otitis externa is not characteristically associated with impairment of hearing except when the meatus is occluded. However, not infrequently an otitis externa must be treated to proceed with the investigation of an auditory disorder.

The treatment of an otitis externa depends upon the type of that disorder. A classification which is relevant to treatment is shown in Fig. 18.1. It should, however, always be borne in mind that such classifications are

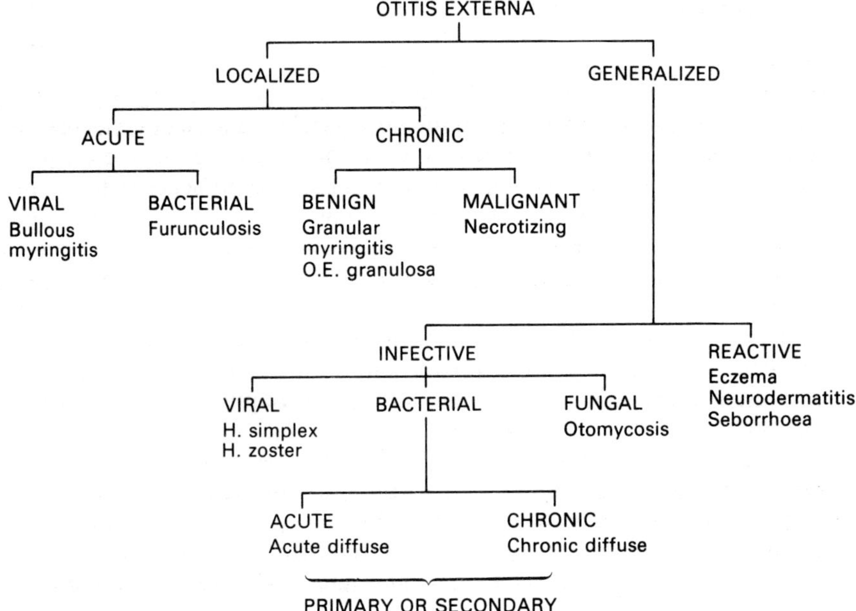

Fig. 18.1. Classification of otitis externa.

invariably arbitrary. As Mawson (1974) points out, the difficulty of precise classification is the blurring of outline by secondary infection, changes in tissue reaction, and spread of the infection. An originally pure bacterial infection may be modified, especially through treatment, to become a predominantly fungal disorder. Similarly, particularly because of treatment, a condition in which infection is dominant can become one in which reactive processes supervene. Nevertheless, consideration must always be given to assessing the three principal factors in the disease, i.e. infective agents, tissue reaction, and psychological factors. Each of these factors may require treating and, if so, with different emphases.

Bullous myringitis (*otitis externa haemorrhagica; acute influenzal otitis*) is characterized by purplish blebs on the tympanic membrane and on the skin of the deep meatus. A serosanguinous discharge follows bursting of the bullae. The condition may be complicated by an otitis media and, less frequently, by cranial nerve involvement (Dawes 1953).

A complaint of hearing loss is not characteristic of bullous myringitis unless there is a supervening otitis media. Severe pain is invariably the initial symptom. Because of the presumed viral aetiology, antibiotics are not indicated. Analgesics will be required and the meatus must be kept clean and dry. Incision of bullae is contraindicated since this will not produce any relief of pain and may, in fact, introduce secondary infection (Clark 1946).

The first symptom of a *furuncle* (*boil*) in the external meatus is frequently a tender spot which produces discomfort, especially on moving the jaw. The tenderness increases to become a severe pain and chewing may be difficult. Occlusion of the meatus by the boil produces a conductive hearing loss.

Intramuscular injection of a penicillin preparation is the treatment of choice (Cheesman 1979). Only if the boil points should it be drained by local incision; otherwise there is a risk of spread of the infection to cartilage. If the boil is not yet pointing, but is occluding the meatus, a pack impregnated with magnesium sulphate, although painful to insert, will relieve the pain. When the boil is beginning to discharge, pus should be mopped away daily and a glycerol pack may be inserted (Hammond 1979).

At least two varieties of meatal granulations unassociated with chronic suppurative otitis media were reported in British soldiers during the Second World War.

Moffett (1943) reported a *granular myringitis* which was not associated with any diffuse inflammation. He reported that the granulations showed 'a high degree of resistance to treatment'. The lead and aluminium acetate solution frequently used successfully for the treatment of desquamative otitis externa was without any marked effect upon granular myringitis. 90 per cent chromic acid was found to be too powerful an escharotic and in one of two cases produced a perforation of the ear drum. The treatment that Moffett subsequently adopted was the application, at intervals of 2–3 days, of 10 per cent silver nitrate, the meatus being thoroughly cleansed before each application. Within three days the granulations lost their bright red appearance, became pink and gradually shrank in size and finally disappeared. It was usually necessary to continue treatment for up to 14 days. A few years later Clark (1946) described a condition characterized by sessile plaques attached to the outer surface of the ear drum or by small pedunculated masses arising from the meatal wall. He recommended removal of the pedunculated granulations with aural forceps. He said that no anaesthetic was necessary for, provided manipulation is gentle and the adjacent meatal wall is not pressed upon, the pain is negligible. Any bleeding was controlled by cotton wool or dry gauze which was introduced for 5 to 10 minutes.

Under the term *otitis externa granulosa*, Punt (1949) described granulations, more often of the pedunculated type, arising from any part of the deep meatus and only in the minority of cases being attached to the ear drum. As he pointed out, this granular otitis must be differentiated from a chronic suppurative otitis media with granulations covering a perforation or a meatal fistula. Punt removed his meatal granulations with aural crocodile forceps, with occasional recourse to a silver nitrate bead fused on to a probe.

Necrotizing otitis is a condition which is being increasingly recognized since it was first described by Meltzer and Kelemen (1959). Although initially considered to affect elderly diabetics, it has been reported in non-diabetics and in children (Joachims 1976). This otitis is characterized by an insidious onset of persistent and progressive pain together with an aural discharge. The condition is due to impaired nutrition of the tissues with infection by *Pseudomonas pyocyaneus* in association with an anaerobic bacterium, particularly *Bacteroides fragilis* (Rees, personal communication). Considerable surgical débridement is required. A few years ago, the mortality was considered to be 58 per cent (Evans 1973). It is thus not surprising that the condition has been referred to as 'malignant otitis externa'. However, distinct from this condition, a squamous cell carcinoma can very rarely develop, apparently secondary to an otitis externa (Robinson 1946).

The introduction of treatment with metronidazole (Fig. 18.2) appears to

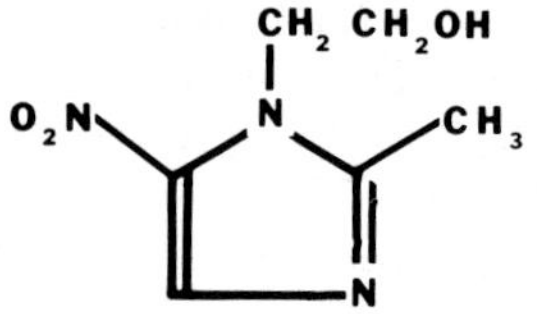

Fig. 18.2. Metronidazole.

have considerably reduced the high mortality rate of necrotizing otitis externa. John and Hopkin (1978) have reported the use of this drug in the successful treatment of a non-diabetic with bilateral involvement and multiple cranial-nerve palsies who had undergone eight surgical procedures. There had been little response to topical antibiotic ear drops, including gentamicin which had been administered both locally and systemically. Moreover, the gentamicin had produced a total bilateral deafness. Before starting the gentamicin, the patient had had a bilateral conductive impairment of about 40 dB HL. In the light of the histopathological report on another case by Morgenstein and Seung (1971), John and Hopkin considered that this conductive loss was probably due to mucosal oedema and granulations together with auditory tubal block. In the treatment of this case John and Hopkin emphasized the value of an extensive incision to create a large wound which was packed daily with gauze soaked in phenoxyethanol (Fig. 18.3).

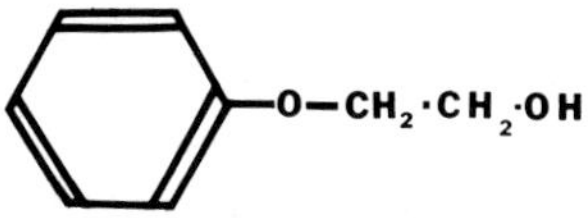

$C_6H_5-O-CH_2 \cdot CH_2 \cdot OH$

Fig. 18.3. Phenoxyethanol.

Herpes simplex may involve the auricle. Experimental comparative studies are yet required to demonstrate that topical idoxuridine preparations are of value in the treatment of this condition. Similarly, the use of systemic steroids may be questioned in herpes zoster involvement of the ear. Herpes zoster is a recrudescence of latent infection with varicella virus in partially immune subjects. There is an acute inflammatory lesion of one or more sensory ganglia. Fully developed herpes zoster oticus comprises the vesicular lesion of the skin of the auricle and external meatus together with a facial nerve palsy and both auditory and vestibular symptoms (Ramsay Hunt syndrome). McNicol (1958) reported herpes zoster oticus developing in a case of ulcerative colitis being treated with steroids. Nevertheless, many otologists, e.g. Morrison (1978), consider the risk of disseminating the virus to be sufficiently slight as not to preclude treatment with systemic steroids. There are, however, the usual risks (exacerbation of hypertension, peptic ulcers, tuberculosis) associated with corticosteroid therapy. Symptomatic treatment of herpes zoster oticus is required for the pain (analgesics), itching (topical calamine cream), and vertigo (vestibular suppressive drugs).

There have been a few double blind ECSs (experimental comparative studies) in respect of the various ear drops available for the treatment of *diffuse otitis externa* (Bain 1976; Barton, Wright, and Gray 1979; Gyde and Randall 1978). However, the problem is not so much one of finding an antibiotic with sufficient potency to combat the bacterial infection as one of finding such an antibiotic which is (a) non-ototoxic, (b) does not produce hypersensitivity reactions, and (c) does not facilitate the development of an otomycosis. The ototoxicity of topical antibiotics has been emphasized by Morizono, Johnstone, and Ng (1974). This is important where a perforated tympanic membrane is associated with an external otitis, or where a chronic suppurative otitis media is being treated. In fact Ajodhia and Dix (1975) say that the use of antibacterial ear drops containing an ototoxic antibiotic should be avoided whenever a suitable alternative is available. Thus suitable topical preparations combine either clioquinol (Fig. 18.4) or halquinol with

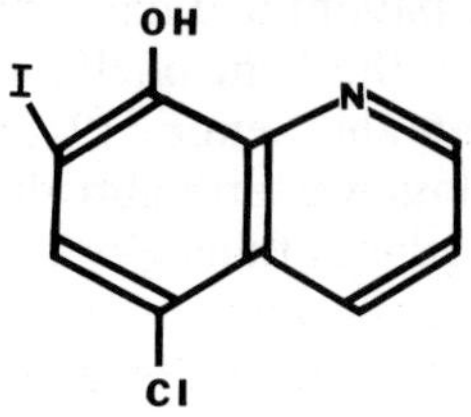

Fig. 18.4. Clioquinol.

a steroid. Such a preparation with 3 per cent clioquinol may contain mildly potent, moderately potent, or potent steroids, e.g. hydrocortisone, flurandrenolene, or fluocinolone respectively. The least potent steroid preparation appropriate to the severity of the external otitis should be used. Prescriptions should not be repeated without assessment of the condition at two weekly intervals.

As Cheesman (1979) points out, in acute diffuse otitis externa, the topical preparation may be conveniently applied on a wick. The wick has three principal functions: (i) removal of exudate by capillary action; (ii) close application of the drug; and (iii) forming a barrier to scratching. One should not lose sight of the fact that the main problem of otitis externa remains as it was stated over 20 years ago, i.e. it is essentially an infected eczema (Keogh and Russell 1956). Indeed, in discussing the external otitides, Mawson (1974) distinguishes not only an *eczematous dermatitis* and a *seborrhoeic dermatitis* but also a *seborrhoeic eczema*.

Treatment of the eczematous group of external otitides includes (a) removing any identifiable external cause, e.g. antibiotic ear drops, (b) attacking the inflammatory action, and (c) attacking infecting organisms. The second and third points can be encompassed with a combined steroid and clioquinol topical preparation, as mentioned previously.

The scaling condition of the scalp (dandruff) which is associated with *seborrhoeic otitis externa* should be treated with initially biweekly cetrimonium shampoos, or those containing selenium disulphide. If aural irritation is severe, the daily installation of drops containing mercuric nitrate may prove beneficial. The use of an arachis oil preparation is said to prevent the accumulation of débris.

In the *neurodermatitis* type of external otitis where a psychological factor is assuming a major role, psychotherapy using such techniques as behaviour modification may be required. The secondary infection associated with repetitive scratching is perhaps best treated with a topical clioquinol–steroid preparation.

Otomycosis has been recognized for over a 100 years. Wreden (1867) reported six cases from which *Aspergillus glaucus* was isolated. The majority of fungi isolated from the lesions of external otitis are generally considered to be saprobic* in nature and can commonly be isolated from normal healthy

* This term is preferred to saprophytic since the latter term implies a plant relationship.

skin (Haley 1950; Lea, Schuster, and Harell 1958). As McKelvie (1976) points out, the part that these organisms play in the production and maintenance of external otitis and the factors which allow them to grow in profusion under certain environmental conditions remain obscure. *Aspergillus niger* is probably the commonest pathogen which is isolated (Sharp, John, and Robinson 1946; Gregson and La Touche 1961). Since, like other external otitides, otomycosis is associated with the accumulation of debris, regular and effective aural toilet is necessary. In view of their action against both bacteria and fungi, quinoline compound preparations are of considerable value. In cases associated with infection with *Candida*, treatment with amphotericin B or with nystatin is recommended (Pyman 1959).

MIDDLE EAR

Acute otitis media

Acute suppurative otitis media undergoes spontaneous recovery in somewhere between 50 per cent (Heller 1940) and 85 per cent (Fry 1958) of cases. The recovery rate after myringotomy alone has been reported to be not greater than 70 per cent (Diamant and Diamant 1974). The recovery rate following treatment with the antibiotic azidocillin (Fig. 18.5) has been

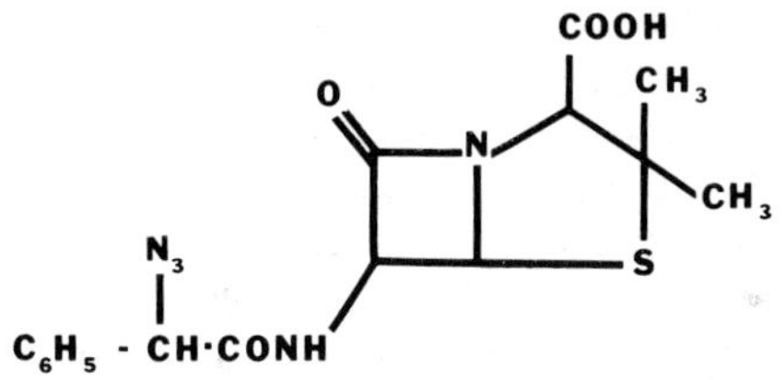

Fig. 18.5. Azidocillin.

reported to be 100 per cent (Bergholtz and Rudberg 1972). Moreover, Heller has suggested that myringotomy constitutes an additional trauma to the tympanic membrane which may prolong resolution time. More severe complications may also, but, fortunately, rarely, occur, e.g. massive haemorrhage due to an abnormally high jugular bulb (Page 1914). The argument against myringotomy has been extended by Lorentzen and Haugsten (1977) who say that the procedure is associated with psychological trauma, especially to children. The procedure is also an expensive way of treatment since an anaesthetist, an otologist, and an operating room may also be required. Nevertheless, there have been statements, such as that by Taylor (1965), that it is 'much more common for a surgeon to regret not performing a myringotomy than to regret performing one'.

In a Norwegian study, Lorentzen and Haugsten (1977) randomly allocated acute otitis media cases to one of three methods of treatment. Diagnosis of the disease was based upon observing a thick, red tympanic membrane with or without bulging or spontaneous perforation. The three methods of treatment were myringotomy, a 10-day course of an oral penicillin, viz. phenoxymethylpenicillin (Fig. 18.6), and a combination of the first two methods. The patients were re-examined on the fifth, tenth, and the twenty-

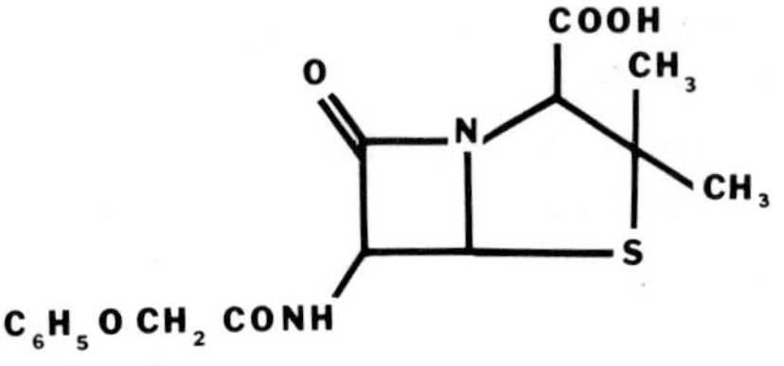

Fig. 18.6. Phenoxymethylpenicillin.

eighth to the thirty-fifth day after the start of treatment. The treatment was considered a failure if either aural discharge or a bulging tympanic membrane were present after 10 days of treatment. After 10 days of treatment, there were significantly more failures in the myringotomy group than in the other two groups. At this time penicillin therapy was started in the failed myringotomy cases. (Diamant and Diamant (1974) have, however, pointed out that 'spontaneous healing' can occur even after a duration of 30 days and without antibiotic treatment.) Lorentzen and Haugsten failed to confirm a previous report (Roddey, Earle, and Haggerty 1966) that more rapid pain relief was obtained by myringotomy than by antibiotic administration.

In considering the success or failure of antibiotic treatment of acute otitis media it is important to consider the concentration of the drug in middle-ear exudate (Silverstein, Bernstein, and Lerner 1966; Coffey 1968; Kamme, Lundgren, and Rundcrantz 1969; Lahikainen 1970) (Figs. 18.7–18.9). Therapeutic failure can often be explained by an inadequate concentration in the middle-ear fluid (Lundgren, Ingvarsson, and Rundcrantz 1979). Nevertheless, both ampicillin and azidocillin stay longer in the effusions of acute otitis media than in blood (Lahikainen, Vuori, and Virtanen 1977).

Using a randomized double-blind study, Howard, Nelson, Clahsen, and Jackson (1976) compared four antimicrobial regimes on 383 infants and children. The infecting organism was monitored by aspirating middle-ear fluid for culture before treatment and during treatment if fluid persisted. The most common causative organisms were *Streptococcus pneumoniae* (31 per cent of cases) and *Haemophilus* spp. (22 per cent). The four treatments were amoxycillin, erythromycin, penicillin V (phenoxymethylpenicillin), and a combination of erythromycin and trisulfapyrimidine (equal parts of sulfadiazine (Fig. 18.10), sulfadimidine (Fig. 18.11), and sulfamerazine (Fig. 18.12)). Amoxycillin was the most effective of the four in treating pneumococcal infections. The amoxycillin and the erythromycin–trisulfapyrimidine mixture produced better response rates than the other two treatments. Recovery rates in the four groups were similar.

The use of a combination of sulphonamide drugs dates back to the days when it was thought that small doses of different sorts of sulphonamides

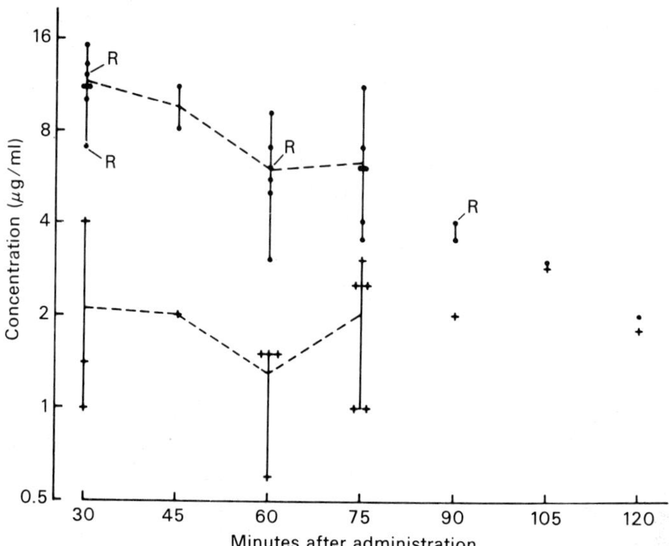

Fig. 18.7. Concentration in serum and ear exudate after a dose of 13 mg (20 000 i.u.) penicillin V per kg body weight (25 patients). ●, concentration in serum; +, concentration in exudate; R, patients with recurrent otitis. The dotted lines connect means. The times given include a margin of ± 5 min. (After Kamme *et al.* 1969.)

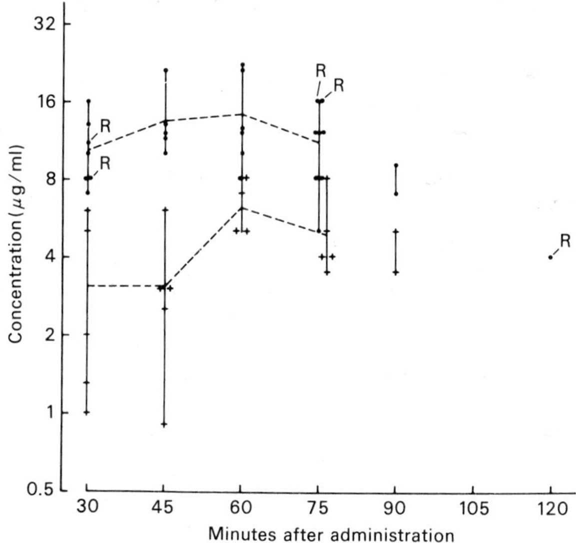

Fig. 18.8. Concentration in serum and ear exudate after a dose of 26 mg (40 000 i.u.) penicillin V per kg body weight (29 patients). ●, concentration in serum; +, concentration in exudate; R, patients with recurrent otitis. The dotted lines connect means. The times given include a margin of ± 5 min. (After Kamme *et al.* 1969.)

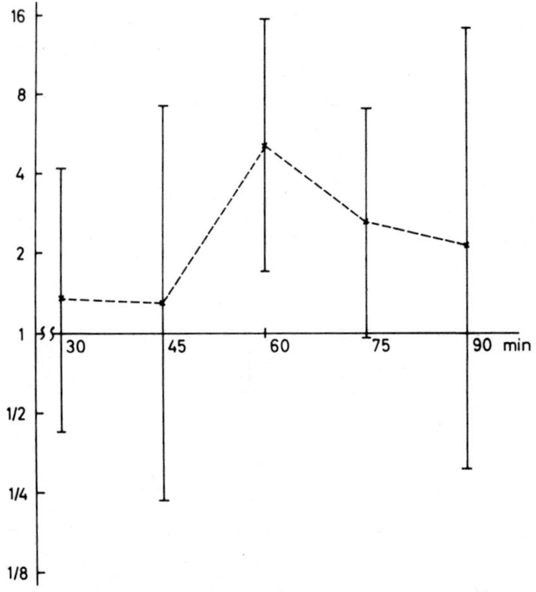

Fig. 18.9. Comparison between concentration of penicillin V in exudate after administration of 13 and 26 mg per kg body weight. The dotted line connects the quotients between the concentration in exudate after a dose of 26 and 13 mg per kg. Quotient is calculated as difference between means of logarithmic values. Confidence interval at 99% level is denoted by vertical lines. (After Kamme *et al.* 1969.)

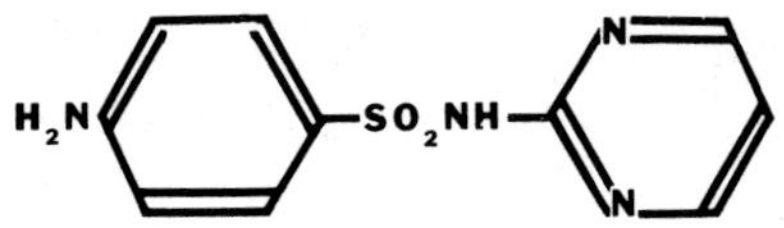

Fig. 18.10. Sulfadiazine.

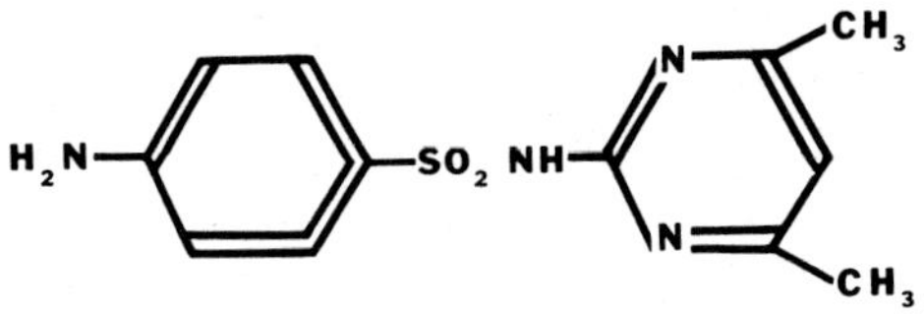

Fig. 18.11. Sulfadimidine.

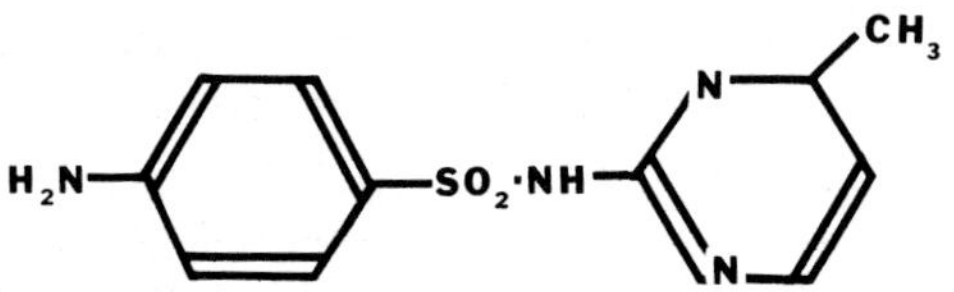

Fig. 18.12. Sulfamerazine.

would decrease the risks of adverse reactions. It is now considered better to use a more soluble sulphonamide and one only. However, even the best tolerated and least toxic of sulphonamides may produce headache, dizziness, nausea, vomiting, drowsiness, and depression (Griffin and D'Arcy 1979) as well as cyanosis, drug fever, rashes, leucopenia, crystalluria, haematuria, and anuria, albeit temporary. Moreover, a rare, but particularly disturbing, adverse effect that has been described in children is the Stevens–Johnson (1922) syndrome, particularly with long-term sulphonamide therapy. This syndrome is characterized by annular maculopapular or vesiculobullous cutaneous lesions involving particularly the dorsa of the hands and feet; mucosal involvement, e.g. conjunctivitis, stomatitis, and balanitis; and constitutional symptoms (Gorlin and Pindborg 1964). Under the term 'erythema multiforme exudativum', von Hebra described the cutaneous and constitutional features in 1860. The mucosal component was reported by Fuchs in 1876. The occurrence of the syndrome as a consequence of sulphonamide administration has been reported by Wright, Gold, and Jennings (1947); by Sidney (1960); and by Carroll, Bryan, and Robinson (1966). The syndrome has also been associated with penicillin administration (Wright *et al.* 1947; Yaffee 1959). The fatality is around 5 to 10 per cent. The treatment of the condition includes calamine lotion to the skin, corticosteroid eye drops, and, perhaps, systemic corticosteroids.

The use of co-trimoxazole, which is a combination of a sulphonamide, sulfamethoxazole, with trimethroprim (Fig. 18.13) has also been studied in

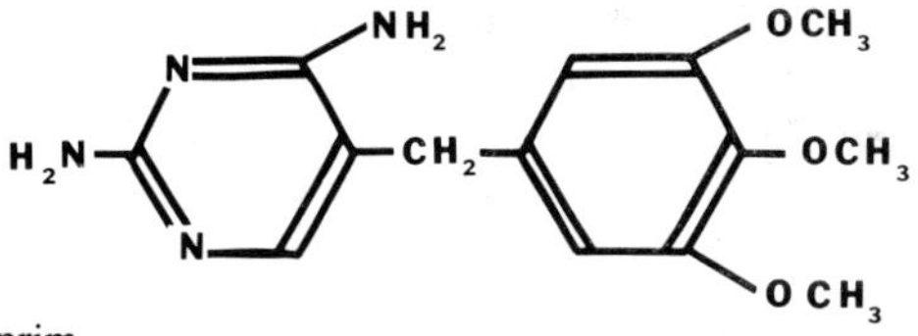

Fig. 18.13. Trimethoprim.

acute otitis media (Cantarelli 1973; Cameron, Pomahac, and Johnston 1975; Cooper, Inman, and Dawson 1976). In the multicentric study by Cooper and his colleagues, eleven primary physicians compared co-trimoxazole with amoxycillin on a group of 61 patients (predominantly in the age range 6 months to 5 years) suffering from otitis media. The condition was diagnosed on the basis of the history and clinical examination. According to a randomization chart, one or other drug was prescribed at a standard dose for a duration of 7 days. The main criterion for recovery was the disappearance of the hearing impairment. Assessment was made initially and 7–10 days after starting treatment. The hearing loss cleared in 7–10 days in 79 per cent of the patients treated with co-trimoxazole and in 77 per cent of these treated with amoxycillin. The average time for the hearing impairment to clear was 6 days for the amoxycillin and 5.6 days for the co-trimoxazole. Thus co-trimoxazole could be considered the preparation of choice for treating otitis media, particularly whenever there was penicillin hypersensitivity or intolerance to that drug.

Trimethoprim is a synthetic pyrimidine derivative unrelated to the sulphonamides. It is effective against *Streptococcus* spp., *Haemophilus* spp., and *Proteus* spp. Thus in conjunction with the sulphonamide, which is, *inter alia*, effective against *Staphylococcus* spp, a much widened and intensified antibacterial spectrum is encompassed. Both drugs block different points on the chain of synthesis leading from *p*-aminobenzoic acid (Fig. 18.14) to the

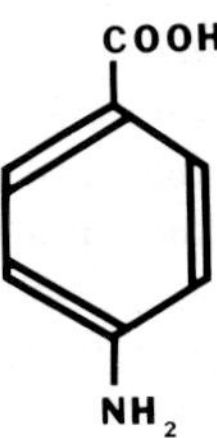

Fig. 18.14. *p*-Aminobenzoic acid.

DNA macromolecule. The first step in the chain, i.e. the synthesis of dihydrofolic acid from aminobenzoic acid, is blocked by the sulphonamide by the method of substrate competitive enzyme inhibition. The second step, i.e. the synthesis of folinic acid from the hydrofolic acid, is blocked by the trimethoprim since it is a competitive inhibitor of dihydrofolic reductase.

Co-trimoxazole is contraindicated in patients with hepatic or renal insufficiency. It should not be given to premature babies nor to full-term infants within the first 6 weeks of life. It is also not recommended to women during pregnancy. With long-term treatment, it is recommended that full blood counts, including thrombocytes, should be done fortnightly for the first month and then monthly. The side effects of co-trimoxazole have included nausea, vomiting, glossitis, skin rashes, thrombocytopenia, purpura, leucopenia, neutropenia, and, rarely, severe skin sensitivity reactions such as the Lyell (1956) syndrome (epidermal necrolysis) and the Stevens–Johnson syndrome.

Increasing importance is now being attached to *Haemophilus* spp. in the causation and delayed resolution of acute otitis media. It has been generally believed that *Haemophilus* spp. is not a common causative organism of acute otitis media in children who are older than five years. Schwartz, Rodriguez, Khan, and Ross (1977) have now shown that, in at least one area of the United States, *Haemophilus* spp. is the causative organism in 36 per cent of cases of acute otitis media in children between five years and nine years of age. Subsequently, Schwartz and his colleagues (1978) reported an increasing incidence of ampicillin-resistant strains of *Haemophilus influenzae* in acute otitis media. At that time, 8 per cent of all cases of acute otitis media in the Washington, DC area were due to such strains. Thirty-one out of thirty-five patients with ampicillin resistant *Haemophilus influenzae* otitis were treated with an erythromycin–sulfafurazole (sulfisoxazole) mixture. There was 'an impressive clinical response'. Twenty-six of these thirty-one cases had failed to have the *Haemophilus influenzae* eradicated by a 10-day course of oral ampicillin in the recommended dose.

Although not based upon a prospective randomized study, Diamant and Diamant (1974) have adduced evidence to indicate that there is a higher rate of *recurrences* in cases of acute otitis media treated with antimicrobial agents than in cases treated with myringotomy alone. Moroever, the data indicated that the recurrence rate is greater the earlier in the course of the disease that the antimicrobial agent is given. Thus Diamant and Diamant's data showed that the recurrence rate was 45.1 per cent when antibiotics were given on the first day of the illness, 34.1 per cent when given after the seventh day and 32.1 per cent if not given at all. These authors hypothesized that the use of antibiotics inhibited the production of antibodies and so interfered with the development of natural immunity. Consequently, they enunciated the 'antibiotic timing treatment' of acute otitis media. This means that treatment with antibiotics should be started only when signs of otitic complications are threatening, or have already presented.

None of the previously cited experimental comparative studies of the treatment of acute otitis media has included a dummy drug. It might be argued that, in view of the information provided on spontaneous cure rates (Heller 1940; Fry 1958), on the 100 per cent response to a penicillin preparation (Bergholtz and Rudberg 1972) and the different response rates to various antimicrobial agents (Howard *et al.* 1976), none was needed. However, Halsted, Lepow, Balassanian, Emmerich, and Wolinsky (1968) conducted an experimental comparative study in which a dummy drug was included. These physicians randomly allocated patients with acute otitis media to one of three treatments (a penicillin preparation, a penicillin together with a sulphonamide, and a dummy drug). In cases where positive bacterial cultures were obtained, there was no significant difference in the response rates to the various methods of treatment. Clearly, further experimental comparative studies are required in which not only a dummy drug is included but, in order to encompass Diamant and Diamant's concept, the timing of treatment is also introduced as an additional variable. The use of a sequential experimental design (Armitage 1960) will dispose of any objections on ethical grounds to the inclusion of dummy drugs.

Recurrent otitis media

In managing this condition, it would appear that attention should be given to nutritional, infective, and allergic factors. Aside from eradicating infective foci in the upper respiratory tract, long-term chemoprophylaxis has its advocates. The otitis media attack rate appears to be significantly lowered by either long-term sulfamethoxypyridazine (Fig. 18.15) (Ensign, Urbanich, and Moran 1960) or long-term sulfafurazole (Fig. 18.16) (Perrin, Charney, McWhinney, McInerny, Miller, and Nazarian 1974). However, newer sulphonamide drugs are now available which might suitably be

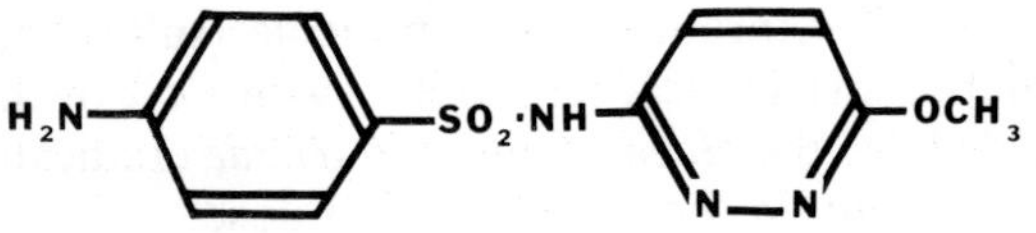

Fig. 18.15. Sulfamethoxypyridazine.

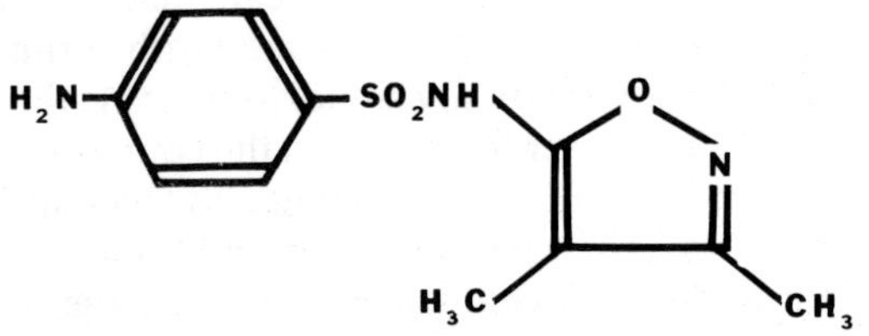

Fig. 18.16. Sulfafurazole.

employed in such long-term chemoprophylaxis. Sulfalene, viz. sulfametopyrazine (Fig. 18.17), can be given orally in weekly doses of 254 μmol (30 mg) per kilogram of body weight. The prolonged effect of sulfalene is not due to a high degree of serum protein binding (actually only about 60 per cent) but to a high degree of renal tubular re-absorption associated with a low rate of hepatic metabolism of the drug. Consequently, if it is necessary to accelerate elimination of the drug, this may be done by making the urine alkaline (about pH 8) by means, for example, of potassium citrate mixture (BPC). The sulfalene will then be retained in the urine in a higher concentration in the form of the alkali metal salt.

Wilson (1971) has drawn attention to the need to consider inhalant and food hypersensitivity in the management of children with recurrent acute otitis media.

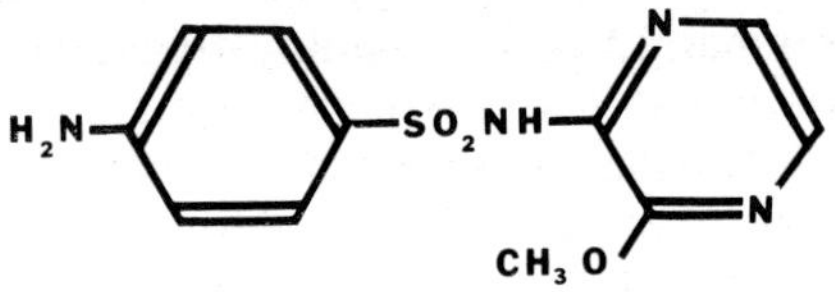

Fig. 18.17. Sulfalene.

Secretory otitis media

As Palva (1979) points out, the plethora of terms relating to the non-suppurative middle-ear effusions frequently restricts the interpretation of published data. Mawson (1974) differentiates acute non-suppurative otitis media from chronic non-suppurative otitis media. The former is associated with thin fluid (serous otitis media) and shows the characteristic 'hairline' on otoscopy. The latter is associated with thick fluid (secretory otitis media) and characteristically shows the dull, poorly mobile tympanic membrane; this is colloquially referred to as the 'glue ear'. A serous otitis media is frequently symptomatic of some other disorder.

Secretory otitis media usually presents as a conductive hearing loss of insidious onset in school children. The histopathological picture is that of hyperplasia of mucus-producing elements and hypersecretion of mucus (Sadé 1966). Although experimental comparative studies have clearly shown the value of tympanostomy tubes (colloquially termed 'grommets') in improving hearing (Shah 1971), the long-term effects have been questioned (Richards, Kilby, Shaw, and Campbell 1971). Brown, Richards, and Ambegaokar (1978) have recently reported a five-year follow-up of an experimental comparative study of tympanostomy tubes in secretory otitis media. Fifty-five children who were between 4 and 10 years of age and who had bilateral secretory otitis media had a tympanostomy tube inserted in one ear; no treatment was given for the other ear. Within the first six months of treatment, hearing gains were better in those ears into which a tube had been inserted. After six months, there was no statistical significant difference in the incidence of fluid in the two middle ears. Moreover, after that elapse of time, the authors reported a 13 per cent incidence of thin tympanic membrane scars and a 42 per cent incidence of tympanosclerosis in the ears which had received the tympanostomy tubes compared with a zero incidence in the comparison ear. Thus, contrary to the initial favourable reports of Hughes, Warder, and Hudson (1974) and others, it would now appear that the use of tympanostomy tubes is not innocuous. Furthermore, cholesteatomas have arisen following the use of such tubes. Consequently, a search has been made for a more rational treatment of secretory otitis media. Unfortunately, oral mucolytics, such as bromhexine, are ineffective (Elcock and Lord 1972). Autoinflation, vasoconstrictor (ephedrine) nasal drops, oral antihistamines (brompheniramine), and oral vasoconstrictors (norephedrine and phenylephrine) are equally ineffective (Fraser, Menta, and Fraser 1977).

A number of amides (Waldron-Edward and Skoryna 1966), including carbamide (urea) (Lieberman 1967) have a mucolytic action on body secretions. Consequently, Bauer (1968, 1970) has cogently argued against the use of tympanostomy tubes and for the intratympanic injection of urea. In 52 out of 60 ears in 37 children followed up from 6 months to 30 months, the results 'were entirely satisfactory with considerable improvement in hearing'. The spontaneous remission rate in this disorder is only 28 per cent.

Since recent microbiological studies (Liu, Lim, Lang, and Birck 1975) have shown that, contrary to previous opinion, the effusion is not sterile, it would appear logical to prescribe antimicrobial drugs. Brockman (1972) had previously claimed a beneficial effect for trisulfapyrimidine. It is to be noted that, as mentioned previously, Howard and his colleagues showed that a combination of this preparation with erythromycin produced a good response in cases of acute otitis media. The previous suggestion of using a long-term drug such as sulfalene in the management of recurrent otitis media might also be repeated in the context of secretory otitis media. Alternatively, a course of co-trimoxazole should be considered.

Both ampicillin and azidocillin orally administered penetrate poorly into the middle-ear fluid in secretory otitis media (Lahikainen *et al.* 1977).

Chronic otitis media

As Gristwood (1979) points out, in treating this condition, the factors predisposing to chronicity of aural infection must be identified and dealt with to make the ear dry and inactive. Then, ideally, all patients should have some form of tympanoplasty both to prevent infection (by repairing the ear drum) and to restore hearing by reconstructing the tympano-ossicular mechanism. This idea is, however, not always realized.

Aural toilet should be done meticulously and at a frequency determined by the quantity of secretion. During washing or swimming, water should be kept out by plugging the meatus with cotton-wool and petroleum jelly (B P).

In between successive aural toilets, ear drops are frequently prescribed. Preparations containing an antimicrobial agent and a corticosteroid to reduce the inflammatory reaction are in vogue. However, Ajodhia and Dix (1975) have called attention to the actual or potential ototoxicity of many of these preparations. In the light of current knowledge it is probable that one is left only with a preparation that contains halquinol and triamcinolone acetonide. Halquinol has a wide range of antimicrobial activity. In contrast to the antibiotics, it is effective against most bacterial and fungal aural surface pathogens. Moreover, it is also effective against many antibiotic-resistant bacteria. However, transient stinging may occur in acute weeping lesions and sensitivity reactions to halquinol may occur. The preparation should be kept away from the eyes. Staining of clothes and plastic materials may also occur; the latter are particularly resistant to cleansing.

Fears have been expressed that the use of topical aural antimicrobial agents might lead to an increase in the number of resistant bacteria. Moreoever, it has been pointed out (Picozzi, Sweeney, Calder, and Browning 1979) that there is no evidence that the use of antimicrobial agents is superior to rigorous aurual toilet in the management of active chronic otitis media. Thus the use of such drugs is yet to be justified by experimental comparative studies.

Two recent reports have questioned the need to consider *cholesteatoma* as an exclusively surgical condition. These are the communications by Duncan (1977) and by Kluyskens, Gillis, and Nsabumukunzi (1979).

Duncan reported the use of topical retinol, viz. vitamin A (Fig. 18.18) in 55 cases of acquired cholesteatoma. The solution had a strength of 150 000 i.u. per ml. The patient was instructed to instil the drops in the ears for at least 20 minutes every night and go to sleep with the treated ear uppermost.

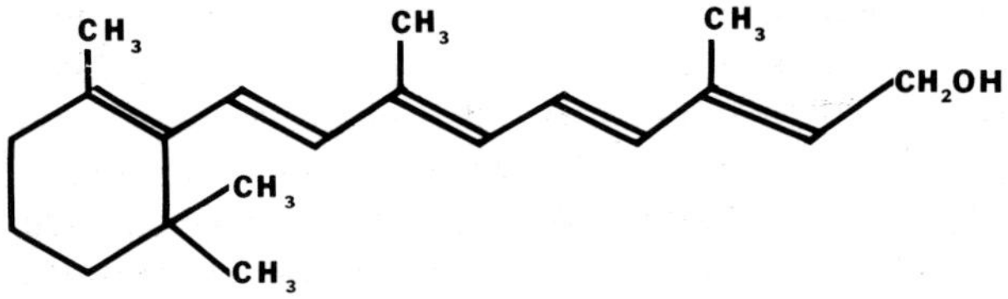

CH_3 CH_3 CH_3 CH_2OH CH_3 CH_3

Fig. 18.18. Retinol.

With bilateral disease, alternate ears were treated daily. About 80 per cent of patients appear to have had some form of surgical operation to facilitate access of the drug. There was disappearance of the cholesteatoma in over half of the cases; probably less than 5 per cent of cases showed no response. Duncan reported that improvement was usually evident in the third to fifth week after starting treatment. The odour associated with such ears disappeared, mucus production increased, and mastoid cavities and tympanic membrane perforations were less painful to clean. The middle-ear mucosa became vascular and thicker. The cholesteatomatous desquamation could be peeled off the underlying tissues without bleeding. It would appear that the only side effects were an oily taste in the nose on waking, itching, excessive mucus production, and, in about 6 per cent of cases, an allergic reaction to the peanut oil which was part of the drug vehicle.

Kluyskens and his colleagues reported the use of topical acetylcysteine (Fig. 18.19) in 29 cases of cholesteatoma. Five of these cases had perforations of the membrana flaccida with cholesteatoma of the epitympanic recess. The 'classic aspiration technique' had not been successful in the treatment of the cases. Acetylcysteine powder was blown into contact with the cholesteatoma. Two or three days later the cholesteatoma was washed out and suction 'resulted in a clean cavity without any cholesteatomatous remains'. Comparison of hearing measurements before and after the procedure showed no hearing loss. One patient failed to return. The other four patients showed very clean cavities when seen 3 to 6 months later.

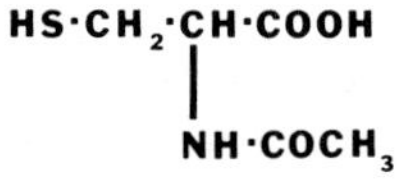

$$HS{\cdot}CH_2{\cdot}\underset{\displaystyle NH{\cdot}COCH_3}{\underset{|}{C}H}{\cdot}COOH$$

Fig. 18.19. Acetylcysteine.

Acetylcysteine is a mucolytic which has been used in the treatment of chronic bronchopulmonary infections. The mucolytic property is attributed to a free sulphydryl group which opens up the disulphide bonds in the mucus. The insolubility of keratin is attributed to the presence of numerous disulphide bonds between its peptide chains.

The only side effect reported by Kluyskens was a 'slight earache which lasted for a few minutes'.

The principal disadvantage of the two methods is that, by foregoing surgery, one is unable to eliminate the serious potential complications of persisting cholesteatoma.

Otosclerosis

Although calcitonin has been shown to be ineffective in hearing disorders associated with Paget's disease (Menzies, Greenberg, and Joplin 1979), there have been suggestions that, nevertheless, the drug might be effective in otosclerosis. This is based upon the observation that the pathological changes in otosclerosis resemble some of those in Pagetic involvement of the ear. Rudman and Parsons (1979) have also shown, experimentally, that calcitonin can inhibit induced osteolysis in guinea pig auditory ossicles.

Calcitonin is a polypeptide hormone secreted by the thyroid gland. Together with the parathyroid hormone it controls the level of the circulating calcium cation. A fall in serum calcium results in the secretion of parathyroid hormone which in turn stimulates an increase in the serum calcium concentration. An increase in blood calcium results in secretion of calcitonin which lowers the level. In each case, the calcium is transferred from, or to, the body calcium depot, i.e. skeletal bone.

Calcitonin may cause nausea, vomiting, facial flushing, paraesthesias, and dysgeusia.

INTERNAL EAR AND NERVE

Cochlear otosclerosis

There have been enthusiastic reports that sodium flouride improves the hearing in cochlear otosclerosis (Shambaugh 1966; Shambaugh, Causse, Petrovic, Chevance, and Valvassori 1974). The experimental basis is the promotion of bone formation and inhibition of bone resorbtion in young rats (Shambaugh and Petrovic 1967). Microchemical analysis of otosclerotic stapes has shown that sodium flouride treatment is associated with a higher calcium/phosphorus ratio (Bretlau, Hansen, Causse, and Causse 1979). This indicates that flouride may stabilize otosclerotic lesions, especially the spongiotic type with unstable mineralization.

Acoustic trauma

Martin and Jakobs (1977) reported a comparison of dextran 40 and xantinol nicotinate on a series of 139 cases. The amelioration of the hearing loss and the tinnitus was statistically better in those patients who received the dextran 40.

Usher's syndrome

Gahlot, Sood, and Khosla (1977) studied the effect of penicillamine on the sensorineural hearing loss associated with pigmentary degeneration of the retina. The hearing improved.

Penicillamine (3,3-dimethylcysteine) is an oral chelating agent which has been recommended for the treatment of hepatolenticular degeneration (Wilson's disease) by promoting the excretion of tissue copper deposits. As well as this chelating property, the drug has the ability to take part in oxidative–reductive reactions, sulphydryl–disulphide interchange, and nucleophilic additions (Friedman 1977). The property of disulphide interchange between penicillamine and cystine is used to control the excessive excretion of cystine in cystinuria.

It is clear that penicillamine affects several enzyme and organ systems.

Moreover, an immunostimulant function has also been suggested. The drug enhances cell-mediated responses (Huskisson 1977).

As a consequence of these many properties, penicillamine has potentially numerous side effects. Indeed, the drug can cause tinnitus and a variety of allergic reactions, including cross-sensitivity between the drug and penicillin. Skin reactions may include a maculopapular or erythematous rash early in the course of treatment, falling hair, a syndrome resembling disseminated lupus erythematosus and pemphigus. Other adverse effects include nausea, anorexia, vomiting, diarrhoea, glossitis, a gingivostomatitis, reversible impairment of taste, a nephrotic syndrome, and, fortunately rarely, Goodpasture's syndrome (severe and ultimately fatal glomerulonephritis and intra-alveolar haemorrhage) (Association of the British Pharmaceutical Industry, 1979). Moreover, Bucknall (1977) has described a syndrome resembling classical myasthenia gravis in patients on long-term treatment with penicillamine.

Ménière's disorder

Using a double-blind technique, Klockhoff and Lindblom (1966) showed that hydrochlorothiazide (Fig. 18.20) is beneficial with respect to the hearing loss, vertigo, and general condition in Ménière's disorder.

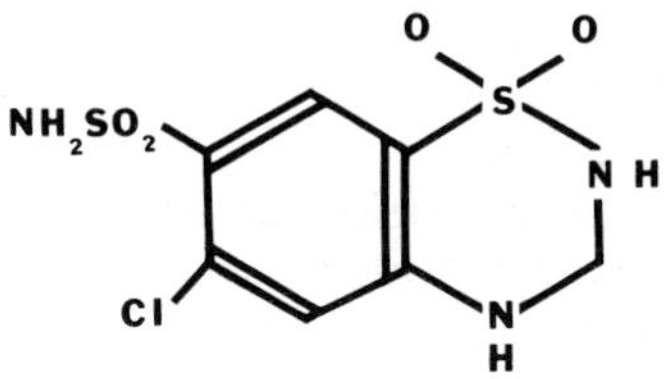

O O S NH NH_2SO_2 Cl N H

Fig. 18.20. Hydrochlorothiazide.

Hydrochlorothiazide may cause mild anorexia, nausea, constipation or diarrhoea, skin rashes, and photosensitivity. There have also been rare reports of blood dyscrasias, including thrombocytopenia. Although the deliberate omission of potassium substitution may be offset by omitting the drug one day out of seven, there is the risk, with prolonged administration of the drug, of producing a hypokalaemia. This hypokalaemia intensifies both the cardiac effect and the toxicity of the cardiac glycosides. The thiazides may also provoke hyperglycaemia and glycosuria in diabetics and other susceptible patients. They may also cause hyperuricaemia and precipitate attacks of gout (Griffin and D'Arcy 1979). Moreover, the action of tricyclic antidepressants and of monoamino-oxidase inhibitors may be potentiated by hydrochlorothiazide. Thus patients who are being treated with hydrochlorothiazide may require regular monitoring of fluid and electrolyte balance particularly when diuresis is marked or in patients suffering from impaired renal function. Particular caution is also required in the elderly since electrolyte balance is more likely to be precarious owing to bowel or renal dysfunction. Urinary retention is also more likely in these patients.

The *modus operandi* for water and salt depletion procedures is uncertain since Perlman, Goldfinger, and Cales (1953) failed to demonstrate any consistent effect by either water depletion and loading or salt depletion and loading in cases of Ménière's disorder. Harrison and Naftalin (1968) have shown that the acute attacks of vertigo occur during a phase of sodium diuresis concomitant with a water gain.

Betahistine, i.e. β-(2-pyridyl) ethylmethylamine (Fig. 18.21), has been shown, in at least three double-blind experimental comparative studies, to be effective in the control of the vertigo (Elia 1966; Hicks, Hicks, and Cooley, 1967) and in improving the hearing (Wilmot and Menon 1976) in Ménière's disorder. The use of this histamine analogue may seem rational if one considers Schayer's (1964) hypothesis that histamine is the intrinsic microcirculatory dilator and the aim is to increase blood circulation to the internal ear.

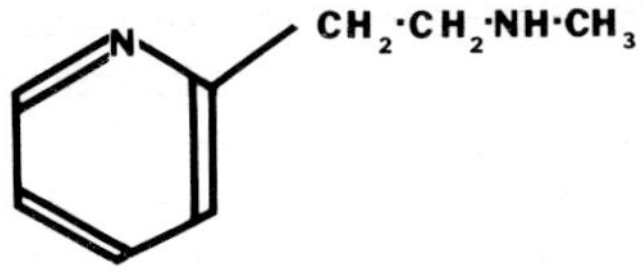

N $CH_2 \cdot CH_2 \cdot NH \cdot CH_3$

Fig. 18.21. Betahistine.

A small number of reports of gastric upset have occurred in patients being treated with betahistine and with a history of peptic ulcer. Although clinical intolerance to betahistine has not been demonstrated in patients with bronchial asthma, caution should be exercised when administering the drug to such patients. The only contraindication would be in patients with phaeochromocytoma.

Syphilis

Wright (1968) found that 3 per cent of cases of sensorineural hearing loss seen at a London hospital were due to late congenital syphilis. Late congenital syphilis is a much more common cause of sensorineural hearing loss than is acquired syphilis. The late onset is emphasized by the ages of presentation in the small series reported by Dawkins, Sharp, and Morrison (1968). The symptomatology of late congenital syphilis may be indistinguishable from that of Ménière's disorder except that it is usually bilateral and severe as regards the hearing loss.

The majority of the cases reported by Wright had developed hearing loss in spite of treatment. There are three possible reasons for this: treatment was inadequate, the organisms persisted in spite of 'adequate' treatment, or an immunopathic process supervened. In both rabbits and Man, treponemes may persist in spite of apparently adequate penicillin treatment (Collart, Borel, and Durel 1962; Collart and Durel 1964). *Treponema pallidum* has also been demonstrated in the temporal bone of a patient who had suffered from congenital syphilis and who had had three courses of penicillin treatment (Mack, Smith, Walter, Rios Montenegro, and Nicol 1969). The association of late congenital syphilitic sensorineural hearing loss with interstitial keratitis where immunopathological factors are considered to be important and which responds to corticosteroids, the preponderance of female patients and the occurrence of lymphocytic aggregations in affected ears would point to an immunopathic process. However, the sera of only two out of 20 patients afflicted with late congenital syphilis were found to contain a rheumatoid or antinuclear factor (Wright 1968). Arising from these considerations, one of the penicillins and/or steroids might be used in the treatment of afflicted individuals. Ampicillin (Fig. 18.22) is the antibiotic of choice for the treatment of labyrinthine syphilis (Kerr, Smyth, and Landau 1970). However, ampicillin may reduce the efficacy of oral contraceptives and patients should be warned accordingly. The drug is, of course, contraindicated in patients with penicillin sensitivity or with glandular fever. The skin reactions that may rarely occur take the form of either an urticarial rash, which is due to penicillin hypersensitivity, or an erythematous rash which is due to a specific ampicillin sensitivity. Occasionally, diarrhoea may occur (Association of the British Pharmaceutical Industry 1979). AAC (antibiotic-associated colitis) is a particularly serious cause of the diarrhoea. This is a pseudomembranous colitis which is due to the toxins of *Clostridium difficile* (Bartlett, Chang, Gurwith, Gurbach, and Onderdonk 1978). The condition responds promptly and unequivocably to oral vancomycin (Tedesco, Markham, Gurwith, Christie, and Bartlett 1978).

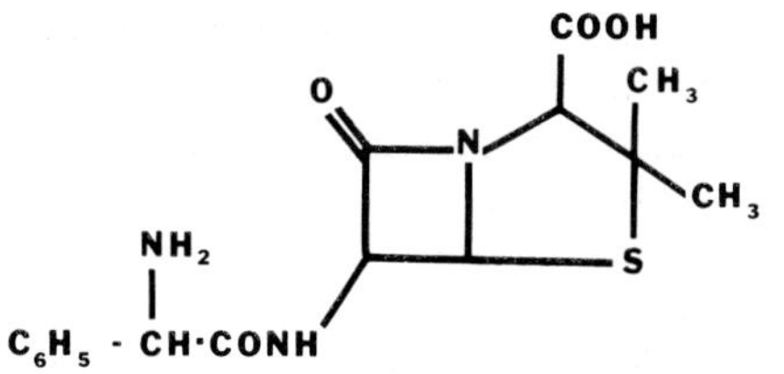

Fig. 18.22. Ampicillin.

Zoller, Wilson, and Nadol (1979) say that hearing loss secondary to congenital or acquired syphilis may be partially reversed by a three-month's course of penicillin and prednisone (Fig. 18.23), although subsequent deterioration of hearing may occur. Continued prednisone treatment can maintain hearing levels in some patients.

Since the use of steroids is not free from serious hazards and one must also consider the syphilitic process in the body as a whole, this treatment should be under the control of a venereologist. In view of the evidence for the persistence of treponemes in spite of apparently adequate antibiotic treatment, the increase in the prevalence of syphilis, changing attitudes to sex and the increasing mobility of affected individuals afforded by modern

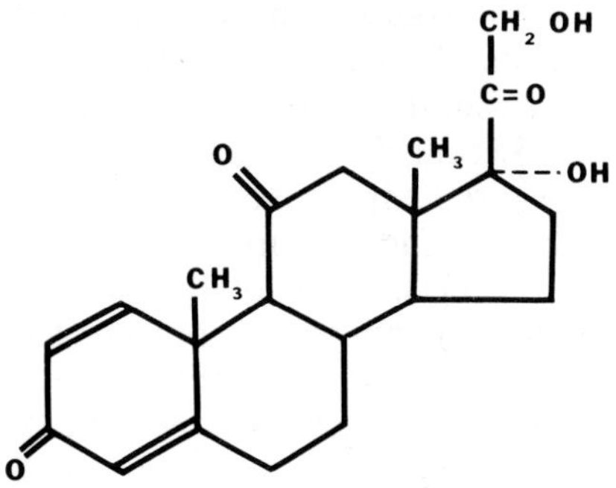

Fig. 18.23. Prednisone.

transportation, it would appear that hope for the future must reside in immunization against the infection.

Sarcoidosis

Although auditory sarcoidosis is rare, this diagnosis should always be borne in mind when confronted with a case of sensorineural hearing loss in conjunction with multiple, fluctuating cranial nerve palsies. The hearing loss in such cases may be of gradual or sudden onset. Gristwood (1958) reported a bilateral sudden hearing loss in a 26-year-old woman which was due to sarcoid and he reviewed thirteen other cases that had been reported in the literature. Although Camp and Frierson (1962) assert that steroids are ineffective in chronic neurosarcoidosis, Matthews (1965) says that the subacute forms respond to steroids but these must be continued for one month after apparent complete cure. The hearing loss in Gristwood's case showed an appreciable improvement with prednisolone (Fig. 18.24), and a combination of aminosalicyclic acid (PAS) (Fig. 18.25) and isoniazid (Fig. 18.26). Reported side effects of both of the last two drugs include headaches, nausea and vomiting, skin rashes, diarrhoea, and, very rarely, blood dyscrasias. A condition resembling infectious mononucleosis has also been reported to be associated with aminosalicylate administration. Dizziness,

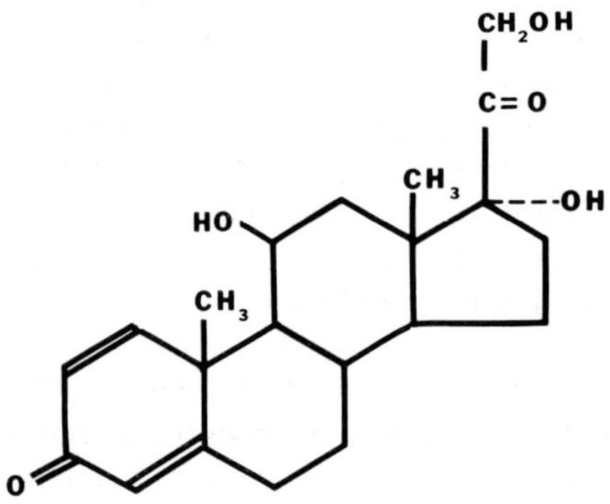

Fig. 18.24. Prednisolone.

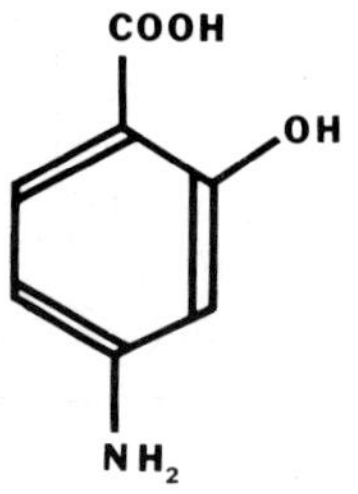

COOH
OH
NH$_2$

Fig. 18.25. *p*-Aminosalicylic acid.

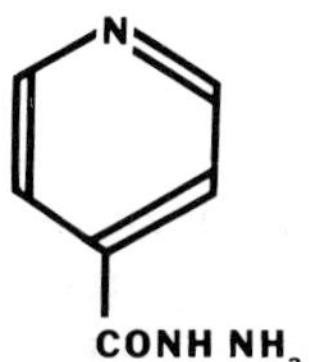

Fig. 18.26. Isoniazid.

ataxia, and tinnitus have figured amongst the reported side effects of isoniazid.

Cogan's syndrome

Cogan's syndrome comprises a Ménière's syndrome in association with a non-luetic interstitial keratitis (Cogan 1945; Smith 1970). The course of the labyrinthine disorder parallels that of the ocular lesions (Teodorescu and Cernea 1962) and the audiometric pattern is that of a receptor organ (end-organ) lesion (Serrins, Harrison, and Chandler 1963). The syndrome is now considered to be a manifestation of polyarteritis nodosa. Consequently, corticosteroids form the main drug for managing the condition.

Vogt–Koyanagi–Harada syndrome

As well as the internal ear dysfunction, this syndrome is characterized by uveitis, alopecia, poliosis (premature greying) of the upper eye lashes, vitiligo (light coloured patches of skin), and meningeal irritation (Johnson 1963). The audiometric pattern in this syndrome is also that of a receptor organ (end-organ) hearing loss (Seals and Rise 1967).

The Vogt–Koyanagi–Harada syndrome shows a certain similarity to sympathetic ophthalmia (Wilson 1962) which has been cured by antilymphocyte serum. This therefore might be used in the treatment of the syndrome if steroids are ineffective. The use of steroids is rational if one accepts that the syndrome represents an immunopathic state.

Jaksch–Wartenhorst syndrome (relapsing polychondritis)

This is a syndrome which is characterized by recurrent inflammation of various cartilaginous structures. It was first described by Jaksh–Wartenhorst in 1923. Although Pearson, Kline, and Newcomer (1960) termed the condition relapsing polychondritis, the disorder is much more widespread than this name would suggest. A varied number of non-cartilaginous structures may be involved in the disease process. Lesions may occur in the arteries, kidneys, and the liver (Dolan, Lemmon, and Teitelbaum 1966) as well as in various parts of the ears (Cody and Sones 1971) and the eyes (Hilding 1952). The condition may involve the external (Jaksch-Wartenhorst 1923), middle (Daly 1966), and internal ear (Kaye and Sones 1964). The middle-ear component may manifest as a secretory otitis media and the internal-ear component as a sensorineural hearing loss. The condition frequently presents as a painful swelling of one or both auricles.

The syndrome is generally considered to belong to the auto-immune group of diseases. Michaels (personal communication) found that both of the two patients whom he investigated showed anticartilage antibodies in the serum. The rational management of the condition would therefore include immunosuppressive treatment. Prednisolone helps about half the cases. However, high dosage is frequently required and complications may result. The addition of immunosuppressive drugs, such as azathioprine, may allow a reduction in the prednisolone dose (Hughes, Berry, Seifert, and Lessof 1972; Mahindraker and Libman 1970). However, Hoshino, Kato, Kodama, and Suzuki (1978) recently reported a case in a 56-year-old woman who, as a result, had become totally deaf in both ears. In spite of (or because of?) the administration of steroids, azathioprine, and antibiotics, the patient took a gradual downward course and died from a gastrointestinal haemorrhage 18 months after the onset of the condition.

Azathioprine is a drug that is particularly toxic for both bone marrow cells and the cells of the small intestine. The drugs should therefore not be prescribed unless the patient can be monitored for toxic effects.

Azathioprine is broken down in the body to 6-mercaptopurine which is then converted to the active agent, 6-mercaptopurine riboside. This competes with the structurally similar inosinic acid for the enzymes involved in the synthesis of guanylic and adenylic acids. There is also inhibition of the inosinic acid precursor 5-phosphoribosylamine. The net result is inhibition of nucleic acid formation and the consequent suppression of actively proliferating antigen-sensitive lymphocytes (Roitt 1971).

Non-specific auto-immune sensorineural hearing loss

McCabe (1979) has reported observing 18 cases of auto-immune internal-ear disorders. Substantial improvement of the hearing was obtained with the combined administration of cyclophosphamide and dexamethasone. In each case, the change in the hearing status reflected changes in the medication. Cyclophosphamide belongs to the nitrogen mustard group of alkylating agents. Its immunosuppressive action probably depends upon attacking the DNA of the actively proliferating antigen-sensitive lymphocytes. Thus correct cell duplication during cell division is prevented (Roitt 1971). Although it is less myelotoxic than most other alkylating agents, it is still sufficiently hazardous that it should be used only under the direction of a medical person experienced in immunosuppressive therapy.

Pellagra

Although the prevalence has dropped precipitously since the last century, pellagra is still seen in Egypt. This nutritional deficiency is associated with a sensorineural hearing loss. Yassin and Taha (1963) report on a study of a sample of 25 pellagrins. All but four of the 25 cases showed a sensorineural hearing loss. Half of the cases received nicotinic acid and the other half nicotinamide. The same dose was used for each drug, i.e. about 800 μmol (100 mg) intramuscularly twice daily for 3 to 4 days followed by an oral maintenance dose of 400 μmol (50 mg) three times a day until all neurological and skin manifestations disappeared. The skin and mucous membrane lesions faded in 3 to 4 days but the neurological deficits did not disappear until 15 to 20 days following the start of treatment. Improvements in the thresholds of hearing seemed to be of the order of 20 dB. However, since the initial hearing losses measured anything up to 40 dB HL it meant that normal or near normal hearing was restored.

Waldenstrom's macroglobulinaemia

Waldenstrom's macroglobulinaemia is a primary plasma cell dyscrasia in which there is excessive production of monoclonal IgM. Consequently, there is an increase in blood viscosity so that the condition is one of the causes of the hyperviscosity syndrome. One of the manifestations of this hyperviscosity syndrome is an acute auditory failure (Ruben, Distenfeld, Berg, and Carr 1969; Afifi and Tawfeek 1971).

Wells, Michaels, and Wells (1977) reported the condition in a 73-year-old man who presented with a 3 years' history of epistaxis, a 2 months' history of haematuria, and a 3 weeks' history of acute auditory failure. The audiometric picture was that of a moderately severe sensorineural hearing loss which was more marked for the higher frequencies. He was treated with chlorambucil, prednisone, and plasmapheresis. Six weeks after starting treatment there was an improvement in the hearing levels in both ears; for the lower frequencies in the poorer ear the improvement was of the order of 50 dB.

Chlorambucil, which is 4-[*p*-bis-(2-chloroethyl) aminophenyl]butyric acid, is a slowly acting, low-toxicity alkylating agent. It belongs, like cyclophosphamide, to the nitrogen mustard group. Alkylation of guanine in DNA is the most likely specific site of its antineoplastic activity. This results in miscoding, clearance of strands and cross-linkage of strands which therefore cannot replicate. Apart from the depressant effect on bone marrow, side effects rarely occur with therapeutic doses.

The aim of the plasmapheresis is to wash out as much as is feasible of the serum proteins, together with their IgM constituent to reduce the hyperviscosity. However, in the case cited, the concentration of the IgM actually increased with treatment.

Leukaemias

Auditory disturbances occur in 27 per cent of leukaemic subjects. Some of these disturbances are due to haemorrhage or infiltration into the middle ear (Druss 1945). Sensorineural hearing losses may be due to leukaemic infiltration of the endolymphatic space (Politzer 1885) or the perilymphatic space (Hallpike and Harrison 1950), or haemorrhage into the internal ear (Schuknecht, Igarashi, and Chasin 1965), or infiltration of the vestibulocochlear nerve trunk.

Current management with chemotherapy and antibiotics prolongs the lives of patients afflicted with the disease and reduces the incidence of infection and, to a certain extent, of haemorrhage, so reducing both the prevalence and the severity of these leukaemic audiological disorders.

Hypothyroidism

Howarth and Lloyd (1956) reported dramatic improvement in the hearing in two out of seven hypothyroid patients with a hearing loss. Aspects of the audiometric picture of hypothyroid hearing loss have been discussed by Stephens and Hinchcliffe (1968).

Acute auditory failure

Initial enthusiastic reports (Hirashima 1978) of the treatment of this condition by intravenous triiodobenzoic acid derivatives have not been supported by the experience of others, e.g. Prasansuk (personal communication). Exacerbations of the loss may occur.

Intravenous heparin is ineffective and may cause priapism (Donaldson 1979).

REST OF AUDITORY NERVOUS SYSTEM

Presbyacusis

The auditory system is afflicted by a number of diverse degenerative processes (Schuknecht 1955; Hinchcliffe 1962; Kirikae, Sato, and Shitara 1964). Consequently the impaired communicative ability of older people is the result of interplay of many factors. These factors range from peripheral ones, such as simple attenuation of the speech signal in the aging ear, to central ones involving attention and short-term memory. Thus the multifaceted picture of presbyacusis is becoming increasingly apparent (Gilad and Glorig 1979; Bergman 1980).

Using a double-blind study, Reinecke (1977) compared vincamine with a dummy drug on 30 patients with presbyacusis. The vincamine was given in a dosage of 170 μmol (60 mg) daily by mouth for a period of six weeks. Although there was no detectable change in the pure-tone threshold of hearing there was a significant change in the monosyllabic speech audiogram at the $p < 0.004$ level. Reinecke said that the vincamine was 'well tolerated'.

Preliminary clinical experience indicates that piracetam (Fig. 18.27) may be of value in the management of auditory disorders in the elderly. Piracetam is 2-oxo-1-pyrrolidine acetamide. It is thus a cyclic derivative of γ-aminobutyric acid (GABA), the neurotransmitter. Piracetam, however, has no GABA-like properties. Its pharamacological properties are reported to be, *inter alia*, the protection of the cerebral cortex against hypoxia (Giurgea, Mouravieff-Lesuisse, and Leemans 1970) and the facilitation of hearing and of memory (Dimond and Brouwers 1976; Wolthuis 1971).

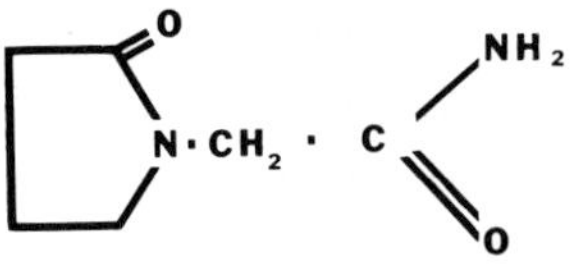

Fig. 18.27. Piracetam.

Mindus, Cronholm, Levander, and Schalling (1976) made a double-blind crossover comparison of the mental performance of 18 'middle-aged non-deteriorated individuals' during two 4-week periods of treatment with piracetam and a dummy preparation. In the majority of the tasks the subject did significantly better when on the piracetam than when on the dummy drug. Stegink (1972) studied the effects of piracetam on 196 patients by a double-blind method. Piracetam was given in a dosage of 17 mmol (2.4 g) daily for 8 weeks. A significant improvement in perception, memory, and alertness was observed with the piracetam. Richardson and Bereen (1977) report that piracetam can be given in a dose of 70 mmol (10 g) daily for 10–21 days without any adverse effects. They also reported that it did not interact with antibiotic, anticonvulsant, analgesic, muscular relaxant, corticosteroid, antifibrinolytic, antidepressant, hormone replacement or hypotensive drugs taken by their patients. Studies made of elderly patients have shown that the drug may be given orally in a dose of 18 to 23 mmol (2.5 to 3.2 g) daily for a period of 3–6 months without there being any changes in any of the usual physiological measures.

Vertebrobasilar insufficiency

Stipon, Doucet, and Blons (1974) studied the effect of cyclandelate on the auditory and vestibular symptoms of vertebrobasilar insufficiency. There was a 'good result' in all of the 11 cases which were studied.

Cyclandelate (3, 3, 5-trimethylcyclohexyl mandelate) is a vasodilator which has been used to improve the cerebral circulation in cerebrovascular and other disorders.

Diffuse cortical encephalitis

This condition is characterized by an acute onset with headaches, drowsiness, 'deaf-mutism', epilepsy, and personality changes. The condition is probably due to a virus.

The 'deaf-mutism' is due to an aphasia since pure-tone audiograms are normal. Morrison (1978) has seen three women with the disorder. From the audiological viewpoint, there was no diagnostic problem since the 'deafness' occurred fairly late in the disorder after the diagnosis had been made. The condition was treated with steroids and ACTH. All three patients made a good recovery although 'one still has occasional episodes of failure to comprehend speech'.

TINNITUS

Tinnitus is a symptom that requires investigation. There are many causes (Fig. 18.28). Tinnitus is broadly classified into subjective (heard only by the

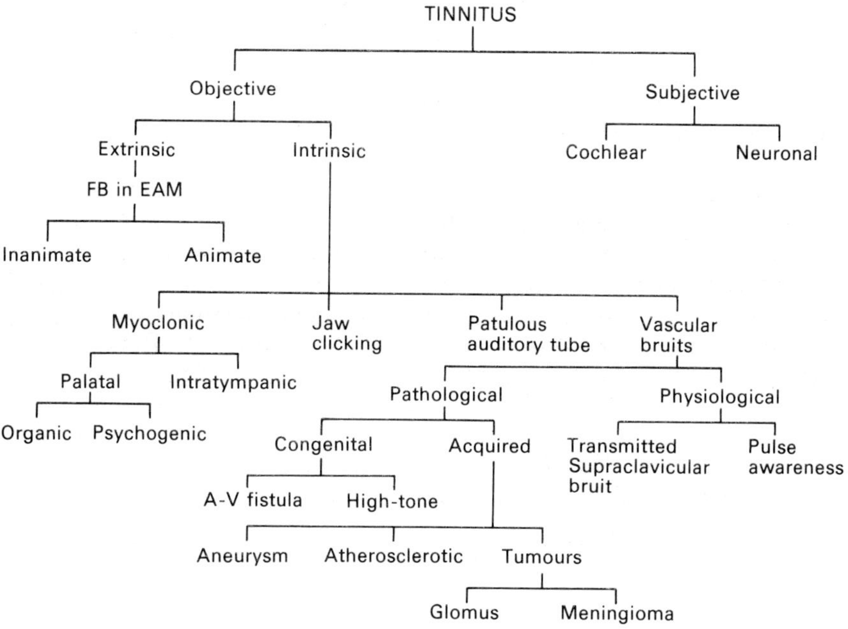

Fig. 18.28. Classification of tinnitus. Note that the 'subjective' group is not classified according to the aetiopathological disorder since they can, in effect, be associated with almost any middle or internal ear disorder.

patient) or objective (heard also by others). The usual distinction between subjective and objective tinnitus is whether or not it can be heard with a stethoscope. However, the level of this dichotomy is dependent upon the degree of sophistication of the sound amplifying methods employed (Kemp 1979). Nevertheless, in clinical practice, the group termed objective tinnitus has a different set of aetiologies and a different set of managements, e.g. the use of therapeutic embolization (Harris, Brismar, and Cronqvist 1979). Specific medical and surgical treatments may also be available for cases of subjective tinnitus where this is symptomatic of distinct aetiopathological disorders, e.g. Ménière's disorder, inflammatory conditions, and tumours. However, no such specific line of treatment is indicated in the majority of cases.

A class of vasodilator-responsive tinnitus has been suggested. Tinnitus was either completely abolished, or almost completely so, in 13 out of 28 cases given an intravenous infusion or naftidrofuryl (Fig. 18.29) (Gibson, personal communication). It is of note that 8 of the 28 cases had congenital syphilis and in every case there was a successful response. However, in no case of tinnitus due to noise damage was there any change.

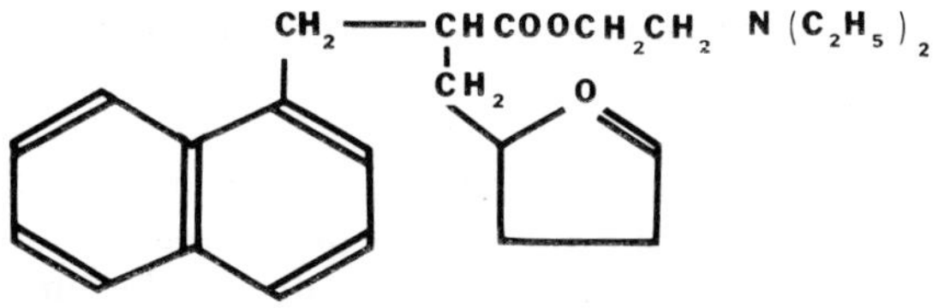

CH_2—$CHCOOCH_2CH_2\ N(C_2H_5)_2$, CH_2, O

Fig. 18.29. Naftidrofuryl.

In 1935 Bárány observed that an intravenous local anaesthetic could temporarily abate tinnitus. Using lidocaine (Fig. 18.30) Gejrot confirmed this observation in 1963 when treating attacks of Ménière's disorder. An Oxford study started by Jackson has been extended by Martin and Colman (1980) who have shown, using a double-blind crossover study, that lidocaine can alleviate tinnitus, albeit temporarily. Bupivacaine (Fig. 18.31) and lorcainide have a more marked effect (Jackson, personal communication).

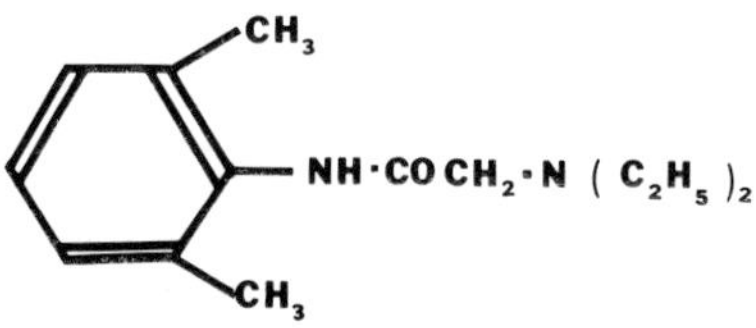

CH_3, $NH{\cdot}COCH_2{\cdot}N(C_2H_5)_2$, CH_3

Fig. 18.30. Lidocaine.

$(CH_2)_3CH_3$, N, CONH, CH_3, CH_3

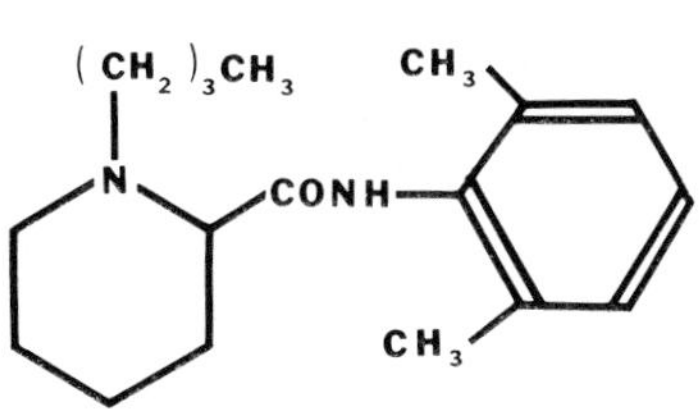

Fig. 18.31. Bupivacaine.

Recently, Emmett and Shea (1980) have suggested tocainide as the drug of choice in the treatment of tinnitus. Tocainide (Fig. 18.32) is a primary amine analogue of lidocaine (Lalka, Meyer, Duce, and Elvin 1976) and was originally developed as an oral antidysrhythmic agent (Coltart, Berndt,

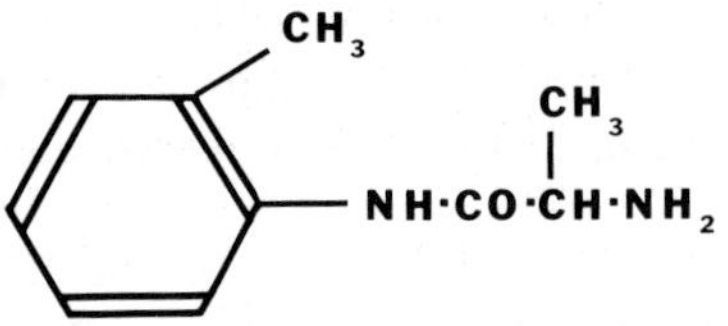

Fig. 18.32. Tocainide.

Kernoff, and Harrison 1974). Because of its primary amine structure, tocainide circumvents the problem of the N-de-ethylation which is the main reason for lidocaine being ineffective by mouth.

Double-blind studies showed that five 6-hourly doses of tocainide effectively abolished tinnitus for periods of up to 48 hours (Emmett and Shea 1980).

Melding and Goodey (1979) reported that lidocaine response is associated with response to oral anticonvulsants, in particular, carbamazepine (Fig. 18.33) and phenytoin. However, patients may be unresponsive or show undesirable side effects to these drugs (Shea 1979). Adverse reactions to carbamazepine include dizziness, ataxia, and drowsiness (Russell 1967) as well as acute renal failure (Nicholls and Yasin 1972). Indeed Arieff and Mier (1966) claim that it is a very dangerous drug and should only be used under careful supervision.

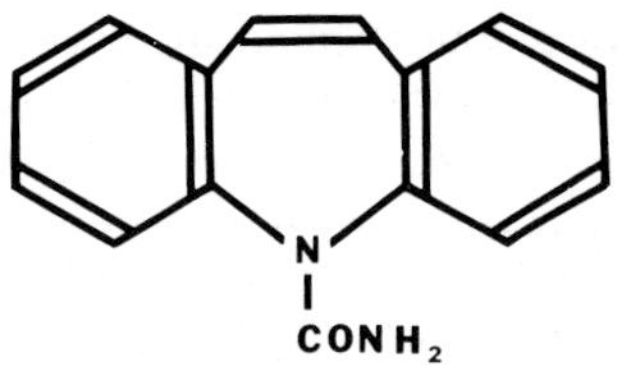

Fig. 18.33. Carbamazepine.

Using a sequential double-blind comparative study, McCormick and Thomas (1979) have shown that mexilitine is ineffective in the relief of tinnitus. However, the most surprising findings were that 'there was no placebo response at all and also that there was no difference between morning and evening assessments' of the intrusiveness of the tinnitus.

Even if the tinnitus cannot be eradicated, a shift in the acoustical characteristics of the tinnitus will bring considerable psychological relief. The possibility of a drug-induced change in the characteristics of the tinnitus was hinted at by Isono, Taguchi, Higuchi, and Sato (1957) in Japan. They studied the effect of intravenous nicotinic acid on 100 tinnitus sufferers. Although they reported no effect in 47 patients, there was 'some response' in 29 per cent, 'marked improvement' in 8 per cent, and a 'cure' in 13 per cent. A change in the character of the tinnitus was noted in 3 per cent. Subsequently, in an experimental study of amobarbital (amylobarbitone), Donaldson (1978) showed that a shift in pitch of the tinnitus occurred after the administration of 725 μmol (180 mg) daily for 12 weeks. The tinnitus pitch returned to its pre-treatment level within a period of 6 months at the end of a course of amobarbital (Donaldson, personal communication).

There appear to be two types of DITPS (drug-induced tinnitus pitch shift). As well as this more persistent effect, Jackson (personal communication) has observed a temporary DITPS after the intravenous administration of local anaesthetics. Moreover, whereas the cases studied by Donaldson showed a fall in pitch, those studied by Jackson showed a rise in pitch. Whether or not this relates to the type of tinnitus studied has yet to be elucidated.

The various psychotropic drugs are invaluable in the management of tinnitus. However, in view of fears about the consequences of the abuse of barbiturates and the increasing influence of CURB (campaign on the use and restriction of barbiturates), there is an increasing preference both among patients and among doctors, for using benzodiazepines (Garrattini, Mussini, and Randall 1973). A number of drugs in this group, including the more recently introduced temazepam, are available. For daytime use, diazepam is perhaps the more widely used, whilst nitrazepam is perhaps the most common for inducing sleep. In connection with their action on tinnitus, it is to be noted that the benzodiazepines also have anticonvulsant properties.

The benzodiazepines are less likely than other groups of psychotropic drugs to result in drug dependence. Moreover, when compared with the barbiturates, they are relatively safe in overdosage since they produce only a slight state of unconsciousness. Nevertheless, they may, like the barbiturates, impair mental concentration, judgment and manual dexterity. They may also release aggression (*British Medical Journal* 1975). Older patients have an increased sensitivity to nitrazepam (Castleden, George, Marcer, and Hallett 1977). Using subjects with an average age of 57 years, Adam, Adamson, Březinová, Hunter, and Oswald (1976) found that 18 μmol (5 mg) nitrazepam every night for ten weeks resulted in longer and more unbroken sleep. No pharmacological tolerance was observed, even after two months of use. However, stopping the drug caused the sleep to be temporarily worse than before the drug had been taken. Thus conditions may be created that lead to perpetuation of intake. Patients should therefore be told that, after giving up nitrazepam, or similar drugs, they may experience an increase in wakefulness for a week or two with one or two nights of little sleep. They should be reassured that this disruption of sleep is only a temporary consequence of the dependence that they had developed on the drug. For these reasons, alternative ways of managing tinnitus are still being sought.

Alternative, or supplementary, methods of managing tinnitus include the use of hearing aids (Saltzman and Ersner 1947; Vernon and Schleuning 1978); maskers (Hazell 1977; Vernon 1977; Longridge 1979); electrosuppression (Portmann, Cazals, Negrevergne, and Aran 1979); biofeedback (House, Miller, and House 1977); hypnosis (Marlowe 1973); and psychotherapy (Goldie 1978). Biofeedback may, however, be a more complicated and more expensive way of providing relaxation treatment (Neuchterlein and Holroyd 1980).

DYSACUSES

Complaint behaviour related to the various dysacuses, e.g. distortion and phonophobia, is correlated with scores on the MPI neuroticism scale (Hinchcliffe 1965). In these cases, there is often no specific underlying disorder for which specific treatment can be given and recourse must be had to the administration of psychotropic drugs. Drugs of the benzodiazepine group are the preparations of choice. Observations made in respect of the use of benzodiazepines in connection with the management of tinnitus are equally applicable here. Particularly pertinent is the need to consider the use of psychological methods of treatment in lieu of using drugs. In the management of the dysacuses and of tinnitus, we could perhaps learn from the application of relaxation techniques (Stone and DeLeo 1976), transcendental meditation (Blackwell, Bloomfield, Gartside, Robinson, Hanenson, Magenheim, Nidich, and Zigler 1976), and yoga (Patel 1975) to the management of the hypertensive patient. Indeed the clinical psychologist's contribution to the management of chronic disorders of sensation has hardly begun to be developed (Rachman and Philips 1980).

CONCLUSIONS

There is already a considerable application of drugs in the field of audiological medicine. There is equally clearly a dearth of experimental comparative studies in this area. Moreover, some studies that have been done have probably not asked the right questions. It is hoped that this unsatisfactory state of affairs will be remedied in the foreseeable future by appropriately-designed experimental comparative studies. The term 'appropriate' must refer not only to the statistical experimental design but also, in view of the studies by Charney, Bynum, Eldredge, Frank, MacWhinney, McNabb, Scheiner, Sumpter, and Iker (1967), to some measurement of the compliance rate and the factors governing this. Their studies showed that oral penicillin prescribed to children for acute otitis media or streptococcal pharyngitis was being taken as prescribed by 81 per cent of the children on the fifth day, and 56 per cent on the ninth day. Moreover, take rate was *inter alia*, correlated with the mother's estimate of the severity of the disorder at the onset and to certain personality traits in the mother.

The studies should also encompass reporting of adverse events, rather than adverse reactions (Skegg and Doll 1977). An adverse event is defined as a particular untoward happening experienced by a patient (Finney 1965). It might be an upper respiratory infection, a rash, or a broken leg. Most adverse events would be unrelated to the treatment being studied. If, however, a particular event was commoner amongst treated patients, suspicion would be aroused and an explanation sought. Together with other methods of monitoring drug use, experimental comparative studies can build up a picture of adverse drug reactions. Such reactions can occur in as many as 26 per cent of in-patients and account for the same proportion of deaths (Ogilvie and Ruedy 1967). For these reasons, no apology is made for stress being made in this chapter on adverse drug reactions.

REFERENCES

ADAM, K., ADAMSON, L., BŘEZINOVA, V., HUNTER, W., and OSWALD, I. (1976). Nitrazepam: lastingly effective but trouble on withdrawal. *Br. med. J.* **i**, 1558–60.

AFIFI, A. M. and TAWFEEK, S. (1971). Deafness due to Waldenstrom macroglobulinaemia. *J. Lar. Otol.* **85**, 275–80.

AJODHIA, J. M. and DIX, M. R. (1975). Ototoxic effects of drugs. *Minerva Otolar.* **25**, 117–31.

ARIEFF, A. J. and MIER, M. (1966). Anticonvulsant action and psychotropic action of Tegretol ®. *Neurology, Minneap.* **16**, 107–10.

ARMITAGE, P. (1960). *Sequential medical trials*. Blackwell, Oxford.

ASSOCIATION OF THE BRITISH PHARMACEUTICAL INDUSTRY (1979). Data Sheet Compendium 1979–1980. Pharmind, London.

BAIN, D. J. G. (1976). A double-blind comparative study of Otoseptil ear drops and Otosporin ear drops in otitis externa. *J. Int. med. Res.* **4**, 79–81.

BÁRÁNY, R. (1935). Die Beeinflussung des Ohrensausens durch intravenös injizierte Lokalanästhetica. *Acta oto-lar.* **23**, 201–3.

BARTLETT, J. G., CHANG, T. W., GURWITH, A., GURBACH, S. L., and ONDERDONK, A. B. (1978). Antibiotic-associated pseudomembranous colitis due to toxin-producing *Clostridia*. *New Engl. J. Med.* **298**, 531–5.

BARTON, R. P. E., WRIGHT, J. L. W., and GRAY, R. F. E. (1978). Clinical evaluation of a new clobetasol preparation in treatment of otitis externa. *J. Lar. Otol.* **93**, 703–6.

BASS, J. W., COHEN, S. H., CORLESS, J. D., and MAMUNESS, P. (1967). Ampicillin compared to other antimicrobials in acute otitis media. *J. Am. med. Ass.* **202**, 697–702.

BAUER, F. (1968). Treatment of 'glue ear' by intratympanic injection of urea. *J. Lar. Otol.* **82**, 717–22.

—— (1970). Glue ear. *Br. med. J.* **i**, 111–12.

BEAGLEY, H. A. (1979). *Auditory investigation: the scientific and technological basis*. Clarendon Press. Oxford.

BERGHOLTZ, L. and RUDBERG, R. (1972). Behandling av otitis media acuta. *Läkartidningen* **69**, 3922–8.

BERGMAN, M. (1980). *Aging and the perception of speech*. University Park Press, Baltimore.

BLACKWELL, B., BLOOMFIELD, S., GARTSIDE, P., ROBINSON, A., HANENSON, I., MAGENHEIM, H., NIDICH, S., and ZIGLER, R. (1976). Transcendental meditation in hypertension. *Lancet* **i**, 223–6.

BRETLAU, P., HANSEN, H. J., CAUSSE, J., and CAUSSE, J. B. (1979). Otosclerosis: morphological and microchemical investigation after NaF treatment. *Dansk Otolar. selskab* Nov. 8.

British Medical Journal (1978). Tranquillizers causing aggression. Leading article. *Br. med. J.* **i**, 113–14.

BROCKMAN, S. J. (1972). The enigma of secretory otitis media. *Trans. Am. Acad. Ophthal. Otolar.* **76**, 1296–304.

BROWN, M. J. K. M., RICHARDS, S. H., and AMBEGAOKAR, A. G. (1978). Grommets and glue ear: a five year follow-up of a controlled trial. *J. R. Soc. Med.* **71**, 353–6.

BUCKNALL, R. C. (1977). Myasthenia associated with D-penicillamine therapy in rheumatoid arthritis. *Proc. R. Soc. Med.* Suppl. 3 **70**, 114–17.

CAMERON, G. G., POMAHAC, A. C., and JOHNSTON, M. T. (1975). Comparative efficacy of ampicillin and trimethoprim-sulphamethoxazole in otitis media. *Can. med. Ass. J.* **112**, 875–85.

CAMP, W. A. and FRIERSON, J. G. (1962). Sarcoidosis of the central nervous system. *Archs Neurol., Chicago* **7**, 432–41.

CANTARELLI, H. (1973). Quoted by Cooper *et al.* (1976).

CARROLL, O. M., BRYAN, P. A., and ROBINSON, R. J. (1966). Stevens–Johnson syndrome associated with long-acting sulfonamides. *J. Am. med. Ass.* **195**, 691–3.

CASTLEDEN, C. M., GEORGE, C. F., MARCER, D., and HALLETT, C. (1977). Increased sensitivity to nitrazepam in old age. *Br. med J.* **i**, 10–12.

CAUSSE, J., CHEVANCE, L. G., and SHAMBAUGH, G. E. J. (1977). Clinical experience and experimental findings with sodium fluoride in otosclerosis (otospongiosis). *Ann. Otol. Rhinol. Lar.* **83**, 643–7.

CHARNEY, E., BYNUM, R., ELDREDGE, D., FRANK, D., MACWHINNEY, J. B., MCNABB, N., SCHEINER, A., SUMPTER, E. A., and IKER, H. (1967). How well do patients take oral penicillin? A collaborative study in private practice. *Pediatrics, Springfield* **40**, 188–95.

CHEESMAN, A. D. (1979). Ear infections In *Clinical otolaryngology* (ed. A. G. D. Maran and P. M. Stell). Blackwell, Oxford.

CLARK, J. V. (1946). Acute otitis externa in India. *J. Lar. Otol.* **61**, 586–93.

CODY, D. T. R. and SONES, D. A. (1971). Relapsing polychondritis: audiovestibular manifestations. *Laryngoscope, St. Louis* **81**, 1208–22.

COFFEY, J. D. JR. (1968). Concentration of ampicillin in exudate from acute otitis media. *J. Pediat.* **72**, 693–5.

COGAN, D. G. (1945). Syndrome of nonsyphilitic interstitial keratitis and vestibuloauditory symptoms. *Archs Ophthal., N.Y.* **33**, 144–9.

COLLART, P. and DUREL, P. (1964). Présence et persistance des tréponèmes dans la L.C.R. au cours de la syphilis expérimentale et humaine après traitement tardif. *Annls Derm. Syph.* **91**, 488–98.

—— BOREL, L.-J., and DUREL, P. (1962). Etude de l'action de la Pénicilline dans la syphilis tardive: Persistance du Tréponème pale après traitement. *Annls Inst. Pasteur, Paris* **102**, 596–615.

COLTART, D. J., BERNDT, T. B., KERNOFF, R., and HARRISON, D. C. (1974). Antiarrhythmic and circulatory effects of Astra W 36095, a new lidocaine-like agent. *Am. J. Cardiol.* **34**, 35–41.

COOPER, J., INMAN, J. S., and DAWSON, A. F. (1976). A comparison between cotrimoxazole and amoxycillin in the treatment of acute otitis media in general practice. *Practitioner* **217**, 804–9.

CULPEPER, N. (1652). *The English Physitian*, pp. 221 and 235. Peter Cole, London.

DALY, J. F. (1966). Relapsing polychondritis of the larynx and trachea. *Archs Otolar.* **84**, 570–7.

DAWES, J. D. K. (1953). Myringitis bullosa haemorrhagica: its relationship to otogenic encephalitis and cranial nerve paralyses. *J. Lar. Otol.* **67**, 313–42.

Dawkins, R. S., Sharpe, M., and Morrison, A. W. (1968). Steroid treatment in congenital syphilitic deafness. *J. Lar. Otol.* **82**, 1095–107.

Diamant, M. and Diamant, B. (1974). Abuse and timing of use of antibiotics in acute otitis media. *Archs Otolar.* **100**, 226–32.

Dimond, S. J. and Brouwers, E. Y. M. (1976). Increase in the power of human memory in normal man through the use of drugs. *Psychopharmacologia* **49**, 307–9.

Dolan, D. L., Lemmon, G. B. J., and Teitelbaum, S. L. (1966). Relapsing polychondritis. Analytical literature review and studies in pathogenesis. *Am. J. Med.* **41**, 285–99.

Donaldson, I. (1978). Tinnitus: a theoretical view and a therapeutic study using amylobarbitone. *J. Lar. Otol.* **92**, 123–30.

Donaldson, J. A. (1979). Heparin therapy for sudden sensorineural hearing loss. *Archs Otolar.* **105**, 351–4.

Druss, J. G. (1945). Aural manifestations of leukaemia. *Archs Otolar.* **42**, 267–74.

Duncan, R. B. (1977). Vitamin A therapy of aural cholesteatoma. In *Cholesteatoma: First International Conference* (ed. B. F. McCabe, J. Sadé, and M. Abramson). Aesculapius, Birmingham, Alabama.

Elcock, H. W. and Lord, I. J. (1972). Bromhexine hydrochloride in chronic secretory otitis media—a clinical trial. *Br. J. clin. Pract.* **26**, 276–8.

Elia, J. C. (1966). Double-blind evaluation of a new treatment for Ménière's syndrome. *J. Am. med. Ass.* **196**, 187–9.

Emmett, J. R. and Shea, J. J. (1980). The treatment of tinnitus with tocaine hydrochloride. In press.

Ensign, P. R., Urbanich, E. M., and Moran, M. (1960). Prophylaxis for otitis media in an Indian population. *Am. J. publ. Hlth* **50**, 195–9.

Evans, I. T. (1973). Malignant (necrotizing) external otitis. *J. Lar. Otol.* **87**, 13–20.

Finney, D. J. (1965). The design and logic of a monitor of drug use. *J. chron. Dis.* **18**, 77–98.

Fraser, J. G. (1970). The efficacy of wax solvents: *in vitro* studies and a clinical trial. *J. Lar. Otol.* **84**, 1055–64.

—— Mehta, M., and Fraser, P. (1977). The medical treatment of secretory otitis media—a clinical trial of three commonly used regimes. *J. Lar. Otol.* **91**, 757–65.

Friedman, M. (1977). Chemical basis for pharmacological and therapeutic actions of penicillamine. *Proc. R. Soc. Med.* Suppl. 3 **70**, 50–60.

Fry, J. (1958). Antibiotics in acute tonsillitis and acute otitis media. *Br. med. J.* **ii**, 883–6.

Fuchs, E. (1876). Herpes iris conjunctivae. *Klin. Mbl. Augenheilk.* **14**, 333–51.

Gahlot, D. K., Sood, V. P., and Khosla, P. K. (1977). Effect of Penicillamine on the sensorineural deafness of retinitis pigmentosa. *J. Lar. Otol.* **91**, 1107–11.

Garrattini, S., Mussini, E., and Randall, L. O. (1973). *The benzodiazepines.* Raven Press, New York.

Gejrot, T. (1963). Intravenous xylocaine in the treatment of attacks of Ménière's disease. *Acta oto-lar.* Suppl. 188, 190–5.

Gilad, O. and Glorig, A. (1979). Presbycusis: the aging ear. *J. Am. audit. Soc.* **4**, 195–217.

Giurgea, C., Mouravieff-Lesuisse, F., and Leemans, R. (1970). Correlations électro-pharmacologiques au cours de l'anoxie oxyprive chez le lapin en respiration libre ou artificielle. *Revue Neurol.* **122**, 484–6.

GOLDIE, L. (1978). Psychiatric aspects of otolaryngology. *Practitioner* **221**, 701–6.

GORLIN, R. J. and PINDBORG, J. J. (1964). *Syndromes of the head and neck.* McGraw-Hill, New York.

GREGSON, A. E. W. and LA TOUCHE, C. J. (1961). Otomycosis: a neglected disease. *J. Lar. Otol.* **75**, 45–69.

GRIFFIN, J. P. and D'ARCY, P. F. (1979). *A manual of adverse drug interactions.* Wright, Bristol.

GRISTWOOD, R. E. (1958). Nerve deafness associated with sarcoidosis. *J. Lar. Otol.* **72**, 479–91.

—— (1979). Management of chronic middle ear disease. In *Clinical otolaryngology* (ed. A. G. P. Maran and P. M. Stell). Blackwell, Oxford.

GYDE, M.-C. and RANDALL, R.-F. (1978). Etude comparative à double insu de la triméthoprime-sulfacétamide-polymyxine B et de la gentamicine dans le traitment de l'otorrhée. *Annls Oto-lar.* **95**, 43–55.

HALEY, L. D. (1950). Etiology of otomycosis. *Archs Otolar.* **52**, 202–24.

HALLPIKE, C. S. and HARRISON, M. J. (1950). Clinical and pathological observations on a case of leukaemia with deafness and vertigo. *J. Lar. Otol.* **64**, 427–30.

HALSTED, C., LEPOW, M. L., BALASSANIAN, N., EMMERICH, J., and WOLINSKY, E. (1968). Otitis media. *Am. J. Dis. Child.* **115**, 542–51.

HAMMOND, V. (1979). Affections of the external ear. In *Diseases of the ear, nose and throat.* Butterworth, London.

HARRIS, S., BRISMAR, J., and CRONQVIST, S. (1979). Pulsatile tinnitus and therapeutic embolization. *Acta oto-lar.* **88**, 220–6.

HARRISON, M. S. and NAFTALIN, L. (1968). *Ménière's disease.* Thomas, Springfield, Ill.

HAZELL, J. W. P. (1977). A tinnitus masker. *Hearing* **32**, 147–8.

—— (1979). Tinnitus. In *Scott-Browne's diseases of the ear, nose and throat*, 4th edn. (ed. J. C. Ballantyne). Butterworth, London.

HEBRA, F. (1860). Acute Exanthema und Hautkrankheiten. In *Handbuch der speziellen Pathologie*, Vol. 3 (ed. R. Virchow). Enke, Stuttgart.

HELLER, G. (1940). A statistical study of otitis media in children. *J. Pediat.* **17**, 322–30.

HICKS, J. J., HICKS, J. N., and COOLEY, H. N. (1967). Ménière's disease. *Archs Otolar.* **86**, 610–13.

HILDING, A. C. (1952). Syndrome of joint and cartilaginous pathologic changes with destructive iridocyclitis. *Archs intern. Med.* **89**, 445–53.

HINCHCLIFFE, R. (1955). Efficacy of current cerumenolytics. *Br. med. J.* **ii**, 722.

—— (1961). Prevalence of the commoner ear, nose and throat conditions in the adult rural population of Great Britain. *Br. J. prev. soc. Med.* **15**, 128–40.

—— (1962). The anatomical locus of presbycusis. *J. Speech Hear. Dis.* **27**, 301–10.

—— (1979). Epidemiology of hearing loss. In *Auditory investigation: the scientific and technological basis* (ed. H. A. Beagley) pp. 552–95. Clarendon Press, Oxford.

HIRASHIMA, N. (1978). Treatment of sudden deafness with sodium salts of Triiodobenzoic acid derivatives. *Ann. Otol. Rhinol. Lar.* **87**, 29–31.

HOSHINO, T., KATO, I., KODAMA, A., and SUZUKI, H. (1978). Sudden deafness in relapsing polychondritis. *Acta oto-lar.* **86**, 418–27.

HOUSE, J. W., MILLER, L., and HOUSE, P. R. (1977). Severe tinnitus: treatment with biofeedback (results in 71 cases). *Trans. Am. Acad. Ophthal. Otolar.* **84**, ORL 697–ORL 703.

HOWARD, J. E., NELSON, J. D., CLAHSEN, J., and JACKSON, L. H. (1976). Otitis media of infancy and early childhood. A double blind study of four treatment regimes. *Am. J. Dis. Child.* **130**, 965–70.

HOWARTH, A. E. and LLOYD, H. E. D. (1956). Perceptive deafness in hypothyroidism. *Br. med. J.* **i**, 431–3.

HUGHES, L. A., WARDER, E. A., and HUDSON, W. R. (1974). Complications of tympanostomy tubes. *Archs Otolar.* **100**, 151–4.

HUGHES, R. A. C., BERRY, C. L., SEIFERT, M., and LESSOF, M. H. (1972). Relapsing polychondritis. *Q. J. Med.* **31**, 363–80.

HUSKISSON, E. C. (1977). Is penicillamine immunostimulant? *Proc. R. Soc. Med.* Suppl. 3 **70**, 142–3.

ISONO, H., TAGUCHI, H., HIGUCHI, A., and SATO, R. (1957). Some experience in use of nicotonic acid in the treatment of tinnitus. *Otolaryngology, Tokyo* **29**, 855–65.

JAKSCH-WARTENHORST, R. (1923). Polychondropathia. *Wien Arch. inn. Med.* **6**, 93–100.

JOACHIMS, H. Z. (1976). Malignant external otitis in children. *Archs Otolar.* **102**, 236–7.

JOHN, A. C. and HOPKIN, N. B. (1978). An unusual case of necrotizing otitis externa. *J. Lar. Otol.* **92**, 259–64.

JOHNSON, W. C. (1963). Vogt–Koyanagi–Harada syndrome. *Archs Derm.* **88**, 146–59.

KAMME, C., LUNDGREN, K., and RUNDCRANTZ, H. (1969). The concentration of Penicillin V in serum and middle ear exudate in acute otitis media in children. *Scand. J. infect. Dis.* **1**, 77–83.

KAYE, R. L. and SONES, D. A. (1964). Relapsing polychondritis: clinical and pathologic features in 14 cases. *Ann. intern. Med.* **60**, 653–64.

KEMP. D. T. (1979). Evidence of mechanical nonlinearity and frequency selective wave amplification in the cochlea. *Archs Oto-rhino-lar.* **224**, 37–45.

KEOGH, C. and RUSSELL, B. (1956). The problem of otitis externa. *Br. med. J.* **i**, 1068–72.

KERR, A. G., SMYTH, G. D. L., and LANDAU, H. D. (1970). Congenital syphilitic labyrinthitis. *Archs Otolar.* **91**, 474–8.

KIRIKAE, I., SATO, T., and SHITARA, T. (1964). Study of hearing in advanced age. *Laryngoscope, St. Louis* **74**, 205–20.

KLOCKHOFF, I. and LINDBLOM, U. (1960). Ménière's disease and hydrocochlorothiazide (Dichlotride ®)—a critical analysis of symptoms and therapeutic effects. *Acta oto-lar.* **63**, 347–65.

KLUYSKENS, P., GILLIS, E., and NSABUMUKUNZI, S. (1979). First observations on treatment of cholesteatoma with (N-acetyl) cysteine. *Acta oto-lar.* **87**, 362–5.

LAHIKAINEN, E. A. (1970). Penicillin concentration in middle ear secretion in otitis. *Acta oto-lar.* **70**, 358–62.

—— VUORI, M., and VIRTANEN, S. (1977). Azidocillin and ampicillin concentrations in middle ear effusion. *Acta oto-lar.* **84**, 227–32.

LALKA, D., MEYER, M. B., DUCE, B. R., and ELVIN, A. T. (1976). Kinetics of the oral antiarrhythmic lidocaine congener tocanide. *Clin. Pharmac. Ther.* **19**, 757–66.

LEA, W. A., SCHUSTER, D. S., and HARRELL, E. R. (1958). Mycological flora of the healthy external auditory canal: a study of 120 human subjects. *J. invest. Derm.* **31**, 137–8.

LIEBERMAN, J. (1967). In vitro evaluation of the mucolytic action of urea. *J. Am. med. Ass.* **202**, 694–6.

LIU, Y. S., LIM, D. J., LANG, R. W., and BIRCK, H. G. (1975). Chronic middle ear effusions. *Archs Otalar.* **101**, 278.

LONGRIDGE, N. S. (1979). A tinnitus clinic. *J. Otolar.* **8**, 390–5.

LORENTZEN, P. and HAUGSTEN, P. (1977). Treatment of acute suppurative otitis media. *J. Lar. Otol.* **91**, 331–40.

LUNDGREN, K., INGVARSSON, L., and RUNDCRANTZ, H. (1979). The concentration of Penicillin–V in middle ear exudate. *J. pediat. Otorhinolar.* **1**, 93–6.

LYELL, A. (1956). Toxic epidermal necrolysis: an eruption resembling scalding of the skin. *Br. J. Derm.* **68**, 335–61.

MCCABE, B. F. (1979). Autoimmune sensorineural hearing loss. *Ann. Otol. Rhinol. Lar.* **88**, 585–9.

MCCORMICK, M. S. and THOMAS, J. N. (1979). A sequential double-blind controlled trial of Mexilitine in the relief of tinnitus. Presented at Third Scientific Meeting of Oto-rhino-laryngological Research Society, 5 October, London.

MACK, L. W. JR., SMITH, J. L., WALTER, E. K., RIOS MONTENEGRO, E. N., and NICOL, W. G. (1969). Temporal bone treponemes. *Archs Otolar.* **90**, 11–14.

MCKELVIE, M. (1976). Mycology. In *Scientific foundations of otolaryngology* (ed. R. Hinchcliffe and D. F. N. Harrison). Heinemann, London.

MCNICOL, G. P. (1958). A note on the Ramsay Hunt syndrome and the place of cortisone in its treatment. *Scott. med. J.* **iii**, 93–4.

MAHINDRAKER, N. H. and LIBMAN, L. J. (1970). Relapsing polychondritis. *J. Lar. Otol.* **84**, 337–42.

MARLOWE, F. I. (1973). Effective treatment of tinnitus through hypnotherapy. *Am. J. clin. Hypnosis* **15**, 162–5.

MARTIN, F. W. and COLMAN, B. H. (1980) Tinnitus: a double-blind crossover controlled trial to evaluate the use of lignocaine. *Clin. Otolar.* **5**, 3–11.

MARTIN, G. and JAKOBS, P. (1977). Klinischer Vergleich der Monosubstanzen Dextran 40 und Xantinol Nicotinat in der Therapie des Knalltraumas. *Lar. Rhinol. Otol. Grenzgeb.* **56**, 860–3.

MATTHEWS, W. B. (1965). Sarcoidosis of the nervous system. *J. Neurol. Neurosurg. Psychiat.* **28**, 23–9.

MAWSON, S. R. (1974). In *Diseases of the ear.* Edward Arnold, London.

MELDING, P. S., and GOODEY, R. J. (1979). The treatment of tinnitus with oral anticonvulsants. *J. Lar. Otol.* **93**, 111–22.

MELTZER, P. E. and KELEMEN, G. (1959). Pyocyaneous osteomyelitis of the temporal bone, mandible and zygoma. *Laryngoscope, St. Louis* **68**, 1300–16.

MENZIES, M. A., GREENBERG, P. B., and JOPLIN, G. F. (1975). Otological studies in patients with deafness due to Paget's disease before and after treatment with synthetic human calcitonin. *Acta oto-lar.* **79**, 378–83.

MINDUS, P., CRONHOLM, B., LEVANDER, S. E., and SCHALLING, D. (1976). Piracetam-induced improvement of mental performance. *Acta psychiat. scand.* **54**, 150–60.

MOFFETT, A. J. (1943). Granulating myringitis: an unusual affection of the ear drum. *J. Lar. Otol.* **58**, 453–6.

MORGENSTEIN, K. M. and SEUNG, H. I. (1971). Pseudomonas mastoiditis. *Laryngoscope, St. Louis* **81**, 200–15.

MORIZONO, T. and JOHNSTONE, B. M. (1978). Ototoxicity of chloramphenicol ear drops with propylene glycol as solvent. *Med. J. Aust.* **ii**, 634–8.

—— —— and NG, P. (1974). Ototoxicity of topical antibiotics. *J. oto-lar. Soc. Aust.* **3**, 666–9.

MORRISON, A. W. (1978). *Management of sensorineural deafness.* Butterworth, London.

NEUCHTERLEIN, K. H. and HOLROYD, JEAN C. (1980). Biofeedback in the treatment of tension headache. *Archs gen. Psychiat.* **37**, 866–73.

NICHOLLS, D. P. and YASIN, M. (1972). Acute renal failure from carbamazepine. *Br. med. J.* **iv**, 496.

OGILVIES, R. I., and RUEDY, J. (1967). Adverse drug reactions during hospitalization. *Can. med. Ass. J.* **97**, 1450–7.

PAGE, J. R. (1914). A case of probable injury to the jugular bulb following myringotomy in an infant 10 months old. *Ann. Otol. Rhinol. Lar.* **23**, 161.

PALVA, T. (1979). Middle ear effusions. In *Clinical otolaryngology* (ed. A. G. D. Maran and P. M. Stell). Blackwell, Oxford.

PATEL, C. (1975). 12-month follow-up of yoga and biofeedback in the management of hypertension. *Lancet* **i**, 62–4.

PEARSON, C. M., KLINE, H. M., and NEWCOMER, V. D. (1960). Relapsing polychondritis. *New Engl. J. Med.* **263**, 51–8.

PERLMAN, H. B., GOLDFINGER, J. N., and CALES, I. A. (1953). Electrolyte studies in Ménière's disease. *Laryngoscope, St. Louis* **63**, 640–51.

PERRIN, J. M., CHARNEY, E., MCWHINNEY, J. B. JR., MCINERNY, T. K., MILLER, R. L., and NAZARIAN, L. F. (1974). Sulfisoxazole as chemoprophylaxis for recurrent otitis media. *New Engl. J. Med.* **291**, 664–7.

PICOZZI, G., SWEENEY, G., CALDER, I., and BROWNING G. G. (1979). Bacteriology and antibiotic sensitivity pattern of active chronic otitis media. Presented at Third Scientific Meeting of Oto-rhino-laryngological Research Society, 5 October, London.

POLITZER, A. (1885). Pathologische Veränderungen im Labyrinthe bei leukämischer Taubheit. *C. r. Congr. int. otolar.* 1884.

PORTMANN, M., CAZALS, Y., NEGREVERGNE, M., and ARAN, J.-M. (1979). Temporary tinnitus suppression in man through electrical stimulation of the cochlea. *Acta oto-lar.* **87**, 294–9.

PUNT, N. A. (1949). Otitis externa granulosa. *Br. med. J.* **i**, 989–90.

PYMAN, C. (1959). Otitis externa. *Med. J. Aust.* **ii**, 534–6.

RACHMAN, S. and PHILIPS, C. (1980). *Psychology and behavioural medicine.* Cambridge University Press.

REINECKE, M. (1977). Doppelblindvergleich von Vincamin gegen Plazebo bei Patienten mit Innenohrschwerhorigkeit. *Arzneimittel-Forsch.* **27**, 1294–8.

RICHARDS, S. H., KILBY, D., SHAW, J. D., and CAMPBELL, H. (1971). Grommets and glue ears: a clinical trial. *J. Lar.* **85**, 17–22.

RICHARDSON, A. E. and BEREEN, F. J. (1977). Effect of Piracetam on level of consciousness after neurosurgery. *Lancet* **ii**, 1110–11.

ROBINSON, D. W., SHIPTON, M. S., and HINCHCLIFFE, R. (1979). Normal hearing threshold and its dependence on clinical rejection criteria. NPL Acoustics Report Ac89., National Physics Laboratory, Middlesex. UK.

ROBINSON, J. T. (1946). External otitis. *Texas St. J. Med.* **42**, 384–6.

RODDEY, O. F., EARLE, R. JR., and HAGGERTY, R. (1966). Myringotomy in acute otitis media. *J. Am. med. Ass.* **197**, 849–53.

ROITT, I. (1971). *Essential immunology.* Blackwell, Oxford.

RUBEN, R. J., DISTENFELD, A., BERG, P., and CARR, R. (1969). Sudden sequential deafness as a presenting symptom of macroglobulinemia. *J. Am. med. Ass.* **209**, 1364–5.

RUDMAN, C. G. and PARSONS, J. A. (1979). Inhibition by calcitonin eardrops of induced osteolysis in guinea-pig ossicles. *Experientia*.

RUSSELL, R. W. R. (1967). Carbamazepine ('Tegretol'). *Prescrib. J.* **7**, 75–7.

SADÉ, J. (1966). Pathology and pathogenesis of serous otitis media. *Archs Otolar.* **84**, 297–305.

—— (1979). *Secretory otitis media and its sequelae*. Churchill Livingstone, London.

SALTZMAN, M. (1949). *Clinical audiology*, p. 125. Grune and Stratton, New York.

—— and ERSNER, M. S. (1947). A hearing aid for the relief of tinnitus aurium. *Laryngoscope, St. Louis* **57**, 538–66.

SCHAYER, R. W. (1964). Histamine and autonomous responses of the microcirculation: relationship to glucocorticoid action. *Ann. N. Y. Acad. Sci.* **116**, 891–9.

SCHUKNECHT, H. F. (1955). Presbycusis. *Laryngoscope, St. Louis* **65**, 402–19.

—— IGARASHI, M., and CHASIN, W. D. (1965). Inner ear haemorrhage in leukaemia: a case report. *Laryngoscope, St. Louis* **75**, 662–8.

SCHWARTZ, R., RODRIGUEZ, W. J., KHAN, W. N., and ROSS, S. (1977). Acute purulent otitis media in children over 5 years. *J. Am. med. Ass.* **238**, 1032–3.

—— —— —— —— (1978). The increasing incidence of ampicillin-resistant *Haemophilus influenzae*: a cause of otitis media. *J. Am. med. Ass.* **239**, 320–3.

SEALS, R. L. and RISE, E. N. (1967). Vogt–Koyanagi–Harada syndrome. *Archs Otolar.* **86**, 419–23.

SERRINS, A. J., HARRISON, R., and CHANDLER, J. R. (1963). Cogan's syndrome. *Archs Otolar.* **78**, 785–9.

SHAH, N. (1971). Use of 'grommets' in glue-ears. *J. Lar. Otol.* **85**, 283–7.

SHAMBAUGH, G. E. JR., (1966). Sodium fluoride for inactivation of the otosclerotic lesion. *Archs. Otolar.* **89**, 381–2.

—— and PETROVIC, A. (1967). The possible value of sodium fluoride for inactivation of the otosclerotic bone lesion. *Acta oto-lar.* **63**, 331–9.

—— CAUSSE, J., PETROVIC, A., CHEVANCE, L. G., and VALVASSORI, G. E. (1974). New concepts in management of otospongiosis. *Archs Otolar.* **100**, 419–26.

SHARP, W. B., JOHN, M. B., and ROBISON, J. M. (1946). Etiology of otomycosis. *Texas St. J. Med.* **42**, 380–4.

SHEA, J. (1979). *Proc. 1st Int. Tinnitus Seminar*, 8–9 June, New York.

SIDNEY, O. C. (1960). Erythema multiforme exudativum associated with the use of sulfamethoxypyridazine. *J. Am. med. Ass.* **173**, 799–800.

SILVERSTEIN, H., BERNSTEIN, J. M., and LERNER, P. (1966). Antibiotic concentrations in middle ear effusions. *Pediatrics, Springfield* **38**, 33–6.

SKEGG, D. C. G. and DOLL, R. (1977). The case for recording events in clinical trials. *Br. med. J.* **ii**, 1523–4.

SMITH, J. L. (1970). Cogan's syndrome. *Laryngoscope, St. Louis* **80**, 121–32.

STEGINK, K. J. (1972). The clinical use of Piracetam, a new nootropic drug. The treatment of senile involution. *Arzneimittel-Forsch.* **22**, 975–7.

STEPHENS, S. D. G. and HINCHCLIFFE, R. (1968). Studies on temporary threshold drift. *Int. Audiol.* **7**, 267–79.

STEVENS, A. M. and JOHNSON, F. C. (1922). A new eruptive fever associated with stomatitis and ophthalmia. *Am. J. Dis. Child.* **24**, 526–33.

STIPON, J. P., DOUCET, F., and BLONS, J. (1974). L'utilisation du cyclospasmol 400 en pathologie cochleo-vestibulaire. *Cah. ORL Chir. cervico-fac.* **9**, 195–202.

STONE, R. A. and DELEO, J. (1976) Psychotherapeutic control of hypertension. *New Engl. J. Med.* **294**, 80–4.

TAYLOR, L. (1965). Acute Inflammation of the middle ear cleft. In *Diseases of the ear, nose and throat*, 2nd edn, Vol. II (eds. W. G. Scott-Brown, J. Ballantyne, and J. Groves). Butterworth, London.

TEDESCO, F., MARKHAM, R., GURWITH, M., CHRISTIE, D., and BARTLETT, J. G. (1978). Oral vancomycin for antibiotic-associated pseudomembranous colitis. *Lancet* **ii**, 226–8.

TEODORESCU, L. and CERNEA, P. (1962). Contributii la studiul sindromului Cogan. *Oto-rino-laringologie* **7**, 49–56.

VERNON, J. (1977). Attempts to relieve tinnitus. *J. Am. Audiol. Soc.* **2**, 124–31.

—— and SCHLEUNING, A. (1978). Tinnitus: a new management. *Laryngoscope, St. Louis* **88**, 413–19.

WALDRON-EDWARD, D. and SKORYNA, S. C. (1966). The mucolytic activities of amides. A new approach to mucus dispersion. *Can. med. Ass. J.* **94**, 1249–56.

WELLS, M., MICHAELS, L., and WELLS, D. G. (1977). Otolaryngological disturbances in Waldenstrom's nacroglobulinaemia. *Clin. Otolar.* **2**, 327–38.

WENTZ, H. S. and SEIPLE, H. H. (1947). Stevens–Johnson syndrome, a variation of erythema multiforma exudativum (Hebra): a report of two cases. *Ann. inter. Med.* **26**, 227–79.

WILMOT, T. J. and MENON, G. N. (1976). Betahistine in Ménière's disease. *J. Lar.* **90**, 833–40.

WILSON, P. (1962). Vogt–Koyanagi–Harada syndrome. *Br. J. Ophthal.* **46**, 626–8.

WILSON, W. H. (1971). Acute suppurative otitis media: a method for terminating recurrent episodes. *Laryngoscope, St. Louis* **81**, 1401–8.

WITTENBORN, J. R. (1979). Effects of diazepines on psychomotor performance. *Br. J. clin. Pharm.* **7**, 615–75.

WOLTHUIS, O. H. (1971). Experiments with UCB 6215, a drug which enhances acquisition in rats: its effects compared with those of methamphetamine. *J. Pharm.* **16**, 283–97.

WREDEN, R. R. (1867). Sechs Fälle von Mryingomykosis (*Aspergillus glaucus Lk.*). *Arch. Ohrenheilk.* **3**, 1–21.

WRIGHT, D. O., GOLD, E. M., and JENNINGS, G. (1947). Stevens–Johnson syndrome. Report of nine patients treated with sulfonamide drugs or penicillin. *Archs intern. Med.* **79**, 510–17.

WRIGHT, I. (1968). Late-onset hearing loss due to congenital syphilis. *Int. Audiol.* **7**, 302–10.

YAFFEE, H. S. (1959). Erythema multiforme (Stevens–Johnson syndrome) caused by penicillin. *Archs Derm.* **79**, 591–2.

YASSIN, A. and TAHA, M. (1963). Sensory neural deafness in pellagra. *J. Lar. Otol.* **77**, 992–1000.

ZOLLER, M., WILSON, W. W., and NADOL, J. B. J. (1979). Treatment of syphilitic hearing loss. *Ann. Otol. Rhinol. Lar.* **88**, 160–5.

19 Surgical management of deafness in adults: the external and middle ear

J. B. BOOTH

Surgical reconstruction of the hearing mechanism consists of remaking or remodelling the external ear and middle-ear mechanism, or both, so that their normal physical properties are restored and conduction of the energy of sound waves to the cochlea is improved. To obtain the best results the external auditory canal must be patent; the tympanic membrane must be intact and coupled to an ossicular chain which is continuous and mobile; and the Eustachian tube must be functioning.

The impedance matching takes place in all three parts of the ear (external, middle, and inner) but this part of the chapter is only concerned with the first two. The surgical attainment of this transformer effect is expressed here from a theoretical viewpoint rather than by detailed analysis of surgical techniques. It is also confined to non-suppurative disease without the presence of cholesteatoma (keratoma).

Figs. 19.1(a) and (b) show two 'views' of the middle ear. The first 1(a) might be termed the 'audiologist's' view relating the anatomical structure to its physical properties. The second (b) is the 'otologist's' view at surgery showing the space for manoeuvre and the constraints imposed upon his expertise in matching those two concepts as best his skill and nature will allow.

The main part of this chapter is devoted to the reconstruction of the middle ear following its partial destruction by infection. The effects of a perforation, including those on audiometry and Eustachian tube function, are discussed rather than the ways in which it may result (see Schuknecht 1974). The last section is devoted to a short review of the effects and surgery of otosclerosis.

Fig. 19.1. (a). b_c friction coefficient of the stapedial cochlear system; b_{d1} a friction coefficient of the eardrum system; b_{d2} a friction coefficient of the eardrum system; b_o friction coefficient of the incudomalleal system; b_s friction coefficient of the incudostapedial system; C_p acoustic compliance of antrum and pneumatic cells; C_t acoustic compliance of the tympanic cavity; k_c spring constant of the stapedial-cochlear system; k_{d1} a spring constant of the eardrum system; k_{d2} a spring constant of the eardrum system; k_o spring constant of the incudomalleal system; k_s spring constant of the incudostapedial system; L_a acoustic inertance of the passage between tympanic cavity and antrum; m_c effective mass of the stapedial cochlear system; m_d effective mass of the eardrum system; m_o effective mass of the incudomalleal system; R_a acoustic resistance of the passage between tympanic cavity and antrum; R_{muc} acoustic resistance of mucosa. (b). Anatomical distances of the middle ear, as seen through a posterior tympanotomy, into the facial recess. (After Banfai (1966).)

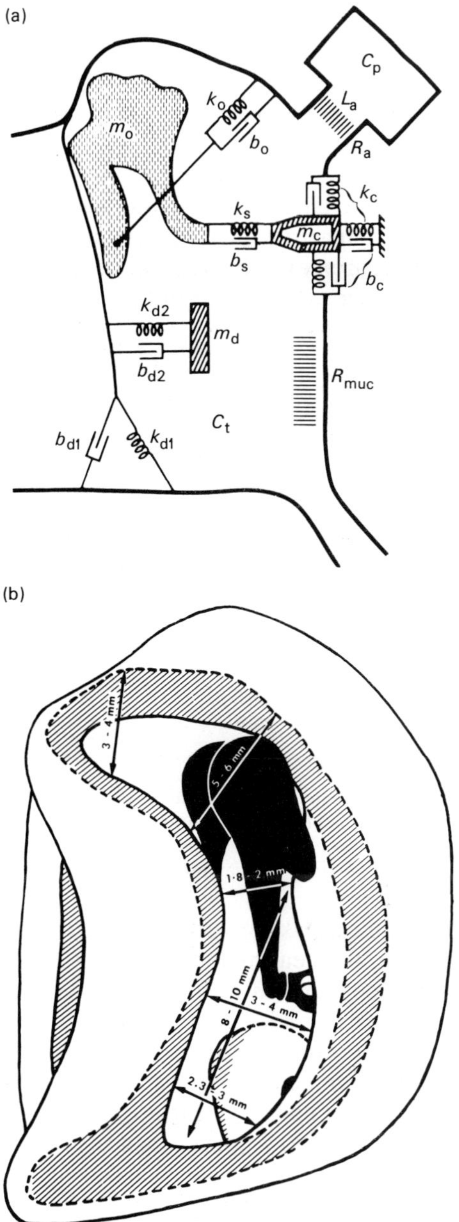
(a)
C_p
L_a
R_a
k_o
b_o
m_o
k_c
k_s
m_c
b_s
b_c
k_{d2}
m_d
b_{d2}
R_{muc}
C_t
b_{d1}
k_{d1}
(b)
3 - 4 mm
5 - 6 mm
1·8 - 2 mm
8 - 10 mm
3 - 4 mm
2.3 - 3 mm

PRE-OPERATIVE TESTS

Pure-tone audiometry and tuning fork tests

Clinically, hearing losses due to tympanic membrane perforations are independent of frequency in the low tones and show little air–bone gap at 2000 Hz or above. This has always contrasted with experimental results which have shown a loss of 12 dB per octave with inverse frequency. Recently Tonndorf, McArdle, and Kruger (1976) have shown in cats that these two apparently conflicting observations are not directly comparable as they derive from different sets of data.

Tuning fork tests are carried out in an *open* system whilst audiometry employs a *closed* system, albeit leaky, that is placing the earphones over the flattened pinna. By comparison most experiments have been on truly closed systems making measurements at the level of the ear drum perforation or middle ear. Fig. 19.2 shows the effect of the variations in recording and, as

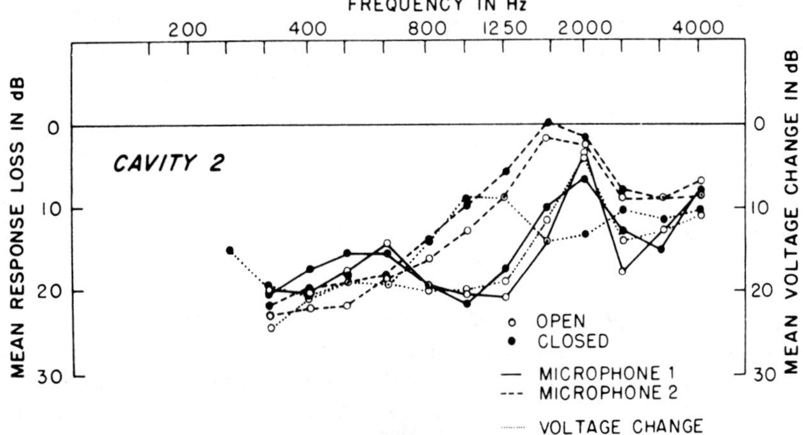

Fig. 19.2. Cochlear microphonic response losses in the cat assessed at the entrance (microphone 1) and at the bottom (microphone 2) of an extended, acoustically leaking, ear canal (polyethylene tubing, 8 cm long) and associated voltage changes across the transducer (average of five animals) (Tonndorf *et al.* 1976).

will be seen, when using a leaking closed system (i.e. pure-tone audiometry) at the canal entrance, the hearing loss from 300–1250 Hz is independent of frequency. This discrepancy may be due to the use of precalibrated SPLs in clinical audiometry (Kruger and Tonndorf 1978). A perforation produces a negative effect in canal resonance and some sound energy leaks through to the medial side of the tympanic membrane which partially cancels out the effect of energy acting on its lateral surface. Such cancellations depend on wavelength, particularly below the resonance point.

Tests of Eustachian tube function

There is some difference of opinion as to the value of such tests but the results are worthless if the patient has discharging ears or inflamed mucosa. The mucosa of the middle ear must be completely normal with no pathological obstruction at the tympanic end of the Eustachian tube; testing during an upper respiratory tract infection also affects the results (Miller 1965). MacKinnon (1970) has shown that pre-operative tubal function tests are helpful in deciding the optimum time for closure of a tympanic perforation. However, it should not be forgotten that many patients desire only a successful graft and a dry ear; although an improvement in hearing is an advantage, the relief of recurrent otorrhoea, even with an atelectatic middle ear, may be wholly acceptable.

A comparison of tubal function tests by Andreasson and Ivarsson (1976) showed good agreement between the *open* and *closed* methods, the latter being the easier to perform. They also found that Toynbee's test was a useful indication of tubal function, whereas Valsalva's manoeuvre had no correlation with tubal function. They noted a close correlation between tubal function and the volume of the air cell system. The size of the mastoid air system has also been shown to be related to the success rate of myringoplasty surgery, being over 90 per cent in those with large systems but reduced to 50 per cent in those with small systems. The critical area appears to be 9 cm^2 as judged on a lateral X-ray film of the ear. If, however, in those with small systems, the mastoid bone is completely drilled out to increase its internal surface area and thereby the air reservoir, then the success rate was raised to 83 per cent (Holmquist and Bergstrom 1976, 1978). Silastic sheeting was used to line the surgically created cavity, the posterior bony canal wall being left intact. This idea was first put forward by Grahne (1964) and reiterated by Booth (1973 a, b).

A correlation has also been shown between the functional volume of the middle ear and mastoid air cell system and tubal function. The volume of the system decreases with the duration of disease though there is no relation to area (Andreasson 1977). Furthermore the displacement of the tympanic membrane increases as the volume of the mastoid air cell system increases and the more efficient the Eustachian tube function, the more pronounced will be the movement of the tympanic membrane (Holmquist 1978). Renvall, Liden, and Bjorkman (1975) have also shown that one of the functions influencing the 'depth' of the tympanogram is the volume of the middle-ear cleft. They also noted that the air pressure in the middle ear follows the air pressure in the ear canal best in ears with a small middle-ear cleft volume leading to a small pressure difference. A recent investigation by Molvaer, Vallersnes and Kringlebotn (1978) has shown a wide variation in the volume of the middle ear and mastoid air cell system ranging from 2–22 ml with an average of approximately 6.5 ml. Nevertheless, Eustachian tube function assessed by tympanometry in patients with intact tympanic membranes has so far failed to produce consistent results (Siedentop, Corrigan, Loewy, and Osenar 1978).

THE EXTERNAL EAR

Surgery may occasionally be required on the external ear (here we shall not consider such operations as those to remove the whole or part of the pinna, as for a malignancy). There are two common procedures that alter the position of the pinna; firstly, for turning back 'bat ears' (pinnaplasty), though no audiometric or acoustic assessment of this procedure seems to have been made, and secondly, in any operation approached from behind the ear where the incision usually divides the posterior auricular muscle. As a result the pinna will have a more forward angle, which ought theoretically to improve its acoustic function according to the direction of the sound. Surgery is also occasionally required to remove obstructing osteomas from the bony meatus.

The external ear consists of three components—the pinna flange, the concha, and the meatal canal. The pinna flange is said to produce a sound pressure gain of 3 dB at 3000–6000 Hz when compared to ears without a flange. The concha acts as a cavity resonator producing a sound pressure increase of 10 dB at 4000–5000 Hz. The acoustic characteristics are closely associated with the geometry of the concha but independent of the shape of the pinna flange (Shaw 1972).

The meatal canal has an average length of 26 mm and a volume of 1 ml. The opening is approximately 9 mm vertically and 6.5 mm horizontally. It functions like a tube closed at one end producing a sound pressure increase of approximately 12 dB 3400–900 Hz. The fundamental resonance occurs at a frequency whose wave length is four times the canal length; with a total external earlength of 35 mm this point is at 4000 Hz. Owing to this resonance the ear canal acts as a transformer over a limited range. The sound pressure gain and resonance varies according to the location of the source, being greatest at an angle of incidence of 45° to the midline of the head (Shaw 1974; Mehrgardt and Mellert 1977).

All the above assumes that any surgery does not alter the shape of the canal or the position of the drum. But the canal may be enlarged at surgery if an extension is made backwards (posteriorly) into the mastoid bone, creating a mastoid cavity. Mastoid cavities have been shown, even when quite large, to have resonances between 2000–4000 Hz with a gain of 15–25 dB. However, ears with lateral displacement of a graft applied to a drum defect produce shorter canals and a relatively higher resonant frequency than normal (Goode, Friedrichs, and Falk 1977). One should remember that a 50 per cent loss of efficiency of the tympanic membrane results in a hearing loss of only 6 dB.

Changes in the anatomy of the external ear produce their acoustic effects in the higher speech frequencies, above 1500 Hz, but they are small and rarely exceed 20 dB. If the ear canal has an opening less than 6 mm in diameter losses occur at 2000–3000 Hz. The actual shape of the canal does not appear to exert much influence except when it connects with the mastoid antrum to form a common cavity with it.

THE TYMPANIC MEMBRANE

The dimensions, width, and thickness respectively, of the intact tympanic membrane are shown in Figs. 19.3(a) and (b) (Kirikae 1960). The natural cone shape and the coupling of the malleus to the manubrium are of great importance if the grafted drum is to have good function. To achieve this shape the graft can either be preformed on a mould or a slit made to accommodate the manubrium, or a specially prepared homograft drum may be used. It must be appreciated that it is the middle layer (lamina propria) of the drum which it is sought to provide by grafting, allowing the squamous epithelium externally and the mucous membrane internally to grow across their respective surfaces. The operation to graft a perforation of the tympanic membrane is termed a myringoplasty (type I tympanoplasty). If, as a result, the grafted drum becomes thicker and heavier then the resonance frequency will be lowered and the sound conduction worsens at high frequencies (Kirikae, Sato, Sato, Funasaka, Kawamura, Sawashima, and Okabe 1964).

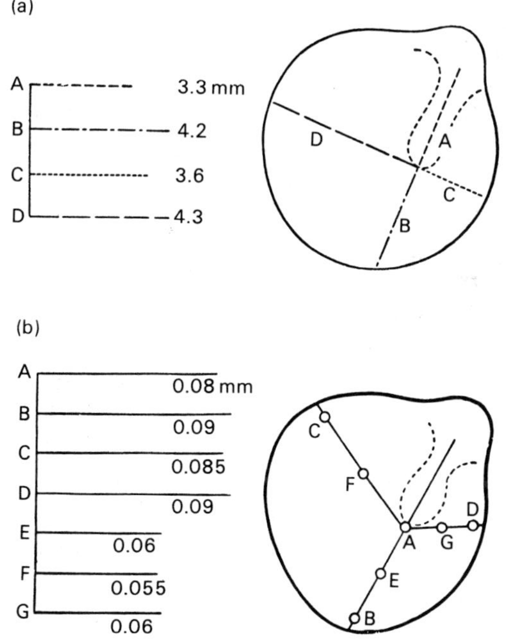

Fig. 19.3. (a). Diameter of the tympanic membrane (Kirikae 1960). (b). Thickness of the tympanic membrane.

The attachment or coupling is important, because by maintaining the curved membrane the larger displacement in the centre of the membrane is exchanged for a smaller displacement of the manubrium itself. The significance of this is explained later. The lamina propria of the tympanic membrane is composed of two groups of fibres—radial and non-radial (Kirikae 1963, 1969); the latter consists of three types: circular, parabolic, and transverse (see Fig. 19.4) (Shimada and Lim 1971). At the umbo the middle fibrous layer divides equally medial and lateral to the malleus handle (Graham *et al.* 1978).

Using time-averaged holography, first in cats and then on human cadaver tympanic membranes, Tonndorf and Khanna (1972) showed that in response to a low frequency the tympanic membrane forms two separate displacement maxima, a lesser one anteriorly and a larger one posteriorly to the manubrium (Fig. 19.5(a) and (b)). This displacement pattern confirms the theory of Helmholtz based on the mechanics of curved membranes. A model of the cat's ear drum as a thin shell using the finite-element method also shows substantial agreement in the vibration pattern and amplitude as determined by laser holography (Fig. 19.5(c)) (Funnell and Laszlo 1978). Holography has also been used to study the tympanic membrane of the frog and this gives support to the curved membrane theory (Mazunda, Bucco, and Hansen 1977). Studies in the guinea pig appear to show a quite different pattern (Manley and Johnstone 1974; Dancer, Franke, Smigielski, Albe, and Fagot 1975).

Because of the curvature of the tympanic membrane the force acting on the malleus is increased over that acting on the tympanic membrane, i.e. larger displacements in the centre of each membrane section on both sides of the manubrium are exchanged for smaller displacements of the manubrium itself (Tonndorf and Khanna 1976). In the transmission of this force from the larger tympanic membrane to the smaller stapes footplate, the pressure at the stapes is increased. The holographic studies have shown that because of the curved membrane principle, the entire tympanic membrane contributes to the ossicular displacement, and therefore the area ratio, tympanic membrane: stapes footplate, is of the greatest importance.

The tympanic membrane as a whole has elastic properties and part of its restoring force is contributed by the air enclosed in the middle ear space (Austin 1977). The collagen fibres of the lamina propria are smooth and when multiply stranded they lie parallel to one another. Tonndorf and Khanna (1972) proposed a mechanism whereby connective tissue fibres slide in respect to one another, with the ground substance acting like a spring, provided that the displacements are relatively small and short lasting, as during vibratory motion. In the tympanic membrane the collagen fibres have their long axis in the plane of the membrane. Accordingly Tonndorf and Khanna proposed the concept that interaction on inward displacement takes place between the radial and circular fibres, and on outward displacement between the radial and parabolic fibres. Unlike the collagen of the homograft tympanic membrane the collagen of fascia is not cross-linked.

Tonndorf, Khanna, and Greenfield (1972) carried out total myringoplasty operations on cats with replacement by fascia grafts. Again using time-averaged holography, they found that the grafted membranes were stiffer

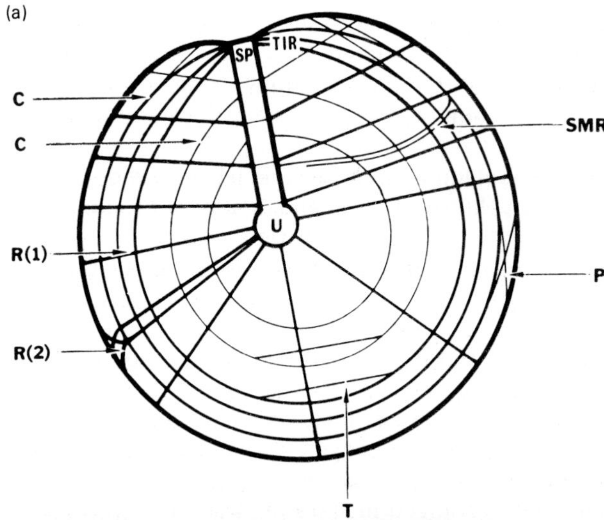

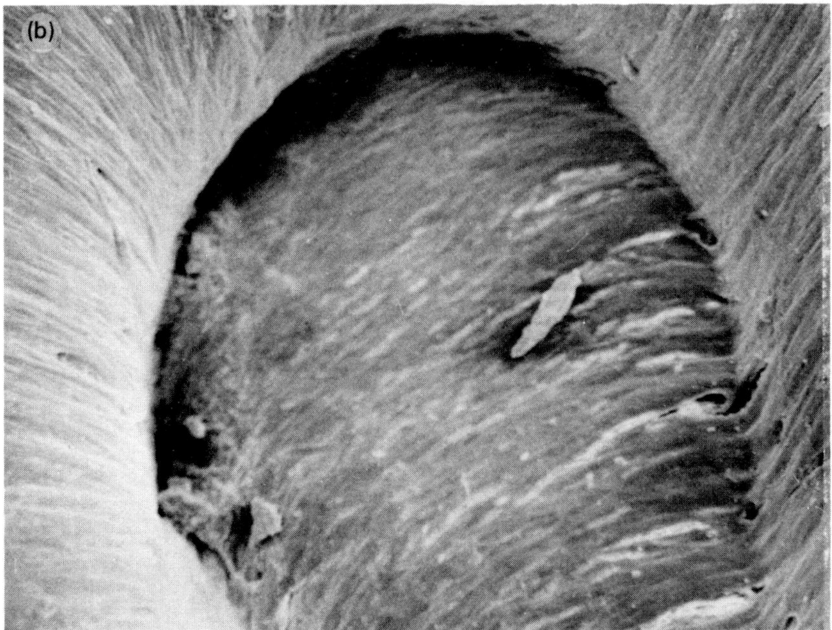

Fig. 19.4. (a). An artist's conception of the fibre arrangement of the human tympanic membrane (Shimada and Lim 1971). SP = short process of malleus. U = umbo. TIR = trigonum interradiale. C = circular fibres. R (1) = radial fibres which attach straight to the annular ring. R(2) = the few radial fibres which diverge and cross over at their terminals. T = transverse fibres. P = parabolic fibres. SMR = submucous fine radial fibres. (b). Scanning electron photomicrograph of the lateral surface radial fibre layer of the tympanic membrane with the squamous epithelial layer removed. Note the attachment of the radial fibres to the umbo. (× 50.) (Courtesy of Professor M. D. Graham, Ann Arbor.)

and the coupling was poor. They found little resemblance between the normal and abnormal patterns at any frequency. The location of the area of maximal displacement differed considerably from normal, failure of coupling with or without thin segments in some location shifted the area of maximal displacement accordingly to that position.

The graft for a myringoplasty may be taken from a wide variety of tissues, including homograft (human tissue) and xenongraft (animal tissue) and at least 20 different materials have been tried (Salen 1968). The tissue most widely used is the fascia overlying the temporalis muscle. Other autogenous tissues still in common use are vein and periosteum. The use of the homograft tympanic membrane provides the tissue most natural in shape but it must be remembered that it requires prior preparation and storage (Marquet, Schepens, and Kuijpers 1973; Marquet 1977; Black and Vercoe 1977).

Of the many different tissues, including vein, dura, and fascia, the primary component is collagen. Collagen is a species-specific protein because of its amino-acid composition. It is an incomplete protein composed of three primary amino-acids arranged in spiral matrix with hydrogen bonding. It will not support bacterial growth, being an incomplete nutritive substance (Abbenhaus 1978). Collagen generally originates from poorly-cellularized tissue and consequently contains few cell-bound T-antigens.

For the sake of simplicity, if fascia is used it may be laid on top of the remnant of the lamina propria (onlay), beneath the mucous membrane of

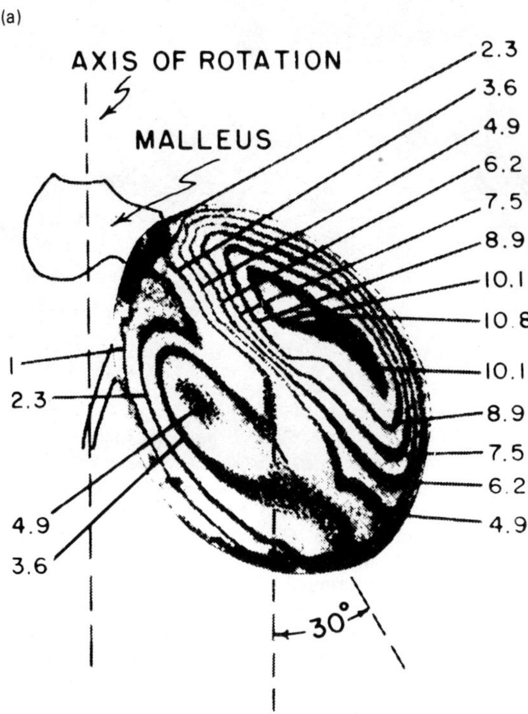

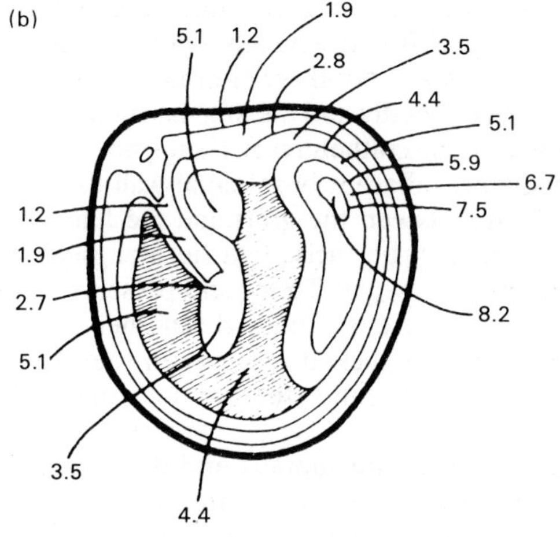

1969
$f = 525$ Hz
Amplitude $= \times 10^{-5}$ cm
SPL = 121 dB

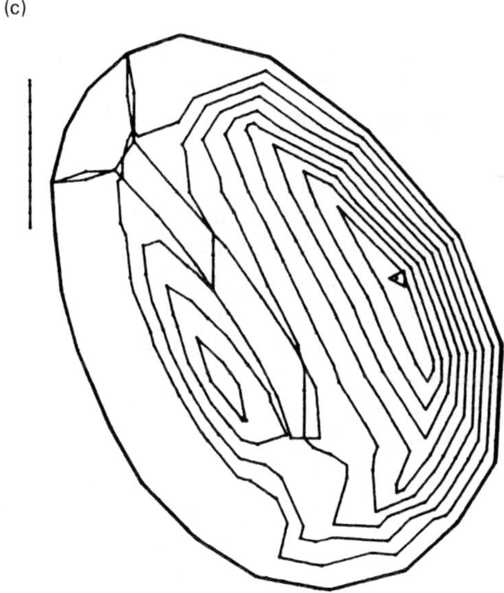

Fig. 19.5. (a). Hologram of a cat's left tympanic membrane. The malleus runs down from the top left (interrupted line); the numbers refer to the sequence of dark figures (600 Hz, 111 dB) (Khanna and Tonndorf 1972). (b). Vibration patterns of the tympanic membrane in man. The displacement amplitudes are given in absolute terms (Tonndorf and Khanna 1972). (c). Vibration pattern calculated for an ear model by the finite-element method (Funnell and Laszlo 1978).

the drum remnant (underlay), or through from the lateral to the medial surface (through) (Booth 1976). It is vitally important that the rim of the perforation is completely removed, thereby breaking the junction between the squamous epithelium laterally and the mucous membrane medially. For an onlay graft, the squamous epithelium is lifted from the laminar remnant and from the immediately adjacent bony canal wall.

To facilitate coupling between the graft and the handle of the malleus after healing, the graft may be incised to lie alongside or beneath the manubrium and umbo (if present). To try and preserve a normal anterior meatal angle and thereby prevent 'blunting' (another cause of poor coupling) the onlaid graft may be tucked in between the fibrous annulus anteriorly and the bone, with a small extension down the tympanic opening of the Eustachian tube.

The underlay graft will require support and this is usually provided by packing the middle ear with pieces of gelatin sponge (see below). Surface tension, while sufficient to keep the underlaid graft in position during the operation, will not do so when the general anaesthesia is discontinued. In operations under general anaesthesia, which is nearly always the case in the UK, but much less often in the rest of Europe or in the USA, nitrous oxide is frequently used. The gas is carried in the blood in physical solution only and will enter any air-filled body cavity including the middle ear (Thomsen, Terklidsen, and Arnfred 1965). At the cessation of anaesthesia, the nitrous oxide leaves the grafted middle ear at a much more rapid rate than it can be replaced by nitrogen, leading to a period of negative pressure.

Starr and Schwartzkroin (1972) showed in the cat that the amplitude of the cochlea microphonic changed inversely with the pressure of the middle ear. They also noted that within five minutes of discontinuing nitrous oxide, the middle ear pressure decreased, stabilizing at approximately −100 mm H_2O and that this negative pressure was maintained for several hours. The use of halothane or ethrane is not accompanied by these changes (Waun, Sweitzer and Hamilton 1967; Patterson and Bartlett 1976).

If the fascial graft is placed beneath, the mucosa does not interfere with hearing as it undergoes atrophy. At the junction of the fascia and mucosa, a layer of flattened mucosa slowly advances to cover the under surface of the graft. On the external surface keratinized epithelium migrates over the fascia (Reeve 1977; Boedts 1978). Within 6–8 weeks, the fascia is covered by epithelium on both surfaces. During this period, vascularization proceeds from the annulus and the mucosa. The transplanted tissue swells and exhibits an increased collagen content. The extent to which newly formed collagen fibres invade the non-viable collagen betwen the epithelial layers determines the success of the graft. However, whereas viable fascia becomes an integral part of the restored drum, denatured fascia (e.g. preserved) though incorporated, remains permanently distinct (Plester and Steinbach 1977).

The surface of fascia is a solid mass of fibrillary elements organized into fibre bundles. It also contains dense connective tissue and collagen fibres.

Fascia may be used fresh ('wet') or dry; neither substance shows any cellular proliferation or growth in tissue culture and whilst wet fascia shows some metabolic activity, dry fascia shows none. By contrast vein shows considerable activity in tissue culture (Patterson, Lockwood and Sheehy 1967). If a homograft tympanic membrane is used the lamina propria is at least partially preserved (Greenfield 1977).

The best preservative for homograft tissue is Cialit, in which the fibrocytes are destroyed at the outset. Homograft tissue is first fixed in 5 per cent buffered formalin for 24 hours and then preserved in a 1 in 5000 aqueous solution of Cialit (the sodium salt of 2-ethylmercurimercaptobenzaoxole, 5 carboxylic acid).

An assessment of various graft techniques and relation to the post-operative hearing result and the compliance of the new 'tympanic membrane' by Booth (1973a, b) showed that a fascia onlay, or underlay with gelfoam in the middle ear, produced one pattern of clinical mobility and hearing result and that fascia onlay plus gelfoam in the middle ear, and periosteum onlay, produced another. The size of the perforation which had been grafted did not affect the mobility. A certain degree of agreement between clinically observed mobility and middle-ear compliance was found but this did not reach statistical significance. Periosteum produced the stiffest grafted tympanic membrane yet the reduced compliance of such a membrane was compatible in a few cases with satisfactory hearing. The relationship between compliance and middle ear pressure in grafted tympanic membranes was also examined; fascia onlay and fascia plus gelfoam either onlay or underlay all produced a uniform pattern. The only exception was periosteum (onlay) which again showed a stiffer result (Booth 1974c).

It is universally agreed that the ear should be 'dry' (free from infection) at the time of grafting, but a long period of freedom from infection prior to surgery does not appear to be essential (Booth 1974b). On some occasions, in spite of meticulous preoperative care, an ear refuses to dry up; successful surgery under these conditions is frequently possible but extra attention must be paid to the Eustachian tube orifice. A mucus-secreting pocket based on the promontory is often found on such occasions.

RESULTS OF SURGERY TO THE TYMPANIC MEMBRANE

A success rate of 90–95 per cent may be achieved by any of the graft techniques. Meticulous attention to detail during the procedure is the important factor rather than any particular method, position, or material used.

THE OSSICULAR CHAIN

The amplitude of vibration in the ossicular chain is very small under physiological conditions, and the amount of energy which is necessary to initiate movement is also small. Gundersen and Hogmoen (1976) have shown by holography that the malleus and incus move like a lever round a common axis, the position of which was somewhat dependent on frequency (Fig. 19.6). Large non-physiological sound pressures are needed in order to produce movement in the joint between them. The axis of rotation remains in the same position when increasing the sound pressure at a fixed frequency

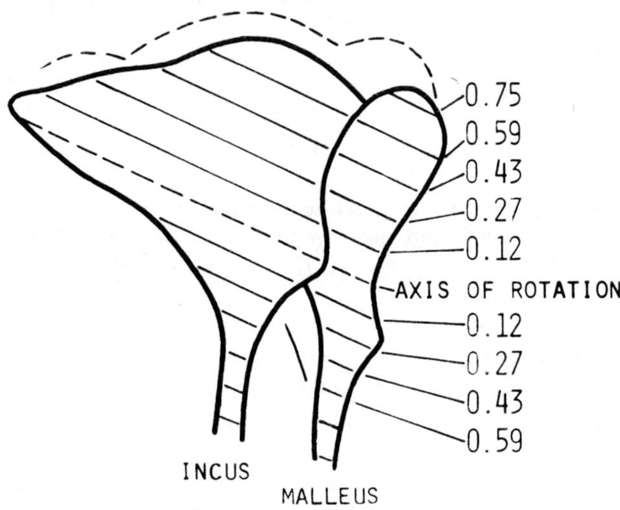

Fig. 19.6. Hologram reconstruction of the malleus and incus showing the position of the axis of rotation and the amplitude of the different fringes) (μm) (1090 Hz, 124 dB) (Gundersen and Hogmoen 1976).

but it shifts a little when the frequency is changed. The ossicular chain has a point of resonance at 800–900 Hz. Shifting the axis position makes the lever ratio of the ossicular chain smaller at the point of resonance and larger at frequencies below and above this point. Experimental studies on sound transmission in the human ear, although somewhat artificial in their conception, do supply some information which is comparable with clinical conditions and provide a guide as to the requirements of ossicular reconstruction. For example, fixation of the stapes produces transmission changes indicating increased stiffness, while subsequent crurotomy causes a high frequency loss (Anderson, Hansen, and Neergaard 1963). Three further situations are shown in Fig. 19.7: (a) shows the effect of experimental fixation of the head of the malleus, (b) the effect of fixation of the incus, and (c) of fixation of the stapedius muscle (Elpern, Greisen, and Anderson 1965). Clinically fixation of the malleus by tympanosclerosis and fusion of the malleus and incus are both well recognized, and require division of the joint. Amputation of the malleus head, may be required to obtain mobility but this in itself produces a negligible acoustic effect (Elpern and Elbrond 1966). As a practical guide it may be taken that a 90 per cent rigidity (fixation) of the malleus will produce a clinical hearing loss of approximately 20 dB and a 95 per cent rigidity, a 40 dB loss.

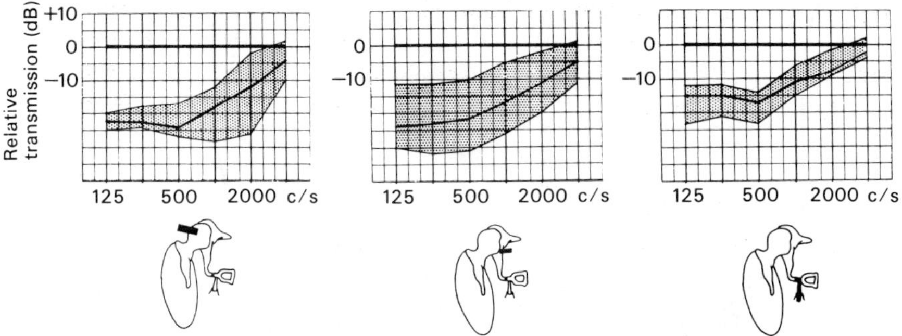

Fig. 19.7. (*left*). Alteration of sound transmission produced by fixation of the head of the malleus. (*centre*) Alteration of sound transmissin produced by fixation of the incus. (*right*) Alteration of sound transmission produced by fixation of the tendon of the stapedius muscle (Elpern *et al.* 1965).

The ossicular chain may become fixed in part or as a whole as the result of disease (e.g. tympanosclerosis), or alternatively some part may become eroded. The latter is by far the commoner clinical situation and it is the long process of the incus which usually suffers. This is considered to be due to its poor blood supply but deep depressions on the surface of the long process may play a part as well (Ghorayer and Graham 1978).

Ossicular replacement between existing ossicles, e.g. handle of malleus and stapes head or footplate, is termed a type II tympanoplasty. This replacement may be achieved either by placing a reshaped ossicle, or using an artificial prosthetic material (Proplast or Plastipore). If the ossicular reconstruction is directly from the tympanic membrane or graft to the stapes head or footplate, it is termed a type III tympanoplasty and involves the construction of a columella as in the avian middle ear (see Fig. 19.8 (a–c)). It also follows that the less destruction or alteration by disease, the more mobile the ossicular reconstruction is likely to be. Generally a type II operation will produce a better hearing results than a type III, and type 1 incus transposition (malleus–incus assembly) will produce better results than a type 2 where the transposed incus extends from the malleus handle to the stapes footplate (Booth 1974a). The ultimate factor is the mobility of the footplate of the stapes. Without this a two-stage procedure will be necessary and a reconstruction between the malleus handle and the oval window using a Teflon or wire prosthesis.

Homograft ossicles are to be preferred to autograft because there is a minimal chance of their containing disease. The ossicle is reshaped using a cutting or diamond burr, and should be of just sufficient length so as to exert a very slight tension on the structures between which it is interposed. Fixation in any form will be self-defeating as it leads to rigidity and without mobility the system will fail to transmit sound vibrations. The usual ossicles used are the incus or malleus but an inverted stapes can also be considered (Tos 1978). Care should also be taken not to increase the mass of the chain.

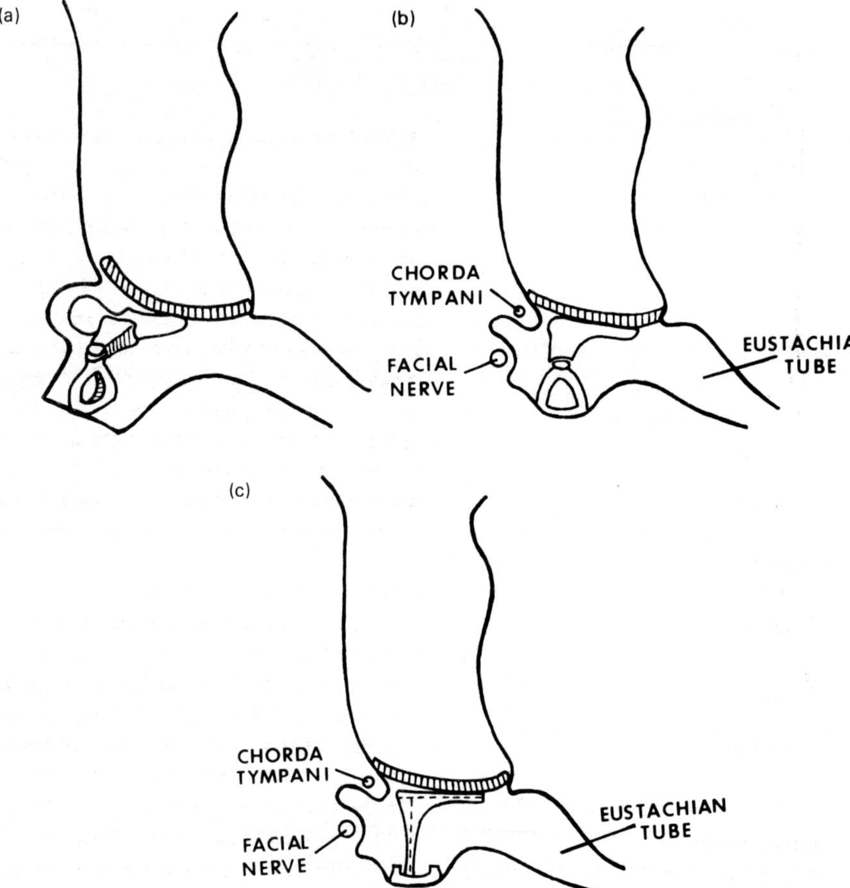

Fig. 19.8. (a). The 'malleus–incus' assembly. Homograft bone is fashioned and transposed to lie between the stapes head and the malleus handle, thereby restoring ossicular continuity—type II tympanoplasty. The graft is laid lateral to the handle of the malleus (onlay). (b). In this situation, the malleus is absent but the stapes remains intact. Transmission is restored by fashioning a homograft ossicle and placing this on the stapes head and beneath the graft—type III tympanoplasty. (c). In this situation, the malleus is again absent but the stapes superstructure is also lost. Transmission now is between the graft and the stapes footplate. The prosthesis shown is a cartilage strut strengthened by wire—type III tympanoplasty.

As an approximate guide, the malleus weighs 20 mg and its centre of gravity is 1 mm above the insertion of the tensor tympani tendon. The incus weighs 27 mg but the stapes only 2.5 mg; the area of the stapes footplate is 3.2 mm^2. It appears that drilling can cause damage to an ossicle, altering the natural defence of the bone, but in spite of this only surface resorption occurs at the damaged margins.

Ossicles contain humoral T-antigens. The bone preserved in Cialit loses most of its antigenic properties but some persist. The mechanism of action of preservation is based on the destruction of the nucleus-bound T-antigen which in turn is provoked by the cell-bound antibodies and it is the latter that cause the transplantation reaction. The Cialit does not alter protein solubility but inactivates a number of enzymes among them the free S-H groups. High molecular weight proteins (e.g. those associated with mucopolysacharides and DNA and collagen) remain in the tissue and are undoubtedly responsible for the antigenicity of the preserved grafts. After two weeks in Cialit the cellular reaction is markedly reduced and the T-antigen effect is minimal. After more than two months bone replacement is observed particularly in the region subjacent to the mucosa (Colman 1976). However, recent work by Veldman and Kuijpers (1978) has demonstrated that the efferent limb of the immune response is intact in the middle-ear complex. While B-cells could hardly be detected in preserved homograft tympanic membrane/ossicular grafts, the T-cells were abundant. They concluded that the middle ear must be an immunologically privileged site for tolerance-induction by such implantation.

Homograft ossicles preserved in Cialit for short periods up to six days show bone replacement on their inner surface. Newly formed osteoid is gradually transformed into lamellar bone and ultimately (after 1–1½ years) replaced by viable bone. However, bone preserved for as long as three weeks showed less bone replacement, which occurred at a slower rate and was limited to perivascular foci (Plester and Steinbach 1977). Regardless of their period in Cialit, all the ossicular grafts retain their original shape and consistency. Within two weeks the ossicular graft starts to become covered with mucous membrane and this is completed by four weeks. Reconstruction of the ossicle starts to appear about 4–6 weeks and this depends on the perivascular connective tissue which produces osteoblasts. Winter and Hohmann (1967) noted in their experiment in cats that whilst the homograft ossicles appeared dead when placed in the host tympanum, they were nevertheless actively undergoing calcium metabolism at least three months later.

As an alternative to transposition of an autograft or preferably a homograft ossicle, a cartilage strut may be used. The cartilage may be taken from the tragus (elastic cartilage), in which case it will usually be an autograft and easily available (Altenau and Sheehy 1978). Autogenous cartilage may remain viable when grafted (Robin, Bennett and Gregory 1976). Alternatively, nasal septal cartilage (hyaline cartilage) may be used; this is usually preserved and will often buckle if not supported by the insertion of wire (38 FG) in the limbs (Smyth, Kerr and Goodey 1971; Smyth, Kerr, and Hassard 1977). The cartilage may be cut into a boomerang shape with an approximate angle of 75°, or T-shape as required. Most recently of all, pre-formed ossicles have been 'grown' by inserting a titanium mould in the proximal tibial metaphysis. The new ossicle 'grew' better when the mould was closest to the endosteal surface (Tjellström, Lindström, Albrektsson, Branemark, and Hallen 1978).

ARTIFICIAL MATERIALS IN TYMPANOPLASTY

Many artificial materials have been used either to maintain an air-filled middle ear space, e.g. Silastic, or as an alternative to natural prosthetic materials. Most recent of such alternatives have been Proplast and Plastipore. Silastic sheeting is a medical grade silicone which may be used in the mesotympanum to prevent the formation of adhesions and promote the regeneration of mucosa and thereby encourage the reformation or preservation of an air-containing middle-ear space. (Colman 1972). (Silastic sponge may be used in the middle ear (Patterson 1968), but in the oval window it failed to provide a satisfactory seal (Colman 1972)).

A gelatin *film* (Gelfilm) is available that is approximately 0.075 mm thick and is non-porous and becomes absorbed (Harris, Barton, Gussen, and Goodhill 1971). Gelatin *sponge* (Gelfoam; Sterispon) in the denuded mesotympanum, however, will induce fibrosis and scarring but there is no report of such a response to the film (Dickson and Hohmann 1971). Kitchens and Gross (1976) found only minimal inflammation and fibrosis with good mucosal regeneration in ears denuded of mucosa. (Gelfilm is not available in the United Kingdom at present.)

Proplast is a polymer of vitreous carbon and Teflon (polytetrofluoroethylene); the carbon ingredient provides a surface that is highly 'wettable' with body fluids, allowing precipitation of proteins, which increases the body's immune tolerance to the implant. It is 70–90 per cent porous and this permits excellent fibrous tissue ingrowth (Mischke, Hyams, Shea and Gross 1977). Loose fibrous tissue and small capillaries will grow in from adjacent mucosa within one week. This fibrous tissue ultimately matures with collagen formation. Multinucleated giant cells may also be seen, especially when bordered by muscle and it is thought that these may be associated with mechanical stress (Kuijpers and Grote 1977). Proplast can become incorporated in the lamina propria of the tympanic membrane without being extruded. Alternatively, a thin covering of fascia or cartilage (e.g. tragal cartilage) can be interposed.

Plastipore is a high-density polyethylene sponge with similar properties to Proplast, in respect of porosity, non-reaction, and the encouragement of fibrous tissue ingrowth, but it is more rigid. It is also available as a manufactured total or partial ossicular replacement, 'TORP' or 'PORP' (Shea and Emmett 1978).

Smyth, Hassard, and Kerr (1978) showed that when Plastipore was used as a TORP, the hearing results were significantly less good than with bone grafts and have discontinued its use. They have also abandoned Proplast in favour of malleus–incus assembly except when the stapes arch is absent. Tragal or septal cartilege etc. should probably be interposed between the TORP and the drum to prevent extrusion of the prosthesis—the fate of many similar materials used earlier (Saraceno, Gray and Blanchard 1978).

RESULTS OF SURGERY TO THE OSSICULAR CHAIN

The reshaped homograft ossicle used to form a malleus–stapes-head connection produces the best hearing result. The latter is assessed by closure of the air–bone gap and producing an air-conduction threshold of 30 dB or better. This will be possible in at least 75 per cent of cases, the mobility of the stapes footplate being the ultimate determining factor. Reconstruction between the malleus and stapes footplate produces less improvement and thus between the grafted tympanic membrane and footplate.

OTOSCLEROSIS

The conductive hearing loss of otosclerosis is due to the fixation of the footplate of the steps. This causes a decreased compliance of the system but the drum still retains full mobility on clinical examination. The normal mature lamellar bone is removed by osteoclasis and replaced by unorganized woven bone of greater thickness, cellularity, and vascularity (Schuknecht 1974). In the first stage, only the anterior part of the stapes footplate and the connecting part of the anterior crus become spongy. In the more advanced stages, the footplate is totally involved by the process but the web-like neoformation is more pronounced. This web-like structure is nearly complete in the third and fourth stages (Kluyskens, Fiermans, Dekeyser, and Vakaet 1976).

Surgery in otosclerosis is designed to mobilize the system by removing the stapes (stapedectomy) and replacing it with a prosthesis. There are two schools of thought regarding the better method, one preferring to remove part or all of the stapes followed by the introduction of a prosthesis of metal or plastic material (e.g. Teflon), the second prefering removal of part or all of the footplate and covering the defect so produced with autogenous tissue (e.g. vein) as a graft and then either repositioning part of the stapes, or using a prosthesis which is allowed to indent the graft covering the oval window. Examples of three of the standard prostheses are shown in Fig. 19.9.

Excellent and essentially similar results are quoted for each method of operation (Schuknecht 1971). Recently two other technical points have received consideration. The first is the size of the hole which should ideally be made in the footplate. It is advocated that a small hole, e.g. 0.7 mm in diameter should be made and a slim-shafted prosthesis (0.6 mm) should be used in preference to removing larger areas of the footplate. This is said to reduce the risk of a perilymph fistula, one of the potential complications of the operation, and whilst it also shows better hearing at 4000 Hz, it is slightly less good at 500 Hz. A still smaller fenestra (0.4 mm in diameter) and a Cawthorne piston (0.3 mm in diameter) is advocated by Smyth and Hassard (1978). Analysis of this smaller fenestra group (Smyth 1978) noted significantly less depression of the bone conduction threshold at 4000 Hz immediately after operation and thought that this indicated less mechanical damage to the basal turn of the cochlea. The second, is the material from

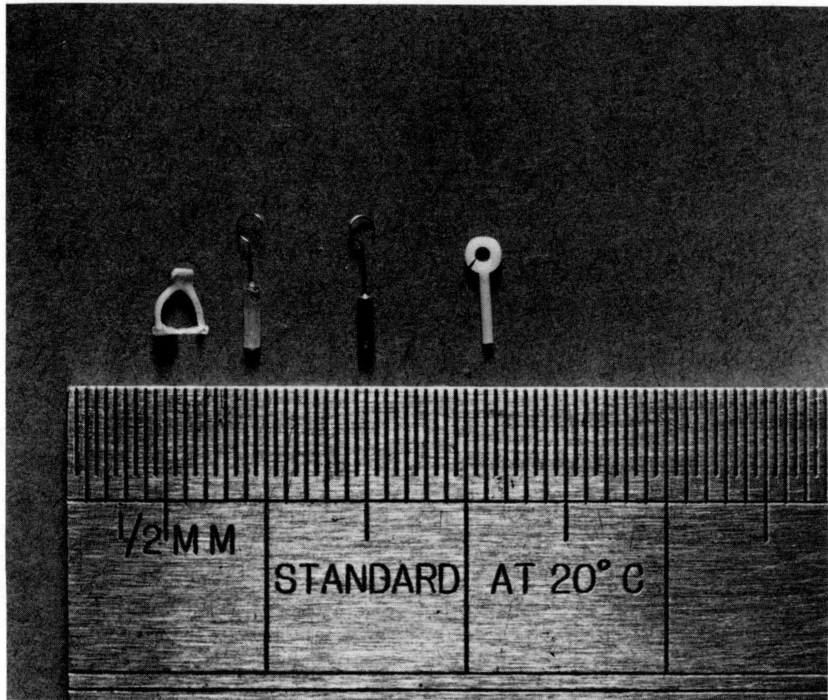

Fig. 19.9. Normal stapes on the left and three prostheses: Teflon/wire piston, McGee stainless steel piston both standard (0.8 mm diameter), and Teflon piston slim shaft (0.6 mm diameter).

which the piston is made. A metal prosthesis is 'wettable' and it allows a perilymph meniscus to form, whereas Teflon is non-wettable. The height of the meniscus will determine the position of the membrane. Fig. 19.10 shows the angle of contact, θ in the two situations; it is the value of θ which determines the most suitable prosthesis. With θ less than 90°, the perilymph will wet and cover the prosthesis and the tissue growing on the miniscus will form a muff. With θ greater than 90°, a more favourable situation is created (Marquet, van Camp, Creten, Decreamer, Wolff, and Schepens 1973) and the tissue will grow level with the piston prosthesis and occlude the opening.

Paradoxically, Feldman (1969) measured the acoustic impedance of ears after stapedectomy using the Zwislocki bridge. He pointed out that the prostheses have different masses and whilst the anterior crurotomy procedure should be the most natural, in fact its use created a low impedance. The best impedance match was produced by a stainless steel piston and the poorest by Teflon, the change of mass tending to shift the resonance point downwards to a lower frequency. It may be helpful to add that neither section of the stapedius muscle nor paralysis of its nerve supply alters the impedance of the normal ear (Feldman 1967), but with the stapes immobil-

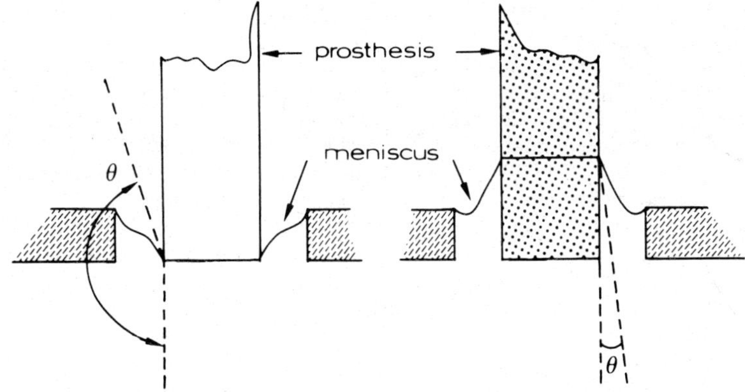

Fig. 19.10. Shape of the perilymph meniscus. (a). Contact angle, θ, of the perilymph on the prosthesis $>90°$. (b). $\theta <90°$.

ized in the oval window, as by otosclerosis, the cochlea is effectively disconnected from the middle-ear system (Zwislocki 1962).

The length of the prosthesis is also important, first for the obvious reason that if too long it may damage structures within the vestibule, e.g. the utricle. Longo and Byers (1971) pointed to two additional reasons: the stiffness of the prosthesis is determined by the elasticity of the material (this is determined by its cross-sectional area divided by the length) and the mass ratio of the strut which is proportional to the length squared.

RESULTS OF SURGERY IN OTOSCLEROSIS

Closure of the air–bone gap, with possibly some improvement in bone conduction, can be produced by stapedectomy in 80–90 per cent of cases. High-tone sensorineural loss is seldom improved. Some 5 per cent will not have any hearing improvement, but can still usefully wear a hearing aid, but approximately 5 per cent will have a total loss of hearing (dead ear).

Acknowledgements

I am indebted to Mr D. J. Connolly, Department of Medical Illustration, Institute of Laryngology and Otology, and to Mr R. Ruddick, Head of the Department of Clinical Photography of the London Hospital for illustrations and to the respective authors and publishers for permission to reproduce their work.

REFERENCES

Abbenhaus, J. I. (1978). The use of reconstituted bovine collagen for tympanic membrane grafting. *Otolaryngology* **86**, 485–7.

Aimi, K. (1978). The tympanic isthmus: its anatomy and clinical significance. *Laryngoscope, St. Louis* **88**, 1067–81.

ALTENAU, M. M. and SHEEHY, J. L. (1978). Tympanoplasty: a report of 564 cases. *Laryngoscope, St. Louis* **88**, 895–904.

ANDERSON, H. C., HANSEN, C. C., and NEERGAARD, E. B. (1963). Experimental studies of sound transmission in the human ear. *Acta oto-lar* **56**, 307–17.

ANDREASSON, L. (1977). Correlation of tubal function and volume of mastoid and middle ear space as related to otitis media. *Acta oto-lar.* **83**, 29–33.

—— and IVARSSON, A. (1976). On tubal function in presence of central perforation of drum in chronic otitis media. *Acta oto-lar.* **82**, 1–10.

AUSTIN, D. F. (1977). On the function of the mastoid. *Otol. Clin. N. Am.* **10**, 541–7.

BANAFAI, P. (1966). Angewandte anatomie bei der radikaloperation mit ehraltung der miteren gehorgangswand. *Arch. Ohr.-, Nas.- KehlkHeilk* **187**, 444–6.

BLACK, B. and VERCOE, G. S. (1977). Experience in homograft membrane tympanoplasty. *Clin. Otolar.* **2**, 311–26.

BOEDTS, D. (1978). Tympanic epithelial migration. *Clin. Otolar.* **3**, 249–53.

BOOTH, J. B. (1973a). Tympanoplasty: factors in post-operative assessment. *J. Lar. Otol.* **87**, 27–67.

—— (1973b). Myringoplasty: factors affecting results. *J. Lar. Otol.* **87**, 1039–84.

—— (1974a). Tympanoplasty. *J. Lar. Otol.* **88**, 625–40.

—— (1974b). Myringoplasty—the lessons of failure. *J. Lar. Otol.* **88**, 1223–36.

—— (1974c). Tympanometry in tympanoplasty. *Acta oto-rhino-lar. belg.* **28**, 510–17.

—— (1976). Closure of perforations of the tympanic membrane. In *Operative Surgery* (ed. J. Ballantyne) pp. 75–81, 3rd edn. Butterworth, London.

—— (1978). Otosclerosis. *Practitioner* **221**, 710–15.

COLMAN, B. H. (1972). Silastic implants in the ears of cats. *Acta oto-lar.* **73**, 296–303.

—— (1976). Experimental aspects of reconstructuve surgery: the ear. In *Scientific foundations of otolaryngology* (ed. R. Hinchcliffe and D. Harrison) pp. 865–81. Heinemann, London.

DANCER, A. L., FRANKE, R. B., SMIGIELSKI, P., ALBE, F., and FAGOT, H. (1975). Holographic interferometry applied to the investigation of tympanic membrane displacements in guinea pig ears subjected to acoustic impulses. *J. acoust. Soc. Am.* **58**, 223–8.

DICKSON, R. and HOHMANN, A. (1971). The fate of exogenous materials placed in the middle ear and frontal sinus of cats. *Laryngoscope* **81**, 216–31.

ELPERN, B. S. and ELBROND, O. (1966). Acoustic effects of removing the malleus head. *Archs Otolar.* **84**, 170–2.

——, GRIESEN, O., and ANDERSON, H. C. (1965). Experimental studies on sound transmission in the human ear. *Acta oto-lar.* **60**, 223–30.

FELDMAN. A. S. (1967). A report of further impedance studies of the acoustic reflex. *J. Speech Hear. Res.* **10**, 616–22.

—— (1969). Acoustic impedance measurement of post-stapedectomised ears. *Laryngoscope, St. Louis* **79**, 1132–55.

FUNNELL, W. R. J. and LASZLO, C. A. (1978). Modelling of the cat ear drum as a thin shell using the finite-element method. *J. acoust. Soc. Am.* **63,** 1461–67.

GHORAYER, B. Y. and GRAHAM, M. D. (1978). Human incus long process. Depressions in the surface of the normal ossicle. *Laryngoscope, St. Louis* **88,** 1184–9.

GOODE, R. L. FRIEDRICHS, R., and FALK, S. (1977). Effect on hearing thresholds of surgical modification of the external ear. *Ann. Otolar.* **86**, 441–50.

GRAHAM, M. D., REAMS, C., and PERKINS, R. (1978). Human tympanic membrane—malleus attachment. *Ann. Otolar.* **87**, 426–31.

GRAHNE, B. (1964). Simple mastoidectomy with air chamber creation in progressive adhesive otitis. *Acta oto-lar.* **58**, 259–70.

GREENFIELD, E. C. (1977). The homograft myringoplasty and the lamina propria of the tympanic membrane. *Laryngoscope, St. Louis* **87**, 1731–9.

GUNDERSEN, T. and HOGMOEN, K. (1976). Holographic vibration analysis of the ossicular chain. *Acta oto-lar.* **82**, 16–25.

HARRIS, I., BARTON. S., GUSSEN, R., and GOODHILL, V. (1971). Gelfilm—induced neotympanic membrane in tympanoplasty. *Laryngoscope, St. Louis* **81**, 1826–37.

HOLMQUIST, J. (1978). Aeration in chronic otitis media. *Clinical Otolar.* **3**, 279–84.

—— and BERGSTROM, B. (1976). Eustachian tube function and size of the mastoid air cell system in middle ear surgery. *Scand. Audio.* **5**, 87–9.

——and —— (1978). The mastoid air cell system in ear surgery. *Archs Otolar.* **104**, 127–9.

JANSEN, C. (1970). Homo- and heterogenous grafts in reconstruction of the sound conduction system. *Acta oto-rhino-lar. belg.* **24**, 60–5.

KHANNA, S. M. and TONNDORF, J. (1972). Tympanic membrane vibrations in cats studied by time-averaged holography. *J. acoust. Soc. Am.* **51**, 1904.

KIRIKAE, I. (1960). *The structure and function of the middle ear,* p. 36. University of Tokyo Press.

—— (1963). Physiology of the middle ear. *Archs Otolar.* **78**, 317–28.

—— (1969). *Physiopathology of the middle ear.* Refresher Audio-visual Course. University of Tokyo Press.

—— SATO, Y., SATO, M., FUNASAKA, S., KAWAMURA, S., SAWASHIMA, M., and OKABE, K. (1964). An experimental study of the patho-physiology of the middle ear mechanics. *Ann. Otolar.* **73**, 124–40.

KITCHENS, G. G. and GROSS, C. W. (1976). Investigations of the mesotympanum's reaction to silastic and gelatin film. *Archs Otolar.* **102**, 547–51.

KLUYSKENS, P., FIERMANS, L., DEKEYSER, W., and VAKAET, L. (1976). Scanning electron microscopic studies of the stapes in normal and in some pathological and experimental conditions. *Acta oto-lar.* **81**, 220–7.

KRUGER, B. and TONNDORF, J. (1978). Tympanic membrane perforations in cats: configurations of loss with and without ear canal extensions. *J. acoust. Soc. Am.* **63**, 436–41.

KUIJPERS, W. and GROTE, J. J. (1977). The use of proplast in experimental middle ear surgery. *Clin. Otolar.* **2**, 5–15.

LONGO, S. E. and BYERS, V. W. (1971). Analog model for stapes prostheses evaluation. *Med. Res. Engng.* **10**, 12–14.

LYONS, G. D., DYER, R. F. and RUBY, J. R. (1977). Morphologic analysis of tympanic membrane grafts. *Laryngoscope, St. Louis* **87**, 1507–9.

MACKINNON, D. M. (1970). Relationship of pre-operative Eustachian tube function to myringoplasty. *Acta oto-lar.* **69**, 100–6.

MANLEY, G. A. and JOHNSTONE, B. M. (1974). Middle ear function in the guinea pig. *J. acoust. Soc. Am.* **56**, 571–6.

MARQUET, J. F. E. (1977). Twelve years experience with homograft tympanoplasty. *Otol. Clin. N. Am.* **10**, 581–93.

—— SCHEPENS, P., and KUIJPERS, W. (1973). Experiences with tympanic transplants. *Arch Otolar.* **97**, 58–66.

—— VAN CAMP, K. J., CRETEN, W. L., DECREAMER, W. F., WOLFF, H. B., and SCHEPENS, P. (1973). Topics in physics and middle ear surgery. *Acta otol-rhino-lar. belg.* **27**, 137–230.

MAZUMDAR, J., BUCCO, D. and HANSEN, C. (1977). Time-averaged holography for the study of the vibrations of the tympanic membrane in frog cadaver. *J. otol. Soc. Aust.* **4**, 149–54.

MEHRGARDT, S. and MELLERT, V. (1977). Transformation characteristics of the external human ear. *J. acoust. Soc. Am.* **61**, 1567–76.

MILLER, G. F. (1965). Eustachian tubal function in normal and diseased ears. *Archs Otolar.* **81**, 41.

MISCHKE, R. E., HYAMS, V., SHEA, J. J. and GROSS, C. W. (1977). Proplast in the middle ear and oval window of cats. *Archs Otolar.* **103**, 489–92.

MOLVAER, O. I., VALLERSNES, F. M., and KRINGLEBOTN, M. (1978). The size of the middle ear and mastoid air cell. *Acta oto-lar.* **85**, 24–32.

PATTERSON, C. N. (1968). Silastic sponge implants in tympanoplasty. *Laryngoscope, St. Louis* **78**, 759–67.

PATTERSON, M. E. and BARTLETT, P. C. (1976). Hearing impairment caused by intratympanic pressure changes during general anaesthesia. *Laryngoscope, St. Louis* **86**, 399–404.

—— LOCKWOOD, R. W., and SHEEHY, J. L. (1967). Temporalis fascia in tympanic membrane grafting. *Archs Otolar.* **85**, 287–91.

PLESTER, D. and STEINBACH, E. (1977). Histologic fate of tympanic membrane and ossicle homografts. *Otol. Clin. N. Am.* **10**, 487–99.

REEVE, D. R. E. (1977). Repair of large experimental perforations of the tympanic membrane. *J. Lar. Otol.* **91**, 767–78.

RENVALL, U., LIDEN, G., and BJORKMAN, G. (1975). Experimental tympanometry in human temporal bones. *Scand. Audiol.* **4**, 135–44.

ROBIN, P. E., BENNETT, R. J., and GREGORY, M. (1976). Study of autogenous transposed ossicles, bone and cartilage. *Clin. Otolar.* **1**, 295–308.

SALEN, B. (1968). Tympanic membrane grafts of full thickness skin, fascia and cartilage with its perichondrium. *Acta oto-lar.* Suppl. 244.

SARACENO, C. A., GRAY, W. C., and BLANCHARD, C. L. (1978). Use of tragal cartilage with the total ossicular replacement prosthesis. *Archs Otolar.* **104**, 213.

SCHUKNECHT, H. F. (1971). *Stapedectomy.* Little Brown, Boston.

—— (1974). *Pathology of the ear.* Havard University Press.

SHAW, E. A. G. (1972). Acoustic response of external ear with progressive wave source. *J. acoust. Soc. Am.* **51**, 150.

—— (1974). Transformation of sound pressure level from the free field to the ear drum in the horizontal plane. *J. acoust. Soc. Am.* **56**, 1848–61.

SHEA, J. J. and EMMETT, J. R. (1978). Biocompatible ossicular implants. *Archs Otolar.* **104**, 191–6.

SHIMADA, T. and LIM, D. J. (1971). The fiber arrangement of the human tympanic membrane. *Ann. Otol.* **80**, 210–17.

SIEDENTOP, K. H. CORRIGAN, R. A., LOEWY, A., and OSENAR, S. B. (1978). Eustachian tube function assessed with tympanometry. *Ann. Otolar.* **87**, 163–9.

SMYTH, G. D. L. (1978). Immediate and delayed alterations in cochlear function following stapedectomy. *Otol. Clin. N. Am.* **11**, 105.

—— and HASSARD, T. H. (1978). Eighteen years experience in stapedectomy. The case for the small fenestra operation. *Ann. Otol.* Suppl. 49, **87.**

—— —— and KERR, A. G. (1978). Ossicular replacement prostheses. *Archs Otolar.* **104,** 345–51.

—— KERR, A. G., and GOODEY, R. J. (1971). Current thoughts on combined approach tympanoplasty. *J. Lar. Otol.* **85**, 417–30.

—— —— and HASSARD, T. H. (1977). Homograft materials in tympanoplasty. *Otol. Clin. N. Am.* **10**, 563–80.

STARR, A. and SCHWARTZKROIN, P. (1972). Cochlear microphonic and middle ear pressure changes during nitrous oxide anaesthesia in cats. *J. acoust. Soc. Am.* **51**, 1367–9.

THOMSEN, K. A., TERKILDSEN, K., and ARNFRED, I. (1965). Middle ear pressure variations during anaesthesia. *Archs Otolar.* **82**, 609–11.

TJELLSTRÖM, A., LINDSTÖM, J., ALBREKTSSON, T., BRANEMARK, P. I. and HALLEN, O. (1978). A clinical pilot study on preformed autologous ossicles. *Acta oto-lar.* **85**, 33–9.

TONNDORF, J. (1977). Modern methods for measurements of basilar membrane displacement. *Acta oto-lar.* **83**, 113–22.

—— and KHANNA, S. M. (1972). Tympanic membrane vibrations in human cadaver ears studied by time-averaged holography. *J. acoust. Soc. Am.* **52**, 1221–33.

—— —— (1976). Mechanics of the auditory system. In *Scientific foundation of otolaryngology* (ed. R. Hinchcliffe and D. Harrison) p. 237. Heinemann, London.

—— —— and GREENFIELD, E. C. (1971). The function of reconstructed tympanic membranes in cats. *Ann. Otolar.* **80**, 861–70.

—— —— —— (1972). Total myringroplasty: functional aspects. *Acta oto-lar.* **73**, 87–93.

—— MCARDLE, F., and KRUGER, B. (1976). Middle ear transmission losses caused by tympanic membrane perforations in cats. *Acta oto-lar.* **81**, 330.

TOS, M. (1978). Allograft stapes—incus assembly. *Archs Otolar.* **104**, 119–21.

VELDMAN, J. E. and KUIJPERS. W. (1978). Experimental and clinical immunopathology of middle ear transplantation. *Clin. Otolar.* **3**, 293–5.

WAUN, J. E., SWEITZER, R. S., and HAMILTON, W. R. (1967). Effect of nitrous oxide on middle ear mechanics and hearing acuity. *Anaesthesiology* **28**, 846–50.

WINTER, L. E. and HOHMANN, A. (1967). Incus homograft viability in cats. *Archs Otolar.* **86**, 44–8.

ZWISLOCKI, J. J. (1962). Analysis of the middle ear function. Part 1. Input impedance. *J. acoust. Soc. Am.* **34**, 1514–23.

20 Surgical management of deafness in adults: the inner ear

A. W. MORRISON

The principles of surgery of the external and middle ear for the relief of conductive deafness are already well established, and the few problems that remain have largely been indentified. Surgical and electrophysiological expertise in the area of sensorineural hearing loss in adults is now being directed towards the inner ear. The surgery is in its infancy and there is still a great deal to be learnt and understood, however, as far as we can foresee it will never have a great part to play in the management of sensorineural lesions; the old adage of prevention being better than cure should continue to apply to such causative factors as noise, ototoxic drugs, chronic local suppuration, and temporal bone trauma in its many guises. Eventually it may be possible to identify and rectify the abnormal enzyme systems associated with the severe forms of hereditary deafness which may occur in adult life, including otosclerosis. Nevertheless, there are a few causes of adult sensorineural deafness which clearly call for surgical treatment, and a number of others where the surgical indications, though more controversial, are at times compelling.

LOCALIZATION OF THE LESION

It is important to undertand that *audiological* is not necessarily synonymous with *pathological* localization. The whole clinical picture must be taken into account in arriving at a diagnosis. For example a fair proportion of patients with acoustic neuromas, especially when the lesion is small or if there are bilateral tumours, exhibit a sensory (end organ) type of hearing loss on audiological testing, irrespective of which tests are employed, Similarly the sudden hearing loss which can be the presenting symptom of a brainstem glioma shows a recruiting type of deafness though speech discrimination tends to be poor. Conversely some peripheral lesions, e.g. labyrinthine window rupture, may mimic a retrocochlear loss; the audiological picture can be confused by the secondary neuronal degeneration which may follow such peripheral lesions. Many examples of these 'false' audiological localizations are given by Morrison (1975).

LABYRINTHINE WINDOW RUPTURE

For a long time, otologists have been conversant with the problems of perilymph fistula following stapedectomy or head injury. In the case of the latter the fracture may traverse the otic capsule causing leakage from the oval or round window or both. In 1971 Goodhill introduced the concept of 'spontaneous' labyrinthine window rupture which may occur after sudden pressure changes experienced during flying or diving, though occasionally after exertion or straining, and rarely without these predisposing factors. Sudden sensorineural hearing loss may be followed by true fluctuations in hearing levels and by variable tinnitus and vertigo. Since 1971 there have been many descriptions of spontaneous window rupture (e.g. Freeman and Edmonds 1972; Pullen 1972; Edmonds, Freeman, Thomas, and Blackwood 1973; Goodhill, Harris, Brockman and Hantz 1973; Fraser and Harborow 1975; Morrison 1975, 1976a, 1978; Tonkin and Fagan 1975; Goodhill 1976). The hearing loss is usually high-tone though it may vary from a fall-off over 2 kHz to subtotal deafness. A fairly consistent audiological feature, despite the predominantly sensory lesion, is the failure to elicit the acoustic (stapedial) reflex by supraliminal pure-tone stimulation of the affected ear above 1 to 1.5 kHz even though there is fair residual hearing to, say, 6 kHz. When the reflex can be elicited at lower frequencies it may show abnormal decay. The features are suggestive of a retrocochlear lesion. In such ears transtympanic electrocochleography usually reveals an objective threshold which is higher than the subjective one, a normally-shaped compound action potential and a distorted cochlear microphonic of a very small voltage, even to stimulation with clicks or sine waves at 100 or 110 dB.

It is important to recognize both the traumatic and spontaneous variants of labyrinthine window rupture since early surgical repair—usually with a fat graft—carries the prospect of reversing the hearing loss. Even in advanced cases with severe loss, repair usually abolishes vertiginous symptoms and the risk of meningitis from CSF leakage.

ACOUSTIC NEUROMA

Preservation of useful hearing following the removal of an acoustic neuroma is possible in only a very small percentage of patients. There are a number of reasons why this aim is seldom achieved. Schuknecht (1974) maintains, quite correctly, that these tumours should be called vestibular Schwannomas since, with few exceptions, they arise from the vestibular nerve(s) in the internal auditory canal. In theory it should be possible to excise these simple tumours while preserving both the facial and the acoustic nerves from the periphery to the brainstem. In practice, however, this is not the case.

Unfortunately many tumours when first diagnosed are already so large that the aim of therapy must be to achieve total removal with as low a mortality and morbidity as possible. Even when the tumour is of medium size, for example 2 to 3 cm in the cerebellopontine angle, the acoustic nerve is frequently so compressed as to be unrecognizable and inseparable from the tumour. When we come to consider small tumours confined to the internal meatus or just budding into the cerebellopontine angle, we find that the hearing is often not worth preserving; furthermore, at surgery, the tumour has often insinuated itself between the facial and acoustic nerves. In such cases dissections and preservation of the former nerve results in trauma to the latter or in damage to the cochlear blood supply. Fortunately there is a pre-operative indication available in respect of tumour separation (at the periphery) from the cochlear nerve. Morrison, Gibson, and Beagley (1976), analysing the electrocochleography findings in patients with retrocochlear tumours, found that a prolonged compound action potential (loss of the P1 wave) was associated with a cochlear nerve which was surgically separable, while a more normally shaped potential was associated with a Schwannoma which could not be surgically separated even peripherally.

Thus, in order even to consider the preservation of hearing in these patients, diagnosis must be early, the lesion must be intracanalicular (or nearly so), and the pre-operative tests must have shown hearing thresholds and discrimination good enough to warrant the different surgical approach which is necessary. Ideally the action potential should also be abnormally prolonged.

Since the pioneering work of House (1964) and of Hitselberger and House (1966), many neurosurgical/otological units have developed throughout the world. In the majority of these units surgery involves the translabyrinthine approach to the internal meatus and cerebellepontine angle (with modifications where necessary). Mortality and morbidity are greatly reduced when compared with the pre-microsurgical days. This surgical route, of course, destroys the function of the ear.

To preserve hearing the approach may be via the middle fossa to uncap the roof of the internal auditory meatus, or via the retrosigmoid (modified suboccipital) route to uncap the posterior wall of the meatus. The middle fossa approach, used mainly for vestibular neurectomy on for exposing the facial nerve, is considered by many to be too limited for the safe removal of acoustic neuromas. There are, however, several reports of this approach being used (e.g. Pulec, House, Britton, and Hitselberger 1971; Portmann 1973; Fisch 1976, 1977). Fisch (1976) emphasizes that only intracanalicular tumours of less than 8 mm may be operated on in this way and even so the hearing is lost in 25 per cent of such cases.

The posterior fossa approach, with the objective of preserving hearing following total tumour removal, has been well described by Smith, Miller, and Cox (1973). Smith and Clancy (1977), and Smith, Clancy, and Lang (1977). Of the 33 patients operated on by this approach ten with tumours of 14–20 mm had useful pre-operative hearing in the affected ear, and of these, useful hearing levels were maintained post-operatively in only three cases. In a period of 18 months in the Department of Otoneurosurgery at The London Hospital, 45 acoustic neuromas and 14 other space-occupying lesions of the cerebellopontine angle were diagnosed and operated.

Of these 59 lesions, only seven small lesions were considered suitable for the posterior fossa approach with the objective of preserving hearing (six acoustic tumours and one meningioma of the internal meatus). Good hearing has been preserved in the meningioma and an island of valueless hearing in two of the acoustic tumours. These figures help to put the subject in perspective.

The posterior fossa operation gives an excellent exposure of the tumour, the brain stem, and the vessels of the angle and of the fifth to ninth cranial nerves, but it is necessary to retract the cerebellum. The post-operative convalescence is usually more prolonged and difficult after the removal of a very small tumour by this route compared with the removal of a much larger lesion through the labyrinth.

OTHER POSTERIOR FOSSA LESIONS

About 80 per cent of space-occupying lesions in the cerebellopontine angle—where varying degrees and types of hearing loss form part of the clinical picture—are acoustic neuromas. Neuromas also arise from other cranial nerves, the facial (VIIth), trigeminal (Vth), and jugular foramen nerves (IXth, Xth, or XIth) and rarely from the abducent (VIth) nerve. Meningiomas of the posterior fossa are not uncommon and pontine gliomas are encountered from time to time. Chordomas of the clivus can involve one or both cerebellopontine angles but secondary malignant tumours and haemangiomas in this site are rare. Developmental cholesteatomas or epidermoids of the angle which grow slowly to involve the brainstem are more common as is fusiform dilatation of the basilar artery (ectasia) which causes all the symptoms and signs of a space-occupying condition.

The advent of computerized axial tomography (the CT scan) has greatly assisted in the differentiation of these lesions, though considerable clinical judgement and neuroradialogical expertise are still required to reach a pre-operative diagnosis. This is not just an academic exercise since the surgical approach should be modified according to the exact site and type of the lesion. For example a very small intrapetrous facial neuroma may be excised, with preservation of hearing, by the middle fossa route (Fisch 1976); jugular Schwannomas may be removed by the sub-occipital approach with preservation or improvement of hearing (Clemis, Noffsinger, and Derlacki 1977); the brainstem and angle may be approached via the middle fossa with division of the tentorium cerebelli for the removal of chordomas, meningiomas, and trigeminal neurinomas without interference to the inner ear or eighth cranial nerve (Morrison and King 1973); and lesions at the petrous apex and clivus may be removed by the infra-temporal approach (Fisch 1978).

Of the 14 other space occupying lesions mentioned above under 'Acoustic Neuroma', hearing has been preserved or improved by the transtentorial operation in two cases of trigeminal neurinomas, one case of chordoma, one case of meningioma, and one case of brainstem glioma, while the suboccipital operation has been employed to preserve hearing in one case of meningioma and one case of jugular neurinoma.

MÉNIÈRE'S DISEASE

Many surgical treatments have been devised to manage Ménière's disease.

Some of them are intentionally destructive such as the transtympanic removal of the utricle (Schuknecht 1956), transmastoid avulsion of the membranous lateral semicircular duct (Cawthorne 1943, 1960), osseous and membranous labyrinthectomy or translabyrinthine eighth nerve section (Morrison 1975), and transtympanic transcochlear eighth nerve section (Silverstein 1977), the latter two procedures offering the prospect of some relief from distracting tinnitus.

Other operations intend to conserve hearing but nevertheless run the risk of further hearing loss. Into this category fall sacculotomy (Fick 1964) and its modifications (Cody 1969; Cody, Simonton and Hallberg 1967), topical osmosis by the application of sodium chloride crystals to the round window (Arslan 1972), cryosurgery of the promontory (House 1962, 1968), and to a lesser extent ultrasonic treatment of the labyrinth (James 1963; Stahle 1976) and middle fossa vestibular neurectomy (House 1961; Fisch 1973). Destructive surgery, ultrasonic treatment, and selective vestibular neurectomy have a definite part to play in the management of Ménière's disease, though mainly for the control of vertigo.

In recent years there has been a revival of interest in surgery of the endolymphatic sac since this offers the prospect not only of stabilizing but of reversing the hearing loss (House and Owens 1973; Turner, Saunders, and Per-Lee 1973; Shambaugh 1975; Morrison 1975, 1976b; Paparella and Hanson 1976; Arenberg and Spector 1977; Glasscock, Miller, Drake, and Kanok 1977; Maddox 1977). Provided the surgery is carried out with great care avoiding possible damage to the posterior semicircular canal, and provided the interference with the sac is minimal, there is virtually no risk of making the hearing worse. This opens the door to surgery on the only hearing or better hearing ear, a situation which is commonly presented to the otologist with a special interest in this problem.

Morrison (1975) and Stahle (1976) have re-examined the nature and history of Ménière's disease and found that although the degree of hearing loss may stabilize for quite long periods of time, the general tendency is for progressive (though occasionally rapid) deterioration in thresholds and discrimination coupled with increasing vestibular hypofunction over the years. Fluctuation in the degree of hearing loss, which is so characteristic of the earlier stages of the disease, tends, with the passage of time to be replaced by irreversibility. Another important feature is the high percentage of bilateral cases; within the first two years of onset some 15 per cent of cases are bilateral; after 20 years almost 45 per cent are bilateral. Stahle, Stahle, and Arenberg (1978), in an important survey, have emphasized the importance of this disease, which affects nearly 1 in 2000 of the population of Sweden.

In many patients with endolymphatic hydrops, whether idiopathic as in Ménière's disease (Gibson, Moffat, and Ramsden 1977; Gibson 1978) or secondary to diseases of the otic capsule such as late syphilis (Ramsden, Moffat, and Gibson 1977), transtympanic electrocochleography reveals an enchanced negative summating potential and a cochlear microphonic potential which varies greatly in amplitude from patient to patient. This negative summating potential may decrease, while the amplitude of the cochlear microphonic potential may increase following glycerol-induced dehydration; proof of the dehydration must be demonstrated by a rise of serum osmolality of at least 10 mOsm kg (Moffat, Gibson, Ramsden, Morrison, and Booth 1978). This latter test appears to be of a more sensitive indicator of changes occurring in the cochlea (and of potential reversibility) than the more commonly practised dehydration study of changes in pure-tone thresholds and speech discrimination.

Morrison (unpublished observations), analysing the results of almost 300 endolymphatic sac operations, has found that the best hearing results following surgery are obtained when Ménière's disease has been present for less than two years, when the vestibular responses are normal or nearly so, when there is a significant improvement in pure-tone thresholds and/or discrimination or a significant change in the electrical potentials following glycerol dehydration, and when electrocochleography prior to surgery has revealed no abnormal negative summating potential and/or a cochlear microphonic of normal amplitude. These results are no more than might be anticipated and they emphasize the importance of considering surgery early in the course of this disease. Though the rationale of operations on the endolymphatic sac (to drain endolymph) seem reasonable, there is no proof as to how the undoubted clinical results are sometimes achieved (Schuknecht 1977). Unfortunately electrocochleography has not yet provided a clue since, with few exceptions, the inner ear potentials before and long after surgery show little if any change irrespective of the hearing result.

Ménière's disease affects primarily and initially the pars inferior (cochlear duct and saccule). Cochlear hydrops presenting as sudden or fluctuant sensory deafness and tinnitus, without vertigo, may be managed in the same way as Ménière's disease itself. The first essential is to recognize the condition.

COCHLEAR IMPLANTATION

The use of electrical auditory stimulation in the management of profound hearing loss is approaching the stage of development when it should soon pass from an experimental to a therapeutic measure. The subject is covered in Chapter 22. The present situation in the United States, and elsewhere, has recently been reviewed by Ballantyne, Evans, and Morrison (1978). There seems little doubt that, following cochlear implantation, the information which can be conveyed by a single-channel stimulation if adequately exploited, can assist the totally or subtotally deaf to achieve partial rehabilitation; there is release from a world of silence, there is an aid to the identification of important environmental sounds, there is an aid to lip reading and to the patient's articulation and intonation, and there can be relief from tinnitus. This is a start.

To restore unaided speech intelligibility multiple-channel implants will be required and, as yet, these are no more effective than single-channel devices; more electrodes, suitably located and with adequate inter-electrode isolation are necessary, together with appropriate coding strategies and reliable transcutaneous transmission systems. It will also be necessary to develop electrode and insulation materials suitable for long-term use. It has yet to be demonstrated what percentage and distribution of surviving auditory neurones are required for multichannel stimulation to be adequately effective. Despite these formidable obstacles encouraging starts have been made to this aspect of the work which is still experimental and which should involve only carefully selected volunteer patients in units with all the appropriate expertise.

DECOMPRESSION OF THE INTERNAL AUDITORY CANAL

The internal auditory meatus varies considerably in its normal dimension and shape from patient to patient, the vertical diameter being sometimes as small as 2.5 mm, sometimes as large as 12 mm. In the absence of congenital defects or tumour pathology the right and left sides in the same individual rarely vary by more than 2.5 mm in this plane. It seems very doubtful if an uncomplicated anatomical narrowing of the canal is responsible for deafness, tinnitus, or vertigo. Nevertheless, there are reports of middle fossa decompression of the canal resulting in slight hearing gain (Glassock 1969; House and Brackmann 1978).

Neuroradiological investigation of patients with unilateral sensorineural deafness occasionally reveals an anterior inferior cerebellar artery coiled within the internal canal. Decompression can be indicated in this situation.

Certain bone diseases, however, may cause some narrowing. House (1961) reported the results of middle fossa decompression of the internal meatus in patients with severe sensorineural deafness owing to otosclerosis. This surgery failed to help but it is historically interesting since it was the stimulus which ushered in the middle fossa approach to the canal. Various cranial nerves, including the seventh and eighth, may be compressed in their exit foraminae by the rare disease osteopetrosis (marble bones). Surgical decompression may be able to prevent the inner ear problems (Hamersma 1973) though it seems likely that, as with other generalized bone diseases (e.g. Paget's disease or osteogenesis imperfecta) compression of nerve fibres is as likely to occur in the modiolus. This surgery must, therefore, be considered as experimental, as must attempts to improve the vascularization of the inner ear by turning muscle flaps into the internal canal from above (Portmann 1973).

REFERENCES

Arenberg, I. K. and Spector, G. J. (1977) Endolymphatic sac surgery for hearing conversation in the Ménière disease. *Archs Otolar.* **103**, 268–70.

Arslan, M. (1972). Treatment of Ménière's disease by apposition of sodium chloride crystals on the round window. *Laryngoscope, St. Louis* **82**, 1736–50.

Ballantyne, J. C. Evans, E. F., and Morrison, A. W. (1978). Electrical auditory stimulation in the management of profound hearing loss. *J. Lar. Otol.* Suppl. **1**, 1–117.

Cawthorne, T. (1943). The treatment of Ménière's disease. *J. Lar. Otol.* **58**, 363–71.

—— (1960). Labyrinthectomy. *Ann. Otol.* **69**, 1170–80.

Clemis, J. D., Noffsinger, D. and Derlacki, E. L. (1977). A Jugular foramen Schwannoma simulating an acoustic tumour with recovery of retro-layrinthine cochleovestibular function. *Trans. Am. Acad. Opthal. Otolar.* **77**, 687–96.

Cody, D. T. R. (1969). Tack operation for endolymphatic hydrops. *Laryngoscope, St. Louis* **79**, 1737–44.

—— Simonton, K. H., and Hallberg, O. E. (1967). Automatic repetitive decompression of the saccule in endolymphatic hydrops. *Laryngoscope, St. Louis* **77**, 1480–1501.

Edmonds, C., Freeman, P., Thomas, J. P., and Blackwood, F. A. (1973). *Otological aspects of diving.* Australasian Medical, Sydney.

Fick, I. A. van M. (1964). Decompression of the labyrinth: a new surgical procedure for Ménière's disease. *Archs Otolar.* **79**, 447–58.

Fisch, U. (1973). Excision of Scarpa's ganglion. *Archs Otolar.* **97**, 147–9.

—— (1976). The middle fossa approach to the internal auditory meatus. In *Rob and Smith's operative surgery—Ear.* (ed. J. C. Ballantyne) pp. 179–92. Butterworth, London.

—— (1977). Vestibular neurectomy. In *Neurological surgery of the ear* (ed. Silverstein and Norell) pp. 144–9. Aesculapius, Birmingham, Alabama.

—— (1978). Infratemporal fossa approach to tumours of the temporal bone and base of the skull. *J. Lar. Otol.* **92**, 949–67.

Fraser, J. G. and Harborow, P. C. (1975). Labyrinthine window rupture. *J. Lar. Otol.* **89**, 1–7.

Freeman, P. and Edmonds, C. (1972). Inner ear barotrauma. *Archs Otolar.* **95**, 556–63.

Gibson, W. P. R. (1978). *Essentials of clinical electric response audiometry.* Churchill Livingstone, Edinburgh.

—— Moffat, D. A., and Ramsden, R. T. (1977). Clinical electrocochleography in the diagnosis and management of Ménière's disorder. *Audiology* **16**, 389–401.

Glasscock, M. E. (1969). Middle fossa approach to the temporal bone: an otologic frontier. *Archs Otolar.* **90**, 15–27.

—— Miller, G. W., Drake, F. D., and Kanok, M. M. (1977). Surgical management of Ménière's disease with the endolymphatic subarachnoid shunt: a five-year study. *Laryngoscope, St. Louis* **87**, 1668–75.

Goodhill, V. (1971). Sudden deafness and round window rupture. *Laryngoscope, St. Louis* **81**, 1462–74.

—— (1976). Sudden sensorineural deafness: labyrinthine membrane ruptures in sudden sensorineural hearing loss. *Proc. R. Soc. Med.* **69**, 565–72.

—— Harris, I., Brockman, S. J., and Hantz, O. (1973). Sudden deafness and labyrinthine window ruptures. Audio-vestibular observations. *Ann. Otol. Rhinol. Lar.* **82**, 2–12.

Hamersha, H. (1974). Total decompression of facial nerve in osteoporosis. *ORL* **36**, 21–32.

Hitselberger, W. E. and House, W. F. (1966). Surgical approaches to acoustic tumors. *Archs Otolar.* **84**, 286–91.

House, W. F. (1961). Surgical exposure of the internal auditory canal and its contents through the middle cranial fossa. *Laryngoscope, St. Louis* **71**, 1363–85.

—— (1962). Subarachnoid shunt for drainage of endolymphatic hydrops: a preliminary report. *Laryngoscope, St. Louis* **72**, 713–29.

—— (1964). Transtemporal bone microsurgical removal of acoustic neuromas. *Archs Otolar.* **80**, 597–756.

—— (1968). Cryosurgery of the promontory. *Otolar. Clin. N. Am.* October, 669–81.

—— and Brackmann, D. E. (1978). Dizziness due to stenosis of the internal auditory canal. In *Neurological surgery of the ear* (eds. Silverstein and Norell) pp. 150–6. Aesculapius, Birmingham Alabama.

—— and Owns, F. D. (1973). Long-term results of endolymphatic subarachnoid shunt energy in Ménière's disease. *J. Lar. Otol.* **87**, 521–7.

James, J. A. (1963). New developments in the ultrasonic therapy of Ménière's disease. *Ann. R. Coll. Surg.* **33**, 226–44.

Maddox, E. (1977). Endolymphatic sac surgery. *Laryngoscope, St. Louis* **87**, 1676–9.

Moffat, D. A., Gibson, W. P. R., Ramsden, R. T., Morrison, A. W., and Booth, J. B. (1978). Transtympanic electrocochleography during glycerol dehydration. *Acta oto-lar.* **85**, 158–66.

Morrison, A. W. (1975). *Management of sensorineural deafness.* Butterworths, London.

—— (1976a). Sudden sensorineural deafness: outline of management. *Proc. R. Soc. Med.* **69**, 572–4.

—— (1976b). The surgery of vertigo: saccus drainage for idiopathic endolymphatic hydrops. *J. Lar. Otol.* **90**, 87–93.

—— (1978). Acute deafness. *Brit. J. hosp. med.* **19**, 237–49.

—— and King, T. T. (1973). Experiences with a translabyrinthine-transtentorial approach to the cerebellopontine angle. Technical note. *J. Neurosurg.* **38**, 382–90.

—— Gibson, W. P. R., and Beagley, H. A. (1976). Transtympanic electrocochleography in the diagnosis of retrocochlear tumours. *Clin. Otolar.* **1**, 153–67.

Paparella, M. M. and Hanson, D. G. (1976). Endolymphatic sac drainage for intractable vertigo (method and experiences). *Laryngoscope, St. Louis* **86**, 697–702.

Portmann, M. (1973). Surgery of the internal auditory canal. *ORL* **35**, 272–7.

Pulec, J. L., House, W. F., Britton, B. H. Jr., and Hitselberger, W. E. (1971). A system of management of acoustic neuroma based on 364 cases. *Trans. Am. Acad. Ophthal. Otolar.* **75**, 48–55.

Pullen, F. W. (1972). Round window membrane rupture: a cause of sudden deafness. *Trans. Am. Acad. Opthal. Otolar.* **76**, 1444–50.

Ramsden, R. T., Moffat, D. A., and Gibson, W. P. R. (1977). Transtympanic electrocochleography in patients with syphilis and hearing loss. *Ann. Otol. Rhinol. Lar.* **86**, 827–35.

Schuknecht, H. F. (1956). Ablation therapy for the relief of Ménière's disease. *Laryngoscope, St. Louis* **66**, 859–70.

—— (1974). *Pathology of the ear.* Harvard University Press, Cambridge, Massachusetts.

—— (1977). Pathology of Ménière's diesease as it relates to the sac and tack procedures. *Ann. Otol.* **86**, 677–82.

Shambaugh, G. E. Jr. (1975). Effects of endolymphatic sac decompression on fluctuant hearing loss. *Otolar. Clin. N. Am.* **8**, 537–40.

SILVERSTEIN, H. (1977). Transmeatal cochleovestibular neurectomy. In *Neurological surgery of the ear* (ed. Silverstein and Norell) pp. 176–89. Aesculapius, Birmingham, Alabama.

SMITH, M. F. W. and CLANCY, T. P. (1977). Conservation of hearing in acoustic neurilemmoma excision. In *Neurological surgery of the ear* (ed. Silverstein and Norell) pp. 261–2. Aesculapius, Birmingham, Alabama.

—— —— and LANG, J. S. (1977). Conservation of hearing in acoustic neurilemmoma excision. *Trans. Am. Acad. Opthal. Otolar.* **84**, 704–9.

—— MILLER, R. N., and COX D. J. (1973). Suboccipital microsurgical removal of acoustic neurinomas of all sizes. *Ann. Otol. Rhinol. Lar.* **82**, 407–14.

STAHLE, J. (1976). Advanced Ménière's disease. A study of 356 severely disabled patients. *Acta oto-lar.* **81**, 113–19.

—— STAHLE, C., and ARENBERG, I. K. (1978). Incidence of Ménière's disease. *Archs Otolar.* **104**, 99–102.

TONKIN, J. P. and FAGAN, P. (1975). Rupture of the round window membrane. *J. Lar. Otol.* **89**, 733–56.

TURNER, J. S., SAUNDERS, A. Z., and PER-LEE, J. H. (1973). A 10-year profile of Ménière's disease and endolymphatic shunt surgery. *Laryngoscope, St. Louis* **83**, 1816–24.

21 Auditory rehabilitation

S. D. G. STEPHENS

INTRODUCTION

Auditory rehabilitation is the process of helping the hearing impaired individual to function as well as possible, given his reduced sensory input. It involves an attempt to minimize the handicap arising from his hearing loss and to reverse any personality changes deriving from the social isolation caused by his sensory deprivation.

Although it is essentially multidisciplinary in its approach and expertise, it may be regarded as that component of audiological medicine concerned with the management of those patients who cannot or can only partially be helped by surgical or medical treatment of their hearing loss.

It may be subdivided into: (i) patient evaluation; (ii) fitting of appropriate prosthesis(es); (iii) counselling and re-education; (iv) environmental aids; and (v) management of employment and social problems. Not all patients will require the same approach. This must clearly be 'tailored' to the specific needs of the individual patient and it is essential at all times to remember that the rehabilitation should be geared to an individual with specific needs and problems rather than to an audiometric configuration. Indeed two people with identical hearing losses may suffer entirely different handicaps and have completely different needs.

PATIENT GROUPS

Patients seen from a rehabilitative standpoint generally fall into four main groups: (i) the elderly with an acquired hearing loss, (ii) the prelingually deaf adult; (iii) the adult with a sudden deafness; and (iv) the working-age adult with an acquired hearing loss.

The elderly hearing impaired

This group comprises by far the largest group of patients presenting for auditory rehabilitation. Most recent studies (e.g. Brooks 1979; Stephens, Barcham, Corcoran, and Parsons (1980) suggest that over 75 per cent of patients being fitted with hearing aids for the first time are over 60 years of age. This is to be expected when the prevalence data of hearing loss is examined as a function of age. Such analyses (e.g. Plomp 1978) indicate that the prevalence of significant hearing loss increases logarithmically with age, with some 50 per cent of patients aged 80 having such a loss. Data from Merluzzi and Hinchcliffe (1973), however, suggest that older patients regard hearing loss as relatively less of a handicap. This may be related partly to the presence of similar hearing problems among many of their contemporaries, but also to other physical problems which increase in prevalence with advancing age and which may be regarded by the patients as being more serious than their hearing difficulties.

Data suggest that the average person in this age group seeking rehabilitative treatment will have had a hearing problem for some 15–20 years before actually seeking help (e.g. Stephens *et al.* 1980). Unfortunately this often means that he is more arthritic and finds it more difficult to learn the new hearing skills than he might have done had he sought treatment earlier.

Most of this group also have a moderate hearing loss of some 40–60 dB HL across the main speech frequencies and hence do not need a great deal of amplification. Many are isolated and about one-third live alone (Stephens *et al.* 1980) so that their communication needs are often limited. It has been argued that, with such individuals, the provision of environmental aids to help them hear the doorbell, the telephone, and the television together with social service involvement to reduce their isolation within the community, may be far more important than the fitting of a hearing aid.

When such a hearing aid is fitted, much emphasis generally needs to be placed on the fitting of the ear mould within the ear and associated general manipulative skills such as handling the controls, changing the battery, etc., and a considerable follow-up service, often on a domiciliary basis, may be necessary.

The prelingually deaf adult

This group may present to the rehabilitation clinic when they leave school and the supportive facilities associated with it, or they may reject amplification on leaving school and seek help some years later when they find a normally hearing spouse, have normally hearing children, or find themselves in a work situation in which they want to make more use of their residual hearing.

The help needed by such individuals varies greatly according to the degree of their hearing loss and communication skills. A recent extensive study on deaf school leavers in the United Kingdom (Conrad 1979) has certainly not been encouraging in this respect, and it is often extremely difficult to help the prelingually deaf adult dramatically at this stage.

It is important, however, to ensure that he is fitted with the hearing aid(s) best suited for his needs. It is essential that close liaison is maintained with social workers with regard to the installation of appropriate environmental aids, with the employment services in the context of job training, and with adult education services to provide on-going education which could lead to an improvement of the patient's employment prospects.

Within the rehabilitation scheme, general audiovisual communication training may be necessary, although in many cases advice on the tactics necessary to use in such circumstances may be all that is needed. In certain cases the patient's communicative skills both oral/aural and manual may be so poor as a result of certain attitudes within the education system that it may be necessary to organize training in manual communication for the patient in order to give him any meaningful social contacts.

The patient with complete acquired hearing loss

This condition affecting both ears is fortunately a rare event. It is estimated that in the whole of Denmark there are less than 100 such patients (Skamris, personal communication) so that extrapolating on a population basis to the United Kingdom, there are probably less than 1000 here. There are rather more such patients who have a severe or profound loss but these can at least derive some benefit from amplification.

Those with bilateral complete loss present with considerable problems in many ways, from communicative, employment, and psychological points of view. What they are experiencing is a complete change in their lifestyle which is entirely different from the problems of the prelingually deaf, who have never known any different situation. Thus, not surprisingly, the psychological problems in particular are markedly different in these two groups of patients.

From a communicative standpoint there has been much controversy as to the orientation of the rehabilitative process. All are agreed on an orientation towards speech-reading (lip-reading) but there is considerable controversy as to what should be used to augment this somewhat limited communication channel. Various sensory communication aids have been tried using vibrotactile or visual stimulation but these have not been particularly successful. Recently much effort has gone into direct electrical stimulation of the cochlear nerve (e.g. Fourcin, Rosen, Moore, Douek, Clarke, Dodson, and Bannister, 1979) but this is at a very early stage of development and presupposes the presence of a significant number of surviving cochlear nerve fibres. Finally manual systems of communication may be used and even here there is controversy as to whether the best approach is a procedure like the Mouth-Hand System which merely supplements speech-reading or whether a system complete in itself should be used, such as the British Sign Language.

The patient of working age with an acquired hearing loss

Patients in this group are often very responsive to prosthetic help with hearing aids and other devices but need considerable support from the employment and psychological standpoints. A recent study (Thomas and Gilhome Herbst 1980) has shown a high prevalence of psychological illness among patients within this group, particularly if they have a fairly severe loss, so that the need for wider use of counselling and group rehabilitative sessions within this group must always be borne in mind.

PATIENT EVALUATION

Before a relevant approach to rehabilitation can be defined there is a great need for a comprehensive evaluation of the patient. This may be divided into three components; (i) medical evaluation; (ii) psychosocial evaluation; and (iii) communicative evaluation.

Medical evaluation

This is necessary to define whether the patient's hearing loss is caused by any condition which may be treatable, at least in part, by medical or surgical intervention. Even if the patient's hearing can be improved only slightly in this way, there may be benefit in that it might be possible to use a more versatile prosthetic approach, and related symptoms such as vertigo and tinnitus may be reduced. Furthermore, the patient coming for auditory rehabilitation may have more general systemic disorders which have not been detected or adequately treated by the primary physician, and for which suitable therapy must be initiated.

The details of the medical evaluation of the hearing-impaired patient have been dealt with elsewhere in this book and will not be considered further at this stage.

Psychosocial evaluation

This is probably the most critical single part of the evaluative procedure and one which will define the various strategies to be adopted in the rehabilitative process. It entails a definition of the real needs and problems of the patient from a personal and social point of view and is something which often cannot be completely elucidated at the first session. Many aspects of a patient's problems may only emerge in the course of the rehabilitative process, and group sessions may be useful in this respect. Thus it is essential to maintain a flexible approach to the rehabilitative strategy adopted and to modify it where relevant new information is presented.

The patient's psychosocial problems may be approached by direct problem evaluation techniques, by the use of purpose-made handicap scales of one kind or another, or by an investigation of personality changes.

DIRECT PROBLEM EVALUATION

This seeks to delimit the difficulties encountered by the patient and the consequences of these difficulties. These may cover a wide range of factors encompassing his everyday life: communication needs, difficulties in the work place, and consequential social and psychological problems. Many of these may emerge at an interview, others may be highlighted by discussions with the patient's 'significant others' (i.e. spouse, companion, close friends, workmates, etc.). However, a visit to hospital, hearing-aid centre, or rehabilitation clinic is a stressful experience for many patients who may find it difficult to express their real difficulties under these circumstances. Consequently, the use of a 'problems questionnaire' sent to the patient with his appointment letter and returned by him by post or when he comes for his appointment, has been found to give much useful information (Barcham and Stephens 1980). This enables the patient to reflect on his true problems in the security of his own environment and achieve a more realistic insight to his situation. The questionnaire used is phrased as follows:

Please make a list of the problems which you have as a result of your hearing loss. List these in order of importance starting with the biggest problem. Write down as many as you can think of.

This approach has provided much useful information for the development of individual rehabilitative strategies and may also provide a starting point for further discussions with the patient to clarify his real problems. It is also of value in the evaluation of the effectiveness of the rehabilitative approach adopted for the particular patient by being repeated after the basic rehabilitative programme has been completed. In some preliminary data on this point (Stephens *et al.* 1980) both quantitative and qualitative changes have been found in the patient's responses, with reductions in the number of problems listed on follow-up, and a change in their nature, often being related to some problems encountered with the hearing aid.

HANDICAP MEASURES

A variety of approaches have been adopted to the assessment of hearing handicap, and these have been discussed at some length by various authors (e.g. Noble 1978; Stephens 1980a). All are designed to provide some quantitative measure of the patient's handicap so that changes resulting from the rehabilitative programme may be evaluated consequently in a quantitative manner.

Various attempts have been made to relate handicap to hearing loss (e.g. Ewertsen and Birk Nielsen 1973; Noble 1978; Habib and Hinchcliffe 1978); however, although all show a positive correlation between hearing loss and handicap, the hearing loss accounts for only a small part of the total inter-subject variance. It may thus be summarized that personal and social factors also contribute to the total handicap measure, although there has been no systematic investigation of this hypothesis.

There have been three types of handicap measure used, self-responding questionnaires sent to or presented to the patient, interviewer-administered questionnaires, and a simple scaling approach. In the last (e.g. Habib and Hinchcliffe 1978) the patient is merely informed that there is a scale of handicap ranging from 0–100 in which 100 is the handicap produced from a complete hearing loss. The patient is then required to place himself on this scale. This approach has not been used extensively in auditory rehabilitation and preliminary results (Stephens 1980a) indicate poor correlation with other handicap measures. Furthermore, many patients find it difficult to grasp the concept involved, and others tend consistently to give a response of 50, bisecting the scale.

Among the more widely used scales most items are orientated towards speech discrimination problems. This is true of the Hearing Handicap Scale (HHS) (High, Fairbanks, and Glorig 1964) the Social Hearing Handicap Index (SHHI) (Ewertsen and Birk Nielsen 1973), and others. Some, such as the HHS give a wide range of response categories but others (e.g. SHHI) require only a yes–no response. Experience with the use of these scales in general rehabilitative practice favours the latter as many patients fail to comply with the more detailed instructions required by the multicategory measure.

The best known interviewer-based questionnaire is the Hearing Measurement Scale (HMS) of Noble and Atherley (1970). This has different measures of speech problems, non-speech problems, sound localization, and emotional response, together with a number of minor categories. Its disadvantage is the time taken for its administration, but it is a valuable scale giving a number of useful measures and many of the questions often provoke responses from the patient giving consderable insight into his real difficulties. The sensitivity of the measure is illustrated by Fig. 21.1, which shows the handicap scale measures in a patient with a symmetrical hearing loss given a monaural hearing-aid fitting. The scores before and after rehabilitation show a general improvement in all the major scales except localization which, as might have been predicted, showed a deterioration in performance.

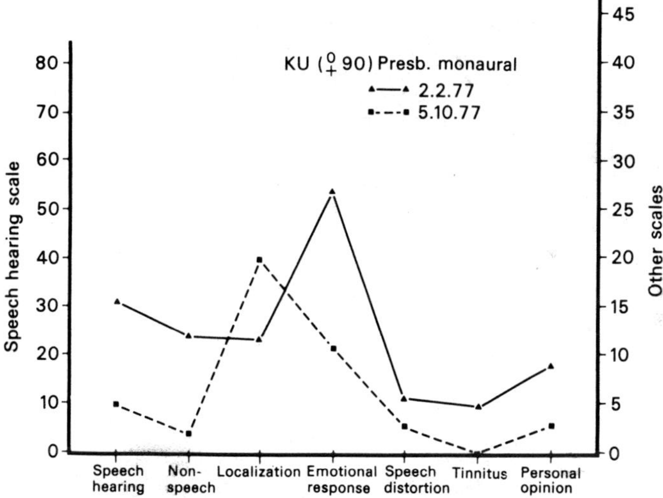

Fig. 21.1. Hearing Measurement Scale scores before and after auditory rehabilitation in a patient with a bilateral symmetrical hearing loss who insisted on having a monaural hearing aid fitted.

PERSONALITY MEASURES

There have been few systematic studies of personality in patients with acquired hearing loss. The work of Thomas and Gilhome Herbst (1980) indicates a high prevalence of psychological disorders as defined by the Bedford and Foulds Screening Scale of anxiety and depression (1978). This high prevalence occurs particularly in patients with hearing losses exceeding

70 dB HL and with poor speech discrimination. Stephens (1980a) found a group of hearing-impaired patients to be more introverted, anxious, and obsessional than a population of ENT out-patients.

There have been so far no extensive follow up studies to determine as to whether the patient's personality profiles became more normal following a course of auditory rehabilitation. This would constitute an interesting study, particularly in view of Gildston and Gildston's demonstration (1972) that the personality of otosclerotic patients becomes significantly closer to normal following a successful stapedectomy.

Communicative evaluation

All means of communication open to the hearing-impaired patient must be used to their fullest extent. This evaluation of a patient's communicative performance must not be restricted to tests of auditory function but must include his visual acuity, speech-reading performance, skills in manual communication, linguistic background, speech production, etc. In addition it is perhaps relevant to determine his manual dexterity.

AUDITORY EVALUATION

The three main audiometric measures traditionally considered important in the evaluation of patients prior to a rehabilitative scheme are pure-tone threshold determination, speech discrimination measures, and uncomfortable loudness levels (e.g. Markides 1977a). The first and last are important in specifying which hearing aid electroacoustic characteristics might be presupposed to be appropriate for the particular patient. Speech discrimination measures may be useful in estimating the optimal auditory discriminative performance which may be achieved with the hearing aid. If a unilateral hearing-aid fitting is being considered it also may give some indication as to which ear might be most appropriately fitted.

The question of the most appropriate speech material to be used is a matter of some controversy and is dependent on the specific question which is being posed. It may be argued that sentence material along the lines of the Speech Intelligibility in Noise (SPIN) test developed by Kalikow, Stevens, and Elliott (1977) might be valuable in that it comprises two components: one dependent on the use of relevant linguistic information and one independent of this. However, at the present stage it is a far from ideal tool but one which may be a pointer in the right direction.

Recently Tyler (1979) has questioned the whole approach to evaluation of the patient using traditionally audiometric measures and argued that a more direct specification of the patient's psychoacoustical deficits might be more appropriate. This approach, however, must be contingent on the development of hearing-aid technology capable of overcoming these specific deficits.

VISUAL AND AUDIOVISUAL EVALUATION

The first stage in this process and one which should not be neglected, is an evaluation of the patient's visual acuity. This should be performed with the patient wearing his normal spectacles, and is performed largely to warn the patient of any corrective action which may be necessary. This is important to ensure that the patient is able to perform optimally from a visual communication point of view when his auditory input is impaired. A number of studies (e.g. Hardick, Oyer, and Irion 1970) have indicated the limiting effect which impaired vision may have an audiovisual performance.

The precise approach which should be subsequently adopted to the assessment of speech reading performance is more controversial. A variety of test materials have been developed in various parts of the world ranging from consonant or vowel discrimination tests, through words to prosodic features, sentences and stories with or without contextual cues. The relationship between the ability to recognize the basic features and the skills with continuous discourse is a matter of some controversy (e.g. Heider and Heider 1940; Risberg and Angelfors 1978) and one which is far from clear.

From the standpoint of a screening test, simple material of different types may be useful and that used by the author (Table 21.1), loosely based on the work of Skamris (1974), has proved useful in practice. This starts with groups of three digits which most patients can discriminate easily. This gives the patient confidence to continue with other aspects of the test. Place names of cities in the United Kingdom are more problematical but presents the situation of contextual cues with the use of single words. The final section, which is introduced to the patient as questions involving 'food, meals, or shopping' in which the patient is required to repeat as much of each question as possible, gives a closer approximation to a real-life situation with contextual cues.

TABLE 21.1. *Material used by the author in a clinical screening test of speech-reading*

561.
312.
479.
854.
906.
Birmingham.
Cardiff.
London.
Edinburgh.
Reading.
What did you have for breakfast?
Have you had any coffee today?
When do you have your lunch?
Do you take sugar in your tea?
Where do you do your shopping?

For most patients, who require only some guidance in general audiovisual tactics, this is probably adequate. For those with more severe communication problems a study of performance with and without acoustical cues and using more sophisticated materials to clearly define their specific problems is indicated.

MANUAL COMMUNICATION SKILLS

These are particularly important for the prelingually deaf. Their role in patients with acquired postlingual hearing loss is at best minimal.

The only extensive testing of such skills in the context of a general rehabilitative/habitative programme is that carried out at the National Technical Institute for the Deaf (Johnson 1978). There, CID sentence material (Silverman and Hirsh 1955) is presented in different forms including a manual presentation alone and a manual presentation together with other audiovisual cues.

In view of Conrad's recent findings (1979) on the poor communicative performance using oral/aural techniques of deaf school leavers, it is essential that more serious consideration be given to manual techniques at least in those prelingually deaf who acquire only limited oral skills. It is important to evaluate such patients in a systematic manner in order to provide them with adequate guidance in this respect.

HANDLING SKILLS

These are of critical importance in the elderly patient when it comes to the selection of the most appropriate hearing aid. As a result of arthritis, tremors, cerebrovascular accidents, Dupuytren's contracture, and other disorders many patients are unable to cope with the small controls of ear-level hearing aids or even of many of the more 'sophisticated' body worn aids. This is particularly important in the patient living alone (approximately 30 per cent of those fitted with hearing aids), who cannot turn to another person for help.

Various approaches have been made to the assessment of handling skills using a variety of psychomotor tasks. However, in practice, it is probably more valuable to determine handling skills using the actual hearing aid or aids which could be fitted. In this way the patient may be more readily convinced that he needs a bodyworn aid rather than the ear level aid which he might prefer for cosmetic reasons.

SPEECH PRODUCTION

This is not the place to discuss in depth the many aspects of the assessment of the speech production skills of the hearing-impaired patient. It is, however, important that those involved in auditory rehabilitation should be aware of the difficulties and problems which can occur.

Here, more than in any other domain, the difference between the prelingually deaf and those with an acquired hearing loss is most marked. This is true not only of the articulatory quality of the speech but also of its linguistic structure. For further discussion of these problems the reader is referred to Conrad (1979).

The patient with an acquired hearing loss may be assumed to have developed normal language before suffering his auditory deficit so that his main problem is the articulatory/acoustical aspects of his speech. It is important to obtain a baseline measure of his speech quality and this may be obtained by the recording of his reading a passage of prose (e.g. the rainbow passage—see Appendix 21.1) which contains all the phonemes in the English language. Simultaneous recordings on the output from a laryngograph (Fourcin and Abberton 1971) on another track of the tape may complement this with fundamental frequency information. This is particularly important in patients with prelingual hearing loss.

The importance of these measures is that they provide baseline information to demonstrate any changes in the patient's speech production performance which may necessitate the intervention of a speech therapist/pathologist.

SELECTION OF THE APPROPRIATE PROSTHESIS(ES)

Technical aspects of hearing aids have been dealt with elsewhere in this book (Chapter 10). At this juncture, however, it is appropriate to consider various aspects of the basis of the selection of hearing aids, and these may be most appropriately defined by a series of questions which must be answered.

Hearing aid or no hearing aid?

This is a question appropriate to those patients with either very mild or very severe hearing losses. In the case of the patient with a very mild loss, the policy to be followed depends very much on the specific handicap and problems which the individual encounters as a consequence of this hearing loss. Thus if the patient's difficulties stem from a need for amplification in certain limited circumstances, for example, the barrister who would rather not risk asking the judge to repeat himself when involved in a difficult case, amplification may be recommended and provided for those specific circumstances. In other cases where the problem is more one of speech-in-noise discrimination which cannot be significantly helped by a hearing aid, counselling on hearing tactics, guiding the patient as to how to optimize his communication ability in the circumstances in which he finds difficulty, might be more appropriate.

In the case of the patient with a profound hearing loss, even if he has no auditory discrimination of speech, a powerful hearing aid may help his speech reading and may also help him to remain in contact with warning sounds. Certain patients with this problem may tend to reject the aid, but it is important to consider the reasons for such a rejection to define whether these are related simply to the aid selected or to inadequate counselling.

Electric or non-electric aids?

In the latter part of the last century Thomas Hawksley's catalogue of aids to hearing included over 300 different non-electric aids. Currently four are available under the United Kingdom National Health Service: a communication tube, two types of ear trumpets, and a pair of auricles. Some 300 are fitted annually.

Although many technologically orientated individuals may question the value of non-electric aids, some elderly patients do not have the same orientation and may more readily accept such an approach rather than use an electric aid. Such acoustic aids are relevant to patients with mild to moderate hearing losses and their acoustical characteristics have been described by Grover (1977).

Bodyworn or ear-level aids?

Although better quality amplification is still available in bodyworn aids in practice cosmetic and practical considerations in favour of ear-level aids tend to outweigh this factor. Bodyworn aids tend, in general, to be fitted to those patients who are incapable of coping with the controls of ear-level aids, or those who require more amplification than can be provided without feedback by such aids. This latter is contingent also on the quality of ear-moulds being made and the material from which they are made. Thus with a carefully made earmould is produced from a soft acrylic, silicone rubber, or vinyl, considerably more gain may be achieved without feedback than with a standard hard acrylic mould.

Ergonomic considerations are the major factors which should influence the fitting of a low or moderate gain bodyworn aid. Thus far more emphasis must be given to those factors in the design of the aid to ensure that it is easy to handle and the batteries easy to change for the patient with limited manipulative skills. This does not mean that the aid should have restricted acoustical characteristics, but rather that more emphasis needs to be given to preset controls as opposed to the controls accessible to the user, which should be a simple as possible. Work by Martin (1973) and others has given some guidance as to appropriate settings which should be used, and further investigations under way at the MRC Institute of Hearing Research (e.g. Foster, Haggard, and Iredale 1980) should provide further refinement of this approach.

Postaural, intra-aural or spectacle aids?

Preference for these different approaches to fitting of postaural aids has varied from time to time over the past 20 years. Postaural aids have advantages in their versatility and the fact that their characteristics are limited only by the restrictions imposed by the earmoulds. Many of the modern postaural aids have a wide range of preset controls which enable their characteristics to be modified as the user adjusts to his new situation of listening with a hearing aid. This is particularly important as the characteristics of an aid which a listener will accept initially often bear little relationship to those which will be optimal from the standpoint of speech discrimination (Barfod 1979). Thus these aids have the advantage that the professional can gradually adjust the characteristics of the aid as the patient adapts to it or as his needs and hearing change.

Spectacle aids have traditionally been limited by the problems of liaison between professionals concerned with the patient's vision and hearing, and that difficulties with one of the sensory modalities may interfere with the use of the appliance by affecting function of the other. Some patients furthermore wear different spectacles under different circumstances, with obvious complications. The drive towards the use of spectacle aids has now also been reduced by the fact that some of the cosmetic emphasis has been switched to intra-aural aids, and also by the growing public acceptance of postaural aids. This has been helped by a reduction in the size of most such appliances.

Recently, however, a simple adapter device has been developed by one hearing aid manufacturer (Siemens) which makes it possible for the professional or even the patient, to convert his spectacle aid into a postaural aid, or to fit it to another pair of spectacles.

Intra-aural 'all in the ear' aids have been extensively fitted in the United States and in the private sector in the United Kingdom. Their advantages are minimal and their disadvantages considerable. From a cosmetic standpoint they are often more obtrusive than a standard postaural aid, they have controls which are generally difficult to manipulate, there are increased feedback problems, and in many cases a lack of flexibility stemming from the fact that the components are usually built into the earmould. Some of the latest aids of this type, however, are produced on a modular basis so that components can be changed to modify the characteristics of the aid.

One aid or two?

The question of binaural fitting of aids to hearing stems from the nineteenth century when binaural ear trumpets (auricles) were produced. In the period immediately after the Second World War two bodyworn aids were fitted to children, and since the introduction of ear-level aids the concept has been applied more and more to both children and adults.

The rationale and advantages have been discussed extensively (e.g. Markides 1977b; Stephens 1980b) and stem mainly from improved speech in noise discrimination, restoration of horizontal directionalization ability, summation of loudness, and the provision for the patient of the concept of a three-dimensional world. The disadvantages stem from the additional handling problems involved, particularly in the elderly who may be multiply handicapped, the more limited benefit in patients with asymmetrical hearing losses, and dangers of recrudescence of infection in patients with chronic middle-ear disease.

Basically the decision as to whether binaural aids should be fitted, as with all rehabilitative procedures, should be based on the needs and difficulties encountered by the patient. The potential benefit must also be balanced against the additional problems which the patient may encounter with the use of two aids. This said, however, it must be emphasized that at the present time in most parts of the world too little consideration is given to the fitting of binaural hearing aids, particularly in adults.

Other hearing aid decisions

At the present time insufficient emphasis is given to certain aspects of hearing-aid technology and probably excessive emphasis to others. Various points which are worth consideration in certain patients include the use of CROS and BICROS hearing aids, the value of an extended frequency response, frequency transposition aids, and various output-limiting devices.

This last has been discussed elsewhere in this book (Chapter 10) and has been a source of considerable dispute and inadequate experimentation. Obviously some output limiting device is necessary to prevent the sounds amplified by the hearing aid from exceeding the patient's uncomfortable loudness level. However, at the present time it is certainly far from clear which approach to this is the most effective for which groups of patients and much more rigorous work is needed in this respect.

The question of frequency responses of the aids is particularly important and more information on this is becoming available. Increasingly results are indicating the importance of a high-frequency emphasis in the output of aids, particularly in patients with cochlear disorders. This helps to counteract the effects of the upward spread of masking found in such damaged ears, and is true even of patients with 'flat' hearing losses (e.g. Schwartz, Surr, Montgomery, Prosek, and Walden 1979). In addition more evidence is accruing (e.g. Lawson and Caffirelli 1978) of the importance of extending the high-frequency response of the hearing aid beyond the normal current limits of about 4 kHz. There are obvious problems with increased feedback arising from such an approach in high-gain hearing aids (e.g. Angård Johanssen 1975), but where such an extended response is used it can result in a marked improvement in auditory performance.

The CROS family of aids are based on the principle of siting the microphone on one side of the head and routing the signal across to the other side (CROS = Contralateral Routing Of Signals). A variety of CROS type aids have been developed (see Pollack 1975) but the two most widely used are the straight CROS and the BICROS. In the CROS system, used in patients with a severe or complete unilateral hearing loss but with normal hearing in the other ear, the sounds are picked up by a microphone on the side of the poor ear and fed to the normally hearing ear through a tube or open mould system so that they do not interfere unduly with the sound impinging that ear. The BICROS system is used when there is some hearing loss in the better ear and provides a double amplification system, one for the signals coming from the worst ear and another for those from the better ear, with both signals being fed into the better ear alone.

The problems with the CROS/BICROS system is that although it results in an improvement in the discrimination of signals coming from the side of the worse ear, it results in a degradation of information coming from the side of the better ear (e.g. Markides 1977b). Thus it requires careful selective use by a highly motivated user and should be fitted only to meet specific needs following careful discussion with and evaluation of the potential user.

Frequency transposition aids, in which sounds of a high-frequency band are reduced in frequency to a band which the patient can hear, were initially introduced for the use of prelingually deaf children with only an island of low-frequency hearing. The results in this group of patients has not been encouraging. More recently, however, Vellmans (1980) has introduced a new system aimed at patients with steep high-frequency hearing losses and the results of this approach seem encouraging. This group of patients is difficult to help by existing approaches, and this new transposition technique may enable such patients to more clearly distinguish the high-frequency components of speech.

Earmoulds

Earmoulds are the critical link in the hearing aid–patient interaction. A poor earmould may entirely negate any advantages derived from a high-quality hearing aid. Careful use and modification of earmoulds can give an enormous degree of versatility to the fitting achieved with a fairly standard hearing aid.

In patients with mild to moderate hearing losses, the material from which a ear mould is made and its fit within the meatus are not critical. Indeed provided it can be achieved without feedback, the use of an open mould or a simple small tube taking the sound into the external acoustic canal may be ideal to reduce or abolish the low-frequency amplification produced by the hearing aid. Smaller modifications in this may be achieved by drilling vents in the earmould, linking the canal with the outside. These should be drilled parallel to the sound tube to minimize the feedback (Angård Johanssen 1975). Further modifications may be achieved by modifying the size of the vents and the dimensions of the tubes. The various effects of these procedures have been discussed at length and modelled by various authors (e.g. Grover and Martin 1979; Egolf 1978).

In patients with more severe hearing loss requiring considerable gain, the occurrence of acoustic feedback is a much more serious problem, particularly when a ear-level hearing aid is being fitted. In these circumstances it is important to make an earmould which provides a very tight fit to the external meatus so minimizing any leakage of sound. This may be best achieved by a soft malleable material such as soft acrylic, one of a variety of synthetic rubber compounds, or by vinyl.

A problem which sometimes arises with such an approach is that the patient may complain of an unpleasant feeling of 'blockage' in his ear. This may be relieved by the insertion of a vent in the mould with a sintered steel or foam rubber filter incorporated in it. Such a procedure allows slow pressure equilibration without acoustical leakage (French St George and Barr-Hamilton 1978).

Alternatives to earmoulds

For many elderly patients fitted with hearing aids for the first time, fitting the earmould to the ear may present the greatest problem. A number of such patients may not be able to overcome this difficulty, even following considerable practise and training. It is thus necessary to consider alternative strategies.

One approach (Navarro 1977) has been to put small handles on the earmould which enables the patient to manipulate it more easily. More commonly, however, temporary rubber tips are used. These tend to present the problem of inadequately retaining the hearing aid in place and often of giving a very poor fit and hence problems with feedback.

Some tremulous or arthritic patients are totally unable to cope with any such linkage and a number of these may be helped by fitting the receiver of a bodyworn aid to a 'stethoclip' as used by audiotypists (Mirza and Stephens). Such an approach (see Fig. 21.2) inevitably introduces some acoustical distortion into the system although even this may be reduced by simple techniques. It does, however, provide a means by which patients with various manipulative problems can control their acoustic input.

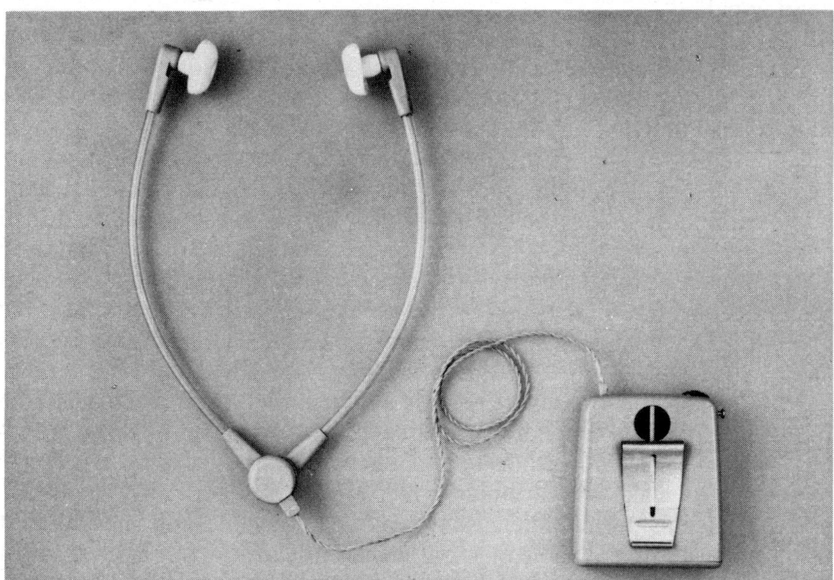

Fig. 21.2. Medresco OL56 hearing aid modified to facilitate its use by an elderly physically handicapped patient. A small screw has been inserted into the switch/volume control to provide an easier control and a stethoclip has been fitted in the place of earmoulds.

COUNSELLING

No hearing aid can be fitted in a vacuum. Many, however, tend to be fitted without due consideration and discussion of the needs and problems of the particular patient. The question of motivation often receives too little attention. Not surprisingly, therefore, many hearing aids are used inadequately if it all (Stephens 1977), a fact completely wasteful of the limited resources available for auditory rehabilitation.

All too often fitting sessions tend to be concerned only with explanation of the controls of the hearing aid and the physical coupling of the aid to the ear with far too little on the coupling of the aid to the psyche.

From the initial evaluation of the patient some indication should have been obtained as to the reasons why the patient came for a hearing aid, and the motivation of the patient must be built up from this. It is apparent that if the patient himself has initiated the process as he feels that he needs help in communication, the task of the rehabilitative team will be much easier than if he has been pressurized into seeking help by his spouse or his children.

At the earliest stage it is essential too that the patient has the correct level of expectancy as to the benefit which he will derive from a hearing aid. If he feels that it will solve all his problems, the probability is that he will reject the prosthesis when he finds that this is not so. Likewise, those with too low expectancy, often pushed into accepting an aid by despairing relatives, will need encouragement or they likewise will reject the aid without any serious attempt to use it. The onus on the rehabilitationist to use all his skills to achieve an appropriate level of motivation at this stage is great. Unfortunately few patients realize that the problem of adapting to a hearing aid may entail the learning or re-learning of new listening skills, a difficulty not appropriate to the falsely analogous situation of spectacles.

Once the aid has been fitted, the professional responsible must give guidance to the patient as to the extent to which it should be used initially and under what circumstances. There is some controversy over this matter although most professionals are agreed that the aid(s) should be used in the quiet initially before being worn in more difficult noisy situations. The degree of practise and build up to this will depend very much on the individual patient, his hearing loss, attitudes, needs, and life style.

Related to this are general aspects of 'hearing tactics'—in other words, how the patient can help himself and his friends to reduce his handicap by taking a positive attitude towards his problems (e.g. Vognsen 1976). This is difficult for many patients and requires continuous encouragement on the part of the professional concerned. He may be considerably helped in this respect by the use of group sessions in which patients can help each other by describing the tactics which they have used to overcome particular difficulties. It is, however, important in this context that the groups should be reasonably homogenous at least with regard to the severity of loss of the patients within the group. Tactics relevant to a mild or moderate hearing loss may be inappropriate to a patient with a severe loss, and vice versa.

COMMUNICATION SKILLS

These entail the development of all possible means of increasing the ability of the individual to communicate with those around him. This involves an integrated approach to audiovisual communication, and the adoption of any other techniques which may be appropriate to patients with a particularly severe hearing loss.

Speech-reading (lip-reading)

Much has been written in the past about the specific skills entailed in speech-reading (lip-reading) and on the effectiveness of auditory training. Most professionals now accept that what is needed is an integrated approach as only a tiny majority of the hearing impaired are unable to derive any benefit from amplification, even if it is only to help speech reading (e.g. McCormick 1979). It is thus essential not to deter patients by presenting mute speech-reading cues when even a very limited amount of acoustic information may dramatically improve the discriminability of the material. Conversely, it is important to emphasize to the patient, even with a mild loss, the importance of visual cues.

For most patients with moderate hearing losses little is required in the way of formal training of speech-reading beyond the discussion of speech-reading tactics. These involve enhancement of the speech-reading cues by ensuring that the speaker is facing the hearing-impaired individual with his face well illuminated and with no undue impediments such as cigarettes dangling from his lips. The speaker should be encouraged to speak moderately slowly and to ensure that the listener has understood the general context of the conversation. As most hearing-impaired patients have sensorineural losses in which the greatest problem is the discrimination of speech in noise, it is essential that the patient organize, where possible, that important conversations take place in a quiet environment with little reverberation. A room with soft furnishings and carpeting is far easier for the hearing-impaired individual than one with many highly reflective surfaces.

The patient with such a loss may practise his speech-reading skills by adjusting the television to a level at which he can barely hear it, and then watch the news programme in which he will have plenty of contextual cues and generally clear speakers. He should be encouraged to pay attention particularly to the place of articulation of various consonantal sounds, although this should not be unduly emphasized in isolation. Indeed, formal tests of speech-reading from those of Heider and Heider (1940) onwards have shown little relationship between the visual discrimination of consonants and that of running speech.

For patients with a more severe hearing loss and poor visual discrimination of speech an analysis must be made initially of where along the discrimination process the difficulty lies, or even whether it is related to uncorrected visual impairment. Without such an analysis, little more than a blundering approach can be made to helping the patient. Indeed, so little is understood as to the most effective way of teaching speechreading (*Clinical Otolarygology* 1979) that little advance is likely, unless such a systematic approach is adopted.

Thus if the individual's problems comprise the discrimination of different phonemes, the source of confusion may be defined and attention given to this. Often the difficulty will be in linking the components together into running speech, and the tactics involved in this must be explained with adequate training and practise. Here the importance of a synthetic approach is essential and the patient must come to accept to that it will be impossible for him to discriminate every word. The great importance of contextual cues must be emphasized here, as it is only by means of these that the patient will be able to distinguish between, for example, PAN–MAN–BAN.

For patients who are already moderately competent at all aspects of speech-reading but who require additional support it is often valuable to define their specific vocabulary needs within the work or particular problem situation and concentrate on these. Such an approach has been shown to be of great value with students of the National Technical Institute for the Deaf in preparing them for specific courses alongside hearing students (Jacobs 1979).

Manual supplements and approaches

Traditionally the use of manual communication or sign language has been the domain of the prelingually hearing impaired patient. In many cases some of these who have a real communication need have been deprived of this by a dogmatic attitude from certain professionals concerned. There have been strong arguments against the application of manual systems to patients with an acquired hearing loss in view of their different linguistic approach and general experience. Most of such patients prefer to maintain, as far as possible, their links with the hearing society as opposed to the prelingually deaf subculture. However, it is essential to help those who wish to become more associated with the prelingually deaf to learn the comprehensive sign languages such as British Sign Language, American Sign Language, or whatever other system is appropriate to the society in which the patient lives. It is also essential to help those prelingually deaf with severe communication problems who have little or no sign language in this way.

For patients with a profound acquired hearing loss who need to supplement their speech-reading, probably the best system, and one which has been extensively used in Denmark, is the Mouth–Hand System. This is a simple system, easy to learn and one which is designed basically to help with the differentiation between voiced and voiceless and nasal consonants with different hand positions. It has no signs for vowels. Recently it has been applied in English-speaking societies and evaluative studies on the benefits derived from it in the United States are very encouraging (Binnie 1978).

Cued speech developed by Cornett at Gallaudet College is a much more complicated system and not appropriate for those who have already acquired language. In fact even Cornett himself is currently concerned with the development of an electronic substitute technique (Cornett, Beadles, and Wilson 1968).

It must be emphasized that these last two techniques are specific supplements to speech-reading and cannot be used alone. They help the patient to discriminate what is not distinguishable on the lips, and in this context some centres have also advocated the use of selective finger spelling in order to clarify words which are difficult to speech-read.

It must be emphasized further that in all these cases, the greatest onus is on the friends and relatives of the hearing-impaired patient learning the manual system, and as such any approach can have only a limited application.

Electronic supplements to speech-reading

The advantage of electronic supplements, when they have reached a sufficient stage of sophistication, not so far achieved, is that there will be no obligation on the speaker to learn a new communication technique. Thus the hearing-impaired individual should, theoretically, be able to communicate as well with strangers as with intimate acquaintances.

Three major approaches have been used in this respect. These have used vibrotactile stimulation, visual stimulation, or electrical stimulation of the cochlear nerve.

The vibrotactile stimulation has generally consisted of one or more vibrators placed on the fingers or other parts of the body providing cues as to voicing, time cues, and intensity information. Another approach, which has been more successful with the blind, has been to use an array of stimulators placed on a large surface of the patient's body with a specific coding system, according to the pattern of stimulation.

Visual substitution is currently being investigated by Cornett as a means of making his cued speech system more universally applicable. This entails a speech analyser linked to special spectacles in which different symbols are illuminated depending on the nature of the signal.

At present the approach which is receiving most attention is that of electrical stimulation of the cochlear nerve. A wide variety of approaches has been used (Thornton 1979) but there is little evidence to suggest that invasive techniques give better results than stimulation by means of a simple electrode on the round window (Fourcin *et al.* 1979). Such an approach coupled with an input from a laryngograph (Fourcin and Abberton 1971) has resulted in a considerable improvement in visual discrimination of voiced/unvoiced consonants and work is under way to replace the laryngograph with an acoustical analyser which can be carried by the patient.

It must be emphasized, that, at present, all these techniques are very much at an experimental stage.

ENVIRONMENTAL AIDS

For all hearing-impaired patients there is a range of aids which can attack specific problems of their daily life in a simple and direct way. For convenience these tend to be lumped together under the title of environmental aids. They may be subdivided into warning devices and communication aids, and the latter may be further subdivided into those which are 'self sufficient' and those such as the Pallantype device, which involve the services of a specific trained operator.

Warning devices

These are to indicate the approach of another person to the room or building in which the patient is located, to indicate that someone is present at the door, that the telephone is ringing, that the baby is crying, or an alarm device to indicate that morning has arrived. The simple indicator of someone approaching consists of a pressure switch which may be put under the door mat and which causes a light to be illuminated when someone steps on the doormat.

More commonplace devices are those which supplement or replace the doorbell. These may give auditory or visual warning and at their simplest comprise merely an extra loud doorbell or a buzzer emitting a high-level of low-frequency noise, clearly audible to the hearing-impaired patients. Such buzzers or loud doorbells are often among the cheapest in the range produced by many manufacturers.

There are a great many varieties of a visual doorbell system. The simplest version comprises a light in the patient's living room which is switched on when the doorbell is rung. More complicated systems cause all the lights in a ring circuit to be switched on during the day, or off momentarily at night. Various patterns of flashing may be used.

Similar approaches may be used for the telephone bell. Many patients may be considerably helped by a simple extension bell, although some may need an extra loud bell. Other approaches consist of a warning light which flashes on and off in the handset of the telephone, and systems similar to the doorbell devices which cause a variety of lights in the patient's home to flash. There may be a combined doorbell/telephone bell flashing system with a different pattern of flashing enabling the patient to differentiate between the two. Perhaps the most sophisticated device entails the whole residence being wired with an electromagnetic induction loop which then activates a pick-up coil carried by the patient differentially according to whether the telephone bell or doorbell is ringing.

Baby alarm devices consist simply of a microphone placed above the infant's cot, linked to a sensor circuit which causes a light to flash when the baby's cries exceed a certain level.

More imagination has been used in alarm clocks. These range from a simple device which causes a bedside lamp to flash on and off, via a bedside fan which blows cold air on the patient's face, to vibrators under the pillow, and even some which shake the whole bed.

Communication aids

These are available to help the patient to be able to use the telephone, to hear the television and radio, and for more sophisticated and specialized purposes.

TELEPHONE AIDS

These may be built into the telephone such as a simple amplifier which provides an extra 15 dB output; they may be optional attachments or they may be devices which can be used as substitutes. The simplest inbuilt telephone aid stemmed from the fact that the output transducer of many old fashioned telephones produced an extensive electromagnetic field which could be picked up by the tele-coil pickup of hearing aids. With increasing telephone sophistication this field strength was reduced, but most recently a device producing a strong field has been incorporated as an 'optional extra' in telephones available in a number of countries including the United Kingdom and parts of the United States. Most telephone systems have the additional amplifier option available in the handset.

Devices to fix on to the telephones have the advantage that the hearing-impaired patient is not restricted to a limited number of adapted phones. These devices consist of a microphone pickup amplifier and output device and generally fixed, on to the telephone by means of elastic bands. They may provide either a simple amplified output or produce a strong electromagnetic field enabling the listener to use the coil pickup of his hearing aid. A variety of approaches to telephone communication for the hearing impaired have been discussed by Birk Nielsen and Gilberg (1978).

The final approach, generally used with the prelingually impaired, has been to replace the standard telephone with a teletype device. In the past this has been too expensive for normal domestic use but with the development of electronic teletypes it is likely to become more accessible to a larger number of users in the near future.

TELEVISION AIDS

Televisions, radios, and other high-fidelity systems have long had headphone options available, initially for enthusiasts but also for the hearing impaired. Fig. 21.3 shows some alternative systems which have various advantages. Fig. 21.3(a) shows a fairly standard insert receiver with an output from the set passing via an isolating transformer to an additional amplifier and then to a suitable transducer such as a hearing aid receiver. The loop system (Fig. 21.3(b)) is likewise wired into the television via an isolating transformer and booster amplifier and thence either to a full-loop system around the room or rooms or to a miniloop system in a chair or in a device which the patient clips over his head adjacent to his hearing aid. Fig. 21.3(c) shows a device which is becoming increasingly popular as it is not limited to one television set or radio, but rather is portable. In this system a microphone is fixed to the front of the loudspeaker grill by an adhesive material. The output of this is then taken via an amplifier to a hearing-aid receiver. The adhesive material is such that the microphone is detachable and can be moved from television to television.

Related to television is the subtitling system and text information system developed by the television companies in the United Kingdom and produced as CEEFAX by the BBC and ORACLE by commercial television. These will become more accessible as the price falls with their wider use. The telephone system in the United Kingdom has also been developing a

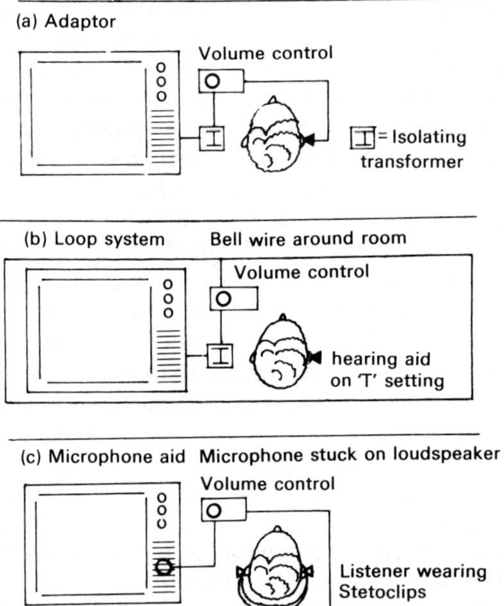

Fig. 21.3. Some approaches which may be used to help the hearing impaired to listen to the television. (a). An additional amplifier with insert receivers which has been wired into the output. (b). A loop system again wired into the output. (c). A system by which a microphone is attached with adhesive material to the loudspeaker. The output from the microphone is taken to an amplifier and hence to an insert receiver.

sophisticated information system using the television screen and called PRESTEL which may also be of value to the hearing impaired.

SPECIAL DEVICES

Finally for certain severely hearing-impaired individuals with considerable needs and support there is the PALANTYPE system refined and developed for the deafened United Kingdom member of Parliament, Jack Ashley. For this device there is a palantypist who types in a running account of ongoing discussions using a phonetic keyboard. This passes through a memory device which covers the 1000 most commonly used words in spoken English are printed out with the correct spelling. Other words are printed out phonetically. At the present stage of development this device has little relevance for the majority of the hearing impaired but as techniques of machine recognition of speech become more sophisticated and the operator becomes redundant, it may find wider use in this context.

REHABILITATION IN A SOCIAL AND EMPLOYMENT CONTEXT

In all countries many individuals of working age who develop a severe hearing loss may experience considerable difficulties with their work and may lose their jobs. It is vital that rehabilitation departments develop and maintain close links with employment retraining centres to ensure that both sides are fully informed as to the potential employment opportunities for such individuals, and ways in which hearing-impaired people may be helped to hold down jobs of various types. This is very much a two-way process and both groups of professionals have much to learn from each other.

In the general social-service context similar links are equally important. This is particularly true in countries like the United Kingdom in which there are specialist social workers for the deaf, and where the social services have responsibility for the provision of environmental aids. It is the author's experience that a close working relationship between the hospital based rehabilitation services and the community-based social workers for the deaf is vital for the provision of an effective and comprehensive service of auditory rehabilitation.

APPENDIX 21.1

The North wind and the sun were arguing one day about which of them was the stronger, when a traveller came along wrapped in a warm coat. They agreed that the one who could make the traveller take his coat off, would be considered stronger than the other one. The North wind blew as hard as he could but the harder he blew, the tighter the traveller wrapped his coat around him and at last the North wind gave up trying. Then the sun began to shine warmly and right away the traveller took his coat off and so the North wind had to admit that the sun was stronger than he was.

REFERENCES

ANGÅRD JOHANSSEN, P. (1975). An evaluation of the acoustic feedback damping for behind the ear hearing aids. Technical Report, Research Laboratory for Technical Audiology, Odense, Denmark.

BARCHAM, L. J. and STEPHENS, S. D. G. (1980). The use of an open-ended problems questionnaire in auditory rehabilitation. *Br. J. Audiol.* **14**, 49–54.

BARFOD, J. (1979). Speech perception processes and fitting of hearing aids. *Audiology* **18**, 430–41.

BEDFORD, A. and FOULDS, G. A. (1978). *Manual of the personal disturbance scale.* National Federation for Education Research, Windsor.

BINNIE, C. A. (1978). The Danish Hand–Mouth system for hearing impaired adults. Presented at Interactive seminar on Communicative Disorders, Purdue University.

BIRK NIELSEN, H. and GILBERG, I. (1978). Telecommunication performance of persons with hearing handicap in relation to speech reception threshold. *Scand. Audiol.* **7**, 3–10.

BROOKS, D. N. (1979). Counselling and its effect on hearing aid use. *Scand. Audiol.* **6**, 101–7.

Clinical Otolaryngology (1980). Can lipreading be taught? *Clin. Otolar.* **4**, 3–4.

CONRAD, R. (1979). *The deaf school child.* Harper and Row, London.

CORNETT, R. D., BEADLES, R., and WILSON, B. (1978). Automatic cued speech. Report, Gallaudet College, Washington, DC.

EGOLF, D. P. (1978). Computer predictions of ear-mould modifications. In *The application of signal processing concepts to hearing aids* (ed. P. Yanick, and S. Freifeld) pp. 61–84. Grune and Stratton, New York.

EWERTSEN, H. W. and BIRK NIELSEN, H. (1973). Social hearing handicap index. *Audiology* **12**, 180–7.

FOSTER, J. R., HAGGARD, M. P., and IREDALE, F. E. (1981). Prescription of gain-setting and prognosis for use and benefit of post-aural hearing aids. *Audiology* **20**, 157–76.

FOURCIN, A. J. and ABBERTON, E. (1971). First applications of a new laryngograph *Med. bio. Illust.* **21**, 172–82.

—— ROSEN, S. M., MOORE, B. C. J., DOUEK, E. E. CLARKE, G. P., DODSON, M., and BANNISTER, L. H. (1979). External electrical stimulation of the cochlea: clinical, psychophysical, speech perceptual and histological findings. *Br. J. Audiol.* **13**, 85–107.

FRENCH ST GEORGE, M. and BARR-HAMILTON, R. (1978). Relief of the occluded ear sensation to improve earmould comfort. *J. Am. aud. Soc.* **4**, 30–5.

GILDSTON, H. and GILDSTON, P. (1972). Personality changes associated with surgically corrected otosclerosis. *Audiology* **11**, 354–67.

GROVER, B. C. (1977). A note on acoustic hearing aids. *Br. J. Audiol.* **11**, 75–6.

—— and MARTIN, M. C. (1979). Physical and subjective correlates of earmould occlusion. *Audiology* **18**, 335–50.

HABIB, R. G. and HINCHCLIFFE, R. (1978). Subjective magnitude of auditory impairment. *Audiology* **17**, 68–76.

HARDICK, E. J. OYER, H. J., and IRION, P. E. (1970). Lipreading performance as related to measurements of vision. *J. Speech Hear. Res.* **13**, 92–100.

HEIDER, F. K. and HEIDER, G. M. (1940). An experimental investigation of lipreading. *Psychol. Monogr.* **22**, 124–53.

HIGH, W. S., FAIRBANKS, G., and GLORIG, A. (1964). Scale for self-assessment of hearing handicap. *J. Speech Hear. Dis.* **29**, 215–30.

JACOBS, M. (1979). Speechreading instruction for the NTID student. Report, National Technical Institute for the Deaf, Rochester, NY.

JOHNSTON, D. D. (1978). The adult deaf client and rehabilitation. In *Handbook of adult rehabilitative audiology* (ed. J. G. Alpiner) pp. 172–221. Williams and Wilkins, Baltimore.

KALIKOW, D. N., STEVENS, K. N., and ELLIOTT, L. L. (1977). Development of a test of speech intelligibility in noise using sentence materials with controlled word predictability. *J. acoust. Soc. Am.* **61**, 1337–51.

LAWTON, B. W. and CAFARELLI, D. L. (1978). The effects of hearing aid frequency response modification upon speech reception. ISVR Memorandum No 588, University of Southampton.

MCCORMICK, B. (1979). Audiovisual discrimination of speech. *Clin. Otolar.* **4**, 355–61.

MARKIDES, A. (1977a). Rehabilitation of people with acquired deafness in adulthood. *Br. J. Audiol.* Suppl. 1.

—— (1977b). *Binaural hearing aids.* Academic Press, London.

MARTIN, M. C. (1973). Hearing aid gain requirements in sensori-neural hearing loss. *Br. J. Audiol.* **7**, 21–4.

MERLUZZI, F. and HINCHCLIFFE, R. (1973). Threshold of subjective auditory handicap. *Audiology* **12**, 65–9.

MIRZA, A. and STEPHENS, S. D. G. The use of stetoclips in hearing aid fitting. In preparation.

NAVARRO, M. R. (1977). An earmould for the geriatric patient. *J. Speech Hear. Dis.* **42**, 44–6.
NOBLE, W. G. (1978). *Assessment of impaired hearing.* Academic Press, New York.
—— and ATHERLEY, G. R. C. (1970). The hearing measurement scale: a questionnaire for the assessment of auditory disability. *J. aud. Res.* **10**, 229–50.
PLOMP, R. (1978). Auditory handicap of hearing impairment and the limited benefit of hearing aids. *J. acoust. Soc. Am.* **63**, 533–49.
POLLACK, M. C. (ed.) (1975). *Amplification for the hearing impaired.* Grune and Stratton, New York.
RISBERG, A. and AGELFORS, E. (1978). Information extraction and information processing in speech reading. STL-QPSR, 62–82.
SCHWARTZ, D. M., SURR, R. K., MONTGOMERY, A. A., PROSEK, R. A., and WALDEN, B. E. (1979). Performance of high frequency impaired listeners with conventional and extended high frequency amplification. *Audiology* **18**, 157–74.
SILVERMAN, S. R. and HIRSH, I. J. (1955). Problems related to the use of speech in clinical audiometry. *Ann. Otol. Rhinol. Lar.* **64**, 1234–44.
SKAMRIS, N. P. (1974). Assessment of lipreading ability of deafened persons. In *Visual and audio-visual perception of speech* (ed. H. Nielsen and E. Kampp) pp. 128–35. Almquist and Wiksell, Stockholm.
STEPHENS, S. D. G. (1977). Hearing aid use by adults: a survey of surveys. *Clin. Otolar.* **2**, 385–402.
—— (1980a). Evaluating the problems of the hearing impaired. *Audiology* **19**, 205–20.
—— (1980b). Binaural hearing aid fitting. *Hear. Aid J.* **33**, 12–13, 36–7.
—— BARCHAM, L. J., CORCORAN, A. L., and PARSONS, N. (1980). Evaluation of an auditory rehabilitation scheme. In *Disorders of auditory function* III (ed. I. G. Taylor and A. Markides). Academic Press, London.
THOMAS, A. J. and GILHOME HERBST, K. (1980). Social and psychological implications of acquired deafness for adults of employment age. *Br. J. Audiol.* 14, 76–85.
THORNTON, A. R. D. (ed.) (1977). *A review of artificial auditory stimulation.* Medical Research Council, Southampton.
TYLER, R. (1979). Measuring hearing loss in the future. *Br. J. Audiol.* Suppl. 2, 29–40.
VELMANS, M. L. (1979). New frequency transposing aid. *Hear. Aid J.* **32**, 51–3.
VOGNSEN, S. (ed.) (1976). *Hearing tactics.* Oticon, Copenhagen.

ADDENDUM

Subsequent to writing this chapter, the author, together with Professor David Goldstein has developed a management model of Auditory Rehabilitation presenting much the same material in the form of flow diagrams. Interested readers are referred to Goldstein, D. P. and Stephens, S. D. G. (1981). Audiological rehabilitation: Management Model I. *Audiology* **20**, in press.

22 Cochlear implants: patho physiological considerations

J. TONNDORF

INTRODUCTION

Otosurgeons have been actively engaged in the restoration of auditory function in patients with various forms of middle-ear disorders for many years. More recently, a few enterprising surgeons (Simmons 1966; House 1976; Michelsen 1971; Chouard and McLeod 1976; Douek *et al.* 1977) began to tackle the problem of profound sensory deafness in an attempt to restore serviceable hearing, i.e. some degree of speech intelligibility. In such patients the cochlear hair cells are lost, while the cochlear nerve is preserved; however, a clinical test to ascertain the latter condition, even in a gross manner, is still lacking. Electrical stimulation has been used in these patients by inserting electrodes either into the scala tympani or directly into the modiolus. Despite some encouraging initial results, progress towards restoration of speech intelligibility has been rather slow (Fig. 22.1). The term

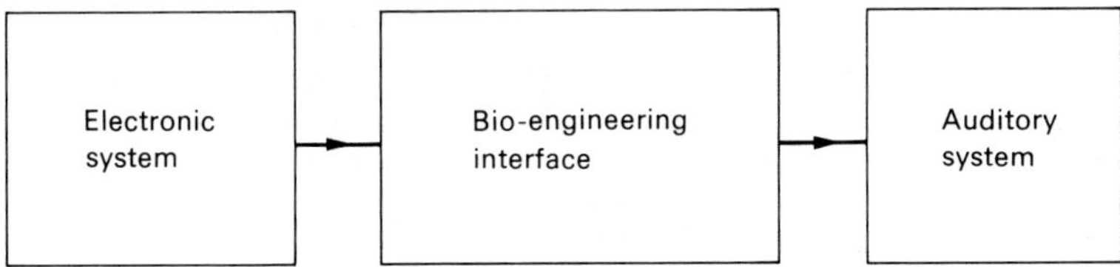

Fig. 22.1. Cochlear prosthesis: schematic representation of its operation.

'electronic system' in the left-hand box stands for the engineering design and physical construction of the electronic equipment that receives the acoustic signals and transforms them into a suitable signal for transmission into the cochlea or the cochlear nerve. I foresee no particular difficulties in this area, and that includes miniaturization, once the requirements have been clearly defined. The term 'auditory system' in the right-hand box refers to the impaired cochlea and the surgical preparation necessary for the implantation of whatever electrode(s) are chosen. Given the present situation of microsurgery of the middle ear, this task is not expected to present unsurmountable difficulties either, once the problems of the compatibility between tissues and the implant materials are completely solved.

Where the difficulties lie—and they are still formidable—is in the area represented by the middle box labelled 'bio-engineering interface'. This represents the connection of the electronic device(s) to the cochlea in such a way that each particular signal will be transmitted precisely where it is intended to go, without further damaging the cochlea or neural tissues by the application of electrical currents over long periods of time. It must be emphasized that the difficulties encountered at the bio-engineering interface are not due to a lack of specific knowledge in the physiology of the peripheral auditory system. As will be shown presently, this is not a problem of what should be done, but rather one of how it should be done.

In the following, I shall first give a brief description of auditory physiology as it applies to the prosthesis problem, then outline the currently used methods, list their achievemements and their inherent limitations, and present some suggestions for future improvements.

PHYSIOLOGICAL CONSIDERATIONS

Normal function of the cochlea and the cochlear nerve

The system the prosthesis is intended to replace consists of a large number of mechano-acoustic/neural transducers, the hair cells (Fig. 22.2). There are

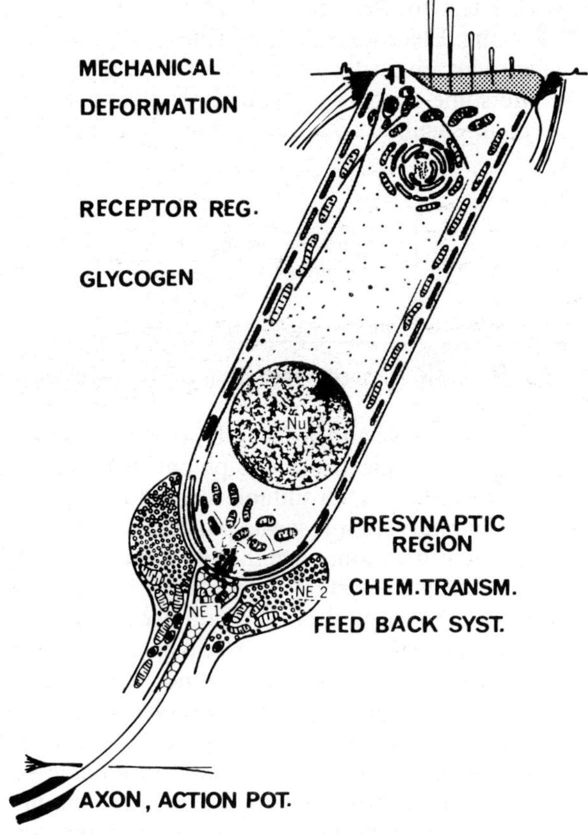

Fig. 22.2. Longitudinal section of an outer hair cell (schematic). At its bottom, one afferent fibre and two efferent ones (labelled 'feedback system') are seen to synapse with the cell. (From Engström and Ades (1973).)

normally about 16 000 of them, arranged in one row of inner hair cells and three rows of outer ones (Fig. 22.3). These cells receive their individual inputs according to a place/time/amplitude distribution that is unique for any type of signal and is due to the travelling waves of Békésy (1960). By way of several intervening steps (Tonndorf 1975), the induced hair cell activity ultimately elicits the action potentials (AP) in the cochlear nerve fibre(s) that are attached to them. APs represent the general code by which information is carried in nerve fibres. Each individual hair cell acts as a biological amplifier (Békésy 1960) thus greatly enchancing neural sensitivity (Khanna and Tonndorf 1977).

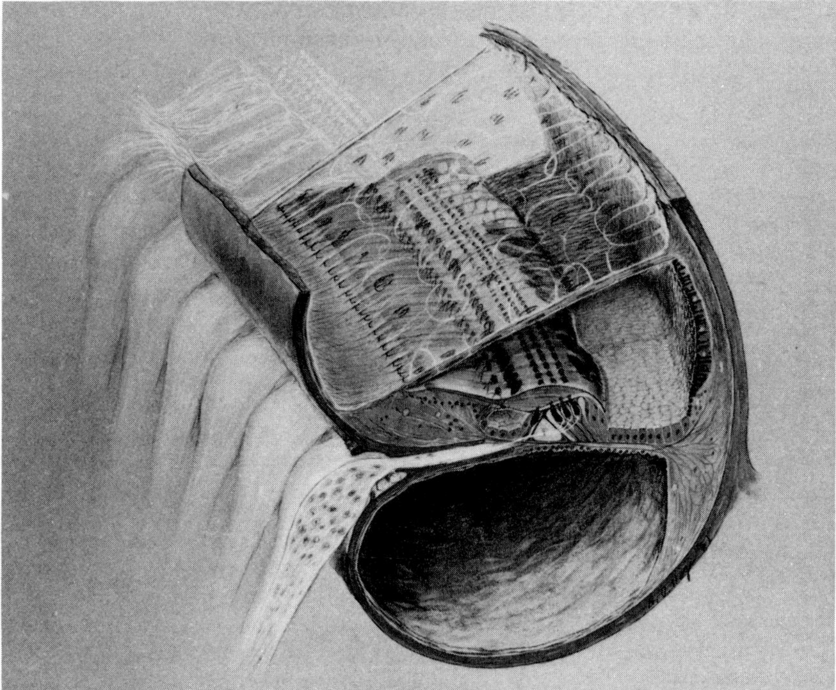

Fig. 22.3. Three-dimensional view of a small segment of a cochlear turn (guinea pig). The inner and outer hair cells and the Hensen cells have been stained by intravital application of methylene blue. (From Tonndorf (1977).)

In addition to the afferent (sensory) nerve fibres, there is a system of efferent fibres that acts as a feedback control both on the hair cells and on their nerve endings.

There are typical synapses between the hair cells and the dendritic nerve-fibre endings (Smith and Sjöstrand 1961). Actually in the bipolar fibres of the cochlear nerve, it is not clear where the dendrites end and where the axons begin. Most neuroanatomists feel that the dendrite is the non-myelinated nerve ending within the organ of Corti and that the axon probably begins at the point where the myelin sheath first appears (Spoendlin, personal communication; Noback, personal communication) a notion I shall adopt for the purpose of the present discussion. The normal complement of afferent nerve fibres is about 30 000; hence, there are about twice as many fibres as hair cells. As is shown schematically in Fig. 22.4, 90–95 per cent of the afferent fibres go to the inner hair cells; the remaining 5–10 per cent go to the outer hair cells. Each inner hair cells receives up to 20 fibres, but each of these fibres goes to only one hair cell. Each outer hair cell fibre, from the point where it merges from the habenula, runs longitudinally backward towards the cochlear base (Fig. 22.4), for a distance of about 0.5 mm, before supplying approximately 8–10 cells in an essentially random manner (Spoendlin 1972; Lorente de Nó 1937). The fibre distribution to the inner hair cells thus represents a classical divergent pattern—divergent in terms of the direction of signal travel—and that to the outer hair cells a convergent pattern.

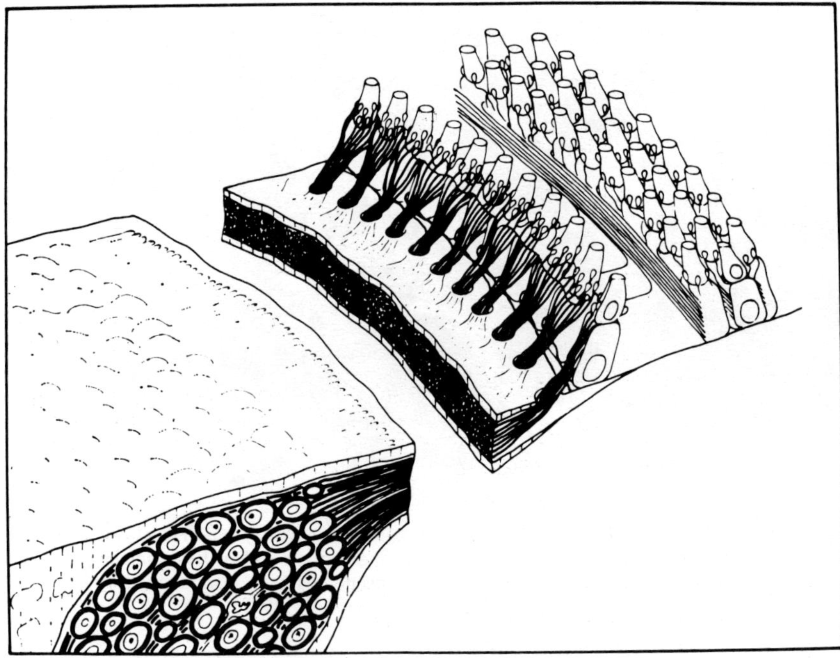

Fig. 22.4. A segment of the organ of Corti, schematically showing the distribution of afferent nerve fibres to inner and outer hair cells. Note the lobulated nucleus of the nerve cell of the single outer-hair cell fibres shown. (From Spoendlin (1972).)

There is a considerable body of knowledge about the mechano-acoustic event that ultimately leads to hair-cell stimulation (Békésy 1960; Dallos 1973; Tonndorf and Khanna 1976) and also about the electrical aspects of the events associated with the absorption of mechano-acoustic energy in hair cells, as well as the resting potentials displayed by these cells (Dallos 1973). However, there is little known about their biochemical counterparts.

The synaptic action at the hair cell–dendritic fibre junction is due to a neurotransmitter. Its exact mechanism and the nature of the transmitting substances are still being disputed (Tonndorf 1977). In nerve fibres the biochemical states and events are much better understood and can be correlated with their electrical counterparts (Ochs 1965), at least as regards the generation of action potentials (Fig. 22.5). As across all other cell membranes, there is a sodium–potassium differential from outside to inside the fibre. Each time an AP is triggered, the cell membrane becomes briefly permeable to both ions, although at different time courses. During the subsequent recovery period, the equilibrial condition is restored owing to the action of a sodium pump.

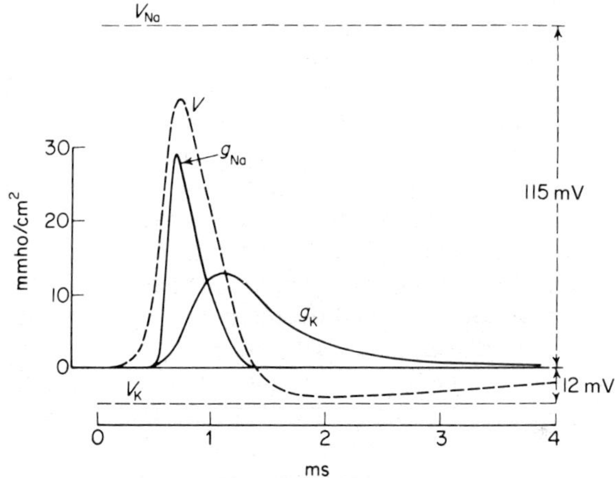

Fig. 22.5. Time courses of the electrical and chemical events making up a nerve action potential; g_{Na} and g_K = computed conductances of sodium and potassium respectively; V_{Na} and V_K = equilibrial potentials of the two substances; V = action potential. (From Ochs (1965); after Hodgkin and Huxley.)

One point must be stressed with respect to the chemo-electrical states and events at all these levels. The chemical and electrical forces keep each other in close check so that run-away forces of either kind cannot exist for any length of time. Let me illustrate this statement by the events that in all likelihood take place in hair cells. The following scheme is in full agreement with general chemo-electric, dynamic considerations (Katchalsky and Curran 1974). As long as the cell is at rest, the inherent chemical and electric forces should hold each other in an intricate equilibrium that is maintained metabolically. This equilibrium will be briefly disturbed on the absorption of mechano-acoustic energy, but it is quickly re-established at its new, elevated level. After the newly acquired energy is expended in a chemo-electric form in initiating the transduction process, the resting equilibrium is once more restored.

As has already been mentioned, the space/time/amplitude distribution of auditory signals along the cochlear partition is produced by the travelling-wave mechanism of Békésy (1960). Specifically, high frequencies form their displacement maxima within the basal region, and when frequency is lowered, there is a systematic shift of this maximum towards more apical places. Furthermore, travel time along the partition is relatively long, about 4 ms from end to end for a low-frequency signal. Therefore the place distribution is accompanied by a time delay that is systematically increasing with inverse frequency, i.e. from base to apex along the partition.

One might ask about the need for this rather elaborate set of events. The answer lies in certain limitation of cochlear nerve fibres—limitations they share with all other nerve fibres. Cochlear nerve fibres are restricted with respect to their time resolution (their ability to carry frequency information), their dynamic range (their ability to carry intensity information), and their way of separating signals from noise (their ability to cope with masking problems). The effects of these limitations are greatly alleviated by the place/time/amplitude distribution. Parallel processing in a number of channels will make up for the limitations of processing in a single channel.

Cochlear nerve fibres, even in the absence of any input, fire spontaneously in a random manner with an average rate that varies considerably from zero to almost 100/s (Kiang, Watanabe, Thomas, and Clarke 1965). The random firing represents a noise which limits the detection of signals by the 'read-out' station, the cochlear nuclei in the present case. Noise constitutes the limit of detection of any signal detector, biological or man-made. The random firing is partially suppressed by evoked activity and it is one of the reasons why cochlear nerve fibres do not respond to a signal in a deterministic manner. Their responses must therefore be analysed statistically. (An example will be shown presently in Fig. 22.7.)

Each cochlear nerve fibre responds only to a limited range of frequencies. Their tuning curves (Fig. 22.6), i.e. the frequency/intensity areas within which they respond, indicate that each fibre acts as a band-pass filter. At near-threshold intensities responses are quite narrowly restricted around a frequency known as the best or characteristic frequency of that fibre. There exists a strict tonotopic relation between these best frequencies and the places along the basilar membrane their fibres are connected to (Kiang *et al.* 1965). The place is also the main determinant of the latency, i.e. the time delay, with which a given fibre responds to an acoustic input. The tonotopic relation with respect to both place *and* time that is caused by the cochlear travelling-wave mechanism is maintained throughout the entire auditory system, up to, and including, cortical levels.

The place/time coding of frequency gives rise to the so-called place pitch. However, cochlear nerve fibres are also capable of carrying frequency information directly by firing their APs in synchrony with the signal, at least up to a limit of 3–4 kHz. This synchronization gives rise to the so called periodicity pitch.

Fig. 22.7 shows a series of post-stimulus time (PST) histograms of various

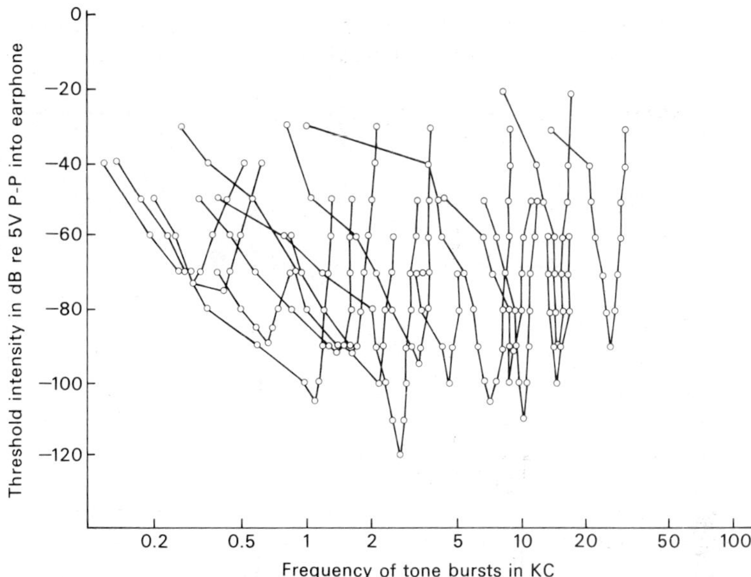

Fig. 22.6. Sample of tuning curves of individual cochlear nerve fibres obtained in one single cat. (From Kiang *et al.* (1965).)

cochlear nerve fibres in response to clicks. (The PST histogram is one of the statistical measures used to assess the activity of cochlear nerve fibres.) It is seen that the responses last much longer than the short-duration click signals. Moreover, at frequencies lower than 3–4 kHz (Fig. 22.7, left-hand side), they clearly occur at preferred post-stimulus times with free intervals between them. These intervals are the reciprocals of the best frequency of each given fibre. It is thus apparent that the fibres 'ring', i.e. they respond to the dampened mechanical vibrations occurring at the places along the basilar membrane to which they are connected. In other words, they synchronize with a signal that is physically present.

At higher frequencies, the synchronization is lost (Fig. 22.7, right-hand side). Russell and Sellick (1977) were recently able to show how this limit in synchronization comes about. Hair cells generate two kinds of receptor potentials, an a.c. component and a d.c. component. (They are the first links in the initiation of the APs.) At low frequencies, the a.c. component is the dominant one, at higher frequencies the d.c. component dominates. The turn-over occurs at about 3 kHz. Thus at higher frequencies, there is no longer a signal the fibre could synchronize with.

Tuning curves narrow somewhat as their best frequency is increased (cf. Fig. 22.6). Hence at high frequencies, tuning is very sharp and frequency information is exclusively carried by place pitch. At low frequencies, however, where tuning is not as sharp, place pitch is complemented by periodicity pitch.

Intensity coding is likewise aided by the place/time/amplitude distribu-

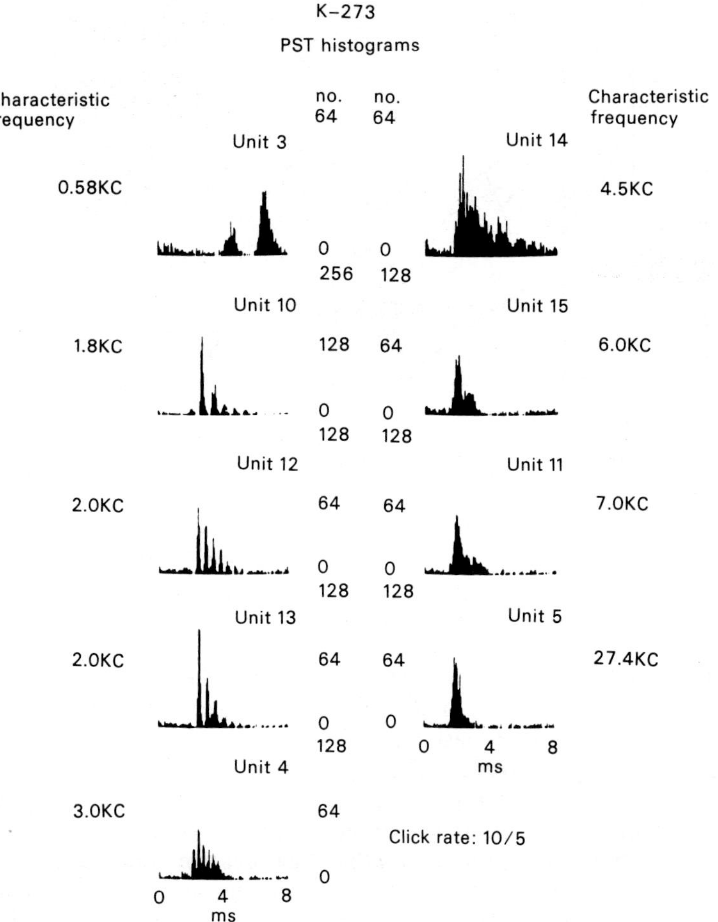

Fig. 22.7. Post-stimulus time (PST) histograms. For explanation see text. (From Kiang *et al.* (1965).)

tion. Cochlear nerve fibres have restricted dynamic ranges, typically not more than 40 dB between threshold and saturation in terms of response rates (Fig. 22.8). Psychophysically, the auditory dynamic range is at least 120 dB, i.e. wider by many order of magnitude. Fig. 22.6 had indicated a widening of tuning curves as intensity is increased, a normal occurence in any narrow-band filter. The corollary of this finding is that with increasing intensity additional fibres must gradually be 'recruited' to participate in the activity of the best-frequency fibre. (As they widen, curves begin to overlap with one another.) However, as can be inferred from Fig. 22.6 and is directly shown in Fig. 22.8, the thresholds of newly recruited fibres for frequencies different from their own best frequency are elevated, and saturation occurs at correspondingly higher levels. This finding strongly suggests that the

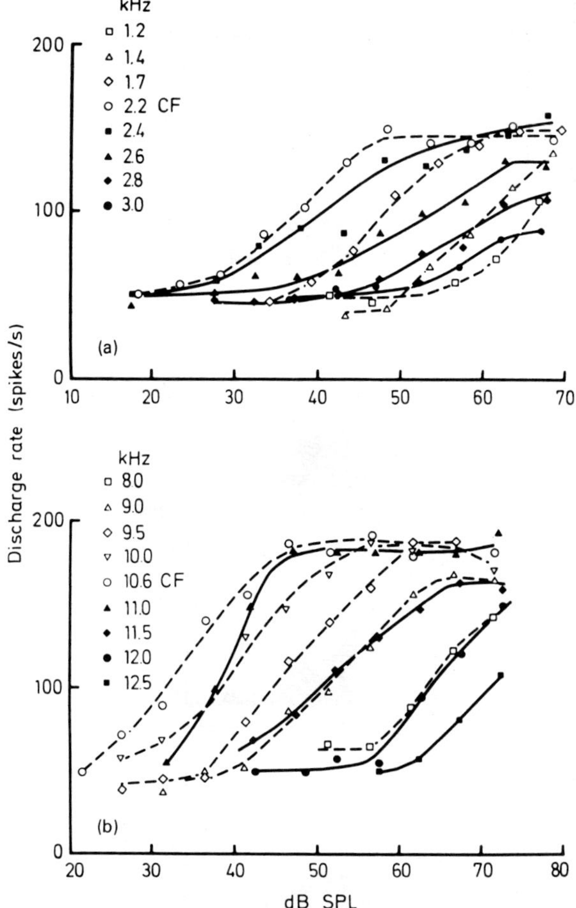

Fig. 22.8. Discharge rates v. stimulus intensity of two cochlear nerve fibres (cat); best frequencies 2.2 and 10.6 kHz respectively. Note the difference in the courses of these curves for frequencies below, at, or above the best frequency. (From Evans (1974).)

restricted intensity range of single fibres responding to their best frequencies is extended by the recruitment of additional, nearby fibres.

The *masking* problem is also alleviated by the place/time/amplitude distribution to some extent. A narrowly-tuned fibre has only to cope with a correspondingly narrower band of noise. In this manner, the signal-to-noise ratio of the fibre is improved over that observed in an otherwise equivalent broad-band system. Fig. 22.9 illustrates the masking effect for a single cochlear nerve fibre in a series of PST histograms with masking level as parameter. It is seen that the rate of nerve discharges evoked by this signal is decreased, the more so the higher the masking level. It is recalled from

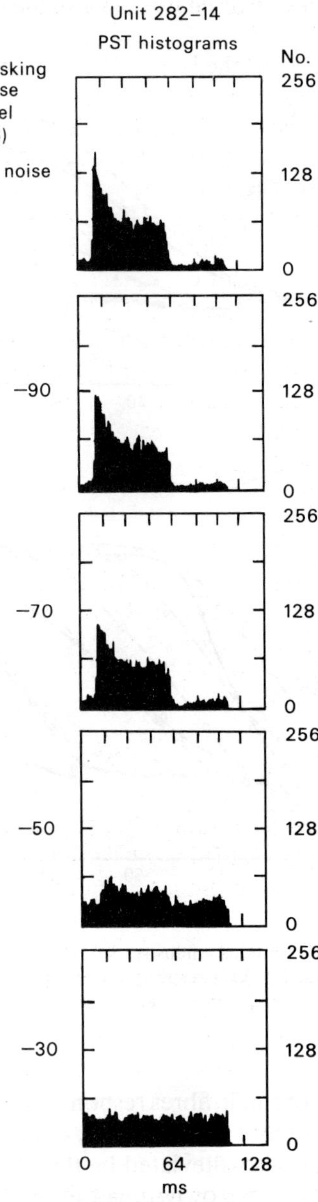

Fig. 22.9. PST histogram for a cochlear nerve fibre in response to tone bursts in the presence of masking noise of various levels. The cochlear nerve is the lowest level of the auditory system at which masking effects can be demonstrated. (From Kiang *et al.* (1965).)

Fig. 22.8 that the rate of nerve discharges in a single fibre is proportional to the intensity.

We have seen above that, at the level of the cochlear nerve, frequency is encoded in a two-fold manner, i.e. (i) as periodicity at low frequencies and (ii) as place for all frequencies; and intensity likewise in a two-fold manner, i.e. (i) as the rate of spike discharges per fibre and (ii) as the number of recruited fibres. However, there is a partial overlap between both codes, specifically between periodicity and the rate of spike discharges. Although we seem to understand the principles of these two coding operations, the partial overlap between frequency and intensity coding might be one of the reasons why its details still eludes us.

One point on which there is currently no concensus of opinion concerns the significance of the innervation pattern of inner and outer hair cells shown in Fig. 22.4. Early ideas that this pattern might aid in the sharpening of mechanical tuning curves (the latter being much broader than those of the cochlear nerve fibres) had to be abandoned after the recent finding that tuning curves of inner hair cells are as sharp as those of the nerve fibres (Russell and Sellick 1977).

What looks more probable at this point is an older notion (Davis 1961), that the inner hair cells and their fibres might provide mainly pitch information, whereas the outer hair cells and their fibres might serve to extend cochlear sensitivity. This is compatible with some recent findings on the effects of Kanamycin poisoning (Kiang, Moxon, and Levine 1970).

The fact that cochlear nerve fibres have properties of band-pass filters of very narrow widths has a practical consequence of particular importance for the processing of speech signals. Such signals vary rapidly in frequency, amplitude, and time duration (Fig. 22.10). When a narrow-band filter receives a signal fitting into its pass band, its output cannot immediately rise to the ultimate, 'steady-state' value in proportion to the input level. The rise in output occurs gradually with time, the more so the narrower the filter width. (This may formally be expressed by saying that the time constant of the filter is inversely related to its bandwidths.)

The recognition of consonant–vowel combinations depends critically on the analysis of short-lasting formant transitions (Figs. 22.10 and 22.11) and consequently on the interaction of a signal properties and those of the analysing filters (Studdert-Kennedy, Liberman, Harris, and Cooper 1970). Alterations of either the signal pattern or the analysing filter must lead to profound changes and/or errors in recognition.

Recently, it has become possible to assess auditory tuning curves psychophysically (Zwicker 1974). They have all the properties of the neurophysiological tuning curves of Fig. 21.6. Strangely enough, when the psychological tuning curves become wider than normal in hearing-impaired individuals, thus by definition making the time constant longer and the onset event correspondingly shorter, the situation is not improved as one might expect. Speech recognition deteriorates markedly in such cases (Martin, Pickett, and Cotton 1972).

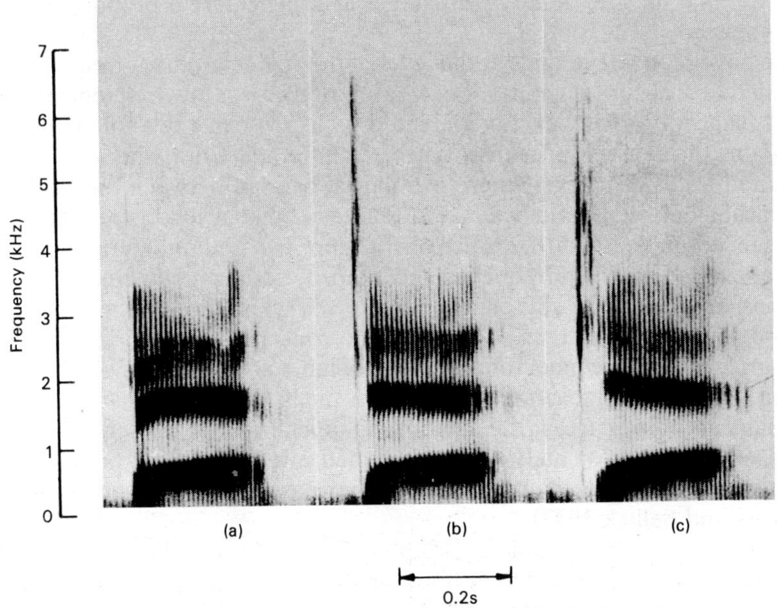

Fig. 22.10. Sound spectrograms (i.e. frequency v. time, with intensity given by the difference in shading) for the three syllables: (a) /bɛ/, (b) /dɛ/, and (c) /gɛ/. Note the formant transitions (upward and/or downward glides) in the transition between consonant and vowel. (From Stevens and House (1972).)

Electrical stimulation of nerve fibres

Nerve fibres, including those of the cochlear nerve, can be stimulated by small electric currents of the order of a few microamperes. On account of their small diameter (1–8 μm in most experimental animals (Gacek and Rasmussen 1961); no data available for man), it is not at present possible to construct permanently-indwelling electrodes that are directly attached to individual nerve fibres. The best that can be done is to bring the electrode into the vicinity of the fibre so that the latter comes to lie within the electric field generated by the electrode within the tissue fluids, with the circuit being completed by a remote ground electrode. To keep the field concentrated, it is advisable to have the electrode insulated save for its very tip. Most commonly, metal electrodes are used for both applications.

In an ideal situation, i.e. within a uniform liquid that is free of obtacles, the current density of such a field decays expotentially with distance away from the active electrode, while the field increases in size. The exitation of a given fibre placed in the field depends on the current density at its location, the conductivity of the medium, and on signal duration. That is to say, other things being equal, slightly distant fibres may start responding after some time (about 1 ms) has elapsed. It is clear that, in an effort to maximize the desired effect, i.e. to keep the stimulating current as low as possible, and to

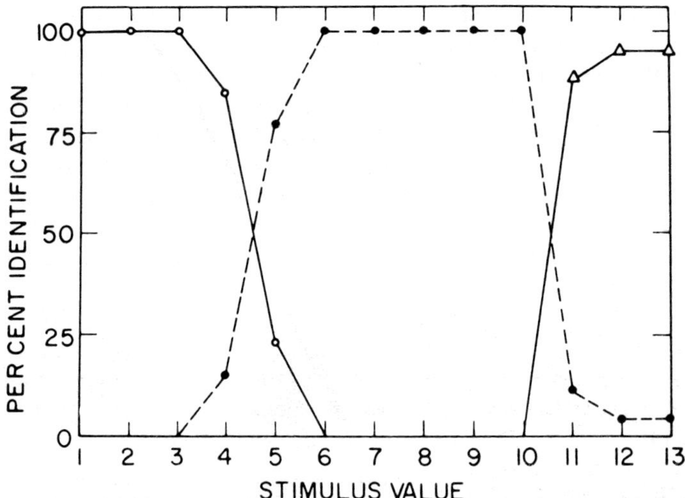

Fig. 22.11. Identification functions for a typical listener obtained for synthetic utterances, consisting of initial rapid formant transitions representing consonants followed by the vowel /ɛ/; open circle: /b/; closed circle: /d/; triangle: /g/. The *stimulus value* represents the starting frequency of the second formant before the glide (cf. Fig. 22.10.). It varied here from 1050 Hz (value 1 on the left) to 2160 Hz (value 13 on the right). Note the sharp, frequency-dependent boundaries between the three functions. (From Stevens and House (1972).)

minimize the undesirable effects, i.e. stimulating other (unwanted) fibres or damaging tissues by generating large stray currents, it is necessary to bring the electrode as close as possible to the fibre to be stimulated.

Application of electric currents by means of electrodes, although a time-tested tool in neurophysiology, is nevertheless a matter somewhat analogous to the injection of a foreign matter—electric energy in this case—and we must examine the general consequences of this mode of energy application.

Tissue fluids are electrolytes, basically 150 millimolar sodium chloride solutions (Bosher 1976). Their detailed composition varies significantly among a number of different tissue compartments. For example, the composition of perilymph is slightly different from that of cerebrospinal fluid, and both of them in turn differ from those found in connective-tissue compartment tissues elsewhere in the body.

When a metal is brought into contact with the electrolyte, the original chemo-electric equilibrium of the electrolyte is disturbed. Negatively-charged ions, mainly chlorides, collect at the metal–fluid interface to balance the positively-charged metal ions. This ionic double layer, first described by Helmholtz, creates an electrical potential; its exact value depends on the type of metal employed and on the electrolyte composition. Additional changes must of course occur within the bulk of the electrolyte to compensate for the negative ions lost that are now bound to the electrode surface. (These facts are explained in considerable detail in any elementary textbook on electricity or electochemistry.)

Essentially the same events take place on the active electrode and on the ground electrode as well. However, if the electrolyte composition is different in the two locations, as is often the case, the two potentials will not be precisely equal to each other; hence, there will be a small potential difference between the two electrodes. The d.c. resistance between them is typically in the order of a few thousand ohms. A d.c. current, admittedly also of small magnitude, will therefore flow, even though no external current has been applied.

The d.c. current has a galvanic effect. It produces an electrolysis, that is electrolyte ions are transported toward the electrodes, and in exchange, metal ions are injected from the electrodes into the electrolyte. Within the solution itself, water molecules are dissociated. Hydrogen gas bubbles collect on the positive electrode, the anode, and oxygen gas bubbles on the negative one, the cathode.

On account of these accumulations, the d.c. resistance between the electrode and the solution rises, and the current flow decreases asymptotically to a low value; the electrode has become 'polarized'. The resistance is now very high, but only for current flowing in the direction of the original polarizing current—still low for currents that would flow in the opposite direction. In actual practice, the polarization process never comes to an end. Its degree is being continually varied by mechanical and/or thermal agitations of the electrolyte. The degree of electrolysis is proportional to the current flow. Even though, in the case under consideration, the flow may be very slow, chronically-implanted electrodes call for consideration of long-range effects.

To avoid any d.c. components present being passed together with an a.c. signal, into the tissue, one employs a stimulus isolation unit, which is simply a transformer that blocks the transmission of d.c. currents. When a.c. currents are applied in this manner, the d.c. 'resting' potential between the electrodes becomes modulated. The modulation magnitude is related to the charge density at the electrode surface. Thus it pays to make the surface of the electrode tip as large as possible, for instance, by roughing its surface, a technique recently applied by Dobelle (personal communication) to his cochlear electrodes.

It is sometimes claimed that, with respect to ion migration, a.c.currents have a net effect of zero, since ions go one way while the current flows in one direction and the other way when the current is reversed. In actual practice, this is once more not correct. Since the ion distribution changes with time, the same ions may not always be available for alternate transport in two directions. Consequently, the pH of the solution may gradually be altered as Dobelle (personal communication) has recently demonstrated. Within living tissue, this may actually be a very minor effect, since, as a rule, tissue fluids are well buffered.

We may consider at this point the fundamental differences between the 'physiological' stimulation of cochlear nerve fibres and 'artificial' electrical stimulation. Under physiological conditions, mechanical energy is applied to elicit in a specific manner a series of well-controlled, chemo-electric events. No foreign materials are brought into the tissues; no unchecked currents are allowed to flow within the tissue at any one time; and a number of specific enzymes are held available to terminate each subevent at its proper time and to restore the disturbed chemo-electric force equilibrium as quickly as possible. In the case of artificial stimulation, the same end result, i.e. nerve fibre stimulation, requires relatively larger expenditures of energy. That is to say, currents cannot be restricted solely to the region of the fibre to be excited. Hence, there may be stray currents of considerable magnitude. Furthermore, foreign materials (metal ions) may enter the tissues, even if only in trace amounts, and the chemical forces required to balance the externally-applied electric ones are non-specific. Yet, for want of a better method, we must try to cope with this situation.

The potentially serious feature of the entire process is the injection of metal ions into the tissues. As a rule, they immediately combine with the chlorides present to form their chloride salts. Metal ions and their salts, especially those of heavy metals, are very toxic to biological tissues, even when present in trace amounts.

In the past, silver electrodes were routinely used in neurophysiological experimentation. When fine silver wires with small exposed tips were employed as indwelling electrodes, they were eroded within a few months. Silver is a material that is very susceptible to electrolysis and is therefore no longer used as an electrode material in chronic neurophysiological experiments.

The problem can be, and is being, minimized in two ways: (i) By the use of noble metals, platinum for example, which do not easily ionize. Certain alloys appear to hold good promise. Chouard and Mcleod (1976) for example, recently reported using electrodes for intracochlear applications made of 90 per cent platinum and 10 per cent irridium. (ii) By the use of 'non-polarizable' electrodes. Metals may be protectively coated by other substances, carbon, for instance. Modern thin-film depositing methods have made this old laboratory method a practical one for protectively coating long-term, indwelling electrodes.

As an indication of the minor nature of the entire electrode problem, cardiac pacemakers with their excellent record as regards the intra-tissue tolerance of their electrodes are sometimes cited. The following comments are, however, necessary: (i) Pacemaker electrodes are coarser by several orders of magnitude than those suitable for cochlear implantation. (ii) Muscular tissue is sturdy, and hence less vulnerable than the delicate cochlear tissues. (iii) A relatively heavy insulation less prone to breakdown can be afforded with pacemakers if only because space is not at a premium as it is within the narrow confines of the cochlea.

Breakdown of the insulating material appears to be the most common cause of long-term failure of cochlear electrodes nowadays. It was this type of failure that ended after only six months the study by Simmons *et al.* (1965), the first really well controlled work of its kind.

Intracochlear electrodes

The mutual tolerance between the cochlear tissues and the metal electrodes and their insulation has been studied by Merzenich, White, Leake, Schindler, and Michelson (1977) and Merzenich, White, Vivian, Leake-Jones, and Walsh (1979) in cats. Electrodes were permanently implanted into the scala tympani via the round window and were kept active, i.e. they were made to receive electrical signals, most of the time. None of the electrodes failed over a span of two years. On histological inspection, tissue damage was found to be slight, generally confined to hair cells, a type of lesion that might be of little importance from the present standpoint. The study happened to include a few animals carrying bipolar electrodes. (More about these animals will be said later on.)

On account of the particular configuration of the current pathway (Fig. 22.12), current density is very high between the two active electrodes, much

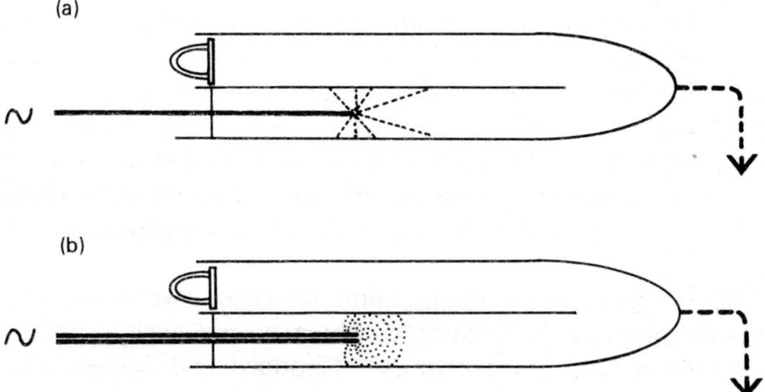

Fig. 22.12. Current pathways between electrodes (highly schematic). (a). Spreading from a single intracochlear electrode toward the remote round electrode. (b). Narrowly confined between bipolar electrodes; for details see text. (From Tonndorf (1977).)

higher than anywhere near a monopolar electrode. With distance away from the electrode, however, it decreases extremely rapidly. No current flows toward the ground electrode which merely serves as a d.c. reference. Damage to tissue is due to current density at a given location and does not depend on the total amount of current flowing through its general region. It is for this reason that the high-current density of bipolar electrodes caused some concern. However, since tissue damage was generally slight, as was already mentioned, no clear difference could be established between the animals carrying monopolar electrodes and those carrying bipolar ones (Merzenich, personal communication). Nevertheless, efforts were made to decrease current density by simply enlarging the surface area of the electrodes, a measure Dobelle (personal communication) had also adopted for minimizing electrolysis.

Taken as a whole, the findings of Merzenich *et al.* (1977; 1979) are certainly encouraging. More systematic studies of this kind, extending over even longer time spans are needed. The following point needs to be emphasized in this connection. In biology, many long-range effects (e.g. those related to aging) are studied to good advantage in short-lived animal species, rats or mice for example, with their accelerated rates of metabolism. With respect to the present problem, this technique is of little help. The effect of chronic tissue poisoning and the wear and tear on the electrodes are not accelerated by the test animals' increased metabolic rate. The factors that determine both of them depend on absolute times.

COCHLEAR NERVE PATHOLOGY

Survival of cochlear nerve fibres following degeneration of the organ of Corti

At present, most surgeons prefer implanting electrodes into the scala tympani via the round window, assuming that in this manner stimulation would readily reach the dendrites of the cochlear nerve in the organ of Corti (cf. Fig. 22.2). Moreover, the placement of electrodes into preselected nerve regions is relatively easy to achieve on account of the systematic spread of fibres side-by-side over the entire length of the cochlea (about 35 mm). The value of the whole procedure rests of course on the assumption that the dendrites, or at least the lower parts of the axons, will survive the degeneration of their attached hair cells.

That the cochlear nerve might quite often be well preserved in the presence of widespread hair-cell degeneration has been known for quite some time (Steurer 1926); also that the chances of survival of these fibres are relatively poor following a generalized labyrinthitis (Steurer 1926)—today fortunately a relatively rare cause of hair cell loss. Following antibiotic poisoning, their survival is dose-dependent (Müsebeck 1964): that is to say on mild intoxication it is mainly the hair cells that are destroyed; on more severe and/or longer lasting intoxication, the fibres of the cochlear nerve may also undergo wide-spread degeneration.

Schuknecht (1976) accounted for the apparent variations in a somewhat different way. As long as only the hair cells are missing, while the supporting cells of the organ of Corti are well preserved, degeneration of the cochlear nerve is minimal. The more severe the destruction of the organ, e.g. following viral or even bacterial labyrinthitis, the more extensive will be the loss of cochlear nerve fibres. Most profound losses of fibres were found following total experimental destruction of the organ of Corti in the cat. In addition to the thinning out of the fibre population, those remaining had lost the unmyelinated dendrites within the organ as well as the myelinated axonal sections up their neuronal cells in the spiral ganglion (cf. Fig. 22.2), with some well-defined changes occurring in the cell bodies themselves.

With respect to the chances of long-term survival of the cochlear nerve dendrites, Schuknecht (personal communication) and several others (Johnsson, personal communication; Kimura, personal communication; Noback, personal communication) expressed grave doubts. Morphologists ought to look once more into this problem in some detail, for if the dendrites do not survive on a long-term basis, and perhaps not even the lower parts of the axons, it may not be the best strategy to employ scala tympani electrodes. It might then be better to place them directly into the modiolus, the method preferred by Simmons *et al.* (1965). Admittedly, scala tympani electrodes have been employed in many patients with profound hearing losses of long standing, and auditory sensations have been elicited by means of these electrodes. However, if there had been no dendrites and if the exitable neural tissues were therefore quite remote from the electrodes, relatively strong currents should have been required. Simmons *et al.* (1965) reported using currents of 1–1000 μA with their modiolar electrodes, whereas Eddington, Dobelle, Brackman, Mladejovsky, and Parkin (1979) using scala-tympani electrodes, employed 50–300 μA. This comparison appears to suggest that the chance of long-term survival of cochlear nerve dendrites may indeed be poor. We shall return to this problem once more from a different angle when discussing the frequency selectivity of implanted cochlear electrodes.

Predictive tests

For the reasons just outlined, there exists a need for a clinical predictive test that would allow one to assess the status of the cochlear nerve in some detail. I personally do not feel that X-ray tomography or similar techniques will provide the answer. Even if they could, there would be no evidence for the functional integrity of the nerve fibres present. One approach that has been suggested (Tonndorf 1977) and has been tried in simplified form (Simmons *et al.* 1965; Simmons, Mathews, Walter, and White 1979; Chouard and McLeod 1976; Pialoux, Chouard, Meyer, and Fugain 1979; Brackmann, personal communication) is to apply electrical signals via a round-window or promontory electrode. So far, only the subjective sensations experienced by the patients have been registered. Whereas Brackmann (personal communication) has stated that testing could not be extended to frequencies higher than 240 Hz on account of pain induced by the spread of current into Jacobson's nerve, Chouard and McLeod (1976) were able to test up to 1000 Hz. Their results might have been expected, i.e. 'pulsing' sensations at frequencies below 300 Hz and 'hissing' ones at higher frequencies. What was disappointing in their report, however, was the fact that all 59 deaf patients tested experienced a definite auditory sensation. There were no exceptions. By the laws of averages, there should have been some among these patients who had no longer a functional cochlear nerve. It appears, therefore, that in the form used the test is too gross.

The original suggestion had actually been to employ brainstem evoked response audiometry (BSER) (Tonndorf 1977) because, in addition to a response waveform, it yields latency-intensity information. However, there is currently a serious technical problem (Brackmann, personal communication), i.e. the presence of long-lasting electrical stimulus artifacts that obscure any BSER registration. If this could be overcome, perhaps by the use of bipolar promontory electrodes, that test might become feasible. However, I think its first evaluation should not be carried out in patients. It requires an animal model so that results obtained in each case could be correlated with the histological status of the cochlear nerve in the same animal.

The value of the predictive test, once it is established, should lie in eliminating cases in which implantation of either the cochlea or the cochlear nerve would be contraindicated, i.e. patients in whom the cochlear nerve would not be functional at all or in whom the number of remaining fibres or their distribution would be insufficient.

One other point must be touched upon briefly in the present context: a patient who is still able to understand amplified speech, even with some difficulty, should not be considered a candidate for cochlear implantation. My reasons for saying so are as follows: there is a tangible risk of severely damaging a cochlea that still possesses a small complement of functioning hair cells. External hearing aids may be expected to be substantially improved in the near future (Villchur 1973; City University of New York 1978). Such improved aids most likely would benefit a marginally functional cochlea more than do current prosthetic devices.

ELECTRODE CONSIDERATIONS

Single-wire electrodes

Single-wire electrodes were employed in most early attempts to apply electrical analogues of acoustic signals (House 1976; Michelsen 1971). The entire procedure, i.e. the design and construction of the electronic circuit and also the surgery, was straightforward. Patients with such indwelling electrodes have been followed for rather long periods of time, some of them for five years and more. There is no doubt that many of these patients have accepted their prostheses because they really feel aided by them. Extensive tests have been conducted on some of these patients (House 1976; Bilger, Black, Hopkinson, Myers, Payne, Stenson, Vega, and Wolf 1977). These patients can hear sounds; they are able to distinguish a number of noises with characteristic time patterns from one another, such as those produced by telephones ringing, doorbells, saws, and the like; they are helped in controlling their own voices; their lip reading abilities are materially aided; and they are able to recognize speech as such, although they cannot understand more than 10 to 15 words, a closed-set vocabulary that is only acquired after some training.

Recognition of simple sounds is obviously based on detection of their time envelopes (Harmon, Guttman, and Lummis 1964), i.e. the characteristic time-varying pattern that is displayed on an oscilloscope following reception of sound by a microphone. However, that is not the whole story. Recently, when the use of multiple, scalatympani electrodes proved disappointing, Burian and also Michelson (personal communication) applied the entire signal simultaneously to all electrodes, eight in number in both cases. This produced a better distribution of the signal in the cochlea. Speech recognition was much improved. Patients did very well with a closed-set word list of about 50 words. Even on an open set, their performance was fairly good. This improvement can be explained in the light of recent neurophysiological experiments employing speech sounds. The synchronization, i.e. phase locking, of neural firings to low-frequency signals has been shown in Fig. 22.7. With synthetic speech sounds, such phase locking to the formants of vowel sounds was definitely observed in experimental animals (Merzenich and Sachs, personal communication). It appears therefore that speech recognition by patients with cochlear protheses occurs on the basis of timing clues, envelope detection (gross structure), and, perhaps more importantly, phase locking to low-frequency formants (fine structure). What is still missing and apparently needed for further improvement is place information.

Multiple-wire electrodes

It was intuitively obvious that the use of multiple electrodes should considerably improve the situation by providing place pitch. A number of such electrode sets have been implanted (Simmons *et al.* 1965, 1979; House 1976; House, Berliner, and Eisenberg 1979; Chouard and McLeod 1976; Pialoux *et al.* 1979; Burian, Hochmair, Hochmair-Desoyer, and Lessel 1979). Although some progress has been made, these attempts have not yet yielded marked improvements in speech perception. The difficulties, as I see them, lie in three areas, all of them related to the bio-engineering interface referred to above (cf. Fig. 22.1): (i) the connection of the electrodes to the cochlear nerve fibres; (ii) space–time distribution; (iii) coding. I will discuss these three points in turn.

CONNECTION TO FIBRES

The way electrodes are able to transmit signals to nerve fibres and the limitations of this technique have already been discussed. Kiang and Moxon (1972) conducted an experimental study in cats that addressed itself specifically to these problems. Comparison was made between cochlear nerve fibre responses elicited by acoustic signals in normal, intact ears and those elicited by electric signals, applied via single-wire electrodes, either in the same animal or in others in which the organ of Corti had been destoyed by Kanamycin.

In response to single clicks applied electrically, fibres did not 'ring' (Fig. 22.13), i.e. they did not fire repeatedly (cf. Fig. 22.7). Neither was there any variation in latency (Fig. 22.14). Both the lack of ringing and of latency variation reflect the absence of mechanical cochlear processing in this situa-

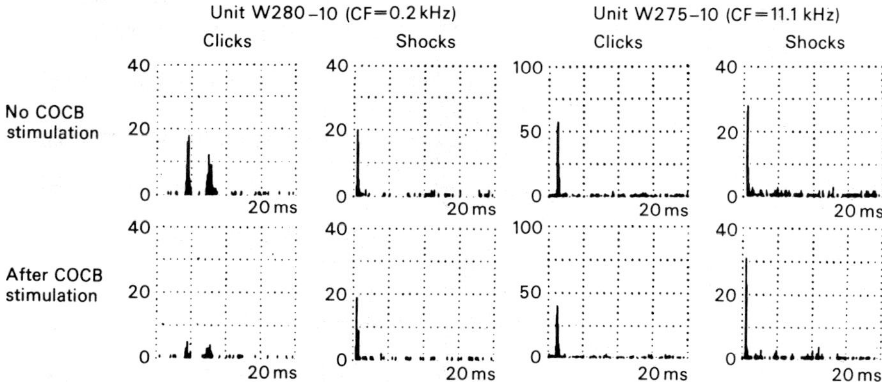

Fig. 22.13. PST histograms of a single cochlear nerve fibre in response to acoustic clicks and electric shocks. (From Kiang and Moxon (1972).)

tion as has already been explained. On electrical stimulation, the input/output function (Fig. 21.15) was very much steeper than usual (cf. Fig. 21.8). This is a common observation with electrical stimulation.

Meanwhile, a loudness matching experiment was conducted between the two ears of a unilaterally-deaf patient for acoustic and electric inputs respectively, the deaf ear being equipped with a set of multiple electrodes (Eddington *et al.* 1979). Equal-loudness points were established such that, when the acoustic signal was varied over a range of 60 dB, the electric signal had to be varied over a range of only 5 dB. This represents a psychophysical confirmation of the earlier physiological findings of Fig. 21.15, both of them pointing to the need of compression amplification in the signal-processing, electronic circuit. This technique is readily available, having been used in the making of phonograph records and in classroom master-hearing-aids for a long time.

On electronic stimulation, fibres were found to be extremely broadly tuned showing no frequency discrimination compatible with the place principle (Fig. 22.16). It was the latter finding that had prompted Merzenich *et al.* (1977) to use bipolar electrodes, as has already been mentioned. Tuning curves were indeed found to be considerably narrower than those shown in Fig. 22.16.

Clinical experience with patients equipped with multiple electrodes are in conflict with thefindings of Fig. 22.16 which were obtained in acute animal experiments. All clinicians working with such patients (Simmons *et al.* 1965, 1979; House 1976; House *et al.* 1979; Chouard and McLeod 1976; Eddington *et al.* 1979) reported the existence of place pitch. How can these two observations be reconciled with each other?

I have recently learned from W. F. House (personal communication) that he prefers to wait for a period of several months after implantation before admitting a patient to his aural rehabilitation and testing programme. During the early period patients are usually unable to give clear-cut responses.

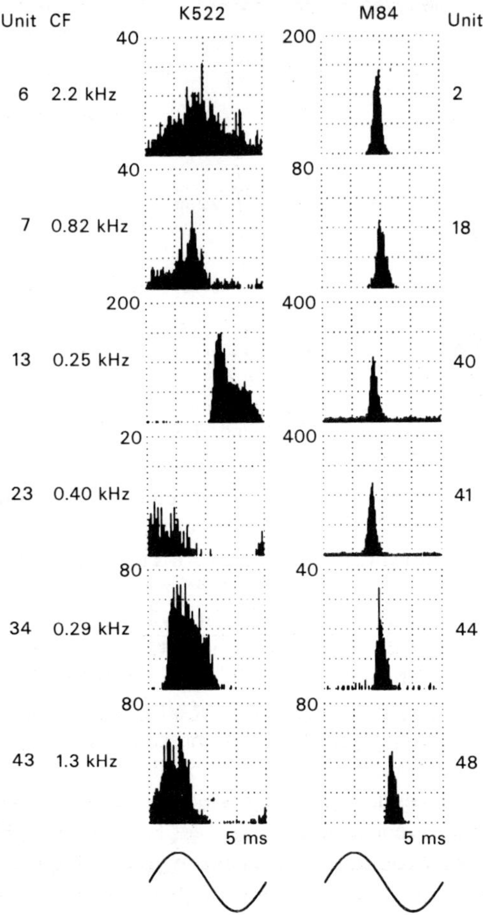

Fig. 22.14. PST histograms in response to acoustic stimulation in a normal cat (K522 on the left) and to electric stimulation in another cat in which the organ of Corti had been destroyed by neomycin (M84 on the right). Bursts of sine-wave signals (200 Hz) were comparable in both cases. Note also that responses durations on the left were much shorter than those of the signal or the responses on the right, making them essentially 'on' responses. (From Kiang and Moxon (1972).)

Dobelle (personal communication) related another experience. He had occasion to test one of House's patients twice, once early after surgery, and the second time several years later. While there was practically no place pitch at the first occasion, it could definitely be elicited at the second one.

These observations indicate that some repair processes go on after surgery, as one might expect, and that they take time before completion. In all likelihood, the surgical intervention is followed by a circumscribed labyrinthitis that first must run its course. In addition, we might ask the related question as to the reaction that might be provided by the implan-

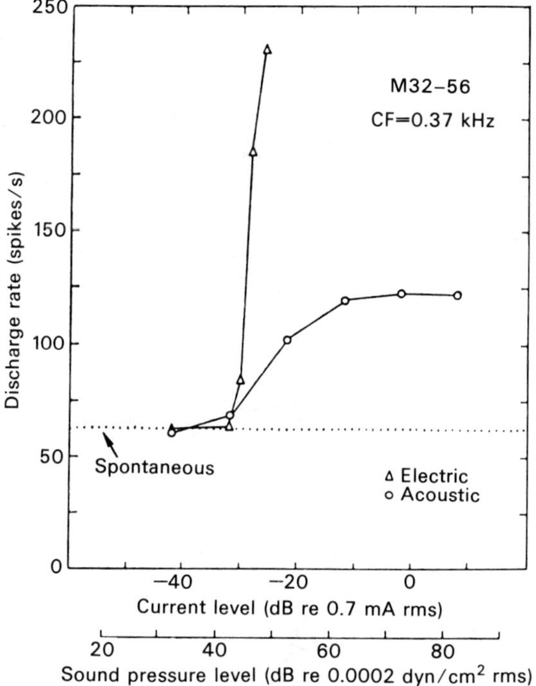

Fig. 22.15. Discharge rates v. signal intensity for acoustic (o) and electric (△) inputs to the same cochlear nerve fibre. (From Kiang and Moxon (1972).)

tation of any electrode, single or multiple. Earlier experiments in cats, with stapedial wire prostheses protruding into the vestibule, had revealed the formation of a mesothelial sleeve around them (Schuknecht 1976). Johnsson (1980) has demonstrated such sleeves in the cochlea of the first patient who came to autopsy after having worn a multiple set of electrodes in one ear for about eight years and a single electrode in the other for a shorter period of time.

Ordinarily, i.e. when left undisturbed, such mesothelial sleeves consist of single-cell layers; they are permeable to tissue fluids and should not present a noticeable barrier to the transmission of electric currents. However, with the passage of time and continual application of a.c. currents, some scarring is bound to develop, and that might restrict the current flow. If the patient examined by Dobelle (personal communication) does not present an isolated case—and the experience of House (personal communication) suggest he might not be one—it could well be that preferred electrical pathways are established in this manner directing current flow in such a way so as to confine stimulation to a limited group of nerve fibres. This point needs clarification in long-duration animal experiments.

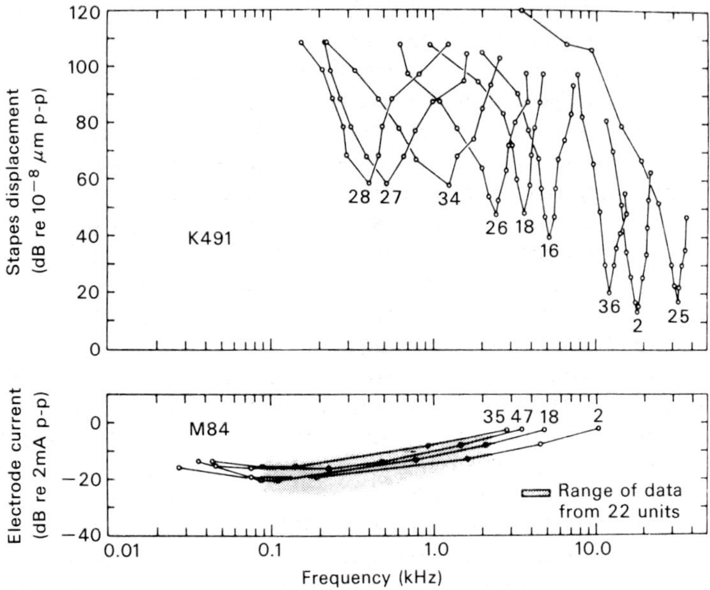

Fig. 22.16. Tuning curves of individual cochlear nerve fibres to acoustic stimulation (top) and to electric stimulation (bottom) in the same two cats that were shown in Fig. 22.14. In the bottom panel only four curves are shown, although 22 units were tested. (From Kiang and Moxom (1972).)

SPACE–TIME DISTRIBUTION

Frequency is distributed in a systematic manner in space and in time. Place pitch, as has been shown by stimulation of cochlear nerve fibres in patients carrying multiple electrodes (Simmons *et al.* 1965; Eddington *et al.* 1979), is an inherent property of such fibres. It is very much doubted that the auditory system would 'learn' to process signals that are severely scrambled in space and/or in time. Recall the difficulties encountered with frequency transposition some years ago (Johansson 1966). Processing an acoustic signal electronically so as to obtain a correct space/time/aplitude distribution is technically not difficult. It is achieved by a so called delay line. Hence, the mere technical part of the problem is solvable.

How many parallel space/time channels will be required for distribution of frequency so as to assure a satisfactory reception of speech signals? Otte, Schuknecht, and Kerr (1978) recently conducted a study in this respect. They correlated the results of speech intelligibility tests with the post-mortem status of the cochlear nerve, arriving at the conclusion 'that for an ear to have some capability of speech discrimination it must have at least 10 000 spiral ganglion cells, and that at least 3000 of these must be located in the apical 10 mm of the cochlea.' (A normal ear has approximately 30 000 cochlear nerve fibres and nerve cells).

Ten thousand channels, i.e. electrodes connected to individual nerve fibres, are simply beyond present-day technical capabilities. Furthermore, if a cochlea has lost most of its hair cells, it is not very likely that such a large number of cochlear nerve fibres are still remaining.

A more realistic goal might be given by the example of a communication device, the *vokoder* (i.e. 'voice coder'; Dudley (1939)). Its principle of operation is as follows: the range of speech frequencies (300 to 3000 Hz) is divided into a number of separate frequency bands, usually eight. (A ninth channel serves for timing purposes.) Only the voltage envelopes are extracted from each channel and are transmitted. At the receiver, carrier frequencies at the centre of each band are held available, and each of them is modulated by its appropriate, incoming voltage envelope. The reconstructed speech sounds quite intelligible.

Kiang and Moxon (1972) arrived at an even smaller number. On the basis of their experimental findings, they came to the conclusion that five channels might already contain all the required information. The experience with vokoders, however, suggests that that number might be too small. Kiang, Eddington, and Delgutte (1979) have employed electronically derived neurograms in a model experiment as an effective means to demonstrate the lost neural information when the number of channels (stimulating electrodes and/or nerve fibres) is being reduced. They came to the conclusion that under favourable stimulus conditions a few hundred neurons stimulated by a relatively small number of electrodes might be all that is needed. Deliberately, they avoided giving exact numbers.

One related problem that also requires attention lies in the fact that real-life speech signals are invariably presented against a background of noise. The differences between a 10 000-channel system as suggested by the study of Otte *et al.* (1978) an an eight-channel, vokoder-type system may lie to some degree in their capabilities of handling adverse signal:noise ratios. How well they could be adapted to the present problem is a question that bears looking into.

One might of course argue that each intracochlear electrode, no matter how far we will be able to restrict its output, will always excite many cochlear nerve fibres. Thus, there should be a built-in multiplication effect; but I do not think that it will be of help with the present problem. When working with their previously mentioned unilaterally-deaf patient, Eddington *et al.* (1975) found that, on electrical, pure-tone stimulation of the deaf ear, he described his sensations as being 'fuzzy' and clearly different from those arising from equivalent acoustic stimulation of his normal ear. One might interpret this finding as follows: in neither ear is the excitation limited to a single fibre. There is recruitment of additional fibres in the normal ear and current spill-over in the other. On acoustic stimulation, the fibres are excited in a given time sequence on account of the travelling-wave delay. Lateral inhibition (Békésy 1960) will then suppress all pitch sensations save for that due to the best-frequency fibre; the result will be a pure-tone percept. On electrical stimulation, by contrast, all fibres are stimulated simultaneously. Therefore, there is no lateral inhibition, and the percept results from the response of many fibres, i.e. it is that of a narrow-band noise, which, while retaining some pitch qualities, will indeed sound 'fuzzy'.

CODING

Even if frequency were properly distributed in space and in time by means of multiple electrodes, a real improvement in speech intelligibility could not be expected. The reason lies in the lack of coding of the input in the cochlear nerve fibres, normally provided by the hair cells. Its principles have already been discussed. Unless such coding is provided, there is little if any chance that a signal will reach the higher processing centres that they can 'read'.

The cochlear nerve code is not yet fully understood. However, Dr Nelson Y.-S. Kiang, with whom I discussed this subject some time ago, and I feel that we have enough information to suggest writing simple speech sounds in neural codes on an experimental basis. That all of our knowledge stems from animal experimentation is no hindrance in this respect. No significant differences exist in the code employed by the cochlear nerve fibres of cat, guinea pig, or monkey; and there is no reason to suspect that man's will be different from theirs. At this low level of the auditory system, the code appears to be universal. The matter might be quite different at the level of the auditory cortex because of its different structural complexity in various animals; but that need not concern us here.

At the beginning, the task of 'translating' acoustic signals into a neural code would have to be performed by a large, multipurpose computer and it could not be done in real time. Once the relevant parameters are understood, small, specialized computers could be designed which should be able to fulfill their task either in real time or at least with a small, acceptable time delay. Some of the experimenters working with multiple electrodes (Chouard and McLeod 1976; Eddington *et al.* 1979) have started preliminary experiments to test this proposition in their patients. However, in my opinion, it is still a long time before the use of running speech or even simple speech signals in such patients will be possible.

I hope the reader will realize from the preceding discussions that there are still a large number of unsolved questions. Many of them are amenable to experimentation in animal models, vokoders, or conceptual models before they should be attacked in patients wearing multi-electrode devices. The ultimate test, i.e. studying methods of coding, has to be done in patients.

We must also realize that in all likelihood the severe restrictions in the number of electrode/nerve-fibre channels will never permit restoration of 'normal hearing'. Even with well-functioning multiple electrodes and with proper coding, patients will still have to learn to cope with a novel and strange auditory situation, in some respect like learning a new language, probably only more difficult.

Maximal number of electrodes: physical considerations

The space in the scala tympani is quite limited, its average cross-section, except in the most basal region, being about 1 mm^2 (Wrightson and Keith

1918). This poses a serious problem, especially with multiple electrodes. The finest diameter in which platinum wire is commercially available is 8 μm. If drawn out thinner, the material loses all of its structural strength. (Even an 8 μm wire is not easy to manipulate.) The insulating material around the wire, for which Teflon currently appears most suitable, will increase the diameter to at least three times that of the uninsulated wire—fortunately also making it stiffer. These considerations indicate that there is a limit as to the number of electrodes, or electrode pairs (bipolar electrodes), the scala tympani can accommodate, when introduced via the round window, without undue cramming and the concomitant danger of dislocating the scala media. Although the scala tympani might have a theoretical capacity of about 80 insulated platinum wires, a safe, practical limit may already be reached with a number that occupies one half of the available cross-sectional area, i.e. approximately 20 single electrodes or ten bipolar ones. Thornton (1977) has gone into considerable details in calculating the effects of electrode diameter, thickness of the insulating material, etc. (It should be added here that in most respects, his review and mine are in very close agreement.)

One possible way out of the present dilemma is to use thin-film techniques, i.e. conducting metal films deposited on plastic, Teflon, or Mylar. This way an array of electrodes can be produced that is quite thin in diameter, yet has sufficient structural strength for the ease of manipulation. The late M. Son (1974) actually developed such an array, i.e. 36 electrodes, with a total diameter of only 0.9 mm; but they have not yet been tested in real ears. I have been told, though, that currently thin films still have problems with maintaining electrical continuity when they are being subjected to bending.

Chouard and McLeod (1976) in recognizing these difficulties, have used an entirely different approach. They drilled eight 'fenestrae' into the scala tympani through the cochlear wall at regular intervals. After stemming the perilymphatic flow by the insertion of small pieces of silastic, one electrode was implanted into each opening and fastened to its rim. Although this approach seems to solve one problem, the questions remain (a) how long these 'fenestrae' may stay open; (b) what might be the fate of the cochlear partition and the nerve fibres in their region; and thus (c) if there is really a long-term gain in this approach. No evidence in these respects is available at this time.

SAFETY OF INTRACOCHLEAR ELECTRODES

The virtual lack of any report on surgical failures or on complications developing at later stages continues to amaze me. As was already mentioned, Johnsson (in press) has just reported on the first case that has come to autopsy. The ears were subjected to his method of microdissection. There was quite severe structural distortion of the cochlear duct, especially in one ear, apparently caused by the buckling of the electrode in its middle section as it was being advanced. In the ears of cats, I have occasionally seen small, sharply pointed, outgrowths from the osseous wall of the scala tympani. Electrodes could conceivably hook onto these protuberances and then buckle before slipping off. I do not know if they also occur in human cochleae.

What worries me in this respect is the technique used by some surgeons, i.e. to alternately advance and withdraw the electrode until a good location is found by means of auditory-electrical testing in the operating room. This, in my opinion, is courting trouble, although there is at the moment no good and safe alternative to this otherwise simple procedure.

Furthermore, many electrodes, on becoming nonfunctional (thus attesting to the fact that the electrode problem is not yet completely solved), have been removed and replaced by new ones. It seems that there is no deterioration in the patient's auditory ability following such replacements. In stapedial surgery, repeated intervention clearly increases the chances of producing a 'dead ear' (Schuknecht 1976). Perhaps it is only the hair cells, and not the nerve fibres, that are endangered in such cases. But then, the changes may be too subtle to be detected by current testing techniques.

Implantation into the cochlear nerve in the modiolus is only being done by Simmons (1966) and Simmons *et al.* (1979). Perhaps his cases are too few in number at this time, but he has not experienced any untoward reaction either. All these points need clarification in animal experiments with subsequent histological confirmation.

ALTERNATE APPROACHES

Arguing that current intracochlear electrodes are not safe enough to justify the relatively small gains derived from them, Douek, Fourcin, Moore, and Clark (1977) have used single round-window or promontory electrodes. Their results are compatible at least with those obtained by means of single intracochlear electrodes.

Others have tried methods of vibrotactile perception of auditory signals (Ifukube, Minato, and Yoshimoto 1975; Sparks and Kuhl 1977; Traumüller 1977). These efforts originated with the earlier work of Geldard (1940); their rationale was given by the skin-analogy studies of Békésy (1960). Although vibrotactile perception of running speech material is still not possible, lip reading ability is definitely improved. From reading some of the published reports (Ifukube *et al.* 1975; Sparks and Kuhl 1977; Traumüller 1977) I have gained the impression that these studies are conducted in quite a sophisticated manner. Vokoder-type devices are being employed combined in some studies with delay-line techniques. The evaluation of patient's performance is also quite advanced.

Taken as a whole, the performance record of current vibrotactile devices appears to be at least on par with that of present single-wire cochlear prostheses and the sophistication of the pertinent studies might even be superior.

As far as I am aware, attempts to elicit auditory sensations have never failed in any of the patients fitted with intracochlear electrodes, although it is safe to assume there must have been some who did no longer possess a functional cochlear nerve. In such cases, the stimulating currents might have reached the cochlear nuclei. However, a direct approach of this kind appears not to be feasible for multiple electrodes at the present time.

An entirely different attempt was made by Dobelle, Steusaas, Mladejowsky, and Smith (1973) some years ago. They conducted exploratory tests on eight patients with direct electrical stimulation of the auditory cortex. Although results at that time were considered promising, Dobelle himself has apparently given up on this approach for the time being. Auditory physiology is not yet ready to make any useful suggestions in this respect or, as N. Y.-S. Kiang put it in discussing Dobelle's paper: '. . . We know very little about what the auditory cortex does and what the appropriate signal should be.'

PERFORMANCE TESTING OF PATIENTS WITH COCHLEAR PROSTHESES

The 1965 study by Simmons *et al.* can still serve as a model on how to test the performance of a patient with his prosthesis. In this respect, the reader must realize the significance of extracting information from these patients for the design of future tests. Most tests currently in use are simple adaptations of standard audiometric and/or psychoacoustic tests. Some of them, threshold tests, for example, are not likely to be replaced. Other tests may have to be redesigned, depending on information derived from today's patients. A good psychophysical test designed for people who hear acoustic signals directly is not necessarily a good test for patients equipped with a cochlear prosthesis. Bilger *et al.* (1977) after having completed their studies, realized this predicament. Bilger has made a statement to the fact that, given the experience he now has, he would design many of his tests differently. The only group of workers to make progress in this respect is that headed by Douek (Douek, Fourcin, Moore, and Clarke 1977). A report by Fourcin *et al.* (1978) indicates that good progress is being made in the training of patients after surgery.

FINAL REMARKS

In closing, I should like to make a plea to the surgeons engaged in cochlear prosthesis work. All of them have apparently realized their need for close co-operation with electronic engineers for the design and construction of the required electronic device and the electrodes (see the left-hand box of Fig. 21.1). They themselves are perfectly capable of handling the surgical task (the right-hand box of Fig. 22.1). When it comes to the problems at the bio-engineering interface (the middle box of Fig. 22.1), most surgeons rely either on their own intuition or on the advice of their engineers. However, some of the problems are clearly physiological ones, and electronic engineers lack training in physiology and are therefore of limited help. (I hasten to add that many of the best auditory physiologists came originally into the field from electrical engineering; their advantages were formal knowledge in network analysis, communication theory, coding theory, etc. Nevertheless, that does not make every electrical engineer automatically, that is, without further training, a good auditory physiologist.) Only a few physiologists have entered the field and they are engaged in research as they properly should. However, their advice on ongoing clinical efforts is urgently needed, as I hope this chapter has demonstrated.

REFERENCES

BÉKÉSY, G. VON (1960). *Experiments in hearing.* McGraw Hill, New York.

BILGER, R. C., BLACK, F. O., HOPKINSON, N. T., MYERS, E. M., PAYNE, J. L., STENSON, N. R., VEGA, A. and WOLF, R. V. (1977). Evaluation of subjects presently fitted with implanted cochlear protheses. *Ann Otolar.* **86**, Suppl. 38.

BOSHER, S. K. (1976). Labyrinthine fluids. In *Scientific foundations of otolaryngology* (ed. D. F. N. Harrison and R. Hinchcliffe) pp. 290–302. Heinemann Medical, London.

BURIAN, M., HOCHMAIR, E., HOCHMAIR-DESOYER, I., and LESSEL, M. R. (1979). Designing and experimenting with multichannel cochlear implants. *Acta oto-lar.* **87**, 190–5.

CHOUARD, C. H. and MCLEOD, P. (1976). Implantation of multiple electrodes for rehabilitation of total deafness: preliminary report. *Laryngoscope, St. Louis* **86**, 1743–51.

CITY UNIVERSITY OF NEW YORK (1978). Conference on acoustic factors affecting hearing aid measurement and performance (Chairmen H. Levitt and G. Studebaker) 14–16 June.

DALLOS, P. (1973). *The auditory periphery.* Academic Press, New York.

DAVIS, H. (1961). Some principles of sensory receptor action. *Physiol. Rev.* **41**, 391–416.

DOBELLE, W. H., STEUSAAS, J. S., MLADEJOWSKY, M. G., and SMITH, J. B. (1973). A prothesis for the deaf based on cortical stimulation. *Ann. Otolar.* **82**, 445–63.

DOUEK, E., FOURCIN, A. J., MOORE, B. C. L., and CLARK, G. P. (1977). A new approach to the cochlear implant. *Proc. R. Soc. Med.* **70**, 379–83.

DUDLEY, H. (1939). The vokoder. *Bell Labs Rec.* **18**, 122–9.

EDDINGTON, D. K., DOBELLE, W. H., BRACKMANN, D. E., MLADEJOVSKY, M. G., and PARKIN, J. L. (1979). Auditory prothesis research with multiple channel intracochlear stimulation in man. *Ann. Otolar.* **87**, Suppl., 53, 1–39.

ENGSTRÖM, H. and ADES, H. W. (1973). The ultrastructure of the organ of Corti. In *The ultrastructure of sensory organs* (ed. I. Friedmann) pp. 85–151. North Holland, Amsterdam.

EVANS, E. F. (1974). Cochlear nerve. In *Handbook of auditory physiology* (eds. W. F. Keidel and W. D. Neff) Fol. V/2, pp. 1–108. Springer, Berlin.

FOURCIN, A. J., ROSEN, S. M., MOORE, B. C. J., *et al.* (1978). Speech and hearing, work in progress. University College, London.

GACEK, R. R. and RASMUSSEN, G. L. (1961). Fiber analysis of the statoacoustic nerve of guinea pig, cat, and monkey. *Anat. Rec.* **139**, 455–63.

GELDARD, G. A. (1940). The perception of mechanical vibrations. *J. gen. Psychol.* **22**, 243–308.

HARMON, L. D., GUTTMAN, H., and LUMMIS, R. S. (1964). Electrophonic "hearing". Tech. Mem. Bell Telephone Labs (unpublished).

HOUSE, W. F. (1976). Cochlear implants. *Ann. Otolar.* **85** Suppl. 27.

—— BERLINER, K. L., and EISENBERG, L. S. (1979). Present status and future directions of the Ear Research Institute cochlear implant program. *Acta oto-lar.* **87**, 176–84.

IFUKUBE, T., MINATO, H., and YOSHIMOTO, C. (1975). Basic studies on tactile vokoders by psychophysical experiments. *J. acoust. Soc. Japan* **31**, 170–80.

JOHANSSON, B. (1966). Use of the transposer for the management of the deaf child. *Int. Audiol.* **5**, 362–72.

JOHNSSON, L. G., HOUSE, W. F., and LINTHICUM, F. H. (1979). Bilateral cochlear implants, histological findings on a pair of temporal bones. *Laryngoscope, St. Louis* **89**, 759–62.

KATCHALSKY, A. and CURRAN, P. F. (1974). *Nonequilibrium thermodynamic in biophysics.* Harvard University Press, Cambridge, Mass.

KHANNA, S. M. and TONNDORF, J. (1977). Hair cells as biological amplifiers? *J. acoust. Soc. Am.* **62**, Suppl. 1, S44.

KIANG, N. Y.-S. and MOXON, E. C. (1972). Physiological considerations on artificial stimulation of the inner ear. *Ann. Otolar.* **81**, 714–30.

—— EDDINGTON, D. K., and DELGUTTE, B. (1979). Fundamental considerations in designing auditory implants. *Acta oto-lar.* **87**, 204–18.

—— MOXON, E. C., and LEVINE, R. A. (1970). Auditory activity in cats with normal and abnormal cochleas. In *Sensorineural hearing loss* (ed. G. E. W. Wolstenholme and J. Knight) pp. 241–68. Churchill, London.

—— WATANABE, T. THOMAS, E. C., and CLARKE, L. F. (1965). *Discharge patterns of single fibers in the cat's auditory nerve.* Res. Monograph 35. MIT Press, Cambridge, Mass.

KLINKE, R. and HARTMANN, R. (1979). Physiologische Grundlagen einer Hörprothese. *Arch. Oto-rhino-lar.* **223**, 77–137.

LORENTE DE NÓ, R. (1937). The neural mechanism of hearing. I. Anatomy and physiology. (b) The sensory endings in the cochlea. *Laryngoscope, St. Louis* **47**, 373–7.

MARTIN, E. S., PICKETT, J. M., and COLTEN, S. (1972). Discrimination of vowel formant transitions by listeners with severe sensorineural hearing loss. In *Speech communication ability* (ed. G. Fant). Arch. Bell Assoc. for the Deaf.

MERZENICH, M. M., WHITE, M. W., LEAKE, P. S., SCHINDLER, R. A., and MICHELSON, R. P. (1977). Further progress in the development of multichannel cochlear implants. *Trans. Am. Acad. Ophthal. Otolar.* **84**, 181–2.

—— —— VIVIAN, M. C., LEAKE-JONES, P. A., and WALSH, S. (1979). Some considerations of multichannel electrical stimulation of the auditory nerve in the profoundly deaf; interfacing electrode arrays with auditory nerve arrays. *Acta oto-lar.* **87**, 196–203.

MICHELSON, R. P. (1971). Electrical stimulation of the human cochlea. *Archs Otolar.* **93**, 317–23.

MÜSEBECK, K. (1964). Histochemische Untersuchungen zur Ototoxität des Streptomyeins. *Annls Univ. sarav. (Med.)* **11**, 159–270.

OCHS, S. (1965). *Elements of neurophysiology*. J. Wiley, New York.

OTTE, J., SCHUKNECHT, H. F., and KERR, A. G. (1978). Ganglion cell population in normal and pathological cochleas, implications for cochlear implantation. *Laryngoscope, St Louis* **88**, 1231–42.

Pialoux, P., Chouard, C. H., Meyer, B., and Fugain, C. (1979). Indications and results of the multichannel cochlear implant. *Acta oto-lar.* **87**, 185–9.

Russell, I. J. and Sellick, P. M. (1977). Tuning properties of cochlear hair cells. *Nature, Lond.* **267**, 858–60.

Schuknecht, H. F. (1976). *Pathology of the ear.* Harvard University Press, Cambridge, Mass.

Simmons, F. B. (1966). Electrical stimulation of the auditory nerve in man. *Archs Otolar.* **84**, 2–54.

—— Epley, J. M., Lummis, R. E., Guttman, N., Frishkopf, L. S., Harmon, L. D., and Zwicker, E. (1965). Auditory nerve: electrical stimulation in man. *Science, N.Y.* **148**, 104–6.

—— Mathews, R. G., Walter, M. G., and White, R. L. (1979). A functioning multichannel auditory nerve stimulator. *Acta oto-lar.* **87**, 170–5.

Smith, C. A. and Sjöstrand, F. S. (1961). A synaptic structure in the hair cells of the guinea pig cochlea. *J. Ultrastruct. Res.* **5**, 184–92.

Sparks, D. W. and Kuhl, P. U. (1977). Recognition of isolated and connected speech elements via the multipoint electro-tactile speech aid. *Gallaudet Conf. Speech Processing Aids for the Deaf*, Washington, DC, 23–6 May.

Son, M. (1974). An artificial cochlea for the sensory deaf: presurgical development. *J. Audit. Res.* **14**, 89–109.

Spoendlin, H. (1972). Innervation densities of the cochlea. *Acta oto-lar.* **73**, 235–48.

—— (1979). Anatomisch-pathologische Aspekte der Elektrostimulation des ertaubten Innenohres. *Archs Oto-rhino-lar.* **223**, 1–75.

Steurer, O. (1926). Die Atrophischen und degenerativen Erkrankungen des inneren Ohres. In *Handbuch der speziellen pathologischen Anatomie und Histologie* (eds. F. Henke und O. Lubarsch) Vol. 12, pp. 445–89. Springer, Berlin.

Stevens, K. N. and House, A. S. Speech perception. In *Foundation of modern auditory theory* (ed. J. Tobias) Vol. II, pp. 3–62. Academic Press, New York.

Studdert-Kennedy, M., Liberman, A. M., Harris, K. S., and Cooper, F. S. (1970). Motor therapy of speech perception: a reply to Lane's critical review. *Psychol. Rev.* **77**, 234–49.

Thornton, A. R. D. (1977). *A review of artificial auditory stimulation.* Institute of Sound and Vibration, University of Southampton.

Tonndorf, J. (1975). Davis—1961 revisited. *Archs Otolar.* **101**, 528–35.

—— (1977). Cochlear prostheses: a state of the art review. *Ann. Otolar.* **86**, Suppl. 44.

—— and Khanna, S. M. (1976). Mechanics of the auditory system. In *Scientific foundations of otolaryngology* (ed. D. F. N. Harrison and R. Hinchcliffe) pp. 237–55. Heinemann Medical, London.

—— and others (1979). Symposium: cochlear protheses. *Acta oto-lar.* **87**, 163–221.

Traunmüller, H. (1977). The Sentiphone, a tactual speech communication aid. *Gallaudet Conf. Speech Processing Aids for the Deaf*, Washington, DC, 23–6 May.

Villchur, E. (1973). Signal processing to improve speech intelligibility in perceptive deafness. *J. acoust. Soc. Am.* **53**, 1646–57.

Wrightson, E. and Keith, A. (1918). *An enquiry into the analytical mechanism of the ear.* Macmillan, London.

Zwicker, E. (1974). On a psychoacoustical equivalent of tuning curves. In *Facts and models in hearing* (ed. E. Zwicker and E. Therhardt) pp. 132–41. Springer, Berlin.

23 Drug ototoxicity

GREGORY J. MATZ and STEPHEN A. LERNER

INTRODUCTION

In discussing drug ototoxicity we intend to describe the methods of assessing inner ear damage, the drugs implicated in this process, and current concepts on the pathogenesis of such damage. Ototoxicity has attracted the attention of investigators from a variety of disciplines: otology, audiology, otoneurology, infectious diseases, histopathology, neurophysiology, and pharmacology/toxicology. Therefore, its understanding includes consideration of material obtained from these various fields.

Ototoxicity is implicated where a decrease in the sensorineural function of the inner ear is associated with the administration of a drug. Such changes have been observed with drugs from a variety of classes, including aminoglycoside antibiotics, vancomycin, loop diuretics, salicylates, and quinine and its derivatives. In this chapter we shall limit our discussion to the aminoglycosides and the loop diuretics. The following aminoglycosides are currently in common parenteral use in the United States: streptomycin (primarily for tuberculosis), kanamycin, gentamicin, tobramycin, and amikacin. In addition, neomycin and some of the drugs mentioned above can be used topically in the eye and ear and on the skin. Of the loop diuretics, ototoxicity is associated primarily with ethacrynic acid. Although high-dose furosemide has been implicated in ototoxicity in animals, its association with permanent ototoxicity in man is rare.

METHODS OF TESTING INNER-EAR FUNCTION

Patients receiving aminoglycoside antibiotics should be alerted to the possibility of ototoxicity and encouraged to report symptoms of cochlear or vestibular dysfunction. These symptoms include decreased hearing, tinnitus, aural fullness or stuffness, dysacusis, vertigo, nausea, instability of gait, and problems with ocular fixation. However, such symptoms of inner-ear dysfunction may be non-specific, so specific tests must be carried out for confirmation. Furthermore, since ototoxicity may be asymptomatic, testing of auditory and vestibular function may be required to detect these side effects.

In our clinical practice we rely primarily on pure-tone audiometry at 0.25, 0.5, 1.0, 2.0, 3.0, 4.0, 6.0, and 8.0 kHz. We have included 6.0 kHz to corroborate deficit at 8.0 kHz, which may be difficult to assess, especially in the presence of high-pitched tinnitus. Also, testing at 6.0 kHz assists us in differentiating ototoxicity from a hearing loss caused by a standing wave in the ear canal which may occur at 8.0 kHz. Whenever possible, audiometry is carried out in a sound-treated room. However, the clinical condition of the patient may necessitate utilization of a portable audiometer at the bedside. Additional tests of cochlear function such as speech discrimination, short increment sensitivity index tests, recruitment, tone decay, and Békésy audiometry have not been used for large scale ototoxicity studies, but they may be useful in the individual patient to determine the exact nature of the auditory dysfunction. Audiometric testing at frequencies above 8.0 kHz would be expected to be extremely sensitive for diagnosis of ototoxicity (Jacobson, Downs, and Fletcher 1969). However, such testing has not been employed because of variability in calibration and test–retest responses.

Our standard test for evaluation of vestibular function is the Fitzgerald–Hallpike (1942) caloric stimulation with electronystagmographic recording of the response. One may also reord optokinetic, spontaneous, and positional nystagmus, since their presence may indicate early vestibular abnormalities. When audiometric and electronystagmographic monitoring is considered desirable for an individual patient, baseline studies should be obtained prior to the initiation of therapy as early in the course as possible. We have defined the period acceptable for baseline studies to be before or within 72 hours of the start of treatment, since we have found only one published account of clinical ototoxicity apparently arising within that period (Moffat and Ramsden 1977). Ototoxicity has not otherwise been reported to appear earlier than five days after initiation of aminoglycoside therapy (Cox 1969; Lowry, May, and Pastore 1973). Further justification for the acceptance of such a baseline period is derived from investigations in animals which show that large doses of aminoglycosides result in demonstrable hearing loss occurring only after the fifth day (Ryan and McGee 1977; Ylikoski, Wersäll, and Björkroth 1973). However, subcellular changes may be seen by electron microscopy before the occurrence of any demonstrable hearing loss (Hawkins 1976; Ylikoski *et al.* 1973).

Auditory toxicity generally manifests itself initially as a high-frequency sensorineural hearing loss (Fig. 23.1). This correlates well with the fact that hair cells in the basal turn of the guinea pig cochlea seem to be most sensitive to aminoglycosides (Hawkins 1976; Ylikoski *et al.* 1973). Vestibular toxicity is normally manifested by a decrease in the average maximum slow-phase velocity, frequency, or duration of the nystagmus after caloric stimulation (Fig. 23.2).

Alternative methods of auditory testing may prove useful in the early detection and evaluation of auditory toxicity, especially in patients who are unable to co-operate with traditional audiometric testing. These techniques record the sound-evoked electrical activity of the auditory system using an averaging computer. (1) Electrocochleography records the action potential of the cochlear nerve (Naunton and Zerlin 1976) and the output of the hair cells of the organ of the Corti (the cochlear microphonic or CM) (Zerlin and Naunton 1978). The electrode is positioned on the promontory of the middle ear, or alternatively, in the ear canal (see Chapter 33). (2) The

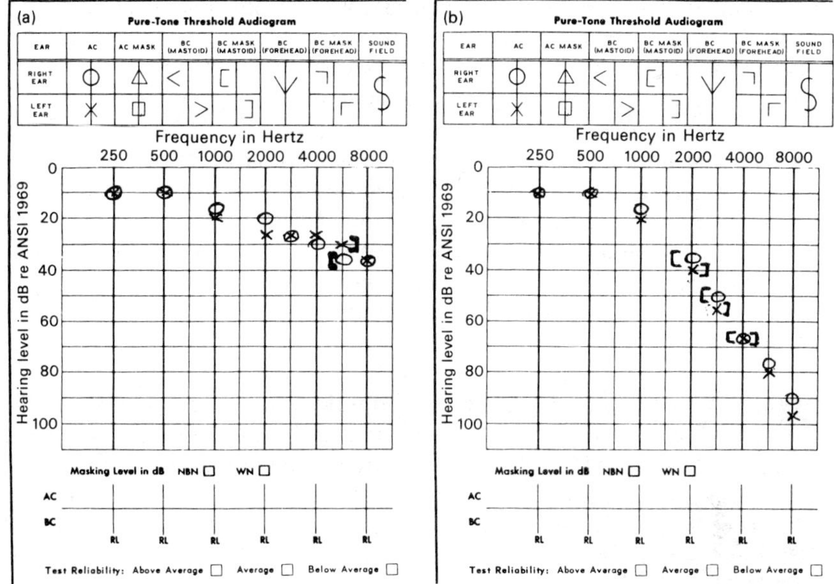

Fig. 23.1. (a) Audiogram of a patient prior to treatment with an aminoglycoside antibiotic. (b) Typical audiogram of a patient with high-frequency sensorineural auditory deficit after three weeks of aminoglycoside therapy.

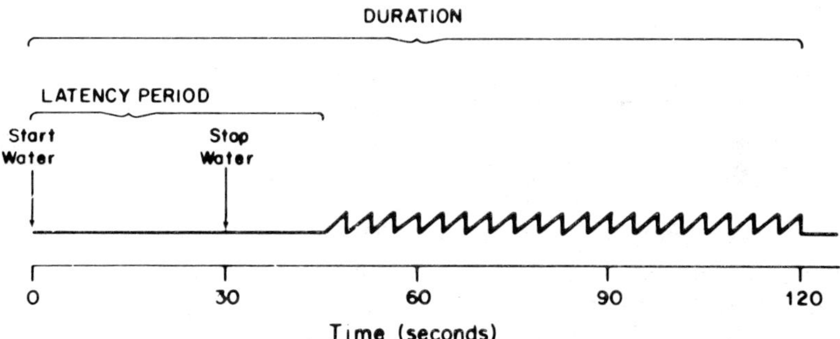

Fig. 23.2. Schematic electronystagmogram from a caloric water stimulation test. The average normal response is nystagmus occurring after a latency period of approximately 45 s and lasting until about two minutes after the beginning of water irrigation. The maximum average slow-phase velocity is determined from the 10-s segment of the tracing that has the highest average velocity of the slow phase of the nystagmus.

brainstem-evoked response is recorded from a scalp electrode and yields the small, synchronized neural activity from ascending structures in the brainstem (Naunton and Zerlin 1976; Zerlin and Naunton 1978). Although, like electrocochleography, this technique can be used to estimate hearing thresholds, it does not provide detailed information concerning the state of the organ of Corti and auditory nerve which is possible to obtain using electrocochleography.

HISTOPATHOLOGY OF AMINOGLYCOSIDE OTOTOXICITY

Experiments designed to examine the histopathology of aminoglycoside ototoxocity have been performed in guinea pigs, cats, chinchillas, and monkeys (Igarashi, Lundquist, Alford, and Miyata 1971; Waitz, Moss, and Weinstein 1971; Ward and Fernandez 1961). In most of these investigations, large doses of the drug were administered daily, and at various times horizontal sections of cochleae were examined by conventional celloidin light and phase-contrast microscopy. (Figs. 23.3 and 23.4) Surface prepara-

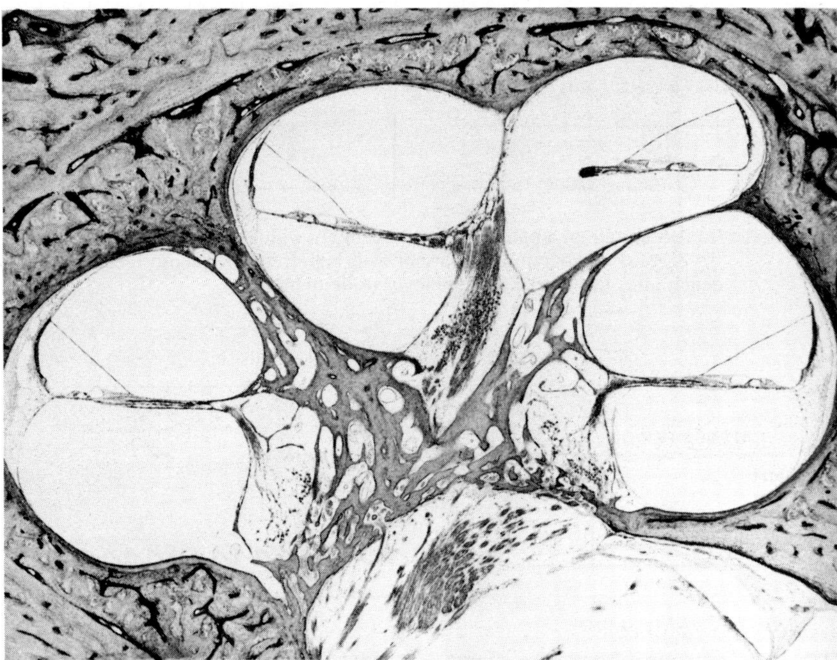

Fig. 23.3. Mid-modiolar section of a human cochlea embedded in celloidin.

tions of cochleas could also be examined by phase-contrast microscopy (Fig. 23.5). The primary manifestation of aminoglycoside ototoxicity is destruction of hair cells of the cochlea. In general, investigators have noted a temporal sequence of destruction, suggesting the following order of decreasing susceptibility: first row outer hair cell (OHC 1), second row outer hair cell (OHC 2), third row outer hair cell (OHC 3), and inner hair cell (IHC) (Fig. 23.5). Figs. 23.6 and 23.7 show examples of aminoglycoside ototoxicity.

The early vestibular abnormality found in animal studies is cellular dam-

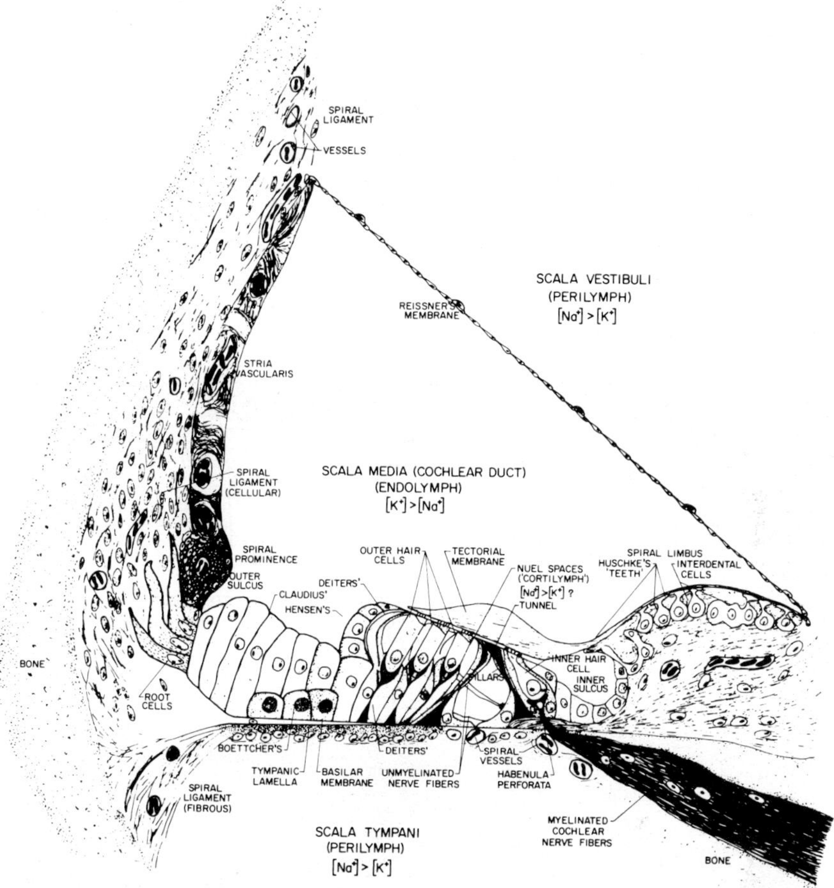

Fig. 23.4. A schematic diagram of the cochlea and organ of Corti. (With permission of the Kresge Hearing Research Institute, Ann Arbor, Mich.)

age to the type I hair cells of the ampulla of the semicircular canals (Wersäll, Björkroth, Flock, and Lundquist 1971). Changes in the maculae of the utricle and saccule have not been well described, since this requires scanning electron microscopic techniques which until recently have not been applied to the inner ear.

As in the animal studies, cochlear hair cell loss associated with aminoglycoside therapy has been demonstrated in a number of human cases in which streptomycin, neomycin (Lindsay, Proctor, and Work 1960), and kanamycin (Matz, Wallace, and Ward 1965) have been used for therapy. Most of the patients received high aminoglycoside dosage, often in the presence of renal failure, and they sustained pronounced hearing loss.

Advanced aminoglycoside ototoxicity, as described above in experimental animals and in patients who have become deaf after high dosage

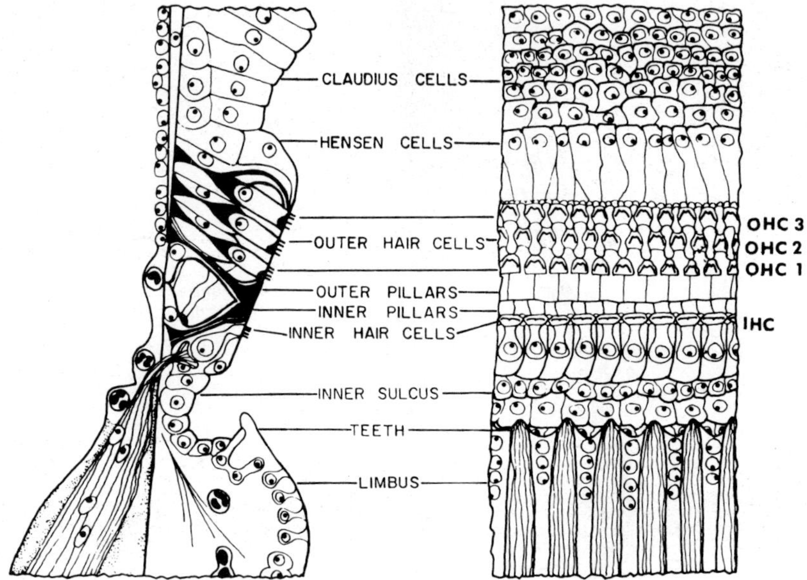

Fig. 23.5. Organ of Corti: diagrams of surface and mid-modiolar cross-sectional views. (With permission of the Kresge Hearing Research Institute, Ann Arbor, Mich.)

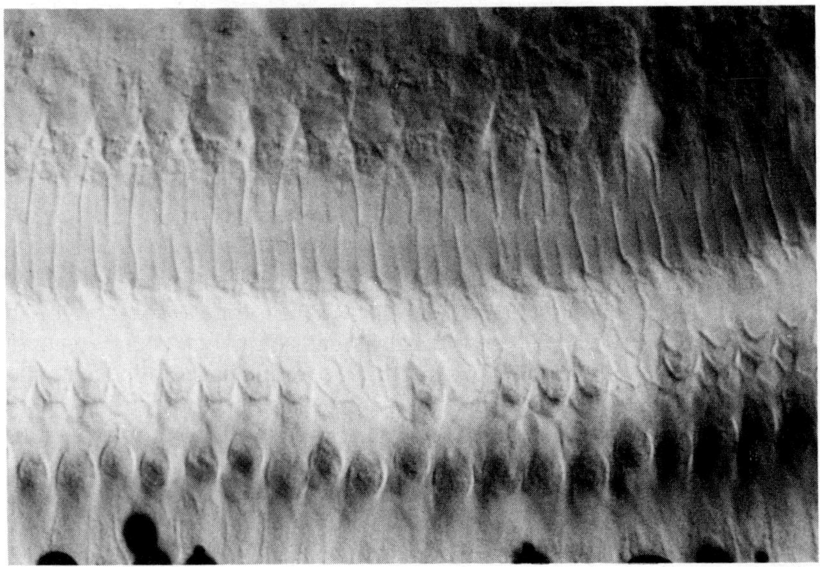

Fig. 23.6. Surface preparation of the cochlea of a guinea pig that received tobramycin (50 mg/kg per day for four weeks). Early outer and inner hair cell destruction and loss is shown. (Courtesy of Robert Brummett, Kresge Hearing Research Institute, Portland, Ore.)

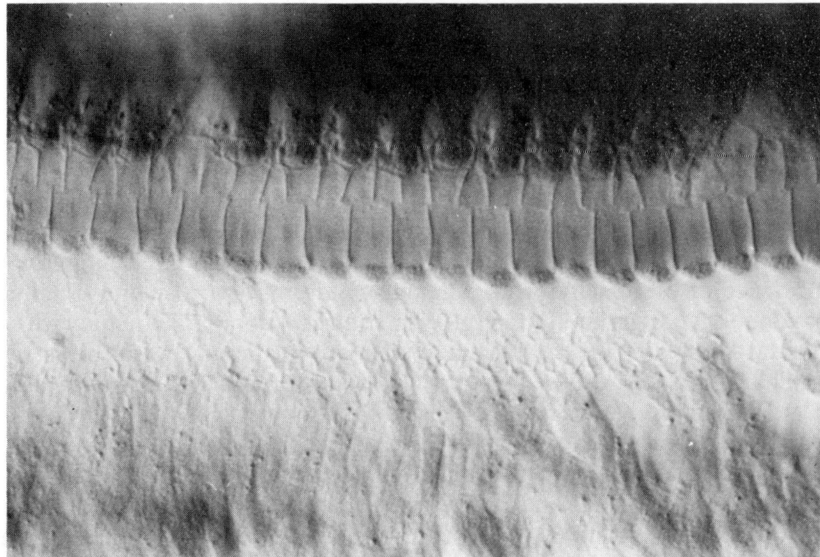

Fig. 23.7. Surface preparation of the cochlea of a guinea pig that received tobramycin (150 mg/kg per day for four weeks). Severe outer and inner hair cell loss is shown. (Courtesy of Robert Brummett, Kresge Hearing Research Institute, Portland, Ore.)

or accumulation of aminoglycosides in the face of renal failure, has been associated with hair-cell damage. Although secondary retrograde neuronal degeneration of the auditory nerve and decrease in RNA content of auditory ganglion cells (Jarlstedt and Bagger-Sjöbäck 1977) has been observed in animals, alterations of ganglion cells have not been reported in the few cases of histopathological examination of human aminoglycoside ototoxicity. Furthermore, there has been no report of the histopathology of early, subtle, subclinical ototoxicity. We have recently had the opportunity to examine the temporal bones of a 29-year-old patient who died after a long course of gentamicin therapy, during which audiometry revealed development of bilateral moderate hearing deficit. Although the cochlear hair cells were morphologically normal, the ganglion cells of the cochlea were significantly reduced in number bilaterally, when compared with those of a series of untreated patients with normal hearing. Temporal bones from other patients with ototoxicity should be examined for similar pathological findings.

PROSPECTIVE CLINICAL STUDIES OF OTOTOXICITY OF NEWER AMINOGLYCOSIDES

Since the introduction of streptomycin in 1944, the pharmaceutical industry has developed a series of aminoglycosides in a quest to broaden the bacterial spectrum of susceptibility and to reduce oto- and nephrotoxicity. In addition to its earlier testing in animals, each new compound that shows promise of clinical efficacy must be tested for ototoxicity in man. Prospective studies are important to define as accurately as possible the incidence of ototoxicity, including asymptomatic cases, to provide accurately documented descriptions of ototoxicity and an examination of its various risk factors, and to serve as a basis for comparative clinical trials.

In order to assess the ototoxic potential of new aminoglycoside antibiotics, a standard aminoglycoside such as gentamicin can be included for comparison in prospective studies with each new drug. Even though the incidence of ototoxicity of an aminoglycoside may vary among different patient populations in different medical centres, a comparative study with a standard drug provides an assessment of relative toxicity that may be useful. Amikacin is a derivative of kanamycin A which has activity against many bacterial strains that are resistant to previously introduced aminoglycosides such as gentamicin and tobramycin. During the investigational phase of the development of amikacin its ototoxicity was assessed clinically (Lane, Wright, and Blair 1977) and careful comparison of its ototoxicity with that of gentamicin was examined in a double-blind study with major emphasis on efficacy (Smith, Baughman, Edwards, Rogers, and Lietman 1977) and in our randomized study that focused on toxicity (Lerner, Seligsohn, and Matz 1977).

We have already completed our randomized comparison of ototoxicity of amikacin and gentamicin. In this study, the serum levels of the respective aminoglycosides were monitored carefully, and dosage was adjusted to maintain peak levels within prescribed ranges. Trough (pre-dose) levels were also monitored. Since amikacin is less potent than gentamicin against most susceptible bacterial strains, amikacin was administered at roughly three times the dosage of gentamicin to achieve serum levels in a range three times higher than the range of gentamicin. Our patients were monitored for objective decline of auditory or vestibular function by periodic audiometry and caloric testing with electronystagmography in the baseline period and during and after aminoglycoside therapy. Patients were alerted to possible inner ear symptoms and were questioned daily. Audiometry or caloric testing was used to confirm symptomatic ototoxicity. Since we were looking for early ototoxicity where no symptoms might be apparent, we relied on objective testing for detection of subclinical changes. Clinical definitions of ototoxicity have not been established. In our study we adopted a conservative definition of auditory toxicity as a decrease in sensorineural threshold of at least 15 dB discernible when tested at two or more frequencies in either ear. Vestibular toxicity was considered to be present when a decrease of 50 per cent from the baseline maximum average slow-phase velocity in the electronystagmogram was evident in either ear.

In the comparative study treated with gentamicin, six (11.1 per cent) of the 54 patients had evidence of ototoxicity, four auditory and two vestibular. Two of the patients with auditory involvement and one with vestibular dysfunction had perceptible syptoms, whereas ototoxicity was detected in the other three by appropriate testing. Amongst the gentamicin-treated patients were examples of unilateral presentation of ototoxicity, delayed onset (after the discontinuation of therapy), and objective as well as subjective reversibility to baseline function. In a previous prospective clinical evaluation of gentamicin, we found ototoxicity in six (15 per cent) of the 40 patients (three auditory, two vestibular, and one combined). As in the comparative study, there were examples of unilateral involvement, delayed onset, and reversibility. Amongst the 54 patients treated with amikacin in the comparative study, seven (13.0 per cent) developed ototoxicity, four auditory, two vestibular, and one combined. Most were asymptomatic. As in our experience with gentamicin, there were examples of unilateral as well as bilateral involvement, delayed onset, and reversibility (Fig. 23.8).

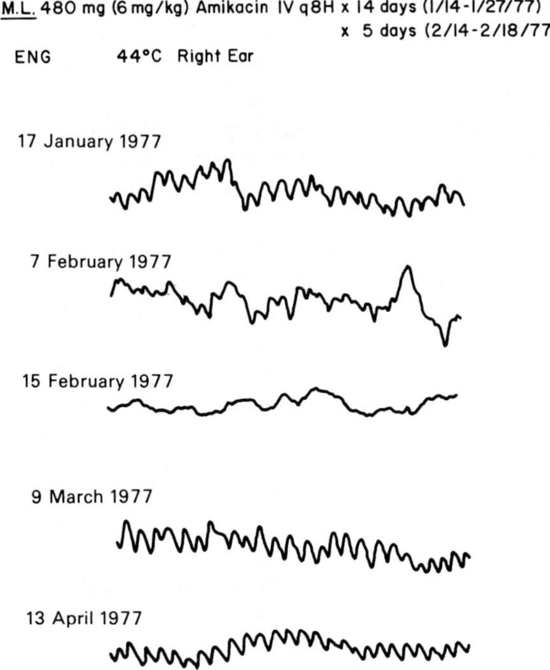

Fig. 23.8. Representative serial electronystagmograms of a patient who developed asymptomatic reversible vestibular toxicity during an interrupted course of amikacin.

Clinical studies on ototoxicity have also been carried out with tobramycin, another recently introduced aminoglycoside antibiotic, although no comparative study including this drug has been published. A small but well-designed prospective study that monitored auditory and vestibular function in 18 patients treated with tobramycin reported no change from baseline audiograms at the completion of therapy or nine months later (Lehmann, Häusler, and Waldvogel 1976). The authors also reported that three of the

18 patients developed systems of vestibular toxicity confirmed by caloric vestibulometry with electronystagmography. In each case the bilateral decline in vestibular response eventually reverted to normal. Cases of auditory toxicity with tobramycin have been reported in uncontrolled studies (Neu and Bendush 1976). Further determination of the incidence and characteristics of auditory toxicity occurring after treatment with tobramycin awaits a study of a larger series of patients treated with this drug in comparison with a well studied drug such as gentamicin.

Recently, a prospective, randomized, double-blind clinical trial comparing the toxicity of tobramycin with that of gentamicin has been reported (Smith *et al.* 1980). Of the 47 gentamicin-treated patients who could be evaluated for auditory toxicity, five (10 per cent) showed evidence of auditory toxicity. Five (11 per cent) of the 44 tobramycin-treated patients evaluated for auditory toxicity had significant audiometric changes.

TOPICAL USE OF AMINOGLYCOSIDE ANTIBIOTICS

Cochlear toxicity may follow the direct application of neomycin to the round window of the cochlea in guinea pigs (Kohonen and Tarkkanen 1969). Hair cell damage similar to that seen after systemic administration of neomycin was reported. The use of drops containing neomycin in patients with perforated or absent tympanic membranes should be considered potentially ototoxic. In reality, the evaluation of ototoxicity in patients with chronic otitis media has been difficult because of associated hearing loss seen with that condition.

Reports in the literature document the occurrence of ototoxicity following the topical application of neomycin to large surfaces, for example the irrigation of pleural (Helm 1960) and peritoneal cavities (Davia, Siemsen, and Anderson 1970) and wounds (Kelly, Nilo, and Berggren 1969), and by oral or rectal administration (Halpern and Heller 1961). Renal failure is usually, but not always, a potentiating factor. Although neomycin is exceptionally oto- and nephrotoxic, similar usage of other aminoglycosides may also impose a risk of toxicity. This caveat may be extended to the use of topical gentamicin cream on large areas of third-degree burns or of kanamycin solutions in peritoneal lavage.

LOOP DIURETICS

Ethacrynic acid, a loop diuretic, initially causes cellular damage in the stria vascularis of laboratory animals (Fig. 23.9) and later in their spiral limbus and cochlear and vestibular hair cells (Matz 1976). Ethacrynic acid also augments the cochlear toxicity of aminoglycosides (West, Brummett, and Himes 1973). This drug has also been associated with cochlear and vestibular toxicity in humans. Most reported cases have been in patients with renal failure who when treated with moderate doses of the drug showed a rapid onset of bilateral transient hearing loss (Meriwether, Mangi, and Serpick

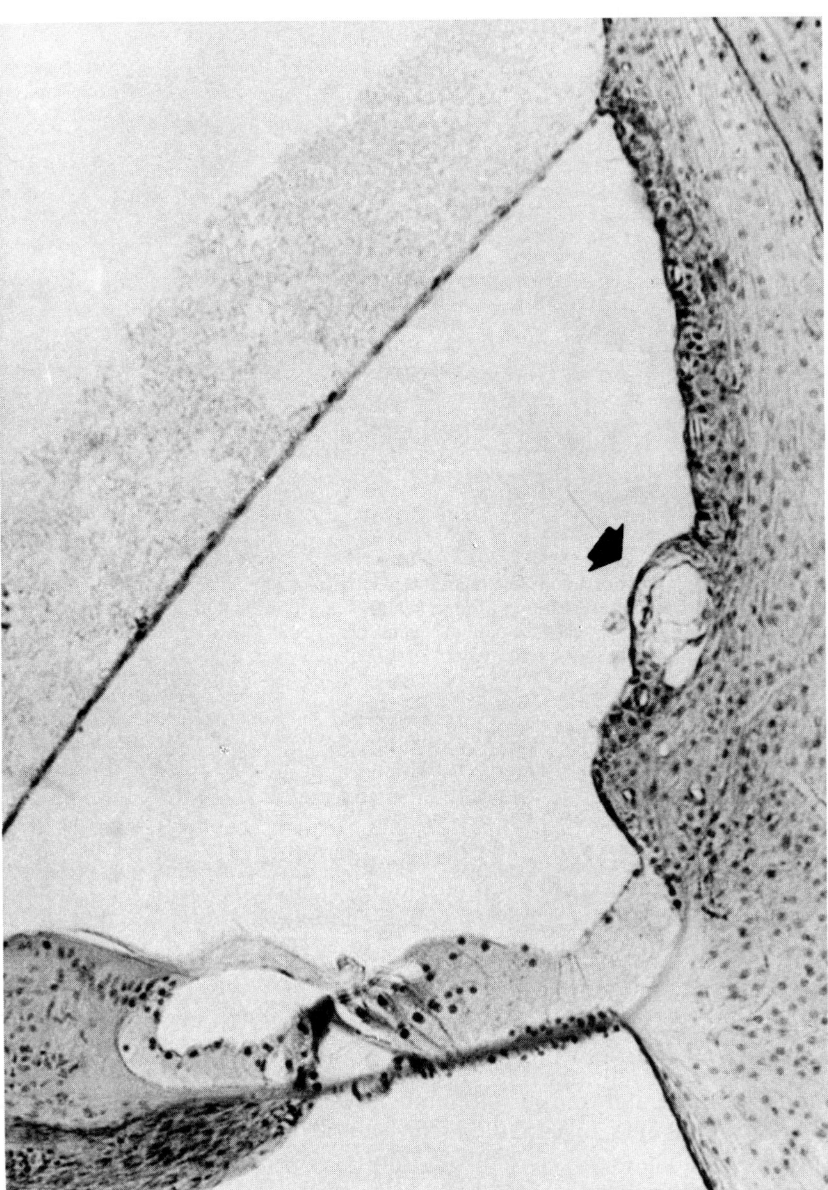

Fig. 23.9. Celloidin horizontal section of a cochlea of a cat treated for 30 days with ethacrynic acid 30 mg/kg per day. The arrow indicates the site of damage in the stria vascularis.

1971). Histopathological studies of patients with permanent hearing loss have shown cochlear hair cell loss (Fig. 23.10) along with damage to the stria vascularis (Matz 1976).

Furosemide, a diuretic with similar pharmacologic properties, has re-

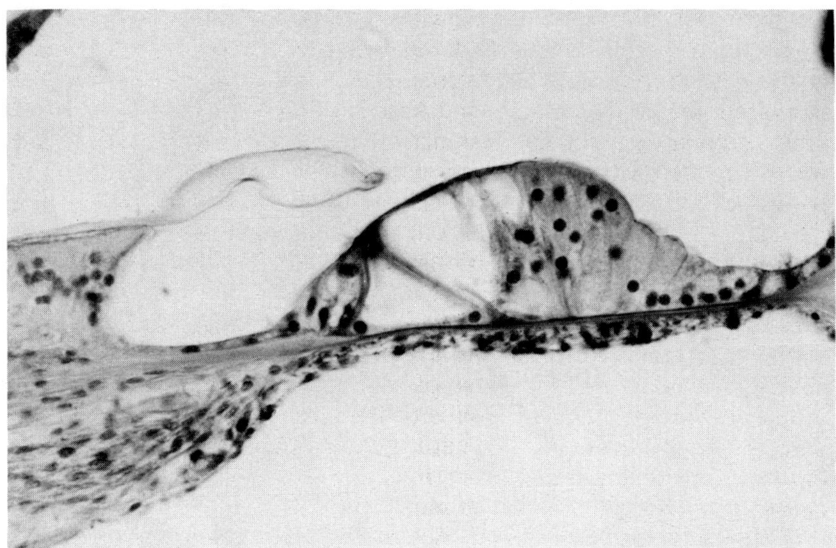

Fig. 23.10. Celloidin horizontal section of the basal turn of a human cochlea. Outer hair cell loss with preservation of the remaining features of the organ of Corti, including the inner hair cell. The patient became deaf 20 min after the infusion of ethacrynic acid during the seventh day of oral neomycin therapy.

placed ethacrynic acid in many medical centres. Transient hearing loss has been reported occasionally after intravenous administration of 1000 mg of this drug or if the infusion rate of the drug exceeds 25 mg/min (Heidland and Wigand 1970). Cases of permanent deafness have been reported (Lloyd-Mostyn and Lord 1971; Quick and Hoppe 1975). At very high doses furosemide augments the electrophysiological effects of aminoglycosides on the guinea pig cochlea (Brown and Feldman 1978), but there is no evidence for enhancement of aminoglycoside ototoxicity in man with the usual dosages of furosemide.

AMINOGLYCOSIDES IN PREGNANCY

Studies of placental transfer of aminoglycosides in humans have reported concentrations in foetal cord blood to be 20–50 per cent of those in maternal serum (Kauffman, Morris, and Azarnoff 1975; McCracken 1974; Weinstein, Gibbs, and Gallagher 1976; Woltz and Wiley 1945; Yoshioka, Monma, and Matsuda 1972). Aminoglycosides might thus be expected to cause either cochlear or vestibular damage, or both, during pregnancy just as postnatally. Furthermore, aminoglycosides given in the period from the beginning of inner ear organogenesis in the third week of gestation up to the end of differentiation in mid-pregnancy might possibly cause teratogenic damage to the structures of the inner ear.

Various studies over the years have examined the inner ear function of children born to mothers treated with aminoglycosides during pregnancy. Virtually all these studies considered pregnant women treated for tuberculosis with streptomycin or dihydrostreptomycin, or both. As summarized in a recent review (Scheinhorn and Angelillo 1977), the incidence of detectable cochlear or vestibular dysfunction in the offspring of such pregnant women treated with streptomycin or dihydrostreptomycin ranged in different series from 7 per cent to 45 per cent. In another similar study (Rasmussen 1969), there was only one case of possible auditory toxicity and no vestibular dysfunction among offspring of 36 mothers treated with streptomycin or dihydrostreptomycin, or both. In these studies, hearing loss was generally mild and at high frequencies, so speech perception was not affected. In some cases hearing loss was unilateral. Such retrospective analyses lack data on the course of therapy (such as serum levels), and pre-treatment inner ear function is obviously untestable in these studies. Since children cannot be tested until years after their prenatal exposure to the drugs, neither worsening nor improvement of inner ear functioning occurring after treatment can be monitored.

Similar studies of intrauterine ototoxicity due to newer aminoglycosides are lacking in the literature. This may be due in part to the fact that newer aminoglycosides are more commonly used for shorter periods of time than is required for the more prolonged treatment of tuberculosis with streptomycin. Intrauterine ototoxicity was described by Jones (1973) in the offspring of a woman treated with kanamycin and cephalothin in her twenty-eighth week of pregnancy. At this point she was noted to be azotemic and oliguric. Antibiotics were discontinued, and she was given two doses of ethacrynic acid. Two weeks later she was totally deaf. When her child was tested at age three, he was totally deaf with normal vestibular function and no other abnormalities. This may reflect toxicity with either kanamycin or ethacrynic acid or a combined effect of both drugs.

Thus, treatment of a pregnant patient with an aminoglycoside may subject the foetus to the risk of ototoxicity similar to that experienced postnatally. This risk, may be enhanced by renal failure in the mother and by concomitant treatment with other ototoxic drugs such as ethacrynic acid. It is not clear whether there is a greater risk of ototoxicity in the foetus than in adults or children. Furthermore, teratogenicity of aminoglycosides has not been demonstrated. In the evaluation of inner ear dysfunction in children, a careful history of administration of these ototoxic drugs during the mother's pregnancy should be obtained.

PATHOGENESIS OF OTOTOXICITY

Aminoglycoside antibiotics are generally administered in man for use by the intravenous or intramuscular route. They do not bind to plasma proteins, but diffuse throughout the extracellular fluid. There is no metabolism of any of the aminoglycosides, and excretion is almost completely by glomerular filtration through the kidney. This organ is also the other major target of aminoglycoside toxicity besides the organ of Corti. During passage through the renal tubules, aminoglycosides bind to proximal tubular epithelial cells in the renal cortex. These may degenerate, producing renal failure, but this is usually reversible as the tubular epithelium regenerates. After the intravenous infusion of an aminoglycoside, there is a rapid decline in its concentration in serum (serum level) as the drug diffuses into the extracellular fluid. This phase is most evident following each of the first few doses. The major phase of decline in serum levels is due to renal excretion, and this follows first-order kinetics (the rate of excretion is proportional to the serum level). For most aminoglycosides, the half-life in serum for this dominant phase is about two hours, but impairment of renal function, as a result of nephrotoxicity or any other cause, lengthens the half-life as it slows excretion. If the usual dosage of aminoglycoside is not decreased in the face of retarded renal excretion, serum levels will rise as the drug accumulates.

Serum levels of aminoglycosides are measured to regulate dosage for two reasons: (i) Since the killing of even susceptible gram-negative bacilli may require relatively high concentrations of aminoglycosides, it is often necessary to assay drug levels in order to ensure that the dosage is sufficiently high for satisfactory antibacterial efficacy. (ii) Increased dosage resulting in higher serum levels raises the incidence of aminoglycoside ototoxicity in animal models (Brummett, Himes, Saine, and Vernon 1972). Higher serum levels also seem to be associated with increased incidence of ototoxicity in man (Black, Lau, Weinstein, Young, and Hewitt 1976; Jackson and Arcieri 1971). Although patients may sustain ototoxicity from aminoglycosides with serum levels of the drug in acceptable therapeutic ranges, serum levels are monitored to reduce the increased risk of ototoxicity from levels elevated above these ranges. Such monitoring for drug accumulation is especially important for patients with reduced renal excretion, but is also carried out in many centres for patients with normal renal function.

Serum is generally drawn for assay of peak (post-dose) and trough (pre-dose) aminoglycoside levels. Dosage is usually adjusted to bring the peak level within an acceptable therapeutic range, with modification based on the clinical setting of the infection and the susceptibility of the infecting pathogen. Trough levels are generally low in patients with normal renal function. A rising trough level may be a sensitive indicator of aminoglycoside accumulation resulting from a decline in renal function. Several methods are utilized to assay aminoglycoside concentrations in serum, cerebrospinal fluid (CSF), and other patient specimens. Materials necessary for microbiological, radioenzymatic, and radioimmunoassay techniques are available in commercial kits.

Several groups have investigated pharmacokinetics of aminoglycoside entry from the serum into the perilymph of the inner ear of guinea pigs given much higher doses than are customarily used in clinical practice. Early studies (Stupp, Rauch, Sous, Brun, and Lagler 1967) suggested that the inner ear can maintain concentrations of aminoglycosides in the perilymph above those in serum and CSF. However, more recent work by Federspil,

Schätzle, and Tiesler (1976) and Brummett, Fox, Bendrick, and Himes (1978) has shown that there is a kinetic barrier to the entry and exit of aminoglycosides into and out of the perilymph. As serum levels rise and fall, the levels in the perilymph are damped and fluctuate in a narrower range within the range of serum levels. Thus, the perilymph levels do not rise to the peak serum level, which is present for only a relatively short period of time, and perilymph levels also fall off more slowly than the decline in serum levels resulting from renal excretion.

We have examined the concentrations of aminoglycosides in the serum and perilymph of patients who died during a course of aminoglycoside therapy. In patients with normal renal function the serum concentrations were at various levels within the usual range. The actual level at death depended on the time since the last dose had been given. However, the concentrations in perilymph were generally very low. This is consistent with the observations in animals that show aminoglycosides not to accumulate in the perilymph when the serum levels rise and fall rapidly. Since the serum levels reached in patients are much less than in animals treated with massive doses, the perilymph levels in patients were generally correspondingly lower than those found in animals. In patients with renal failure, however, the perilymph levels were generally higher than in patients with normal renal function, although still within the range of their serum levels. This is not surprising, since in such patients with renal impairment the serum levels may be sustained for long periods because of slow excretion. Furthermore, the levels are generally not allowed to fall as low as in normal patients before the next dose is given. Whether the entry of higher concentrations of aminoglycosides into the perilymph of patients with renal impairment increases their risk of developing ototoxicity is not certain.

In humans and other mammals a bony channel, the cochlear aqueduct, connects the scala tympani (perilymph compartment) with the subarachnoid space. The patency of this channel is in doubt (Rask-Anderson, Stahle, and Wilbrand (1977)). In particular, it is not known whether there is exchange between the CSF and the perilymph. Aminoglycosides may be administered directly into the lumbar subarachnoid space or the intracerebral ventricles, causing sustained concentrations much higher than in serum. These elevated levels in the CSF might lead to a rise in the perilymph levels if there is direct communication via the aqueduct. However, studies of treatment of patients with gram-negative meningitis with intrathecal or intraventricular gentamicin have indicated that there is no increased incidence of ototoxicity in these patients (Kaiser and McGee 1975; Rahal, Hyams, Simberkoff, and Rubinstein 1974).

A patient treated in our hospital with repeated daily doses of tobramycin intrathecally and then intraventricularly, as well as with usual intravenous doses, had levels of tobramycin in the CSF elevated above the range of serum levels. At death, although the concentration of tobramycin in the CSF was still well above the serum level, the perilymph level was in the usual low range for patients with normal renal function. Thus, in this patient tobramycin apparently did not diffuse from CSF into perilymph. Whether the cochlear aqueduct is patent in other patients remains to be established.

Little is known of the actual mechanisms by which aminoglycosides damage the cochlear hair cells. Recently, however, Schacht (1976) has investigated the effects of neomycin and other aminoglycosides on membrane phospholipids in the organ of Corti of the guinea pig cochlea. These drugs appeared to interfere with the metabolism of polyphosphoinositides in the organ of Corti (and in the kidney as well). The binding of calcium was also reduced, perhaps by its displacement from the membrane phosphoinositides, and this might have altered the membrane permeability to other cations. Alternatively, it has been proposed that the alteration of the membranes in the organ of Corti caused by such treatments might allow increased penetration of the aminoglycoside so that it could exert inhibitory effects on intracellular structures such as mitochondria.

Ethacrynic acid causes changes in the sodium and potassium concentrations of the inner ear fluids, and, dependent on the species of animal studied, the ionic changes may be correlated with the hearing loss. This drug also causes depression of the endocochlear potentials, cochlear microphonics, and action potentials (Matz 1976). Early oedematous changes in the stria vascularis may be associated with inhibition of cochlear carbonic anhydrase and strial Na^+–K^+ ATPase. In larger doses, ethacrynic acid causes depression of succinic dehydrogenase and nucleotide adenine diphosphate diaphorase, enzymes of the outer hair cells (Brown and Feldman 1978; Matz 1976). The relevance to ototoxicity of these subcellular events which occur in the cochlea after administration of aminoglycosides or ethacrynic acid is not clear.

COMMENTS

The evaluation and utilization of each new aminoglycoside has benefited from studies and general experience with other members of the same class of drug introduced earlier. Thus, experience of ototoxicity with kanamycin influenced the monitoring for ototoxicity during the clinical trials of gentamicin in the 1960s. In these clinical trials inner ear function was recorded for many patients, dosage was used conservatively with consideration of the influence of renal function on aminoglycoside accumulation, and attempts were made to assay serum levels (Jackson and Arcieri 1971). As we have described, experience with gentamicin has prompted even more careful studies with the newer drugs and an attempt to carry out prospective comparative studies. For these reasons, newer drugs may seem less toxic than older drugs such as kanamycin, but only careful comparative studies under current conditions could resolve that question. Similarly, experience of ototoxicity with ethacrynic acid and furosemide in humans and later in animals would indicate a need for careful studies in animals and man on ototoxicity with such loop diuretics as may be introduced in the future.

Each aminoglycoside has been considered to affect primarily either the auditory or the vestibular system. Thus, kanamycin has been considered cochleotoxic (Finegold 1966) and gentamicin primarily vestibulotoxic (Jackson and Arcieri 1971). Our experience, however, suggests that gentamicin may cause auditory as well as vestibular changes, and amikacin, a semi-synthetic derivative of kanamycin, produces vestibular as well as auditory effects. It may well be that if kanamycin were subjected to careful prospective study in man, significant vestibulotoxic potential would be revealed. Thus, each new aminoglycoside antibiotic should be examined in man for effects on both the auditory and vestibular systems.

A number of potential risk factors for aminoglycoside ototoxicity have been proposed, namely old age, length of therapy or total dose, previous treatment with aminoglycosides, concomitant treatment with a loop diuretic, impaired renal function, and elevated peak or trough serum levels. Older patients have reduced hair cell reserve, so that further loss from aminoglycoside insult may be more evident. In our studies there has been no correlation of ototoxicity with duration of treatment or total dose; an earlier survey (Jackson and Arcieri 1971) showed a correlation of gentamicin ototoxicity with total dosage and with previous treatment with gentamicin and other ototoxic antibiotics. Prolonged treatment with aminoglycosides or a previous course might be expected to impose sub-threshold damage and thereby potentiate development of overt toxic effects. In fact, we found patients who developed ototoxicity with gentamicin were significantly more likely to have previously had a course of aminoglycosides than patients who did not develop ototoxicity with gentamicin. As discussed previously, loop diuretics can augment aminoglycoside ototoxicity in animals and man, although such effects of furosemide have not been reported in patients. Impaired renal excretion can lead to accumulation of aminoglycosides with resulting ototoxicity. However, we feel that if renal function and serum levels are monitored closely, administration of an aminoglycoside can be adjusted appropriately to reduce the risk of ototoxicity. Dosage of the aminoglycoside should be adjusted to keep serum levels in an acceptable range, as high doses of the drug, associated with elevated serum levels, have been shown to increase the risk of ototoxicity (Black, Lau, Wienstein, Young, and Hewitt 1976; Jackson and Arcieri 1971). However, it is clear that ototoxicity can occur in patients whose aminoglycoside treatment is well monitored and regulated. Furthermore, although for convenience we follow peak and trough serum levels, it is not clear which parameter is preferable, or whether some other more comprehensive function, such as 'area under the curve', would be more accurate in predicting risk of ototoxicity.

The otolaryngologist and audiologist generally see patients treated with aminoglycosides after ototoxicity has occurred, since aminoglycosides are usually administered by medical, surgical, and paediatric physicians. It is, therefore, important for audiological specialists to provide education and information on ototoxicity and its risks to these medical colleagues. Despite these risks, aminoglycoside antibiotics are critically important in treating serious infections, justifying much of their common usage. Since it is likely that awareness of potential oto- and nephrotoxicity and monitoring of renal function and serum aminoglycoside levels can help to reduce the incidence of serious ototoxicity, physicians treating patients with aminoglycoside antibiotics should be encouraged to follow these parameters and to adjust dosage of the drug accordingly. It is impractical to subject all patients treated with aminoglycosides to routine audiometric and vestibular function testing. If possible, these patients should be alerted to inner ear symptoms, and then tested if these symptoms arise. In addition, the physician might consider periodic inner-ear testing in selected patients for whom subtle inner-ear toxicity would be catastrophic (e.g. piano tuners and high-wire aerialists).

REFERENCES

Black, R. E., Lau, W. K., Weinstein, R. J., Young, L. S., and Hewitt, W. L. (1976). Ototoxicity of amikacin. *Antimicrob. Agents Chemother.* **9**, 956.

Brown, R. D. and Feldman, A. M. (1978). Pharmacology of hearing and ototoxicity. *A. Rev. Pharmac. Toxic.* **18**, 233.

Brummett, R. E., Fox, K. E., Bendrick, T. W., and Himes, D. L. (1978). Ototoxicity of tobramycin, gentamicin, amikacin, and sisomicin in the guinea pig. *J. Antimicrob. Chemother.* **4** Suppl. A, 73.

—— Himes, D., Saine, B., and Vernon, J. (1972). A comparative study on the ototoxicity of tobramycin and gentamicin. *Archs Otolar.* **96**, 505.

Cox, C. E. (1969). Discussion on gentamicin ototoxicity. *J. infect. Dis.* **119**, 427.

Davia, J. E., Siemsen, A. W., and Anderson, R. W. (1970). Uremia, deafness, and paralysis due to irrigating antibiotic solutions. *Archs intern. Med.* **125**, 135.

Federspil, P., Schätzle, W., and Tiesler, E. (1976). Pharmacokinetics and ototoxicity of gentamicin, tobramycin, and amikacin. *J. infect. Dis.* **134** Suppl., S200.

Finegold, S. M. (1966). Toxicity of kanamycin in adults. *Ann. NY Acad. Sci.* **132**, 942.

Fitzgerald, G. and Hallpike, C. S. (1942). Studies in human vestibular function: 1. Observations on the directional preponderance of caloric nystagmus resulting from cerebral lesions. *Brain* **65**, 115.

Halpern. E. B. and Heller, M. F. (1961). Ototoxicity of orally administered neomycin. *Archs Otolar.* **73**, 73.

Hawkins, J. E. Jr (1976). Drug ototoxicity. In *Handbook of sensory physiology* (ed. W. D. Keidel and W. D. Neff) Vol. 5, p. 707. Springer-Verlag, Berlin.

Heidland, A. and Wigand, M. E. (1970). Einfluss höher Furosemiddosen auf die Gerhörfunktion bei Urämie. *Klin. Wschr.* **48**, 1052.

Helm, W. H. (1960). Ototoxicity of neomycin aerosol. *Lancet* **i**, 1294.

Igarashi, M., Lundquist, P. G., Alford, B. R., and Miyata, H. (1971). Experimental ototoxicity of gentamicin in squirrel monkeys. *J. infect. Dis.* **124**, Suppl., S114.

Jackson, G. G. and Arcieri, G. (1971). Ototoxicity of gentamicin in man; a survey and controlled analysis of clinical experience in the United States. *J. infect. Dis.* **124** Suppl., S130.

JACOBSON, E. J., DOWNS, M. P., and FLETCHER, J. L. (1969). Clinical findings in high-frequency thresholds during known ototoxic drug usage. *J. audit. Res.* **9**, 379.

JARLSTEDT, J. and BAGGER-SJÖBÄCK, D. (1977). Gentamicin induced changes in the RNA content in sensory and ganglion cells in the hearing organ of the lizzard *Calotes versicolor. Acta oto-lar.* **84**, 361.

JONES, H. C. (1973). Intrauterine ototoxicity. *J. natn. Med. Ass.* **65**, 201.

KAISER, A. B. and MCGEE, Z. A. (1975). Aminoglycoside therapy of gram-negative bacillary meningitis. *New Engl. J. Med.* **293**, 1215.

KAUFFMAN, R. E. MORRIS, J. A. and AZARNOFF, D. L. (1975). Placental transfer and fetal urinary excretion of gentamicin during constant rate maternal infusion. *Pediat. Res.* **9**, 104.

KELLY, D. R., NILO, E. R., and BERGGREN, R. B. (1969). Deafness after topical neomycin wound irrigation. *New Engl. J. Med.* **280**, 1338.

KOHONEN, A. and TARKKANEN, J. (1969). Cochlear damage from ototoxic antibiotics by intratympanic application. *Acta oto-lar.* **68**, 90.

LANE, A. Z., WRIGHT, G. E., and BLAIR, D. C. (1977). Otoxocity and nephrotoxicity of amakacin: an overview of phase II and phase III experience in the United States. *Am. J. Med.* **62**, 911.

LEHMANN, W., HÄUSLER, R., and WALDVOGEL, F. A. (1976). A clinical study on the ototoxic effects of tobramycin. *Archs oto-rhino-lar.* **212**, 203.

LERNER, S. A., SELIGSOHN, R., and MATZ, G. J. (1977). Comparative clinical studies of ototoxicity and nephrotoxicity of amikacin and gentamicin. *Am. J. Med.* **62**, 919.

LINDSAY, J. R., PROCTOR, L. R., and WORK, W. P. (1960). Histopathologic inner ear changes in deafness due to neomycin in a human. *Laryngoscope, St. Louis* **70**, 382.

LLOYD-MOSTYN, R. H. and LORD, I. J. (1971). Ototoxicity of intravenous frusemide. *Lancet* **ii**, 1156.

LOWRY, L. D., MAY, M., and PASTORE, P. (1973). Acute histopathologic inner ear changes in deafness due to neomycin: a case report. *Ann. Otol. Rhinol. Lar.* **82**, 876.

MCCRACKEN, G. H., Jr. (1974). Pharmacological basis for antimicrobial therapy in newborn infants. *Am. J. Dis. Child.* **128**, 407.

MATZ, G. J. (1976). Ototoxic effect of ethacrynic acid in man and animals. *Laryngoscope, St. Louis* **86**, 1065.

—— WALLACE, T. H., and WARD, P. H. (1965). The ototoxicity of kanamycin: a comparative histopathologic study. *Laryngoscope, St. Louis* **75**, 1690.

MERIWETHER, W. D., MANGI, R. J., and SERPICK, A. A. (1971). Deafness following standard intravenous dose of ethacrynic acid. *J. Am. med. Ass.* **216**, 795.

MOFFAT, D. A. and RAMSDEN, R. T. (1977). Profound bilateral sensorineural hearing loss during gentamicin therapy. *J. Lar. Otol.* **91**, 511.

NAUNTON, R. F. and ZERLIN, S. (1976). Basis and some diagnostic implications of electrocochleography. *Laryngoscope, St. Louis* **86**, 475.

NEU. H. C. and BENDUSH, C. L. (1976). Ototoxicity of tobramycin: a clinical overview. *J. infect. Dis.* **134** Suppl., S206.

QUICK, C. A. and HOPPE, W. (1975). Permanent deafness associated with furosemide administration. *Ann. Otol. Rhino. Lar.* **84**, 94.

RAHAL, J. J., HYAMS, P. J., SIMBERKOFF, M. S., and RUBINSTEIN, E. (1974). Combined intrathecal and intramuscular gentamicin for gram-negative meningitis. *New Engl. J. Med.* **290**, 1394.

RASK-ANDERSON, H., STAHLE, J., and WILBRAND, H. (1977). Human cochlear aqueduct and its accessory canals. *Ann. Otol. Rhinol. Lar.* **86** Suppl. 42, (No. 5, Part 2), 1.

RASMUSSEN, F. (1969). The oto-toxic effect of streptomycin and dihydrostreptomycin on the foetus. *Scand. J. resp. Dis.* **50**, 61.

RYAN, A. and MCGEE, T. J. (1977). Development of hearing loss in kanamycin treated chincillas. *Ann. Otol. Rhinol. Lar.* **86**, 176.

SCHACHT, J. (1976). Biochemistry of neomycin ototoxicity. *J. acoust. Soc. Am.* **59**, 940.

SCHEINHORN, D. J. and ANGELILLO, V. A. (1977). Antituberculous therapy in pregnancy. *West. J. Med.* **127**, 195.

SMITH, C. R., BAUGHMAN, K. L., EDWARDS, C. Q., ROGERS, J. F., and LIETMAN, P. S. (1977). A controlled comparison of amikacin and gentamicin. *New Engl. J. Med.* **296**, 349.

SMITH, C. R., LIPSKY, J. J., LASKIN, O. L., HELLMANN, D. B., MELLITS, E. D., LONGSTRETH, J., and LIETMAN, P. S. (1980). Double-blind comparison of the nephrotoxicity and auditory toxicity of gentamicin and tobramycin. *New Engl. J. Med.* **302**, 1106.

STUPP, H., RAUCH, S., SOUS, H., BRUN, J. P., and LAGLER, F. (1967). Kanamycin dosage and levels in ear and other organs. *Archs Otolar.* **86**, 515.

WAITZ, J. A., MOSS, E. L., and WEINSTEIN, M. J. (1971). Aspects of the chronic toxicity of gentamicin sulfate in cats. *J. infect. Dis.* **124**, Suppl., S125.

WARD, P. H., and FERNANDEZ, C. (1961). The ototoxicity of kanamycin in guinea pigs. *Ann. Otol. Rhinol. Lar.* **70**, 132.

WEINSTEIN, A. J., GIBBS, A. J., and GALLAGHER, M. (1976). Placental transfer of clindamycin and gentamicin in term pregnancy. *Am. J. Obstet. Gynec.* **124**, 688.

WERSÄLL, J., BJORKROTH, R., FLOCK, A., and LUNDQUIST, P. G. (1971). Sensory hair fusion in vestibular sensory cells after gentamicin exposure. *Arch. Klin. exp. Ohr.-, Nas.-u. Kehlk. Heilk.* **200**, 1.

WEST, B. A., BRUMMETT, R. E., and HIMES, D. L. (1973). Interaction of kanamycin and ethacrynic acid. *Archs Otolar.* **98**, 30.

WOLTZ, J. H. and WILEY, M. M. (1945). Transmission of streptomycin from maternal blood to the fetal circulation and the amniotic fluid. *Proc. Soc. exp. Biol.* **60**, 106.

YLIKOSKI, WERSÄLL, J., and BJÖRKROTH, B. (1973). Hearing loss and cochlear pathology in gentamicin intoxicated guinea pigs. *Acta path. microbiol. scand.* Sec. **B81**, Suppl. 30, 241.

YOSHIOKA, H., MONMA, T., and MATSUDA, S. (1972). Placental transfer of gentamicin. *J. Pediat.* **80**, 121.

ZERLIN, S. and NAUNTON, R. F. (1978). CM in clinical diagnosis. In *Evoked electrical activity in the auditory nervous system* (ed. R. F. Naunton and C. Fernandez) p. 275. Academic Press, New York.